To my parents, for teaching me the meaning of hard work and reminding me when to slow down. To Mason and Colin, you bring me all the joy and happiness that a father could imagine. To Michelle, for your constant love and support.
Scott C. Sherman, MD

To my parents for a lifetime of encouragement; to Bridget, Elsie, and Jane, who give meaning to my life; and to our patients, who give us the opportunity to learn something new every shift.
Joseph M. Weber, MD

To my beautiful wife, loving parents, and gracious sisters, without whose compassion and support my career would not be possible. And to teachers everywhere, helping the next generation achieve their dreams.
Mike Schindlbeck, MD

To my students, who continually show me how much more I have to learn.
Rahul Patwari, MD

Clinical Emergency Medicine

Scott C. Sherman, MD

Medical Student Clerkship Director
PA Residency Director
Associate Residency Director
Department of Emergency Medicine
Cook County (Stroger) Hospital
Rush Medical College
Chicago, Illinois

Joseph M. Weber, MD

EMS Medical Director
Department of Emergency Medicine
Cook County (Stroger) Hospital
Assistant Professor of Emergency Medicine
Rush Medical College
Chicago, Illinois

Michael A. Schindlbeck, MD

Assistant Professor
Department of Emergency Medicine
Rush Medical College
Assistant Residency Director
Cook County (Stroger) Hospital
Chicago, Illinois

Rahul G. Patwari, MD

Medical Student Clerkship Director
Assistant Professor
Attending Physician
Department of Emergency Medicine
Rush Medical College
Chicago, Illinois

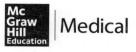

Mc Graw Hill Education | Medical

New York   Chicago   San Francisco   Athens   London   Madrid   Mexico City
Milan   New Delhi   Singapore   Sydney   Toronto

Clinical Emergency Medicine

1 2 3 4 5 6 7 8 9 0   DOC/DOC 18 17 16 15 14 13

ISBN 978-0-07-179460-2
MHID 0-07-179460-3

Notice

Medicine is an ever-changing science. As new research and clinical experience broaden our knowledge, changes in treatment and drug therapy are required. The authors and the publisher of this work have checked with sources believed to be reliable in their efforts to provide information that is complete and generally in accord with the standards accepted at the time of publication. However, in view of the possibility of human error or changes in medical sciences, neither the authors nor the publisher nor any other party who has been involved in the preparation or publication of this work warrants that the information contained herein is in every respect accurate or complete, and they disclaim all responsibility for any errors or omissions or for the results obtained from use of the information contained in this work. Readers are encouraged to confirm the information contained herein with other sources. For example and in particular, readers are advised to check the product information sheet included in the package of each drug they plan to administer to be certain that the information contained in this work is accurate and that changes have not been made in the recommended dose or in the contraindications for administration. This recommendation is of particular importance in connection with new or infrequently used drugs.

This book was set in Minion by MPS Limited.
The editors were Anne M. Sydor and Cindy Yoo.
The production supervisor was Catherine Saggese.
Project management was provided by Charu Khanna at MPS Limited.
RR Donnelley was printer and binder.
This book is printed on acid-free paper.

Library of Congress Cataloging-in-Publication Data
Clinical emergency medicine (Sherman)
   Clinical emergency medicine / [edited] by Scott Sherman, Joseph Weber, Michael Schindlbeck, Rahul Patwari.
        p. ; cm.
 . Includes bibliographical references.
   ISBN 978-0-07-179460-2—ISBN 0-07-179460-3
   I. Sherman, Scott C., editor of compilation. II. Weber, Joseph M., editor of compilation. III. Schindlbeck, Michael, 1978- editor of compilation. IV. Patwari, Rahul, editor of compilation. V. Title.
   [DNLM: 1. Emergencies. 2. Emergency Medicine—methods. 3. Diagnosis, Differential. WB 105]
   RC86.8
   616.02'5—dc23

2013043236

McGraw-Hill Education books are available at special quantity discounts to use as premiums and sales promotions or for use in corporate training programs. To contact a representative, please visit the Contact us pages at www.mhprofessional.com.

Contents

Contributors

Negean Afifi, DO
Department of Emergency Medicine
Cook County (Stroger) Hospital
Chicago, Illinois

Steven E. Aks, DO
Director, The Toxikon Consortium
Division of Toxicology, Department of Emergency Medicine
Cook County (Stroger) Hospital
Associate Professor
Department of Emergency Medicine
Rush Medical College
Chicago, Illinois

Amer Zia Aldeen, MD
Assistant Professor
Department of Emergency Medicine
Northwestern University Feinberg School of Medicine
Attending Physician
Department of Emergency Medicine
Northwestern Memorial Hospital
Chicago, Illinois

Kim L. Askew, MD
Assistant Professor
Department of Emergency Medicine
Wake Forest University School of Medicine
Winston-Salem, North Carolina

John Bailitz, MD, RDMS
Emergency Ultrasound Director
Department of Emergency Medicine
Cook County (Stroger) Hospital
Assistant Professor of Emergency Medicine
Department of Emergency Medicine
Rush Medical College
Chicago, Illinois

Jeffery A. Baker, MD
Attending Physician
Department of Emergency Medicine
Ochsner Health System
Clinical Instructor
University of Queensland, Ochsner Clinical School
New Orleans, Louisiana

Jonathan Bankoff, MD, FACEP
Medical Director
Emergency Department
Middlesex Hospital
Middletown, Connecticut

Eric H. Beck, DO, NREMT-P
Assistant Professor
Section of Emergency Medicine
The University of Chicago
EMS Medical Director
Chicago EMS
Illinois EMS Region 11, Medical Directors Consortium
Chicago, Illinois

Lauren Emily Bence, MD
Department of Emergency Medicine
University of Chicago Hospital
Chicago, Illinois

Steven H. Bowman, MD, FACEP
Assistant Professor
Department of Emergency Medicine
Rush Medical College
Program Director
Department of Emergency Medicine
Cook County (Stroger) Hospital
Chicago, Illinois

Sean M. Bryant, MD
Associate Professor
Emergency Medicine
Assistant Fellowship Director
Toxikon Consortium
Cook County (Stroger) Hospital
Associate Medical Director
Illinois Poison Center
Chicago, Illinois

Ann Buchanan, MD
Assistant Director/Trauma Medical Director
Department of Emergency Medicine
St. David's Medical Center
Austin, Texas

Paul E. Casey, MD
Instructor in Clinical Medicine
Department of Emergency Medicine
Rush University Medical Center
Chicago, Illinois

Esther H. Chen, MD
Associate Professor
Emergency Medicine
University of California, San Francisco General Hospital
San Francisco, California

George Chiampas, DO
Assistant Professor, Department of Emergency Medicine
Northwestern University Feinberg School of Medicine
Team Physician, Northwestern University
Medical Director, Bank of America Chicago Marathon
Chicago, Illinois

Kristine Cieslak, MD
Assistant Professor
Department of Pediatrics
Northwestern University Feinberg School of Medicine
Chicago, Illinois
Director, Pediatric Emergency Medicine
Department of Pediatric Emergency Medicine
Children's Memorial at Central DuPage Hospital
Winfield, Illinois

Michael T. Cudnik, MD, MPH
Assistant Professor
Department of Emergency Medicine
The Ohio State University Medical Center
Columbus, Ohio

Joanna Wieczorek Davidson, MD
Department of Emergency Medicine
Cook County (Stroger) Hospital
Chicago, Illinois

John Davis, MD, PhD
Assistant Professor
Department of Medicine
The Ohio State University
Attending Physician
Department of Medicine
Wexner Medical Center at The Ohio State University
Columbus, Ohio

Alex de la Fuente, MD
Private Practice
Everett, Washington

Nicole M. Deiorio, MD
Associate Professor
Department of Emergency Medicine
Director, Medical Student Education
Oregon Health and Science University
Portland, Oregon

E. Paul DeKoning, MD, MS
Assistant Professor
Emergency Medicine
Dartmouth-Hitchcock Medical Center
Medical Student Education Director
Emergency Medicine
Dartmouth Medical School
Lebanon, New Hampshire

Bradley L. Demeter, MD
EMS Physician
Emergency Medicine
University of Chicago
Chicago, Illinois

Vinodinee L. Dissanayake, MD
Global Toxicology Fellow Emergency Medicine
University of Illinois at Chicago and Cook County (Stroger) Hospital
Clinical Instructor
University of Illinois at Chicago
Chicago, Illinois

Marc Doucette, MD
Associate Professor
Emergency Medicine
University of Colorado School of Medicine
Attending Physician
Emergency Medicine
St. Anthony Hospital System
Denver, Colorado

Matthew T. Emery, MD
Assistant Professor
Emergency Medicine
Michigan State University College of Human Medicine
Attending Physician
Department of Emergency Medicine
Spectrum Health Hospital-Butterworth Campus
Grand Rapids, Michigan

Rakesh S. Engineer, MD
Assistant Professor
Emergency Medicine
Case School of Medicine
Attending Physician
Emergency Services Institute
Cleveland Clinic
Cleveland, Ohio

Jorge Fernandez, MD
Assistant Professor of Clinical Emergency Medicine
Department of Emergency Medicine
University of Southern California
Director of Medical Student Education
Department of Emergency Medicine
LA County + USC Medical Center
Los Angeles, California

Michael T. Fitch, MD, PhD, FACEP, FAAEM
Associate Professor
Department of Emergency Medicine
Wake Forest School of Medicine
Winston-Salem, North Carolina

Alison R. Foster, MD
Department of Emergency Medicine
Northwestern University
Chicago, Illinois

Douglas Franzen, MD, M.Ed, FACEP
Assistant Professor
Department of Emergency Medicine
Virginia Commonwealth University Medical Center
Richmond, Virginia

Casey Glass, MD
Assistant Professor
Department of Emergency Medicine
Wake Forest Health Sciences
Winston-Salem, North Carolina

David C. Gordon, MD
Assistant Professor
Division of Emergency Medicine, Department of Surgery
Duke University
Durham, North Carolina

Nihja O. Gordon, MD
Department of Emergency Medicine
Cook County (Stroger) Hospital
Chicago, Illinois

Krista A. Grandey, DO
Department of Emergencey Medicine
Cook County (Stroger) Hospital
Chicago, Illinois

Pilar Guerrero, MD
Assistant Professor
Department of Emergency Medicine
Cook County (Stroger) Hospital
Chicago, Illinois

Marianne Haughey, MD
Associate Professor of Emergency Medicine
Department of Emergency Medicine
Jacobi Medical Center, Albert Einstein College of Medicine
Bronx, New York

Tarlan Hedayati, MD
Assistant Program Director
Department of Emergency Medicine
Cook County (Stroger) Hospital
Assistant Professor
Department of Emergency Medicine
Rush Medical College
Chicago, Illinois

Corey R. Heitz, MD
Assistant Professor
Department of Emergency Medicine
Virginia Tech Carilion School of Medicine
Roanoke, Virginia

Ross A. Heller, MD, MBA
Associate Professor
Department of Surgery/Division of Emergency Medicine
Saint Louis University School of Medicine
Saint Louis, Missouri

Colleen N. Hickey, MD
Assistant Professor
Department of Emergency Medicine
Northwestern University Feinberg School of Medicine
Attending Physician
Department of Emergency Medicine
Northwestern Memorial Hospital
Chicago, Illinois

Katherine M. Hiller, MD, MPH, FACEP
Associate Professor
Department of Emergency Medicine
University of Arizona College of Medicine
Tucson, Arizona

Russ Horowitz, MD, RDMS
Assistant Professor
Department of Pediatrics
Northwestern University Feinberg School of Medicine
Attending Physician, Director Emergency Ultrasound
Division of Emergency Medicine
Children's Memorial Hospital
Chicago, Illinois

Craig Huston, MD
Emergency Physician
Department of Emergency Medicine
Blessing Hospital
Quincy, Illinois

Harry C. Karydes, DO
Assistant Professor
Attending Physician
Department of Emergency Medicine
Rush Medical College
Chicago, Illinois

Elizabeth W. Kelly, MD
Assistant Professor
Department of Emergency Medicine
Wake Forest School of Medicine
Winston-Salem, North Carolina

Chad S. Kessler, MD
Section Chief, Emergency Medicine
Department of Medicine
Jesse Brown VA Medical Center
Chicago, Illinois

Sorabh Khandelwal, MD
Associate Professor
Department of Emergency Medicine
Assistant Dean for Clinical Sciences
College of Medicine
The Ohio State University
Columbus, Ohio

Basem F. Khishfe, MD
Department of Emergency Medicine
Cook County (Stroger) Hospital
Chicago, Illinois

Brian C. Kitamura, MD
Emergency Medicine
Maricopa Integrated Health System
Phoenix, Arizona

Nicholas E. Kman, MD, FACEP
Assistant Professor
Department of Emergency Medicine
The Ohio State University College of Medicine
Columbus, Ohio

Amy V. Kontrick, MD
Assistant Professor
Emergency Medicine
Northwestern University Feinberg School of Medicine
Chicago, Illinois

Carl M. Kraemer, MD, FAAEM, FACEP
Assistant Professor
Department of Emergency Medicine
Saint Louis University School of Medicine
St. Louis, Missouri

Brian Krieger, MD
Department of Emergency Medicine
Cook County (Stroger) Hospital
Chicago, Illinois

Rashid E. Kysia, MD, MPH
Attending Physician
Department of Emergency Medicine
Cook County (Stroger) Hospital
Assistant Professor
Rush Medical College
Chicago, Illinois

Patrick M. Lank, MD
Fellow
Division of Medical Toxicology
Toxikon Consortium
Cook County (Stroger) Hospital
Attending Physician
Department of Emergency Medicine
Northwestern Memorial Hospital
Chicago, Illinois

William B. Lauth, MD, FACEP
Clinical Professor
Department of Emergency Medicine
Rosalind Franklin University, The Chicago Medical School
Attending Physician
Department of Emergency Medicine
Captain James A. Lovell Federal Health Care Center
North Chicago, Illinois

Moses S. Lee, MD, FAAEM, FACEP
Assistant Professor
Emergency Medicine
Rush Medical College
Attending Physician
Emergency Medicine
Cook County (Stroger) Hospital
Chicago, Illinois

Trevor J. Lewis, MD
Associate Professor
Department of Emergency Medicine
Rush Medical College
Medical Director Emergency Department
Cook County (Stroger) Hospital
Chicago, Illinois

Nathan Lewis, MD
Assistant Professor
Department of Emergency Medicine
Virginia Commonwealth University School of Medicine
Richmond, Virginia

Chuang-yuan Lin, MD
Department of Emergency Medicine
Cook County (Stroger) Hospital
Chicago, Illinois

Jenny J. Lu, MD, MS
Assistant Professor
Department of Emergency Medicine, Division of Medical Toxicology
Cook County (Stroger) Hospital
Chicago, Illinois

David E. Manthey, MD
Professor
Emergency Medicine
Wake Forest School of Medicine
Winston-Salem, North Carolina

Anitha E. Mathew, MD
Clinical Instructor
Department of Emergency Medicine
Emory University School of Medicine
Attending Physician
Department of Emergency Medicine
Emory University Hospital and Grady Memorial Hospital
Atlanta, Georgia

Alisa A. McQueen, MD
Assistant Professor
Department of Pediatrics, Section of Pediatric Emergency
Medicine
University of Chicago Pritzker School of Medicine
Attending Physician
Pediatric Emergency Medicine
University of Chicago Comer's Children Hospital
Chicago, Illinois

Biswadev Mitra, MBBS, MHSM, PhD, FACEM
Emergency & Trauma Centre
The Alfred Hospital
Melbourne, Australia

Brooks L. Moore, MD
Assistant Professor
Department of Emergency Medicine
Emory University School of Medicine
Attending Physician
Department of Emergency Medicine
Emory University Hospital and Grady Memorial Hospital
Atlanta, Georgia

Tom Morrissey, MD, PhD
Associate Professor
Department Emergency Medicine
University of Florida-Jacksonville
Jacksonville, Florida

Jordan B. Moskoff, MD
Associate Medical Director
Department of Emergency Medicine
Cook County (Stroger) Hospital
Assistant Professor
Department of Emergency Medicine
Rush Medical College
Chicago, Illinois

Mark B. Mycyk, MD, FACEP, FACMT
Associate Professor
Department of Emergency Medicine
Rush Medical College
Northwestern University Feinberg School of Medicine
Attending Physician
Department of Emergency Medicine
Cook County (Stroger) Hospital
Chicago, Illinois

Isam F. Nasr, MD, FACEP
Assistant Professor
Department of Emergency Medicine
Rush Medical College
Attending Physician
Department of Emergency Medicine
Cook County (Stroger) Hospital
Chicago, Illinois

Michael E. Nelson, MD, MS
Attending Physician, Medical Toxicology Fellow
Department of Emergency Medicine
Cook County (Stroger) Hospital
Chicago, Illinois
Attending Physician
Department of Emergency Medicine
Northshore University Health System
Evanston, Illinois

Erik K. Nordquist, MD
Assistant Professor
Department of Emergency Medicine
Cook County (Stroger) Hospital
Chicago, Illinois

Paula E. Oldeg, MD, FACEP
Attending Physician
Department of Emergency Medicine
West Suburban Medical Center
Oak Park, Illinois
Adjunct Clinical Instructor
Department of Emergency Medicine
Rush Medical College
Chicago, Illinois

S. Margaret Paik, MD
Assistant Professor of Pediatrics
Department of Pediatrics
Associate Section Chief, Pediatric Emergency Medicine
The University of Chicago Comer Children's Hospital
Chicago, Illinois

Lisa R. Palivos, MD
Assistant Professor
Department of Emergency Medicine
Rush Medical College
Attending Physician
Department of Emergency Medicine
Cook County (Stroger) Hospital
Chicago, Illinois

Jonathon D. Palmer, MD
Assistant Professor
Department of Emergency Medicine
University of Arkansas for Medical Sciences
Little Rock, Arkansas

Matthew S. Patton, MD
Department of Emergency Medicine
Northwestern University Feinberg School of Medicine
Chicago, Illinois

Rahul G. Patwari, MD
Medical Student Clerkship Director
Assistant Professor
Attending Physician
Department of Emergency Medicine
Rush Medical College
Chicago, Illinois

Monika Pitzele, MD, PhD
Attending Physician
Department of Emergency Medicine
Mount Sinai Hospital
Chicago, Illinois

Henry Z. Pitzele, MD, FACEP
Deputy Director
Emergency Medicine
Jesse Brown VA Medical Center
Clinical Assistant Professor
Department of Emergency Medicine
University of Illinois at Chicago
Chicago, Illinois

Natalie Radford, MD
Associate Professor
Department of Clinical Medicine
Florida State University
Attending Physician
Bixler Emergency Department
Tallahassee Memorial Hospital
Tallahassee, Florida

Christopher Reverte, MD
Chief Resident
Department of Emergency Medicine
LA County + USC Medical Center
Los Angeles, California
Attending Physician
Department of Emergency Medicine
St. Luke's-Roosevelt
New York, New York

Neil Rifenbark, MD
Department of Emergency Medicine
University of Southern California
Department of Emergency Medicine
LA County + USC Medical Center
Los Angeles, California

Rebecca R. Roberts, MD
Director, Research Division
Attending Physician
Department of Emergency Medicine
Cook County (Stroger) Hospital
Chicago, Illinois

Sarah E. Ronan-Bentle, MD, MS, FACEP
Assistant Professor
Department of Emergency Medicine
University of Cincinnati College of Medicine
Attending Physician
Center for Emergency Care
University Hospital
Cincinnati, Ohio

David H. Rosenbaum, MD, FAAEM
Attending Physician
Department of Emergency Medicine
WakeMed Health and Hospitals
Raleigh, North Carolina
Adjunct Professor
Department of Emergency Medicine
University of North Carolina School of Medicine
Chapel Hill, North Carolina

Christopher Ross, MD, FRCPC, FACEP, FAAEM
Assistant Professor
Department of Emergency Medicine
Associate Chair
Planning, Education, and Research
Cook County (Stroger) Hospital
Chicago, Illinois

John Sarko, MD
Attending Physician
Department of Emergency Medicine
Maricopa Medical Center
Assistant Professor
Department of Emergency Medicine
University of Arizona Phoenix School of Medicine
Phoenix, Arizona

Shari Schabowski, MD
Assistant Professor
Department of Emergency Medicine
Rush Medical College
Attending Physician
Department of Emergency Medicine
Cook County (Stroger) Hospital
Chicago, Illinois

Conor D. Schaye, MD, MPH
Department of Emergency Medicine
Northwestern Memorial Hospital
Chicago, Illinois

Michael A. Schindlbeck, MD, FACEP
Assistant Professor
Department of Emergency Medicine
Rush Medical College
Assistant Residency Director
Cook County (Stroger) Hospital
Chicago, Illinois

Suzanne M. Schmidt, MD, FAAP
Clinical Instructor
Department of Pediatrics
Northwestern University Feinberg School of Medicine
Attending Physician
Department of Pediatrics
Ann & Robert H. Lurie Children's Hospital of Chicago
Chicago, Illinois

Theresa M. Schwab, MD
Attending Physician
Department of Emergency Medicine
Advocate Christ Medical Center
Oak Lawn, Illinois
Assistant Professor
Department of Emergency Medicine
University of Illinois at Chicago
Chicago, Illinois

Brian R. Sellers, MD
Department of Emergency Medicine
Northwestern University Feinberg School of Medicine
Chicago, Illinois

Emily L. Senecal, MD
Clinical Instructor
Department of Emergency Medicine
Harvard Medical School
Attending Physician
Department of Emergency Medicine
Massachusetts General Hospital
Boston, Massachusetts

Michelle Sergel, MD
Assistant Professor
Department of Emergency Medicine
Rush Medical College
Attending Physician
Department of Emergency Medicine
Cook County (Stroger) Hospital
Chicago, Illinois

Scott C. Sherman, MD
Medical Student Clerkship Director
PA Residency Director
Associate Residency Director
Department of Emergency Medicine
Cook County (Stroger) Hospital
Rush Medical College
Chicago, Illinois

Jeffrey N. Siegelman, MD
Assistant Professor
Department of Emergency Medicine
Emory University
Atlanta, Georgia

Jessica Sime, MD
Department of Emergency Medicine
Union Memorial Hospital
Baltimore, Maryland

Lauren M. Smith, MD
Assistant Professor
Department of Emergency Medicine
Rush Medical College
Attending Physician
Department of Emergency Medicine
Cook County (Stroger) Hospital
Chicago, Illinois

William Thomas Smith, MD
Emergency Medicine
Oregon Health and Sciences University
Portland, Oregon

Shannon E. Staley, MD
Pediatric Emergency Medicine Fellow
Department of Pediatrics
University of Chicago Comer Children's Hospital
Chicago, Illinois

Christine R. Stehman, MD
Clinical Fellow
Department of Surgery, Division of Trauma, Burn, and Surgical Critical Care
Associate Physician
Department of Emergency Medicine
Brigham and Women's Hospital, Harvard Medical School
Boston, Massachusetts

Harsh Sule, MD, FAAEM, FACEP
Assistant Professor
Department of Emergency Medicine
Thomas Jefferson University & Hospitals
Philadelphia, Pennsylvania

Gim A. Tan, MBBS, FACEM
Adjunct Lecturer
Department of Emergency Medicine
Monash University
Senior Emergency Physician
Emergency and Trauma Centre
The Alfred Hospital
Melbourne, Australia

Katie L. Tataris, MD
Department of Emergency Medicine
Cook County (Stroger) Hospital
Chicago, Illinois

Matthew C. Tews, DO
Associate Professor
Department of Emergency Medicine
Medical College of Wisconsin
Milwaukee, Wisconsin

S. Spencer Topp, MD
Assistant Professor
Department of Emergency Medicine
University of Florida Health Science Center-Jacksonville
Jacksonville, Florida

Brandon C. Tudor, MD
Private Practice
Everett, Washington

Katrina R. Wade, MD, FAAEM, FAAP
Associate Professor
Department of Surgery, Emergency Medicine Division
Assistant Professor, Pediatrics
Department of Pediatrics
Saint Louis University School of Medicine
St. Louis, Missouri

David A. Wald, DO
Professor of Emergency Medicine
Medical Director, William Maul Measey Institute for Clinical
Simulation and Patient Safety
Temple University School of Medicine
Philadelphia, Pennsylvania

Joseph Walline, MD
Assistant Professor
Department of Surgery, Division of Emergency Medicine
Saint Louis University School of Medicine
Saint Louis, Missouri

Joseph M. Weber, MD
EMS Medical Director
Department of Emergency Medicine
Cook County (Stroger) Hospital
Assistant Professor of Emergency Medicine
Rush Medical College
Chicago, Illinois

Joanne C. Witsil, PharmD, RN, BCPS
Adjunct Clinical Assistant Professor
Department of Pharmacy Practice
University of Illinois at Chicago
Clinical Pharmacist
Department of Emergency Medicine
Cook County (Stroger) Hospital
Chicago, Illinois

Kathleen A. Wittels, MD
Instructor in Medicine
Department of Emergency Medicine
Harvard Medical School
Associate Clerkship Director
Department of Emergency Medicine
Brigham and Women's Hospital, Harvard Medical School
Boston, Massachusetts

Lynne M. Yancey, MD, FACEP
Associate Professor
Department of Emergency Medicine
University of Colorado School of Medicine
Denver, Colorado
Attending Physician
Department of Emergency Medicine
University of Colorado Hospital
Aurora, Colorado

Leslie S. Zun, MD
Professor
Emergency Medicine
Chicago Medical School
Chair
Emergency Medicine
Mount Sinai Hospital
Chicago, Illinois

Preface

We wrote this book because we remember our own experiences as medical students and junior residents working in the emergency department (ED). The ED is a unique environment that requires knowledge and skills often not covered in medical or physician assistant school. In this book, we attempt to create a resource for the medical student, physician assistant, nurse practitioner, and junior-level resident to use to get a grasp on the issues and scope of problems that they will confront while working in the ED.

The book's length and format are designed to allow the student and practitioner to begin to digest the broad range of topics inherent to emergency medicine (EM). Each chapter begins with a section on Key Points, followed by an Introduction, Clinical Presentation (History and Physical Examination), Diagnostic Studies, Medical Decision Making, Treatment, and Disposition. Whenever possible, we tried to give practical information regarding drug dosing, medical decision-making thought processes, treatment plans, and dispositions that will actually allow you to function more comfortably in the clinical environment. The diagnostic algorithms are a unique feature that attempt to simplify the problem and point the clinician in the right direction.

The book has 19 sections and 98 chapters that cover the entire contents of the EM clerkship curriculum (*Acad Emerg Med.* 2010;17:638-643). The authors are all practicing emergency physicians and EM educators from throughout the country. For medical student clerkship directors, we believe that this text is the perfect book for the student to pick up and digest during a 4-week rotation.

In summary, we hope this book will enhance the emergency medicine experience of all its users.

Scott C. Sherman, MD
Joseph M. Weber, MD
Michael Schindlbeck, MD
Rahul Patwari, MD

Acknowledgments

We have many people to thank in helping us bring this project to fruition. First and foremost, this text would have never made it to print without the support and encouragement of our McGraw-Hill editor, Anne Sydor. Anne is a friend as much as an editor. She took a chance on us and for that we will always be grateful. One of Anne's many gifts has been providing us with such great editorial support in the form of Sarah M. Granlund. She has been the quarterback of this project from the onset, and without her planning and attention to detail, we would not be here today. We would also like to acknowledge our project manager, Charu Khanna, for her attention to detail during page proofs and willingness to go the extra mile.

We also want to thank our "bosses," Jeff Schaider and Steve Bowman. Jeff is a constant source of enthusiasm for the academic project in whatever form makes his faculty happy. He is a mentor, role model, and friend to us all. Steve, our residency director, also deserves so much credit. He shoulders the burden of one of the largest residencies in the country in a way that allows his assistants to pursue the true pleasures of the academic job in emergency medicine. Thank you both.

Estella Bravo, Ethel Lee, Mishelle Taylor, Deloris Johnson, and Hilda Nino also deserve a load of credit for the support they provide in the offices. Estella has been the dream clerkship coordinator, managing 24 students per month with grace and determination. She sets the bar high and makes our students feel comfortable during their time with us. For those who consider becoming a clerkship director one day, the most important consideration is making sure you have someone like Estella at the reins of the coordinator position.

Several groups of people also deserve high praise. Our authors have turned in an outstanding product, making the job of editing so much easier. We have tried to assemble an "all-star" group of contributors, and based on what came back to us, we were not disappointed. We all benefit from the hard work and expertise of our authors after "too many years to count" spent working in emergency departments and educating eager learners in the field. We also want to acknowledge our students and residents. You folks are the driving force behind all of our efforts. You inspire, test, and humble us on a daily basis. Lastly, and most importantly, we would like to thank our patients. We learn what our patients teach us, and so any learning we have accomplished over the years is attributed to them. They are the true educators of emergency medicine, and we owe them a debt of gratitude.

Incision and Drainage

David E. Manthey, MD

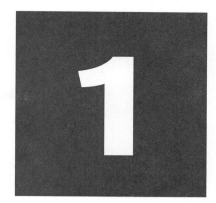

INDICATIONS

Incision and drainage (I&D) is the definitive treatment for any subcutaneous abscess. Abscesses should be drained if larger than 5 mm and accessible to percutaneous incision. Antibiotics alone are not adequate treatment of an abscess. In fact, skin abscesses without surrounding cellulitis, once drained, do not require any further treatment with antibiotics.

Abscesses can be diagnosed by physical examination based on swelling, pain, redness, and fluctuance (Figure 1-1). Some abscesses will spontaneously drain, leaving little diagnostic doubt. Bedside ultrasound may aid in diagnosis by identifying a hypoechoic area of fluid just under the skin. Needle aspiration may also be employed to prove the presence of pus.

Abscesses are often denoted by various names depending on their location and/or structure involved. The treatment remains the same. Paronychia and eponychia form around the nail (Figure 1-2). Felons occur with infection of the volar pad of the finger and require a specific approach for drainage. Bartholin gland abscesses occur in the paired glands that provide moisture to the vestibule of the vaginal mucosa. When the opening becomes occluded, either an abscess or a cyst can develop. After I&D, a Word catheter is placed to insure continued drainage of the gland. Removal or marsupialization of the gland may be required to prevent recurrence.

Hidradenitis suppurativa is a chronic relapsing inflammatory process affecting the apocrine glands in the axilla, inguinal area, or both. Multiple abscesses can form and eventually lead to draining fistulous tracts that require surgical management. I&D of these abscesses is frequently necessary and performed in the emergency department.

Incision and drainage may also be used to treat infected pilonidal or sebaceous cysts. Further treatment by a

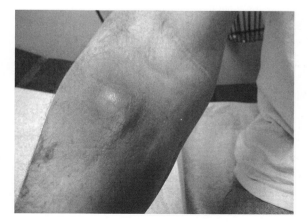

▲ **Figure 1-1.** A subcutaneous abscess in an intravenous drug user.

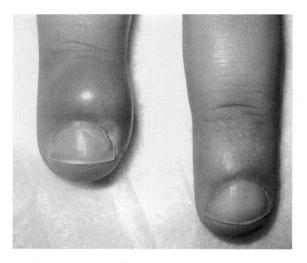

▲ **Figure 1-2.** Paronychia.

surgeon will often include removing the capsule to prevent recurrence.

Perirectal abscesses include superficial abscesses (ie, perianal), which can be drained by emergency physicians, and deeper abscesses (ie, ischiorectal, intersphincteric, supralevator), which require operative surgical drainage. Perianal abscesses present as tender, fluctuant masses palpated around the anal verge. Deeper abscesses often present with rectal pain, pain with defecation, rectal and buttock erythema and tenderness, and systemic symptoms (ie, fever, lethargy).

CONTRAINDICATIONS

Cellulitis without evidence of underlying abscess should not be incised. Pulsatile masses that may be infected pseudoaneuryms should not be incised.

Extremely large or deep abscesses should be considered for drainage under anesthesia. As a result of transient bacteremia, those patients at risk for endocarditis owing to an artificial or abnormal heart valve should be given appropriate perioperative antibiotics.

Abscesses of the palms, soles, nasolabial fold, breasts, finger pads (felons), face, and deeper perirectal region can be associated with complications. Consider consultation with the appropriate surgical subspecialty.

EQUIPMENT

Povidone-iodine solution or chlorhexidine solution to cleanse the skin

Anesthetic of 1% lidocaine or 0.25% bupivacaine with epinephrine

18-gauge needle (to aspirate anesthetic)

27-gauge needle and syringe (to inject local anesthesia)

Splash guard or 18-gauge angiocatheter (without needle)

30-mL syringe for irrigation

Sterile water or normal saline

11-blade scalpel

Swab for bacterial culture

Curved hemostat

¼-inch iodoform packing

Scissors

Gloves, gown, and facemask with shield (universal precautions)

Gauze and tape

PROCEDURE

Discuss the risks and benefits of the procedure with the patient before obtaining consent. Verify abscess location with ultrasound if necessary. Wash your hands and wear gloves, gown, and a face shield, as many abscesses are under pressure. Position the patient and lighting to allow for the best visualization and access to the abscess. Prepare the area with povidone-iodine solution or chlorhexidine.

Utilizing a 27-gauge needle, inject the anesthetic just under the dermis parallel to the surface of the skin. Blanching of the tissue will occur as the anesthetic spreads out through the skin. Cover the entire area to be incised. Avoid injecting lidocaine into the abscess cavity. This may increase the pressure in the cavity causing more pain. For larger abscesses, local field blocks, parenteral analgesics, and/or procedural sedation may be necessary.

If it is unclear whether an abscess exists, attempt aspiration of pus with a syringe and an 18- or 20-gauge needle. If confirmed, use an 11-blade scalpel to make a single incision in the skin. The incision should be at the point of maximal fluctuance oriented in the long axis of the abscess. In general, the incision should extend two thirds of the diameter of the abscess cavity (except when draining Bartholin gland abscesses, for which only an incision 0.5–1 cm should be made). Attempt to incise parallel to existing skin tension lines to promote cosmetic results.

Use gentle and steady pressure around the abscess to express pus from the cavity. Insert a curved hemostat to break loculations by working in a clockwise fashion around the entire abscess cavity. This will also help identify any deeper tracks. If desired, obtain a culture of the wound at this time.

Consider gentle irrigation of the wound until the fluid returning is clear. Pack the wound with enough iodoform gauze to keep the sides of the abscess from touching. This will allow for further drainage. Cover the wound with gauze.

When treating a Bartholin gland abscess, a small catheter (Word catheter) is placed in the opening instead of iodoform. The catheter should remain in place for several weeks to allow for the development of a fistula for continued drainage.

The patient is instructed to follow up in 48 hours to have the packing removed. If pus is no longer present and symptoms are resolving, the wound is allowed to heal by secondary intention.

COMPLICATIONS

Scarring from the abscess and incision will occur. Numbness from cutaneous nerve injury may occur. Seeding of the blood with bacteria may transiently occur.

SUGGESTED READING

Fitch MT, Manthey DE, McGinnis HD, et al. Abscess incision and drainage. *N Engl J Med* 2007;357:e20.

Hankin A, Everett WW. Are antibiotics necessary after incision and drainage of a cutaneous abscess? *Ann Emerg Med.* 2007;50: 49–51.

Kelly EW, Magilner D. Soft tissue infections. In: Tintinalli JE, Stapczynski JS, Ma OJ, Cline DM, Cydulka RK, Meckler GD. *Tintinalli's Emergency Medicine: A Comprehensive Study Guide.* 7th ed. New York, NY: McGraw-Hill, 2011: Pages 1014–1024.

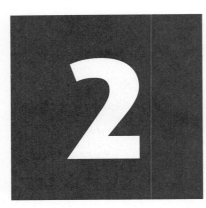

2

Arterial Blood Gas

Brian C. Kitamura, MD

John Sarko, MD

Key Points

- Arterial puncture for blood gas analysis is a common procedure performed in the emergency department (ED).
- Blood obtained from the radial artery can be used to quickly provide quantitative information on the patient's acid–base status and carboxyhemoglobin, methemoglobin, and electrolyte levels.
- Arterial puncture is a useful way to obtain blood for analysis when traditional phlebotomy is limited or difficult on the basis of patient characteristics.

INDICATIONS

The primary indication for obtaining an arterial blood sample is for the assessment of the partial pressures of oxygen and carbon dioxide and accurate assessment of arterial pH. Secondarily, arterial blood can be analyzed for carboxyhemoglobin, methemoglobin, and basic electrolytes depending on the capabilities of the laboratory. Under certain circumstances it may be necessary to obtain a sample of arterial blood for other routine laboratory tests, such as in patients who are obese or have a history of intravenous drug abuse, in whom the radial artery is palpable, but venous access is difficult or may be delayed.

CONTRAINDICATIONS

There are few absolute contraindications for arterial puncture for blood gas analysis. Trauma, infection, or abnormalities of the overlying skin such as a burn are contraindications because of concern for infection or further damage to the vascular structures. Patients with known coagulopathies, taking anticoagulants, or who may require thrombolytic agents should be approached with caution because of the increased risk of bleeding, hematoma formation, or rarely, compartment syndrome. Finally, a known history of insufficient blood flow through the palmar arch or previous surgery to the radial or ulnar arteries should also be considered a contraindication. The Allen test, described later, has been used as a way to determine adequacy of collateral circulation, however, its necessity has been questioned.

EQUIPMENT

Many commercially prepared kits for arterial puncture are available, and if a commercial kit is not available, then equipment is easily found in most EDs. The following equipment is typically used to perform the procedure (Figure 2-1).

▶ Required Equipment

Alcohol, chlorhexidine, or iodine prep pads

2- to 3-mL heparinized syringe with a 23- to 25-gauge needle

Syringe cap

Appropriate personal protective equipment

Gauze or other dressing

▶ Suggested Equipment

Anesthetic (eg, lidocaine)

Ultrasound or Doppler (if the artery is difficult to palpate)

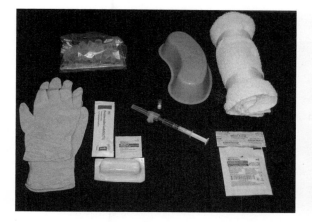

Figure 2-1. Equipment used for an arterial puncture.

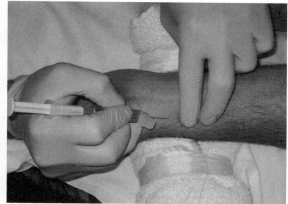

Figure 2-2. Position of the forearm for puncture of the radial artery. A kidney basin or rolled towel may be helpful to hold the patient's wrist in this position.

Rolled towel or kidney basin (to stabilize and extend the wrist)

Ice (for specimen process times > 10 minutes)

Local anesthesia is not strictly required for the procedure; however, studies have shown that pain, as well as the number of attempts required to obtain a sample, are reduced when appropriate anesthesia is provided. Traditionally, 1% lidocaine is used, avoiding epinephrine because of concern for vasospasm. Recent studies have suggested that jet-injected 2% lidocaine also provides reasonable anesthesia.

PROCEDURE

Before selecting an appropriate wrist, the Allen test may be used to assess collateral circulation. Manually occlude the radial and ulnar arteries using your fingers. Ask the patient to clench the fist to increase venous drainage from the hand for approximately 30 seconds. Ask the patient to open the hand, which should be noticeably pale. At this point, release only the ulnar artery. Rapid return of color signifies adequate collateral flow. Although the necessity of the test for arterial puncture is questioned, common sense dictates that if collateral flow in one wrist is noticeably decreased compared with the other, the wrist with better collateral flow should be accessed. In the absence of good collateral flow in both wrists, the necessity of the procedure should be weighed against the remote risk of serious vascular injury and distal extremity ischemia.

The radial artery is easily palpated in a majority of patients. It runs down the radial aspect of the forearm, generally located between the styloid process of the radius and the flexor carpi radialis tendon at the proximal crease of the wrist. The patient's wrist should be extended to bring the artery to a more superficial position. A kidney basin or rolled towel as well as tape may be helpful to hold the patient's wrist in this position (Figure 2-2). The skin overlying the artery should be cleaned. The skin and immediate subcutaneous tissue should then be appropriately anesthetized. The authors recommend massaging the area or letting it rest for 1–2 minutes for the anesthetic to take complete effect. This time may be used to prepare your other equipment.

After locating the impulse of the artery with the non-dominate hand, take the syringe and needle in your dominate hand and slowly advance the needle toward the impulse at a 30- to 45-degree angle proximally toward the patient. If the impulse is difficult to detect, an ultrasound or Doppler may be helpful to locate the artery (Figure 2-3). Some practitioners use a direct 90-degree angle to the skin, but this is largely a matter of preference. When the artery is accessed, blood will passively fill the syringe. It should not be necessary to draw back on the syringe. Pulsatile or bright red blood signals the correct vessel has been accessed; however, this may not be apparent in the critically ill patient. If blood is not obtained, withdraw the needle to just below the skin and reattempt the procedure after slight adjustments have been made. Do not move the needle in an arc deep in the skin, as this risks damage to the vascular structures.

After blood is collected, the needle should be removed and disposed of appropriately. Remove air from the syringe and place the syringe cap, ensuring that blood contacts the cap. Maintain pressure over the arterial site for approximately 5 minutes to prevent development of a hematoma, and dress the wound appropriately.

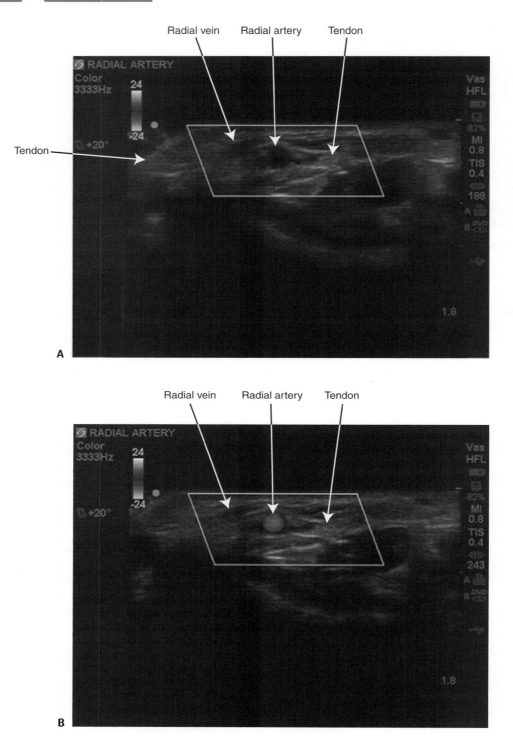

▲ **Figure 2-3.** The radial artery on ultrasonography. **A.** A high-frequency linear transducer is used to locate the vessel based on anatomic landmarks. The ultrasound probe is oriented toward the patient's thumb. **B.** If there are other vascular structures in the image, color Doppler can be used to locate the artery by identifying pulsatile flow.

COMPLICATIONS

Complications from this procedure are rare but include infection, bleeding, arterial laceration, pseudoaneurysm or arteriovenous malformation, and nerve injury.

SUGGESTED READING

Dev SP, Hillmer MD, Ferri M. Arterial puncture for blood gas analysis. *N Engl J Med.* 2011; 364:e7.

Giner J, et al. Pain during arterial puncture. *Chest.* 1996;110: 1443–1445.

Hajiseyedjavady H, et al. Less painful arterial blood gas sampling using jet injection of 2% lidocaine: a randomized controlled clinical trial. *Am J Emerg Med.* 2012;30:1100–1104.

Haynes JM, Mitchell H. Ultrasound-guided arterial puncture. *Resp Care.* 2010;55:1754–1756.

Shiver S, Blaivas M, Lyon M. A prospective comparison of ultrasound-guided and blindly placed radial arterial catheters. *Acad Emerg Med.* 2006;13:1275–1279.

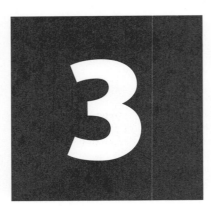

3

Central Venous Access

Basem F. Khishfe, MD

Rashid E. Kysia, MD

Key Points

- The ability to access the central venous circulation is an imperative skill for emergency physicians and is often needed for life-saving measures.
- The central venous circulation can be accessed both above and below the diaphragm. The site should be chosen based on reason for access as well as body habitus and pattern of injury for trauma patients.
- Although the overall complication rate for central line placement is low for experienced providers, serious complications may occur.

INDICATIONS

The most common reason for placement of a central venous catheter in the emergency department (ED) is for resuscitation of the critically ill medical or trauma patient. Medical patients may require central access for large volume fluid resuscitation, central venous pressure monitoring, IV pressors or other medications caustic to the peripheral veins (dextrose, hypertonic saline, total parenteral nutrition), transvenous pacing, or emergent dialysis. Trauma patients most often require central access for large-volume resuscitation with both fluids and blood. Central access is also used in ED patients with difficult peripheral IV access.

CONTRAINDICATIONS

Central access should not be attempted when peripheral access is obtainable and no other indication is present. Central access should be avoided at sites with overlying cellulitis or other anatomic abnormalities such as extensive trauma that may cause distorted anatomic landmarks. Known coagulopathy is an absolute contraindication to subclavian vein cannulation (noncompressible site) and a relative contraindication for internal jugular and femoral cannulation. Finally, patients must be able to cooperate during the procedure by remaining still. An uncooperative patient is a relative contraindication that may require sedation before the procedure.

EQUIPMENT

Most of the equipment needed to perform central venous cannulation can be found in commercially available central line kits (Figure 3-1). Kits include povidone-iodine swabs, guidewire introducer needle, J-tip guidewire, multiple 5-mL syringes, 1% lidocaine, 22- and 25-gauge needles for local anesthesia, #11 blade scalpel, dilator, central line, and silk suture on a cutting needle.

There are multiple types of central lines. In general, 1 of 2 types is used in the ED (Figure 3-2). A triple-lumen catheter is used for patients who require multiple different medication drips or when there is difficulty obtaining peripheral venous access. A sheath introducer (Cordis) catheter is shorter and wider and is used for introducing transvenous pacers, Swan-Ganz catheters, and for rapid infusion of fluid and blood products in the hypotensive patient. These larger catheters can achieve flow rates up to 1 L/min.

PROCEDURE

The procedure including risks and benefits should be completely explained to the patient or their representative. Informed consent should be obtained unless the

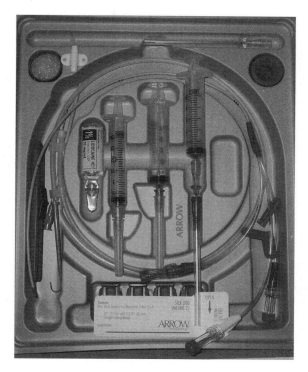

Figure 3-1. Triple lumen kit.

procedure is performed emergently. First locate the appropriate anatomical landmarks for the chosen site (see later). Next, apply povidone-iodine to the area of needle insertion followed by the sterile drape. Then

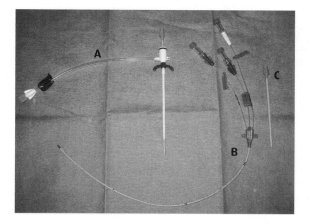

Figure 3-2. From left to right: **A.** sheath introducer kit (Cordis) with dilator. **B.** Triple lumen catheter. **C.** triple lumen dilator.

anesthetize the area of needle insertion with lidocaine. Once the preparation is complete, Seldinger technique should be followed in a stepwise fashion to complete the procedure.

▶ Seldinger Technique

1. Use a large-bore needle with syringe to cannulate the vein. There should be free flow of dark nonpulsatile blood into the syringe with traction on plunger (Figure 3-3A).
2. Thread the guidewire through the needle until 3–5 cm of the guidewire remains (Figure 3-3B). If resistance is met, withdraw the wire and confirm that the needle is in the vessel. Attempt to rethread the wire.
3. When the guidewire is in place, remove the needle (Figure 3-3C). ***Never let go of the guidewire during any part of the procedure because it can migrate fully into the vessel.***
4. Using a #11 blade scalpel, make a superficial stab incision in the skin at the site that the guidewire enters (Figure 3-3D).
5. Pass the dilator over the wire and thread into the vessel (Figure 3-3E). (For the Cordis catheter, the dilator and catheter are inserted together.)
6. Remove the dilator and thread the triple lumen over the wire, backing out the wire until it protrudes 2-3 cm out of the brown port.
7. Holding the free wire with one hand, thread the line into the vein (Figure 3-3F).
8. Remove the wire and confirm placement with aspiration of blood (Figure 3-3G). Secure the catheter in place with suture.

Internal jugular vein cannulation can be achieved by multiple approaches. The central approach is described here (Figure 3-4). Position the patient supine and in slight Trendelenburg position, with the head rotated 75 degrees to the opposite side. Palpate the triangle formed by the 2 heads of the sternocleidomastoid muscle. Palpate the carotid artery pulse within this triangle. The vein is lateral to the artery in this location and is widest just below the level of the cricoid cartilage. Insert the needle at the apex of the triangle, aiming toward the ipsilateral nipple with 30 degrees of angulation. The vein should be entered within 2–3 cm of needle advancement. If unsuccessful, withdraw slowly, as the vessel, if punctured, may have been compressed during advancement and will be pulled open on withdrawal. Do not palpate the carotid pulse while attempting to cannulate the internal jugular vein. The slight compression that results can compress the vein, making it more difficult to access. Cannulation of the right internal jugular is preferred over the left because of the straight line into the right atrium

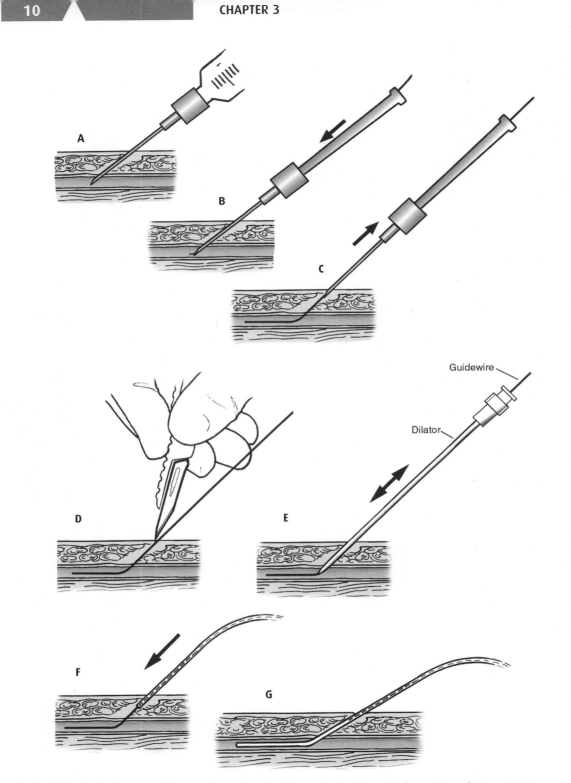

Figure 3-3. The Seldinger technique. (Reproduced with permission from Reichman EF and Simon RR. *Emergency Medicine Procedures*. New York: McGraw-Hill, 2004. Figure 38-10.)

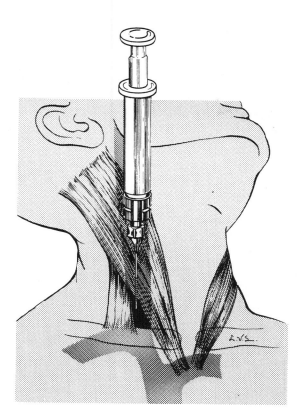

▲ **Figure 3-4.** Internal jugular vein catheterization. (Reproduced with permission from Dunphy JE, Way LW. *Current Surgical Diagnosis & Treatment*. 5th ed. Lange, 1981.)

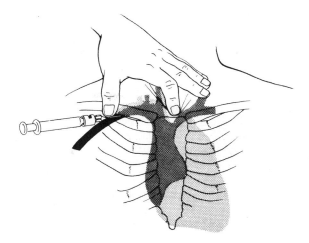

▲ **Figure 3-5.** Subclavian vein catheterization. (Reproduced with permission from Stone CK and Humphries RL. *Lange: Current Emergency Diagnosis and Treatment*. 57th ed. New York: McGraw-Hill, 2004–2011. Figure 7-7.)

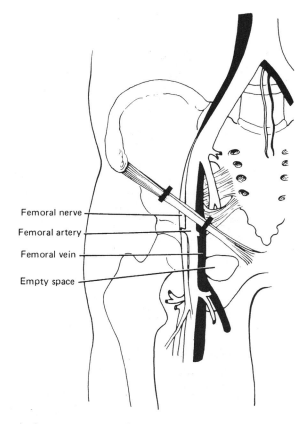

Femoral nerve
Femoral artery
Femoral vein
Empty space

▲ **Figure 3-6.** Femoral vein anatomy. (Reprinted with permission from Stone CK and Humphries RL. *Lange: Current Emergency Diagnosis and Treatment*. 57th ed. New York: McGraw-Hill, 2004–2011. Figure 7-8.)

and the presence of the thoracic duct and a higher pleural dome on the left side.

The **subclavian vein** can also be cannulated by multiple approaches. The infraclavicular approach is described here (Figure 3-5). Position the patient supine and in slight Trendelenburg position. Place a rolled sheet or towel between the patient's scapulas to allow the shoulders to fall backward and flatten the clavicles. Insert the needle 1 cm inferior to the clavicle, at the junction of the middle and medial thirds. Direct the needle under the clavicle and toward the suprasternal notch, with the needle parallel to the chest wall. The vein should be entered within 4 cm of needle advancement.

The **femoral vein** has a single approach. Palpate the femoral artery 2 cm below the inguinal crease. The vein is usually 1 cm medial to the artery at this location. Insert the needle at a 45-degree angle to the skin, medial to the femoral pulse, in a cephalad direction. In the pulseless patient, palpate the anterior superior iliac spine and the pubic tubercle. Draw an imaginary line connecting these 2 points. If this line is divided into thirds, the vein will be located where the medial and middle thirds intersect (Figure 3-6).

COMPLICATIONS

Central venous access has multiple complications common to each site, including bleeding, infection, arterial or venous laceration, and air embolism. Site specific complications include the following: for internal jugular, airway compression from expanding hematoma, carotid artery dissection, pneumothorax, and arrhythmia from cardiac irritation; for subclavian, pneumothorax and arrhythmia; for femoral, deep venous thrombosis, line sepsis, retroperitoneal bleeding, and bowel perforation.

SUGGESTED READING

Weber J, Schindlbeck M, Bailitz J. Vascular procedures. In: Simon RR, Ross C, Bowman S, Wakim P. *Cook County Manual of Emergency Procedures.* 1st ed. Philadelphia, PA: Lippincott Williams & Wilkins, 2012.

Wyatt CR. Venous and intraosseous access in adults. In: Tintinalli JE, Stapczynski JS, Ma OJ, Cline DM, Cydulka RK, Meckler GD. *Tintinalli's Emergency Medicine: A Comprehensive Study Guide.* 7th ed. New York, NY: McGraw-Hill, 2011.

Procedural Sedation

Paula E. Oldeg, MD

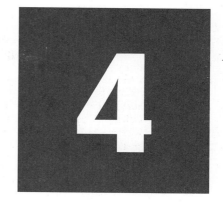

Key Points

- Procedural sedation is the administration of analgesic and sedative agents to induce a depressed level of consciousness so that a medical procedure can be performed without patient movement or memory.

- Procedural sedation should maintain cardiorespiratory function without requiring advanced airway adjuncts.
- Preprocedure patient assessment and proper selection of pharmacologic agents are the keys to patient safety.

INDICATIONS

Procedural sedation is a clinical technique that creates a decreased level of awareness, but allows maintenance of protective airway reflexes and adequate spontaneous ventilation. The goals of procedural sedation are to provide analgesia, amnesia, and anxiolysis during a potentially painful or frightening procedure. Pharmacologic agents used in procedural sedation are of 3 general classes: sedatives, analgesics, and dissociative agents. The use of such medications in the emergency setting is common and has been shown to be safe. Before the procedure, the physician should assess the patient for systemic disease and for a potential difficult airway. The patient's fitness for sedation can be quantified using the American Society of Anesthesiologists (ASA) physical status classification system (Table 4-1). The risk of a complication from emergency department (ED) procedural sedation and analgesia in ASA class I and II patients is low, usually <5%.

Examples of clinical scenarios appropriate for procedural sedation include painful or anxiety-provoking situations such as joint or fracture reduction, lumbar puncture, pediatric radiologic studies, incision and drainage, or cardioversion.

CONTRAINDICATIONS

Contraindications include ASA class III/IV, altered mental status, hemodynamic instability, known medication allergy, and lack of equipment or qualified personnel. Oral

Table 4-1. The American Society of Anesthesiologists physical status classification.

I.	Healthy patient
II.	Mild systemic disease—no functional limitation
III.	Severe system disease—definite functional limitation
IV.	Severe systemic disease—constant threat to life
V.	Moribund patient—not expected to survive without the operation

Data from American Society of Anesthesiologists. ASA Physical Status Classification System. http://www.asahq.org

intake within 3 hours is a relative contraindication. Higher risk cases may be more safely performed with anesthesia consultation or in the operating room.

EQUIPMENT

Patients should be closely monitored to recognize any change in vital signs and avert complications, most notably respiratory depression. Continuous pulse oximetry, cardiac monitor, and end-tidal CO_2 capnography (if available) should be applied. Intravenous (IV) access, an oxygen source and delivery method (eg, nasal canula), suction, airway management equipment (ie, bag-valve-mask, supraglottic airway, laryngoscope, endotracheal tube), resuscitation cart, and reversal drugs should be readily available. Personnel should be skilled in airway management and patient monitoring and recovery.

PROCEDURE

Appropriate preprocedure history includes allergies to or adverse effects from anesthetic agents, medical conditions, and time of last oral intake. Physical exam should include a thorough airway assessment to predict difficulty with bag-valve-mask ventilation or endotracheal intubation. Consider the presence of dentures, neck mobility, obesity, and Mallampati scale (Figure 4-1). Sedation in the emergency department should generally be limited to ASA class I and II patients. A fasting period of 3 hours is recommended; however, studies have shown that a shorter period does not increase the incidence of aspiration. The urgency of the procedure often dictates acceptable preprocedure fasting period. Obtain informed consent and document the conversation in the record. Many institutions have a standardized procedural sedation record for recording consent as well as pertinent history and physical.

Appropriate personnel to perform the procedure, administer medications, and monitor the patient should assemble at the bedside. The medications are administered and titrated to effect. Medication selection is guided by the type of procedure being performed (Table 4-2). Using a combination of a sedative/analgesic (eg, midazolam/fentanyl) generally gives consistent clinical results. Other commonly used regimens include ketamine alone or with atropine (0.01 mg/kg IV or IM) for pediatric cases, propofol plus an analgesic (fentanyl), or midazolam plus an analgesic.

The physician should perform the procedure as a nurse or other physician monitors the patient. After completion of the procedure, the patient should be monitored until mental status returns to baseline. Discharge criteria include stable vital signs, return to baseline mental status,

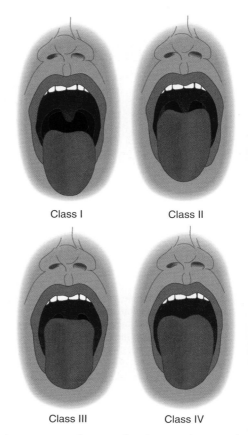

Class I   Class II

Class III   Class IV

▲ **Figure 4-1.** Mallampati classification. (Reprinted with permission from Vissers RJ. Chapter 30. Tracheal Intubation and Mechanical Ventilation. In: Tintinalli JE, Stapczynski JS, Cline DM, Ma OJ, Cydulka RK, Meckler GD, eds. *Tintinalli's Emergency Medicine: A Comprehensive Study Guide.* 7th ed. New York: McGraw-Hill, 2011.)

Table 4-2. Common medications used for procedural sedation in the ED.

Drug (Class)	Dose	Effects	Onset	Duration	Side Effects	Reversal Agent
Midazolam (benzodiazepine)	0.02–0.1 mg/kg IV	Sedation, amnesia, anxiolysis	2 min	20–30 min	Apnea, hypotension	Flumazenil
Morphine (opioid)	0.1–0.2 mg/kg IV	Analgesia	2 min	3–4 hr	Histamine release	Naloxone
Fentanyl (opioid)	0.5–1 mcg/kg to total dose of 2–3 mcg/kg IV	Analgesia, mild sedation	2 min	30 min	Respiratory depression and rigid chest syndrome	Naloxone
Ketamine (PCP derivative)	0.5–1 mg/kg IV or 3–5 mg/kg IM	Sedation, amnesia, analgesia, anxiolysis	1 min	1–2 hr	Secretions, tachycardia, emergence reactions, increased intracranial pressure	None
Etomidate (imidazole derivative)	0.1–0.2 mg/kg IV	Sedation, amnesia, anxiolysis	30 sec	10–30 min	Myoclonus, apnea	None
Propofol (phenol compound)	1–2 mg/kg IV	Sedation, amnesia	40 sec	3–5 min	Hypotension, bradycardia, injection site pain	None

Table 4-3. Reversal agents.

Drug	Dose	Effect	Onset	Duration	Side effects
Flumazenil	0.2 mg IV may be repeated to max 1 mg	benzodiazepine antagonist	1–2 min	45 min	Seizures, symptoms of benzo withdrawal
Naloxone	0.1–2 mg IV	opioid antagonist	Seconds	30 min	Can precipitate withdrawal in chronic users

ability to tolerate liquids, and an understanding of discharge instructions.

COMPLICATIONS

Respiratory depression is the most common adverse reaction. Close observation of the patient's pulse oximetry and respiratory effort can alert the physician to potential airway compromise. Support respirations by positioning the airway and providing bag-valve-mask ventilations if needed. Recent data have supported the use of continuous end-tidal CO_2 monitoring to recognize hypoventilation before hypoxia is seen on pulse oximetry. If respiratory depression persists, consider administration of a reversal agent (Table 4-3). Nausea and vomiting is another possible side effect. Prevent aspiration and ensure the airway is clear by turning the patient, suctioning, and supporting respirations. Inadequate amnesia or analgesia can make a procedure more difficult; conversely, prolonged sedation can occur with repeated doses of sedative agents. Careful medication titration and monitoring for effect can avoid these complications.

SUGGESTED READING

American College of Emergency Physicians. Clinical policy for procedural sedation and analgesia in the emergency department. *Ann Emerg Med.* 1998;31:663–677.

Deitch K, Miner J, Chudnofsky CR, Dominici P, Latta D. Does end tidal CO2 monitoring during emergency department procedural sedation and analgesia with propofol decrease the incidence of hypoxic events? A randomized, controlled trial. *Ann Emerg Med.* 2010;55:258–264.

Green SM, Roback MG, Miner JR, Burton JH, Krauss B. Fasting and emergency department procedural sedation and analgesia: a consensus-based clinical practice advisory. *Ann Emerg Med.* 2007;49:454–461.

Miner JR. Procedural sedation and analgesia. In: Tintinalli JE, Stapczynski JS, Ma OJ, Cline DM, Cydulka, RK, Meckler GD. *Tintinalli's Emergency Medicine: A Comprehensive Study Guide.* 7th ed. New York, NY: McGraw-Hill, 2011:283–291.

Lumbar Puncture

Pilar Guerrero, MD

Key Points

- Knowledge of anatomical landmarks and proper sterile technique are important when performing a lumbar puncture (LP).

- Absolute contraindications to LP are skin infection over puncture site and a brain mass causing increased intracranial pressure.

- Herniation is the most serious complication of a LP, whereas post-LP headache is most common.

INDICATIONS

Lumbar puncture (LP) is performed in the emergency department (ED) primarily to diagnose central nervous system (CNS) infections (ie, meningitis) and subarachnoid hemorrhage (SAH). It may also be performed to relieve cerebrospinal fluid (CSF) pressure and to confirm the diagnosis of idiopathic intracranial hypertension (pseudotumor cerebri). Other indications include the diagnosis of demyelinating or inflammatory CNS processes and carcinomatous/metastatic disease.

CONTRAINDICATIONS

Absolute contraindications for performing a LP include infected skin over the puncture site, increased intracranial pressure (ICP) from any space-occupying lesion (mass, abscess), and trauma or mass to lumbar vertebrae. A non-contrast head computed tomography (CT) scan should be performed to rule out an intracranial mass before performing an LP in the following clinical situations: altered mental status, focal neurologic deficits, signs of increased ICP (papilledema), immunocompromise, age >60 years, or recent seizure. Relative contraindications include patients who have bleeding diathesis or coagulopathy (Table 5-1).

Table 5-1. Contraindications to lumbar puncture.

Skin infection near the site of lumbar puncture
Central nervous system lesion causing increased intracranial pressure or spinal mass
Platelet count <20,000 mm³ is an absolute contraindication; platelet counts >50,000 mm³ are safe for lumbar puncture*
International normalized ratio ≥1.5*
Administration of unfiltered heparin or low-molecular-weight heparin in past 24 hours*
Hemophilia, von Willebrand disease, other coagulopathies*
Trauma to lumbar vertebrae

*Correct clotting factor and/or platelet levels before lumbar puncture.

Reprinted with permission from Ladde JG. Chapter 169. Central Nervous System Procedures and Devices. In: Tintinalli JE, Stapczynski JS, Cline DM, Ma OJ, Cydulka RK, Meckler GD, eds. *Tintinalli's Emergency Medicine: A Comprehensive Study Guide.* 7th ed. New York: McGraw-Hill, 2011.

EQUIPMENT

Most EDs have a commercially available LP kit, which contains a 20-gauge spinal needle, 22- and 25-gauge needles for lidocaine administration, 4 collection tubes, stopcock

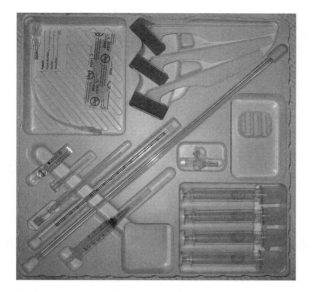

Figure 5-1. Lumbar puncture kit.

and manometer with extension tubing, sterile drapes, skin-cleansing sponges, and lidocaine (Figure 5-1). Smaller spinal needles may be used (22, 25 gauge) and may decrease the incidence of post-LP headache; however, a 22 or larger gauge needle must be used to determine an accurate opening pressure. Other required supplies include additional 1% lidocaine without epinephrine, povidone-iodine (Betadine), and sterile gloves.

PROCEDURE

Lumbar puncture is an invasive procedure. Always perform a neurologic examination before LP. Explain the procedure, risks and benefits, and potential complications and obtain written consent.

Assemble all equipment and have it within easy reach. Position the patient in a lateral decubitus position with hips and knees flexed and the upper back arched. This will allow better opening of the interlaminar spaces. Make sure the patient's shoulders, back, and hips are perpendicular to the stretcher. Alternatively, the patient may be in a sitting position, leaning forward and resting their arms on a tray stand. The latter may work well for patients who are obese, have degenerative joint disease, or have problems breathing. However, an accurate opening pressures can only be obtained with the patient in the lateral decubitus position.

Next, identify your landmarks by palpating the top of the posterior superior iliac crests, moving your fingers medially, as if drawing an imaginary line toward the spine. This should be at the L4 interspace level. Palpate the spinous processes and identify the L3–L4 and the L4–L5 interspace. Either of these spaces can be used for the procedure (Figure 5-2).

Open the sterile tray and pour Betadine into the empty receptacle in the kit. Put on the sterile gloves. Draw up your lidocaine and place the collection tubes in sequential order (numbers are written on the tubes, #1–4). Connect the manometer to the stopcock. Clean the area with Betadine-soaked handheld sponges in a circular motion, from the site of planned puncture outward. Include a spinal level above and below L4. Allow the area to completely dry. Place the unfenestrated drape on the patient's bed and the fenestrated drape (with the opening) over the procedure site. Palpate landmarks again. Using the 25-gauge needle, raise a skin wheal of lidocaine over the interspace. Then, use a 20- or 22-gauge needle to anesthetize the deeper subcutaneous tissue along the approximate line that the spinal needle will pass. Aspirate before injecting to make sure you are avoiding intravascular administration.

Identify your landmarks again by palpating the interspinous space with your nondominant hand. With the

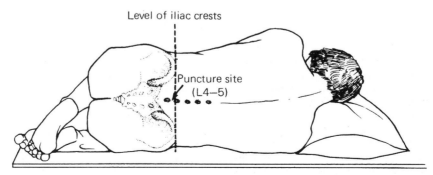

Level of iliac crests

Puncture site (L4–5)

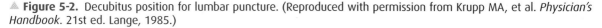

Figure 5-2. Decubitus position for lumbar puncture. (Reproduced with permission from Krupp MA, et al. *Physician's Handbook.* 21st ed. Lange, 1985.)

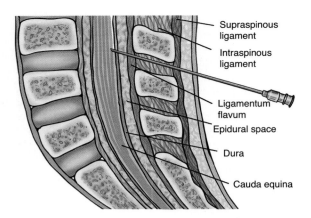

Supraspinous
ligament

Intraspinous
ligament

Ligamentum
flavum

Epidural space

Dura

Cauda equina

▲ **Figure 5-3.** Anatomy of the lumbar spinal interspaces for LP. (Reprinted with permission from Ladde JG. Chapter 169. Central Nervous System Procedures and Devices. In: Tintinalli JE, Stapczynski JS, Cline DM, Ma OJ, Cydulka RK, Meckler GD, eds. *Tintinalli's Emergency Medicine: A Comprehensive Study Guide.* 7th ed. New York: McGraw-Hill, 2011.)

needle parallel to the stretcher, slowly insert in the midline aiming 10 degrees cephalad. The needle will cross 3 ligaments (supraspinous, interspinous, and the strong elastic ligamentum flavum) before entering the dura and subarachnoid space (Figure 5-3). You may feel a "pop" as you transverse the ligamentum flavum. The bevel of the needle should be pointed to the patient's side (left or right) to prevent it from cutting the longitudinally oriented fibers of the dura. Theoretically, this will reduce the risk of persistent CSF leak and subsequent post-LP headache. After inserting the needle 4–5 cm or after feeling a "pop," remove the stylet and look for the efflux of CSF at the base of your needle. If no fluid returns, replace the stylet and advance or withdraw the needle and recheck. You may have to withdraw the needle to the subcutaneous tissue and redirect it more cephalad. The depth of insertion before getting into the subarachnoid space depends on the size of the patient. Never advance or remove the needle without the stylet in place to avoid it from becoming obstructed.

When the subarachnoid space is entered and CSF begins to flow, assess the opening pressure. Attach the manometer to the needle and direct the lever of the 3-way stopcock away from the needle to create a communication between the needle and glass column. At the point when fluid stops flowing into the manometer, the pressure is recorded. Normal opening pressure is between 7–18 cmH$_2$O. Deposit the CSF from the manometer into tube #1 and disconnect the manometer. In adults, proceed to collect 1–2 mL of CSF per tube. More tubes may be needed for additional tests or special situations

(VDRL, viral titer, Cryptococcus antigen, etc). When the fluid has been collected in all 4 tubes, the needle is removed with the stylet in place. This too has been shown to reduce the incidence of post-LP headache. The theoretical explanation for this effect is that the stylet pushes back any pia mater that may be sticking out from the hole made in the dura. Any tissue in the dura puncture can act to keep the hole from closing and result in a persistent CSF leak.

Tubes #1 and 4 should be sent for cell counts with differential. Tube #2 is sent for protein and glucose. Tube #3 should be sent for culture and Gram stain. Patients with an obese body habitus or with degenerative joints may present a challenge when performing an LP. Fluoroscopy (performed by a radiologist) or the use of ultrasound may aid in identifying the anatomical landmarks, making it possible to perform the procedure.

COMPLICATIONS

A "traumatic" LP (from injury to the dura or arachnoid vessels) is a common occurrence, with more than 50% of all LP procedures having from 1 to 50 red blood cells (RBCs) in the CSF. The incidence of traumatic LP may be minimized by proper patient and needle positioning. The best method to differentiate a traumatic LP from an SAH is noting that the number of RBCs significantly decrease from tube #1 to tube #4 in a traumatic LP. Tube #4 should have close to zero RBCs. The presence of xanthochromia indicates a SAH.

Spinal hematomas (epidural, subdural, and subarachnoid) are rare complications of LP, which are more likely to occur in patients with coagulation disorders. Correcting coagulation disorders (eg, Factor for a hemophiliac) is required before LP is performed.

Herniation can occur when CSF is removed from a patient with increased ICP from a mass, emphasizing the importance of performing a head CT if a mass lesion is suspected.

Post-LP headaches are the most common complication of LP and are thought to be from continued CSF leakage through the dura at the puncture site. A post-LP headache is observed in 20–70% of patients and is more common in young adults. Post-LP headaches are usually fronto-occipital and may have associated nausea, vomiting, and tinnitus. In most cases, the headache begins within 24–48 hours of the LP and is usually postural (worse in the upright position or with valsalva maneuvers). Post-LP headaches usually last 1–2 days, but occasionally can persist up to 14 days. Treatment consists of IV fluids, caffeine (IV or oral), antiemetics, analgesics, barbiturates, diphenhydramine, and ergots. Headaches lasting >24 hours may be alleviated by an epidural blood patch performed by an anesthesiologist. If the headache does not have a postural component, lasts more than 1 week, or recurs after initially resolving, consider the possibility of a subdural hematoma. Subdural hematomas are due to tearing of bridging veins from decreased CSF volume.

Patients may also complain of mild backache after an LP. This is common from trauma of the spinal needle and is usually self-limited, resolving in a few days. Other potential complications include iatrogenic infection caused by improper sterile technique, a contaminated field, or contaminated needle. Infectious complications include cellulitis, skin abscess, epidural or spinal abscess, discitis, or osteomyelitis.

SUGGESTED READING

Fong B, VanBendegom J. Lumbar puncture. In: Reichman EF, Simon RR. *Emergency Medicine Procedures*. 1st ed. New York, NY: McGraw-Hill, 2004.

Ladde JG. Central nervous system procedures and devices. In: Tintinalli JE, Stapczynski JS, Ma OJ, Cline DM, Cydulka RK, Meckler GD. *Tintinalli's Emergency Medicine: A Comprehensive Study Guide*. 7th ed. New York, NY: McGraw-Hill, 2011:1178–1180.

Miles S. Ellenby, et al. Lumbar puncture. *N Engl J Med*. 2006;335:12.

Wright BL, Lai JT, Sinclair AJ. Cerebrospinal fluid and lumbar puncture: a practical review. *J Neurol*. 2012;259:1530–1545.

6

Laceration Repair

Jeffrey N. Siegelman, MD

Key Points

- The timing of wound closure is determined by balancing the risk of infection with the likelihood of scarring.
- Identify and remove foreign bodies before wound closure.

- Evert wound edges for better aesthetic outcomes.
- Wound irrigation and debridement prevent wound infections.

INDICATIONS

Any wound deeper than a superficial abrasion should be considered for closure to improve the cosmetic result, preserve viable tissue, and restore tensile strength. This can be accomplished with sutures, tissue adhesive, or staples. Tissue adhesive may be indicated for hemostatic wounds in low tension areas that are at low risk for infection. Staples are appropriate for relatively linear lacerations located on the extremities, trunk, or scalp.

CONTRAINDICATIONS

The decision about whether and when to repair a laceration is based on many factors, which can be divided broadly into host and wound factors. Host factors include age (elderly patients have 3–4 times higher rate of infection and slower wound healing), malnutrition, and immunocompromise (eg, diabetes mellitus). Wound factors include timing, location, mechanism, and contamination. Bacterial counts begin to increase 3–6 hours post-injury, and every attempt is made to achieve primary wound closure as expeditiously as possible. However, there is no evidenced-based definitive time by which wounds must be closed. Wounds of the face and scalp rarely become infected (1–2%) because the face and scalp have an excellent blood supply; such wounds may be closed safely 24 hours or more after injury. Infection rates of upper (4%) and lower (7%) extremity wounds are higher, and many practitioners

use 6–12 hours as a guideline for closing these wounds. Lacerations sustained by a blunt, crushing force produce more local tissue damage and therefore have a higher rate of infection than lacerations caused by a sharp instrument (ie, knife). A puncture wound also has a high rate of infection because bacteria are driven into the tissue and are difficult to remove. Visible contamination within a wound doubles the likelihood of infection. Bite wounds (eg, dog, cat, human) have a very high rate of infection owing to bacterial colonization within the mouth. Generally, bite wounds are not closed primarily unless the wound is gaping or in a cosmetically sensitive area (eg, face).

Staples and tissue adhesive should not be used on deep wounds that would require multiple layered closure. Tissue adhesives should not be used near mucosal surfaces, within the scalp, or over joints (without immobilization), and care must be taken when used near the eyes.

EQUIPMENT

When preparing the wound for closure, the following are needed: povidone-iodine solution, local anesthetic (1% lidocaine with or without 1:100,000 epinephrine), 25- or 27-gauge needle, and a syringe. Irrigation is typically performed with normal saline or sterile water, a 60-mL syringe, and an irrigation shield or 18-gauge angiocatheter; however, some authors have argued that tap water is sufficient for uncomplicated wounds. Similarly, sterile gloves are typically used, although one study did not show

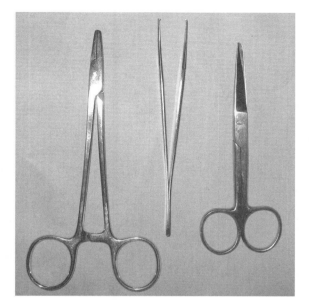

▲ **Figure 6-1.** Suture instruments. From left to right: needle driver, tissue forceps (pick-ups), and scissors.

a decreased infection rate when sterile gloves were used compared with clean gloves in the repair of clean wounds less than 6 hours old. Instruments needed include a needle driver, tissue forceps (pick-ups), and scissors (Figure 6-1). Use the smallest monofilament suture available that will adequately appose the ends of the laceration, because thinner suture causes less scarring. Usually 4-0 (largest, for torso and extremities) to 6-0 (smallest, for face) will suffice. Antibacterial ointment, gauze, and tape are needed for aftercare.

PROCEDURE

▶ Timing

Wound healing occurs by primary, secondary, or tertiary intention. Primary intention is the most common method of repair and involves the approximation of wound edges soon after the injury with the use of sutures, staples, tape, or tissue adhesive. In secondary intention, the wound is cleaned but left open and allowed to heal spontaneously. This method is used when the risk of infection after primary closure is high. Tertiary intention (delayed primary closure) decreases infection rate in highly contaminated wounds. It is performed by cleaning and débriding contaminated wounds acutely, then suturing the wound after 3–5 days.

▶ Wound Preparation

First, ensure adequate lighting and hemostasis to allow for a complete evaluation. A thorough neurovascular examination is required for all wounds before administration of

local anesthesia. Tendon function must also be assessed, when appropriate. Wound exploration may detect foreign bodies and diagnose injuries to deeper structures. If the depth of the wound is not easily appreciated and a foreign body is suspected (ie, patient fell on broken glass), then a plain radiograph is recommended. Glass fragments >2 mm are almost universally visualized on plain radiographs. Plastic and wood foreign bodies are not radiopaque and may require further imaging (computed tomography scan, ultrasound, or magnetic resonance imaging).

Lacerations through hair-covered surfaces require further preparation before proceeding with repair. Clipping hair to 1–2 mm (but not shaving) or applying antibacterial ointment to part hair away from wound edges will allow better visualization during wound closure and decrease risk of infection. Do not remove hair from eyebrows or the hairline, as this can lead to impaired or abnormal regrowth.

The edges of the wound are prepped with povidone-iodine solution. Care should be taken not to get the solution in the wound itself, as this inhibits healing. Draw up 1% lidocaine into a syringe and prepare to infiltrate using a 25- or 27-gauge needle. Pain of injection can be reduced by buffering the lidocaine with bicarbonate. To do this, mix 1 mL of sodium bicarbonate with 9 mL of 1% lidocaine; this solution must be used promptly. Lidocaine is infiltrated within the wound edges and around the entire wound (field block). In contaminated wounds, puncture the skin around the laceration (theoretical lower risk of infection); in clean wounds, puncture the wound edge within the wound itself (decreases pain of injection). Remember, the maximum dose of lidocaine without epinephrine is 4 mg/kg. This equates to 280 mg in a 70-kg (154 lb) man or 28 mL of 1% lidocaine (10 mg/mL). Lidocaine with epinephrine has a maximum dose of 7 mg/kg. Other advantages of adding epinephrine include decreased bleeding and increased duration of anesthetic. Traditional teaching dictates that caution should be used with epinephrine in end-arterial fields (eg, fingers, toes) for patients with vascular injury or a history of vascular disease; however, little evidence exists supporting this practice.

Wound irrigation and debridement of devitalized tissues are the two most important ways to decrease the incidence of wound infection. When irrigating a wound, use a commercially available shield to avoid accidental exposure to the health care worker and create the required pressure to decrease bacterial counts. If unavailable, an 18-gauge angiocatheter with a 60-mL syringe can be used. Irrigation with a saline bag or bottle with holes punched into the top does not create enough pressure to adequately reduce bacterial counts. The amount of saline required to irrigate a wound is not known, but a basic guideline is to use 50–100 mL for each 1 cm of laceration.

▶ Wound Closure

A few principles should be considered when placing simple interrupted sutures (Figure 6-2). Clamp the needle driver

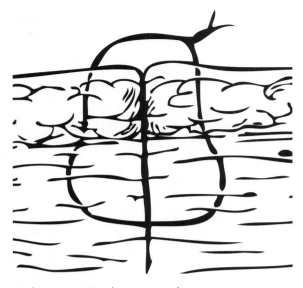

▲ **Figure 6-2.** Simple interrupted suture.

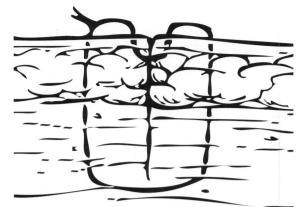

▲ **Figure 6-3.** Vertical mattress.

in the middle of the needle. Grasping the end of the needle will damage the cutting edge and make suturing more difficult. Insert the needle at 90 degrees to help evert the tissue. Eversion permits more rapid epithelialization than inversion and avoids a scar that is depressed after contraction. The tissue forceps are used to lift up the skin on one side of the laceration. Grasping the tissue too tightly (especially when using forceps with teeth) may damage the tissue and should be avoided. Instead use the teeth or a skin hook to lift the subcutaneous tissues. When the needle is inserted, maintain the same depth as the other side. Use 4–5 instrument ties to secure the knot. Avoid pulling the wound edges too tightly (indicated by blanching) because this may strangulate the wound edges, reducing blood supply. Begin in the middle of the wound, and then bisect the resulting segments with subsequent sutures until the wound is sufficiently approximated. As a rule, the distance from the needle insertion to the wound edge should be the same on both sides, as well as the same depth. The distance between stitches should also be equal. On the face, this will be 1–3 mm and can be farther apart elsewhere.

Vertical and horizontal mattress sutures both provide excellent wound eversion and help to better approximate wound edges that are under tension and difficult to pull together (Figures 6-3 and 6-4). Vertical mattress sutures are especially useful in lacerations in which there is minimal subcutaneous tissue for deep sutures such as the hands or over joints. In addition, these sutures will help stop bleeding from a scalp laceration. The disadvantage of these sutures is that they may strangulate the tissues.

Deep sutures are indicated in wounds with multiple layers of tissue to close (eg, full thickness lip lacerations) and to minimize tension on superficial skin for gaping wounds. Deep sutures should be placed with absorbable suture material. To get the knot to the depth of the wound, make the first pass of the needle from the deep portion of the wound to the superficial portion (Figure 6-5). Avoid infection by placing only enough deep sutures to effectively bring the wound edges together and cut the suture as close to the knot as possible.

Staples are placed by first everting the edges of the wound and then firing the automatic stapler with the same principles of spacing as above.

Tissue adhesive is applied using 4–5 layers on a hemostatic, cleaned, dry wound, which the provider approximates while applying the adhesive. Avoid getting the adhesive into the wound itself. Wound tape may be applied to the wound before placing the adhesive to provide improved approximation.

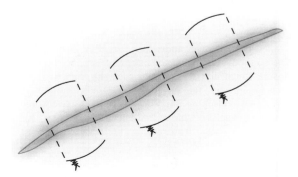

▲ **Figure 6-4.** Horizontal mattress.

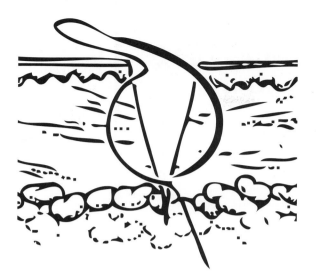

Figure 6-5. Deep dermal stitch. On the first pass, the needle enters at the depth of the wound so that the knot will end up at the bottom of the wound.

► Wound Aftercare

Topical antibiotic ointments provide a moist environment that assists epithelization and reduces the rate of infection. They should not be used after the use of tissue adhesive. Prophylactic oral antibiotics are recommended for heavily contaminated wounds, significant animal or human bites, areas prone to infection (mouth, plantar aspect of the foot), open fractures, tendon or joint involvement, immunocompromised patients, a prosthetic heart valve, or deep puncture wounds.

In patients with full childhood immunizations, tetanus toxoid, given with diphtheria toxoid (Td 0.5 mL administered intramuscularly [IM]), is administered after a minor, clean wound if the last booster was >10 years ago. In all other wounds (contaminated, puncture, crush), tetanus toxoid is given if the last booster was >5 years ago. Tetanus immune globulin (TIG) 3,000–5,000U IM and around the wound is administered to patients with a history of <3 immunizations and a contaminated wound.

Apply a topical ointment (eg, bacitracin) and then a sterile dressing. The dressing may be removed in 24 hours and the wound can be gently cleansed with soap and water, using caution to blot the sutures dry.

Suture removal is recommended in 3–5 days for face and neck; 7–10 days for upper extremity, chest, legs, and scalp; and 10–14 days for hand, back, buttocks, foot, and overlying joints.

COMPLICATIONS

Complications may include infection and scarring. Despite all efforts to reduce the risk of infection, this complication can still occur. The patient should be instructed to return at the first signs of infection (ie, fever, purulent drainage, or erythema). Patients with high-risk wounds should be asked to return to their physician or the emergency department within 24–48 hours to have the wound reexamined by a physician. Patients should also be instructed that a scar will form with healing. Scarring is more significant after deeper wounds, or those that do not run parallel to natural skin lines, and when absorbable sutures are used. There are insufficient data to recommend routine use of topical healing creams such as vitamin E, aloe vera, or other commercially available products.

▼ SUGGESTED READING

Desai S, Stone SC, Carter WA. Wound preparation. In: Tintinalli JE, Stapczynski JS, Ma OJ, Clince DM, Cydulka, RK, Meckler GD. *Tintinalli's Emergency Medicine: A Comprehensive Study Guide.* 7th ed. New York, NY: McGraw-Hill, 2011, pp. 301-306.

Singer AJ, Hollander JE. Methods for wound closure. In: Tintinalli JE, Stapczynski JS, Ma OJ, Clince DM, Cydulka, RK, Meckler GD. *Tintinalli's Emergency Medicine: A Comprehensive Study Guide.* 7th ed. New York, NY: McGraw-Hill, 2011, pp. 306–315.

Singer AJ, Hollander JE, Quinn JV. Evaluation and management of traumatic lacerations. *N Engl J Med.* 1997;337:1142–1148.

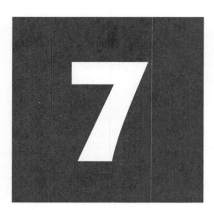

Needle and Tube Thoracostomy

Ann Buchanan, MD

Key Points

- Do not confuse a pulmonary bleb or bullae for a pneumothorax.
- The neurovascular bundle runs inferior to each rib. Always enter the thoracic cavity over the rib, never under.
- Never advance or replace a tube that has migrated out of the chest. Always place a new one.

INDICATIONS

Needle thoracostomy is indicated for emergent decompression of suspected tension pneumothorax. Tube thoracotomy is indicated after needle thoracostomy, for simple pneumothorax, traumatic hemothorax, or large pleural effusions with evidence of respiratory compromise.

CONTRAINDICATIONS

A pneumothorax on chest x-ray may be confused with a pulmonary bleb or bullae. Bullae and blebs are large gas-filled spaces with thin walls where pulmonary parenchyma has been destroyed, therefore greatly increasing alveolar size and mimicking pneumothorax. These are frequently located in the lung apices and are often seen in patients with severe chronic obstructive pulmonary disease. It is essential to confirm the presence of a pneumothorax before placement of a thoracostomy tube. See Chapter 24 for further clinical scenarios in which tube thoracostomy can be substituted for less invasive or conservative management of pneumothoraces.

EQUIPMENT

Needle thoracostomy requires a 12- to 16-gauge angiocatheter, 3 to 4.5 inches in length, and a 5–10 mL syringe. Tube thoracostomy requires a 36- to 40-F tube for hemothorax in adults or 20- to 24-F tube in children. For a simple pneumothorax, an 18- to 28-F tube in adults or 14- to 16-F tube in children is sufficient. Additional supplies required for tube thoracostomy placement include povidone-iodine (Betadine)

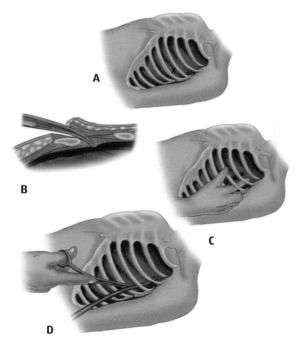

▲ **Figure 7-1. A-D.** Steps in tube thoracostomy placement. (Reprinted with permission from Cothren C, Biffl WL, Moore EE. Chapter 7. Trauma. In: Brunicardi FC, Andersen DK, Billiar TR, Dunn DL, Hunter JG, Matthews JB, Pollock RE, eds. *Schwartz's Principles of Surgery*. 9th ed. New York: McGraw-Hill, 2010.)

24

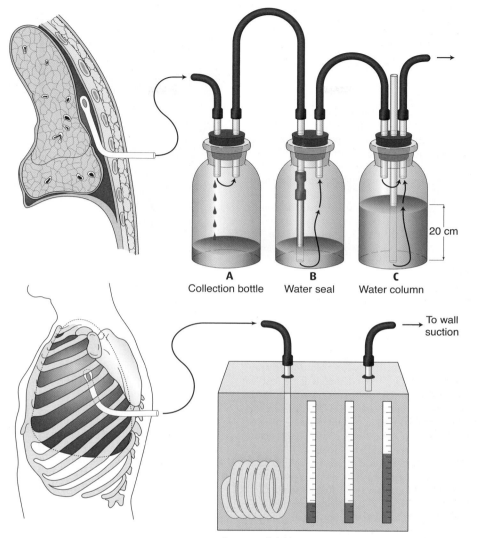

20 cm

A
Collection bottle

B
Water seal

C
Water column

To wall
suction

Commercial thoracostomy tube drainage system

▲ **Figure 7-2.** Diagram of tube thoracostomy and 3-bottle suction apparatus. **Bottle A** is connected to the thoracostomy tube and collects pleural drainage for inspection and volume measurement. **Bottle B** acts as a simple valve to prevent collapse of the lung if tubing distal to this point is open to atmospheric pressure. Pulmonary air leak can be detected by escape of bubbles from the submerged tube. **Bottle C** is a system to regulate the negative pressure delivered to the pleural space. Wall suction should be regulated to maintain continuous vigorous bubbling from the middle open tube in bottle C. The resulting negative pressure in cm H20 is equal to the difference in the height of the fluid levels in bottles B and C. The commercial Pleur-Evac system works in a similar manner. One end is attached to the chest tube and the other to wall suction. Each chamber of the Pleur-Evac is filled with sterile water to the level noted in the manufacturer's instructions. (Stone CK and Humphries RL: *Lange: Current Diagnosis and Treatment Emergency Medicine,* 7th edition. McGraw-Hill, New York, 2011.)

solution, sterile drapes, sterile gloves, 20 mL of 1% lidocaine with epinephrine, scalpel with #10 blade, large curved and straight clamps, a needle driver, 2-0 silk suture, and a commercial or 3-bottle suction apparatus.

PROCEDURE

Needle thoracostomy is accomplished by cleansing the skin in the upper chest and inserting the catheter over needle into the second intercostal space (just over the third rib) at the midclavicular line. Tension pneumothorax is confirmed with a sudden rush of air followed by improvement in the patient's vital signs. Tube thoracostomy placement should follow this procedure.

Tube thoracostomy is performed by first positioning the patient with the arm of the affected side above the patient's head and securing it with a soft restraint. The chest wall is prepared with povidone-iodine solution and a sterile field in the area of the fourth intercostal space (below the fourth rib) at the mid to anterior axillary line. The skin is then anesthetized with lidocaine, followed by anesthesia of the deeper structures tunneling above the fifth rib. Next, inject the intercostal muscles of the fourth to fifth intercostal space, extending into the parietal pleura. Additionally, procedural sedation or intercostal nerve blocks may be used. After adequate anesthesia, a 2- to 3-cm incision is made at the fifth rib between the mid and anterior axillary lines (Figure 7-1A). Using a large curved clamp, tunnel up through the soft tissues over the fifth rib to the fourth to fifth intercostal space. Then, using the same clamp, puncture through the intercostal muscles, using care not to enter the pleural space too deeply (Figure 7-1B). Open the jaws of the clamp to widen the hole in the intercostal muscles. Insert a gloved finger through the tract into the pleural cavity, using the curved clamp as a guide, and then remove the clamp. Using your finger, ensure there are no lung adhesions (Figure 7-1C). Using your finger or the curved clamp, insert the chest tube into the thorax, directing the tube posterior and superior, ensuring that all the evacuation holes of the tube are within the thorax (Figure 7-1D). The tube is then attached to a suction device (Figure 7-2). Secure the tube by placing a simple interrupted suture inferior to the tube. After tying a knot, the remaining suture should be wrapped around the tube several times and a second knot tied. The skin above the tube should then be closed with simple interrupted sutures. Cover the wound with Vaseline gauze and a bandage. A postprocedure chest x-ray should be ordered to check tube position and confirm lung reexpansion (Figure 7-3).

COMPLICATIONS

The most common complication of needle thoracostomy is failure to decompress. The patient's body habitus should dictate the size of the catheter over needle being used. If a

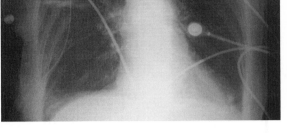

▲ **Figure 7-3.** Chest x-ray showing the proper position of a chest tube in the right lung.

3-cm catheter over needle fails to reach the pleural space, the procedure should be immediately repeated with a 4.5-cm catheter over needle.

Infection remains a serious complication of tube thoracostomy for patients with chest trauma, with incidences ranging from 2% to 25%. Thus strict sterile technique should always be followed. Tubes should never be advanced back into the thoracic cavity if they have migrated out. A new tube should be placed. Bleeding can also complicate tube thoracostomy. It may occur from superficial venules or arterioles at the incision site or from iatrogenic injury to the lung or abdominal organs. Incorrect tube placement may cause kinking, subcutaneous placement, or evacuation holes remaining outside the thoracic cavity, which results in either a nondraining tube or one with a persistent air leak. Reexpansion pulmonary edema, a rare but life-threatening complication, is more common when the lung has been completely collapsed for several days. Avoid this complication by placing the tube to water seal after insertion if the lung has been collapsed for a prolonged period. This allows for a more gradual reexpansion.

▼ SUGGESTED READING

Brunett PH, et al. Pulmonary trauma. In: Tintinalli JE, Stapczynski JS, Ma OJ, Cline DM, Cydulka RK, Meckler GD. *Tintinalli's Emergency Medicine: A Comprehensive Study Guide.* 7th ed. New York, NY: McGraw-Hill, 2011, pp. 1744–1758.

Joseph KT. Tube thoracostomy. In: Reichman EF, Simon RR. *Emergency Medicine Procedures.* 1st ed. New York, NY: McGraw-Hill, 2004, pp. 226–236.

Introduction to Emergency Ultrasonography

John Bailitz, MD

Basem F. Khishfe, MD

Key Points

- Use of ultrasound by emergency physicians has grown significantly in the last decade.
- Emergent applications include the setting of trauma, abdominal aortic aneurysm, ectopic pregnancy, gall bladder, and kidney and as an aid to procedures (eg, intravenous access).

- The 2008 American College of Emergency Physicians ultrasound guidelines describe the history and training process for the now 11 core applications of emergency ultrasound.

INDICATIONS

Emergency ultrasound (EUS) is preformed by emergency physicians at the patient's bedside to rapidly answer an increasing number of focused diagnostic questions, safely guide invasive procedures, and monitor the response to treatment. The 2008 American College of Emergency Physicians ultrasound guidelines describe the history and training process for the now 11 core EUS applications. EUS is most commonly used to evaluate and manage patients with the following clinical presentations:

Abdominal and chest trauma. The Focused Assessment with Sonography for Trauma (FAST) exam evaluates for blood in the pericardial, pleural, and peritoneal compartments in a rapid, reproducible, portable, and noninvasive approach. The extended FAST exam evaluates for evidence of pneumothorax.

Ectopic pregnancy. Abdominal/pelvic pain or vaginal bleeding are common presentations in the first trimester. An intrauterine pregnancy on EUS effectively rules out an ectopic pregnancy in the majority of patients.

Abdominal aortic aneurysm. EUS can quickly rule out abdominal aortic aneurysm (AAA) in patients presenting with nonspecific abdominal or low back pain, avoiding the need for a computed tomography

(CT) scan. At the other end of the clinical spectrum, in a hypotensive patient with abdominal or back pain, EUS may rapidly rule in the diagnosis of AAA, facilitating life-saving transport to the operating room instead of threatening decompensation during CT.

Acute cholecystitis. Physical examination and laboratory findings are often nonspecific in acute cholecystitis. EUS often helps rule in or out the diagnosis, prompting faster intervention or disposition.

Renal colic. In the uncomplicated patient with flank pain and hematuria, mild to moderate hydronephrosis often further supports the diagnosis of nephrolithiasis without the need for additional imaging.

Procedural applications. Use of ultrasound to aid in performing procedures includes placement of peripheral and central lines, abscess and foreign body localization, interspace visualization for lumbar puncture, and US guidance of pericardiocentesis, thoracentesis, and paracentesis.

CONTRAINDICATIONS

Relative contraindications to EUS include patient factors such as obesity and excessive bowel gas, as well as physician inexperience. If the specific clinical question is not answered or unexpected findings are encountered, then always proceed to the next test. EUS is another advanced diagnostic and procedural tool, but is not always a replacement for more definitive testing.

EQUIPMENT

US is analogous to a submarine's sonar system. Sound waves are emitted by the US probe, travel through tissue, are reflected off structures, and then return to the probe. Travel time is translated by the computer into depth within the body. Strength of returning echoes is translated into brightness or intensity of the structure on the display.

Sound is a series of repeating pressure waves. Audible sound is in 16–20,000 cycle/sec or Hz range, whereas diagnostic US uses sound waves in the 2–12 MHz range (million cycles/sec).

Probes send out and receive information via the piezoelectric or the pressure-electricity effect. The probe relies on a complex, delicate, and expensive arrangement of crystals. These crystals convert electrical energy to mechanical energy in the form of sound waves. Returning sound waves are translated back into electricity by the probe. Probe maintenance is of utmost importance; a probe must never be used if cracked or otherwise significantly damaged.

Frequency. The higher the frequency of sound waves emitted by the probe, the greater the tissue resolution, but the lower the depth of penetration. Different types of probes exist for different clinical questions. Low-frequency probes (2–5 MHz) are used in thoracic and abdominal imaging to visualize deeper structures. High-frequency probes (8–10 MHz) are used in procedural applications, such as central line placement and nerve blocks, to visualize more superficial structures with more detailed resolution.

Echogenicity. Images are described in terms of echogenicity. Dense bone is highly reflective, appearing bright or hyperechogenic. Less dense organ parenchyma appears grainy or echogenic. Fluid-filled structures or acute bleeding do not reflect, appearing black or anechogenic. Air has an irregular reflective surface and appears as bright scatter with dirty posterior shadows.

Orientation. A marker on the US probe corresponds to an indicator on the screen. By accepted standard in emergency medicine and radiology, the indicator is always on the physician's left side of the screen. In the sagittal (longitudinal) anatomic plane, the probe marker is pointed at the patient's head, resulting in the head being displayed toward the left side of the screen and the feet toward the right (Figure 8-1A). In the coronal (transverse) anatomic plane, the probe marker is pointed at the patient's right, resulting in the patient's right side being displayed on the left side of the screen, similar to viewing a CT scan image (Figure 8-1B).

Modes. The most commonly used mode is the brightness (B) mode on the US machine. Other modes include the motion (M) mode, often used to measure the fetal heartbeat, as well as the Doppler and color flow modes to measure blood flow.

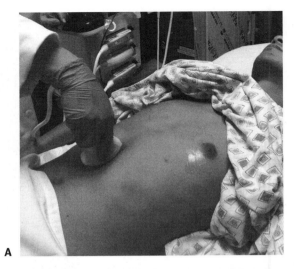

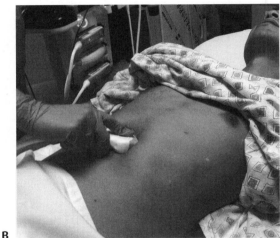

▲ **Figure 8-1. A.** Longitudinal probe orientation. The probe marker points to the head of the patient. **B.** Transverse probe orientation. The probe marker points to the right of the patient.

PROCEDURE

The basic FAST examination consists of multiple ultrasound views of the abdomen and lower thorax. The patient should be in the supine position with the physician and machine on the patient's right side of the bed.

Subxiphoid view. The probe is placed in the subxiphoid area with the marker in the transverse anatomic plane aimed at the patient's left scapula. Blood between the visceral and pleural pericardial layers will appear anechogenic (Figure 8-2).

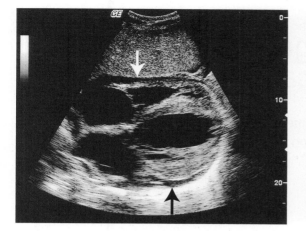

▲ **Figure 8-2.** Subxiphoid view showing a pericardial effusion.

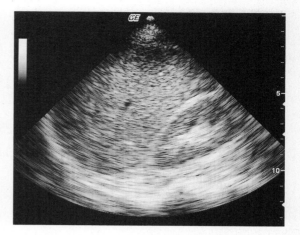

▲ **Figure 8-3.** Right upper quadrant view showing Morison's pouch between the liver and kidney. No free fluid is present.

Right upper quadrant (RUQ) view. The probe is placed in the midaxillary line in the ninth to 12th interspace with the marker to the patient's head in the coronal plane. Examine for blood in the right hemithorax, the hepatorenal fossae (Morison's pouch), and the inferior paracolic gutter. Morison's pouch is the most dependent portion of the abdomen above the pelvis and therefore the most common site to visualize large amounts of free intraperitoneal fluid (ie, blood) (Figure 8-3).

Left upper quadrant (LUQ) view. The probe is placed in the posterior axillary line in the eighth to 11th interspace with the marker to the patient's head in the coronal plane. Examine for blood in the left hemithorax, the subphrenic space, the splenorenal space, and the left inferior paracolic gutter.

Pelvic view. The probe is initially placed longitudinally in the midline just above the pubic symphysis. Examine for blood in the retrouterine pouch of Douglas in the female or in the retrovesicular space in the male.

COMPLICATIONS

Complications may arise from inadequate visualization of structures or image misinterpretation, but usually do not occur because of the procedure itself.

▼ SUGGESTED READING

American College of Emergency Physicians Emergency ultrasound guidelines. *Ann Emerg Med.* 2009;53:550–570.

Hoffmann R, Pohlemann T, Wippermann B, et al. Management of sonography in blunt abdominal trauma. *Unfallchirurg.* 1989;92:471–476.

Ma OJ, Mateer JR, Ogata M, et al. Prospective analysis of a rapid trauma ultrasound examination performed by emergency physicians. *J Trauma.* 1995;38:879–885.

Melniker LA, Leibner E, McKenney MG, et al. Randomized controlled clinical trial of point-of-care, limited ultrasonography for trauma in the emergency department: The first sonography outcomes assessment program trial. *Ann Emerg Med.* 2006;48:227–235.

Emergency Medical Services

Bradley L. Demeter, MD

Eric H. Beck, DO

Key Points

- Emergency medical services (EMS) is the extension of emergency medical care into the prehospital setting.
- The U.S. EMS Systems Act of 1973 established key elements for EMS systems to receive funding.
- In 2012, the American Board of Medical Specialties approved EMS as a subspecialty.

INTRODUCTION

Emergency medical services (EMS) is the medical specialty that involves the delivery of prehospital care. The use of the term "EMS" may refer solely to the prehospital element of care or be part of an integrated system, including the main care provider, such as a hospital.

Federal funding for emergency medical services came with the U.S. EMS Systems Act of 1973, which established 15 key elements that must be addressed by systems to receive funding. The elements are used here as an outline for discussion.

▶ Manpower

The workforce providing prehospital care varies largely based on population density. Urban areas typically have paid providers serving through government agencies or as public safety officers in large public venues (airports, amusement parks, etc). Volunteers are more commonly found in suburban, rural, and wilderness areas.

▶ Training

The U.S. Department of Transportation (DOT) National Highway Traffic Safety Administration (NHTSA) National Standard Curriculum for prehospital care providers historically outlined 4 levels of training: first responder, EMT-basic, EMT-intermediate, and EMT-paramedic. Currently, these levels are being transitioned to 4 nationally standardized levels of certification: emergency medical responder (EMR), emergency medical technician (EMT), advanced EMT (AEMT), and paramedic. Each level of training infers a specific role, skill set, and knowledge base (Table 9-1). EMS provider training at all levels emphasizes airway, breathing, and circulation (ABCs) and provider scene safety as priorities in patient care. Although significant efforts have been made to standardize education and certification throughout the United States, variability exists from state to state in scope of practice and specific medication usage by each level of prehospital provider.

▶ Communications/Access to Care

In the early 1970s, "9-1-1" became the now ubiquitous common point of access to emergency services. Call centers are typically staffed by trained dispatchers who practice priority dispatching. Their job is to gather sufficient information to triage and allocate the most appropriate resources for a given response. It is becoming increasingly common for dispatchers to provide pre-arrival instructions to the caller, such as how to perform layperson CPR.

▶ Transportation

Transport vehicles vary in equipment based on the intended response model and provider scope of practice.

Table 9-1. Prehospital care providers.

Certification Level	Description
Emergency medical responder (EMR)	The first responders to arrive on scene, they are trained to perform immediate lifesaving care with limited resources until additional EMS responders arrive. Their skill set includes CPR, spinal immobilization, oxygen administration, hemorrhage control, and use of an automated external defibrillator (AED).
Emergency medical technician (EMT)	This is the basic level of training necessary for ambulance operations. EMTs' skill set includes that of the EMR, with the addition of transport operations and the assistance of patients in taking some of their own prescription medications, such as metered-dose inhalers or nitroglycerine tablets. They may also provide several medications including oral glucose, aspirin, albuterol, and epinephrine for anaphylaxis.
Advanced emergency medical technician (AEMT)	Under medical direction, the AEMT may initiate intravenous or intraosseous access, perform manual defibrillation, interpret electrocardiograms, and administer an expanded range of medications.
Paramedic	Traditionally the highest prehospital level of training with the broadest scope of practice. Their expanded skill set includes endotracheal intubation, cricothyrotomy, needle thoracostomy. Drug administration includes vasoactive agents, benzodiazepines, and opiates for pain control. They are also trained to perform higher level ECG analysis and to provide antiarrhythmic therapy with medications, electrical cardioversion, manual defibrillation, and transcutaneous pacing.
Critical care paramedic	This is a provider level that reflects additional training, knowledge, and scope of practice that is needed for initiating or maintaining advanced level intervention during transport. Critical care paramedics often have training in chest tube placement and management, balloon pump management, neonatal care, central venous catheters, arterial lines, and hemodynamic monitoring. Additional medications including neuromuscular blockers and sedation agents are commonly used at this level of care.

Basic life support (BLS) ground units have automated external defibrillators (AED) and supplies necessary for basic wound care and airway management, including oxygen, bag-valve-masks, suction equipment, and oral and nasal airways. Advanced life support (ALS) units have equipment necessary for a paramedic's scope of practice, including equipment for IV access, medications, and a cardiac monitor/defibrillator for rhythm analysis and intervention. Some systems have uniquely equipped critical care transport units that are designed to accommodate patients with continuous IV infusions, ventilators, or other specialized medical equipment such as intra-aortic balloon pumps or neonatal incubators. Air medical transport comprises both fixed-wing (airplane) and rotary-wing (helicopter) vehicles. General indications for air medical transport are outlined in Table 9-2.

Table 9-2. Relative indications for air medical transport.

Distance by ground to the closest appropriate medical facility is too great for safe and timely transport.
A delay during ground transport would likely worsen the patient's clinical condition.
Specialized care is not available from local ground response agencies.
An area is inaccessible to ground traffic.
The use of local ground resources would leave an area temporarily without adequate resources.

Facilities/Critical Care Units

In general, prehospital patients are transported to the closest appropriate medical facility. There are some situations in which a patient's preference may dictate hospital destination. One issue that has emerged as a product of hospital overcrowding is ambulance diversion, where ambulances may need to bypass the closest appropriate facility to transport to another center that has capacity. Another factor in hospital destination is availability of specialty care for time-critical diagnoses. Examples of field triage and transport for time-critical illnesses include designated "trauma centers," facilities with surgical teams and operating rooms on standby; "stroke centers," with immediately available neurology and neurosurgical capabilities; and "cardiac centers," with cardiac catheterization laboratories and therapeutic hypothermia resources readily available for patients with acute coronary syndromes or cardiac arrest. Obstetrical, pediatric, and burn centers are recognized in some regions as specially designated receiving facilities.

Public Safety Agencies

Prehospital responses are often coordinated efforts between police, fire, and EMS personnel. Various paradigms for the division of labor within a given municipality exist. Some of the more common EMS structures include fire-based, third-service, private, and hospital-based. Fire-based ambulances are staffed and operated by the local fire department, whereas in third-service systems, EMS are separate from both police and fire departments. Private ambulance companies may provide nonurgent transports or may operate under contract with local governments to supplement or provide all emergency care for a municipality. Lastly, hospital-based ambulances have crews of hospital-employed personnel dispatched on ambulances owned by the hospital.

Consumer Participation/Public Information and Education

An important aspect of most EMS operations is community service, ranging from public relations expositions to educational initiatives like CPR training. It is also common for public representatives to participate in the oversight and decision making that takes place within a public EMS organization. EMS is often described as existing at the intersection of public safety and public health; EMS data and personnel are a critical link in public health infrastructure and preventative interventions.

Patient Transfer

One of the primary purposes of EMS is to deliver patients to the care that they need. In many cases, this involves transport from the scene of an injury or medical event to a receiving hospital, but it may also involve the transport of a patient from one medical facility to another. A key legislative mandate set forth in the Emergency Medical Treatment and Active Labor Act (EMTALA) is that an appropriate medical screening exam must be performed to identify emergent medical conditions that must be stabilized before a patient can be considered for transfer to another facility. Receiving hospitals must explicitly accept a transfer before a patient is transported.

Coordinated Patient Record Keeping

The method of charting varies from one system to another, with many systems now implementing an electronic medical record. A significant barrier to prehospital research is the tremendous variation that exists in charting methods, data definitions, and reporting requirements. There is also difficulty linking prehospital data to hospital or outcomes data.

Review and Evaluation

The care rendered by prehospital providers is overseen by a physician medical director. Day-to-day operations generally function using either "standing orders" (offline medical control—protocols developed to guide patient care) or online medical control (real-time telephone/radio communication with hospital personnel to answer clinical questions or to receive orders). Protocols undergo periodic review for updates based on changing system needs and current science. Proactive systems have robust continuous quality

Table 9-3. The "Simple Triage and Rapid Treatment" (START) system.

Green (minor)	Care may be delayed (eg, non-limb-threatening extremity trauma)
Yellow (delayed)	Will require urgent care (eg, hemorrhage with signs of adequate perfusion)
Red (immediate)	Requires immediate care for life-threatening injury (eg, severe hemorrhage or airway compromise)
Black (deceased)	Either dead or mortally wounded, such that dedication of any additional resources is unlikely to alter outcome

improvement processes, by which EMS data are used to identify areas of the system in need of improvement.

Disaster Plan/Preparedness

Emergency response plans exist at local, state, and national levels. Key features include provisions for interagency communication and agreements regarding the optimal allocation of limited resources when a system's capacity is exceeded—a situation referred to as a mass casualty incident. In these situations, the "Simple Triage and Rapid Treatment" (START) algorithm is a commonly employed triage protocol used to assess severity of injury and to assign transport priority. Providers assign 1 of 4 colors to victims during an initial assessment focused on the ABCs (Table 9-3).

Mutual Aid

Agreements among neighboring municipalities or EMS services are common to bolster the capacity of a given agency's emergency response system. Interagency communication and equipment interoperability are potential challenges that need to be addressed in establishing such relationships.

SUGGESTED READING

Emergency Medical Services: Clinical Practice and Systems Oversight. National Association of EMS Physicians. Dubuque, IA: Kendal/Hunt, 2009.

Mechem CC. Emergency medical services. In: Tintinalli JE, Stapczynski JS, Ma OJ, Cline DM, Cydulka RK, Meckler GD. *Tintinalli's Emergency Medicine: A Comprehensive Study Guide.* 7th ed. New York, NY: McGraw-Hill, 2011, pp. 1–4.

National Highway Traffic Safety Administration. *The National EMS Scope of Practice Model.* DOT HS 810 657. Washington, DC: National Highway Traffic Safety Administration, 2007.

Cardiopulmonary Arrest

Katherine M. Hiller, MD

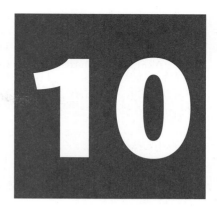

Key Points

- Cardiac disease is the most common cause of nontraumatic death in the United States.

- There are more than 300,000 sudden cardiac deaths (SCD) each year in the United States. The survival rate of

- SCD is dependent on the length of time without a pulse, the underlying cardiac rhythm, and comorbidities.

- Early and uninterrupted chest compressions and early defibrillation are the keys to successful resuscitation.

INTRODUCTION

Cardiopulmonary arrest is defined by unconsciousness, apnea, and pulselessness. Sudden cardiac death (SCD) is associated with an underlying history of coronary artery disease (CAD), but an acute thrombotic event is causal in only 20-40% of cardiac arrests. Twenty-five percent of cardiac arrests may have a noncardiac origin (eg, pulmonary embolus, respiratory arrest, drowning, overdose). The most common initial rhythm is ventricular fibrillation (VF), found in approximately 30% of patients. Asystole and pulseless electrical activity (PEA) are the next most common presenting rhythms.

The risk of SCD is 4 times higher in patients with coronary artery disease risk factors and 6–10 times higher in patients with known heart disease. Structural heart disease (eg, cardiomyopathy, heart failure, left ventricular hypertrophy, myocarditis) accounts for 10% of cases of SCD. Another 10% of SCD cases occur in patients with no structural heart disease or CAD. These cases are thought to originate from Brugada syndrome, commotio cordis, prolonged QT syndrome, and familial ventricular tachycardia (VT), which all cause dysrhythmias leading to SCD.

Other risk factors associated with an increased risk of SCD include smoking, diabetes mellitus, hypertension, dyslipidemia, and a family history of cardiac disease. Moderate alcohol consumption (1–2 drinks per day) is considered protective, whereas heavy alcohol consumption (>6 drinks per day) is a risk factor for SCD.

Despite advances in the field of cardiac resuscitation, the survival rate of out-of-hospital SCD is estimated to be 3–8%. Survival to discharge in out-of-hospital SCD is largely determined by the presenting rhythm. Patients with VF are 15 times more likely to survive to discharge than patients in asystole (34% vs 0–2%).

CLINICAL PRESENTATION

History

Obtain history from paramedics, bystanders, or any available family members. Inquire about medications, past medical history, allergies, trauma, and events leading up to SCD.

Physical Examination

Do not halt treatment (including chest compressions and bag-valve-mask ventilation) to perform a complete physical exam. If the patient has an endotracheal tube in place, verify position by using end-tidal CO_2 capnography or capnometry.

DIAGNOSTIC STUDIES

▶ Laboratory

If the patient has a return of spontaneous circulation (ROSC), order a complete blood count, electrolytes, renal function, and myocardial markers (ie, troponin). Coagulation studies, an arterial blood gas, and a lactate may also be useful.

▶ Imaging

If the patient has a ROSC, obtain a chest x-ray to evaluate endotracheal tube placement and an electrocardiogram to evaluate for cardiac ischemia.

PROCEDURES

Pericardiocentesis is indicated if there is a suspicion of cardiac tamponade in the setting of PEA. Bedside ultrasound can be useful if tamponade is suspected. A long spinal needle is inserted subxiphoid into the pericardial sac aimed toward the left shoulder. Pull back on a 60-mL syringe while advancing the needle until blood is obtained.

A needle thoracostomy is indicated if there is a suspicion of tension pneumothorax in the setting of PEA. Insert an 18-gauge needle into the second intercostals space in the midclavicular line. A needle thoracostomy must always be followed by a tube thoracostomy in patients with ROSC.

MEDICAL DECISION MAKING

The differential diagnosis for SCD is broad. Management of SCD depends on the presenting rhythm; however, every patient should receive continuous high-quality uninterrupted chest compressions. Defibrillate VF/pulseless VT. Administer epinephrine for asystole and PEA. Attempt to correct reversible causes of PEA, the H's, and T's (Table 10-1). Once ROSC occurs, initiate postresuscitative care, including therapeutic hypothermia, which improves neurologic outcome.

Table 10-1. The H's and T's of PEA.

H's
Hypoxia
Hypovolemia
Hydrogen ion (acidosis)
Hypo-/hyperkalemia
Hypothermia

T's
Toxins
Tamponade (cardiac)
Tension pneumothorax
Thrombosis (pulmonary, cardiac)

TREATMENT

If there is a clear, written, advanced directive signed by the patient or medical power of attorney stating that resuscitative efforts should not be instituted, or if the resuscitation would be futile because of clear signs of irreversible death (decapitation, rigor mortis), resuscitative efforts should not be initiated or continued.

The resuscitative team must orchestrate simultaneous assessment and management of patients in cardiopulmonary arrest.

1. Defibrillation. Indicated for patients in VF or pulseless VT. The rate of successful defibrillation when attempted within 1 minute of VT is >90%, but falls 10% with each subsequent minute.

2. Chest compressions. The carotid pulse is the most reliable in low-flow states. If no pulse is detected, chest compressions should be initiated. Survival is greatly increased when chest compressions are performed properly (depth 1.5–2 inches, >100/min) and greatly decreased when there are delays or interruptions in chest compressions. Chest compressions should be performed continuously and should not be interrupted for ventilation. A brief rhythm check should be undertaken after every 2 minutes of chest compressions. When defibrillation is indicated, compressions should be continued while the manual defibrillator or AED is charging. Chest compressions should only be briefly halted (<10 seconds) to deliver the shock and immediately resumed after delivery.

3. Airway. The most common airway obstruction in the unconscious patient is the tongue falling back against the posterior pharynx. This can be managed immediately with a jaw thrust or chin lift maneuver. Bag-valve-mask ventilation should then be used until enough providers are available to allow continued compressions and defibrillation while advanced airway adjuncts are assembled. Endotracheal intubation is the definitive airway management technique used for patients in cardiac arrest. Attempts at intubation should be brief so as not to hinder delivery of high-quality continuous chest compressions.

4. Pharmacologic therapy.
   a. Vasopressors. The current recommended dose of epinephrine is 1 mg initially, with repeated doses every 3–5 minutes. "High-dose" epinephrine confers no benefit and may be harmful. When there is no IV access, epinephrine can be given in the endotracheal tube at a dose 2–2.5 times the IV dose. Alternatively, vasopressin 40 units IV may be given once.
   b. Antidysrhythmics. Amiodarone, 300 mg IV push, repeated as a second dose of 150 mg IV push may be useful for defibrillation refractory VT/VF. Magnesium, 2 g IV, may be useful in patients with torsade de points.

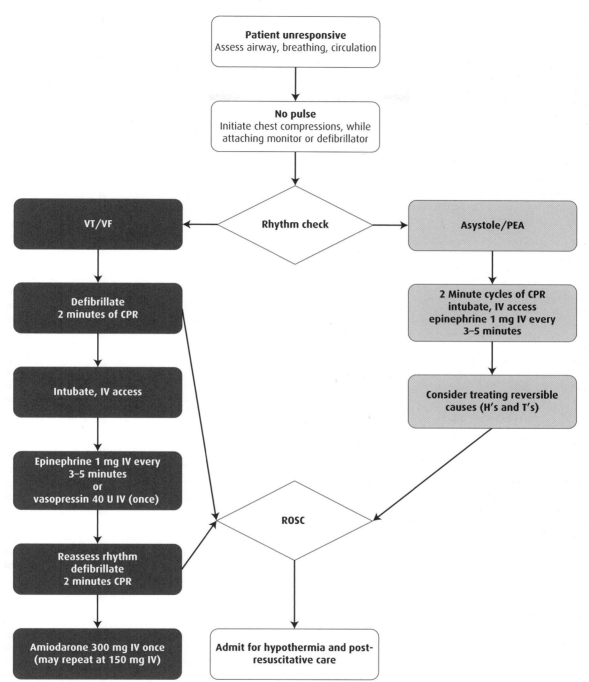

▲ **Figure 10-1.** Cardiac arrest algorithm. U, Units; VT/VF, ventricular tachycardia/ventricular fibrillation; PEA, pulseless electrical activity.

5. Postresuscitation care. All patients who remain comatose with an ROSC should receive therapeutic hypothermia (33°C for 24 hours, then rewarm over 24 hours).

DISPOSITION

▶ Admission

All patients with ROSC should be admitted to the intensive care unit or cardiac care unit for postresuscitative care as well as management of underlying conditions leading to the arrest. If CAD/acute coronary syndrome is the presumed cause of SCD, all therapies, especially percutaneous coronary intervention, should be considered.

▼ SUGGESTED READING

Field JM, Hazinski MF, Sayre MR, Chameides L, Schexnayder SM, et al. Part 1: Executive Summary: 2010 American Heart Association Guidelines for Cardiopulmonary Resuscitation and Emergency Cardiovascular Care. *Circulation.* 2010;122: S640–S656.

Neumar RW, Otto CW, Link MS, Kronick SL, Shuster M, et al. Part 8: Adult Advanced Cardiovascular Life Support: 2010 American Heart Association Guidelines for Cardiopulmonary Resuscitation and Emergency Cardiovascular Care. *Circulation.* 2010;122:S729–S767.

Ornato, JP. Sudden cardiac death. In: Tintinalli JE, Stapczynski JS, Ma OJ, Cline DM, Cydulka RK, Meckler GD. *Tintinalli's Emergency Medicine: A Comprehensive Study Guide.* 7th ed. New York, NY: McGraw-Hill, 2011, pp. 63–67.

Airway Management

Theresa M. Schwab, MD

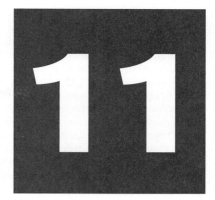

Key Points

- Rapid-sequence intubation (RSI) is the preferred method for endotracheal tube placement in the emergency department.
- The decision to intubate should always be made on clinical grounds. Time permitting, assess for factors predictive of a difficult airway before RSI.
- General criteria for endotracheal intubation include a failure to protect the airway, a failure to adequately oxygenate, and a failure to expire accumulating CO_2.
- Pursue alternative techniques (eg, cricothyrotomy) in patients when the initial airway intervention has failed and the patient cannot be adequately ventilated.

INTRODUCTION

Successful airway management depends on the prompt recognition of an inadequate airway, the identification of risk factors that may impair successful bag-valve-mask (BVM) ventilation or endotracheal tube (ETT) placement, and the use of an appropriate technique to properly secure the airway. The decision to intubate is a clinical one and should be based on the presence of any 1 of 3 major conditions: an inability to successfully protect one's airway against aspiration/occlusion, an inability to successfully oxygenate the blood (hypoxemia), or an inability to successfully clear the respiratory byproducts of cellular metabolism (hypercapnia). Additional indications including the desire to decrease the work of breathing (sepsis), the need for therapeutic hyperventilation (increased intracranial pressure [ICP]), and the need to obtain diagnostic imaging in noncooperative individuals (altered mental status) should be taken into account on a patient-by-patient basis.

Techniques for the management of unstable airways range from basic shifts in patient positioning to invasive surgical intervention. Standard basic life support recommendations such as the head-tilt chin-lift maneuver may open a previously occluded airway. Oropharyngeal and nasal airway adjuncts are both simple to use and highly effective in this setting, but are unfortunately often under-utilized. Failure to respond to these measures warrants the placement of an ETT. Rapid-sequence intubation (RSI) combines the careful use of pretreatment interventions with the administration of induction and paralytic agents to create the ideal environment for ETT placement and is the preferred method in the emergency department (ED).

A patient who cannot be intubated within 3 attempts is considered a failed airway. This scenario occurs in ~3–5% of all cases. Numerous alternative devices including laryngeal mask airways (LMA), introducer bougies, and fiberoptic instruments have been developed to facilitate airway management in these situations. That said, these methods are not failsafe, and roughly 0.6% of patients will require a surgical airway. Emergent cricothyrotomy is the preferred surgical technique for most ED patients.

CLINICAL PRESENTATION

▶ History

The need for immediate airway intervention in emergency situations always supersedes the need for a comprehensive history and physical exam. Time permitting, perform a rapid airway assessment to identify any risk factors predictive of a difficult airway, inquire about any current medication use and known drug allergies, and try to ascertain the immediate events leading up to ED presentation.

Risk factors predictive of a difficult airway include those that impair adequate BVM ventilation and those that preclude successful placement of an ETT. Examples of the former include patients with facial trauma and distorted anatomy, obese patients with excessive cervical soft tissue, and asthmatic patents with excessively high airway resistances. Examples of the latter include patients with a history of degenerative changes of the spine that limit cervical mobility (eg, rheumatoid arthritis, ankylosing spondylitis), patients with underlying head and neck cancers that distort the normal cervical anatomy, and those with excessive swelling of the airway and surrounding tissues (eg, angioedema).

▶ Physical Examination

Rapidly examine the airways of all critically ill patients. Always consider the presence of concurrent cervical spine injury in victims of trauma and immobilize as appropriate. Carefully examine the face, noting any signs of significant facial trauma and the presence of a beard, both of which frequently impair adequate BVM ventilation. Inspect the oropharynx, noting the presence of dentures; the size of the teeth and presence of a significant overbite; visibility of the soft palate, uvula, and tonsillar pillars (ie, Mallampati classification); and the presence of significant airway swelling. The pooling of blood or secretions in the oropharynx indicates an inability to properly protect the airway. A good adage to remember when assessing the airway is the 3-3-2 rule. The inability to open the mouth 3 finger breaths, a distance from the tip of the chin to the base of the neck less than 3 finger breaths, or a distance between the mandibular floor and the prominence of the thyroid cartilage of less than 2 finger breaths all predict more difficult ETT placement. Assess the range of motion of the cervical spine, provided there is no concern for occult injury.

DIAGNOSTIC STUDIES

▶ Laboratory

Although abnormalities on either blood gas analysis (hypercapnia) or pulse oximetry (hypoxemia) may be indicative of an inadequate airway, normal values on either of these studies should not justify the delay of definitive intervention in the appropriate clinical scenario. Progressive abnormalities on serial testing (increasing $PaCO_2$, decreasing PaO_2) in patients who are clinically decompensating indicates the need for airway intervention.

▶ Imaging

Imaging studies should not be used to predict the need for airway intervention. Obtain a chest x-ray (CXR) in all patients after intubation to confirm proper ETT placement. The tip of the ETT should be visualized approximately 2 cm above the carina. Deeper insertion results in placement into the right mainstem bronchus.

MEDICAL DECISION MAKING

Consider all rapidly reversible causes of airway compromise (eg, hypoglycemia, opioid overdose) before pursuing endotracheal intubation. Proper intervention may transform a comatose patient with a rather tenuous airway into an awake coherent individual with adequate airway protection. Identify patients who are likely to present a difficult airway and those who require specialized approaches (eg, head trauma precautions, hypotension, cervical spine injury) and proceed accordingly (Figure 11-1).

PROCEDURES

▶ Bag-Valve-Mask Ventilation

Proper BVM ventilation requires an open airway and an airtight seal between the mask and the patient's face. Use the head-tilt chin-lift technique (jaw-thrust maneuver in trauma victims) to open the airway and insert oropharyngeal or nasal adjuncts as necessary to maintain patency. Avoid the use of oral adjuncts in patients with intact gag reflexes and nasal adjuncts in patients with significant mid-face trauma. With proper technique and a high-flow oxygen source, this method can provide an FiO_2 of approximately 90% (Figure 11-2).

▶ Rapid-Sequence Intubation

Preoxygenate all patients with a high-flow oxygen source (eg, nonrebreather [NRB] mask) for several minutes as time permits before RSI. Avoid positive pressure ventilation (eg, BVM) to prevent insufflation of the stomach, which can increase the patient's risk for aspiration. Use this time to prepare and check your equipment. Ensure adequate IV access and proper function of the suction device. Remove patient dentures, significant loose teeth, and any oral debris. Choose the appropriate size ETT. Tube sizes range in diameter from 2.5–9 mm. A size 7.5- or 8.0-mm tube is appropriate for most adult female and male patients respectively. Inflate the balloon to check for leaks and insert a stylet. Uncuffed ETTs have been historically preferred in patients younger than 8 years of age as the narrowest portion of their airways lies inferior to the vocal cords at the level of the cricoid ring. That said, most practitioners now prefer cuffed ETTs for all patients. To determine the appropriate size of the ETT in pediatric patients, either use the formula Size = (Age/4) + 4 for uncuffed tubes or (Age/4) + 3 for the cuffed variety, or use a tube that is equal in diameter to the child's fifth finger.

Check the light on your laryngoscope blade to ensure that it works. Laryngoscope blades range in size from 0–4 and come in 2 major varieties. The Macintosh blade is curved in shape and meant to indirectly lift the epiglottis away from the vocal cords. It is also designed with a special

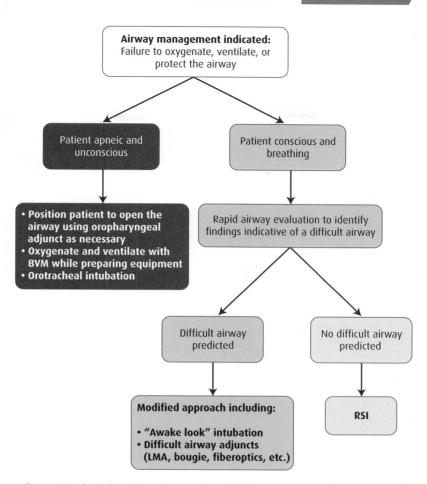

Figure 11-1. Airway diagnostic algorithm. LMA, laryngeal mask airways; RSI, rapid-sequence intubation.

ridge meant to sweep the tongue to the side during insertion to improve visualization of the vocal cords. The Miller blade is straight in appearance and meant to directly lift the epiglottis away from the vocal cords. It is of particular benefit in patients with very anterior airways and those with a large "floppy" epiglottis. A size 3 or 4 Macintosh blade is appropriate for most adult ED patients (Figure 11-3).

Certain clinical scenarios warrant unique modifications to standard RSI to attenuate the adverse physiologic responses to endotracheal intubation. Pretreat head injury patients with lidocaine (1.5 mg/kg) and a "defasciculating" dose of a nondepolarizing neuromuscular blocker (eg, pancuronium 0.01 mg/kg) to limit the potential spike in ICP that may accompany ETT placement. Pretreat most pediatric patients with an anticholinergic agent (eg, atropine 0.02 mg/kg) to prevent reflex bradycardia. Pretreat patients in whom rapid elevations in either blood pressure or heart rate would be catastrophic (eg, aortic dissection) with an opioid analgesic (eg, fentanyl 3 mcg/kg) to limit excessive catecholamine surges. Of note, the clinical utility of many of these pretreatment regimens has recently come under considerable debate.

Outside of the pretreatment agents listed previously, the remaining RSI medications can be divided into either

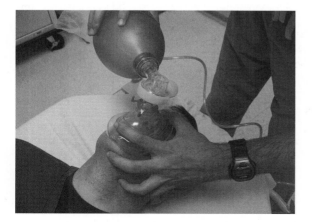

Figure 11-2. Proper method of BVM ventilation.

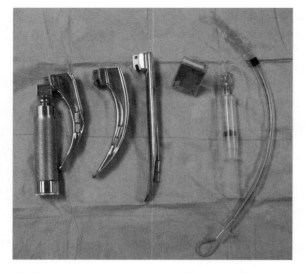

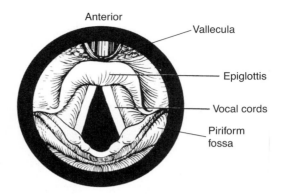

Figure 11-4. Laryngoscopic view. (Reproduced with permission from Kempe CH, Silver HK, O'Brien D, (editors): *Current Pediatric Diagnosis & Treatment.* 4th ed. Lange, 1976.)

Figure 11-3. Equipment needed for orotracheal intubation in an adult. From left to right, laryngoscope handle attached to Macintosh 3 blade, Macintosh 4 blade, Miller 4 blade, end-tidal CO_2 detector, 10-mL syringe, and endotracheal tube with stylet.

induction agents or paralyzing agents. Induction agents are designed to elicit extremely rapid sedation to facilitate ETT placement. A variety of medications are available, including etomidate (0.3 mg/kg), propofol (1 mg/kg), ketamine (2–3 mg/kg), and midazolam (0.05–0.1 mg/kg). Of these, etomidate is used most frequently in the ED because of its rapid onset and offset and relative hemodynamic neutrality. Avoid the use of benzodiazepines and propofol in hypotensive patients and ketamine in patients with potential traumatic brain injury.

Paralytic agents can be divided into depolarizing and nondepolarizing categories. Succinylcholine (1.5 mg/kg) is the lone agent in the depolarizing class and the most commonly used paralytic for RSI because of its rapid onset and short duration of activity. Most patients achieve relaxation within 1 minute, complete paralysis by the 2- to 3-minute mark, and a return of motor function within 10 minutes. Avoid succinylcholine in patients with known hyperkalemia and those with pathologically denervated tissues (eg, spinal cord injuries, burns) as it can precipitate life-threatening ventricular dysrhythmias. Given the longer duration of paralysis for most nondepolarizing agents (eg, atracurium), their use is generally avoided in RSI.

Certain patients predicted to have difficult airways may benefit from intubation via the use of lower than normal doses of induction agents without concurrent paralytics. Also known as the "awake look," this limits the all too real potential for creating the scenario of a paralyzed and, therefore, not breathing patient who cannot be intubated. Finally, apneic patients or those in cardiac arrest are not candidates for RSI. Their condition does not allow time for either preoxygenation or pretreatment, and being unconscious, they do not require RSI medications to facilitate ETT placement. Temporize these patients with BVM ventilation pending their emergent intubation.

To visualize the vocal cords, hold the laryngoscope in the left hand and carefully insert the blade into the oropharynx directed downward along the tongue and into the throat. Gentle upward traction should lift the epiglottis from the larynx and reveal the vocal cords (Figure 11–4). Concurrent external laryngeal manipulation may shift the patient's vocal cords into better view. Keep in mind that pediatric airways are typically more anterior than those of adults and that their relatively large tongues and floppy epiglottis often necessitate the use of a Miller blade.

Insert the ETT and maintain visualization until the balloon has clearly passed the vocal cords. Advance the ETT until the depth (at the teeth) is at 3 times the diameter of the tube. Keep in mind this is only an estimate, and all patients require a postprocedural CXR to document the depth of ETT placement. Proper insertion can be immediately confirmed at the bedside by auscultating for symmetric bilateral breath sounds and via the use of color-change capnography.

Gentle downward pressure applied to the cricoid cartilage (Sellick's maneuver) at the onset of induction and paralysis has been historically advocated to limit the potential for aspiration. A growing body of literature has begun to question the utility of this maneuver as it not only fails to prevent aspiration but can limit adequate visualization of the vocal cords and impair successful insertion of the ETT. If cricoid pressure is applied, release immediately if the patient begins to vomit to prevent secondary esophageal rupture.

▶ Difficult Airway Adjuncts

Multiple devices have been designed to assist with the management of difficult airways. Laryngeal mask airways

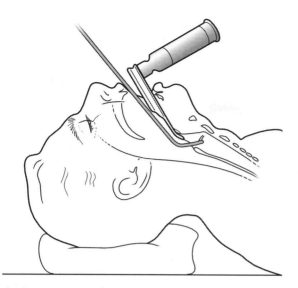

▲ **Figure 11-5.** Schematic demonstrating use of bougie.

(LMA) conform to the natural curvature of the oropharynx and are designed for blind insertion into the supraglottic region. Proper insertion creates an airtight seal over the larynx, allowing for mechanical ventilation. LMA insertion does not prevent aspiration, though, and is not considered a definitive airway.

Introducer bougies are very useful in patients whose vocal cords cannot be adequately visualized. They are essentially long flexible rubber stylets with a distal curve at their tip, which, when blindly inserted along the inferior margin of the epiglottis, will naturally angle upward into the larynx and through the vocal cords. Successful endotracheal placement can be detected as the tip of the bougie skips along the tracheal rings. The ETT is then inserted blindly over the bougie and into the airway (Figure 11-5).

Cricothyrotomy is performed by making a percutaneous incision in the cricothyroid membrane through which a tracheostomy or small ETT can be placed (Figure 11-6). This can be a life-saving intervention in the crashing patient when less invasive techniques to secure the airway have failed. Common indications include massive facial trauma and angioedema. Cricothyrotomy is contraindicated in children <8 years of age and should be replaced with needle cricothyrotomy.

Additional difficult airway adjuncts include blind nasotracheal intubation, lighted stylets, Combitubes, fiberoptic intubation, retrograde wire-guided tracheal intubation, and percutaneous translaryngeal ventilation.

DISPOSITION

Admit all patients who require airway management to an intensive care unit setting.

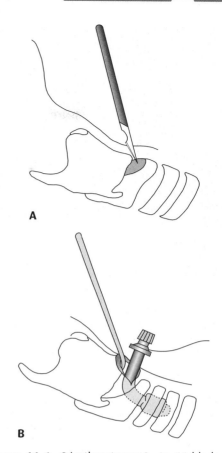

▲ **Figure 11-6.** Cricothyrotomy. **A.** An 11 blade scalpel is used to cut the cricothyroid membrane. **B.** A skin hook opens the incision and lifts the thyroid cartilage superiorly so that the tracheostomy tube or ETT can be inserted into the airway. (Reprinted with permission from Bailitz J, Bokhari F, Scaletta TA, et al. *Emergent Management of Trauma.* 3rd ed. New York: McGraw-Hill Education, 2011.)

▼ SUGGESTED READINGS

Hedayati T, Ross C, Nasr N. Airway procedures. Rapid sequence intubation. In: Simon RR, Ross CR, Bowman SH, Wakim PE. *Cook County Manual of Emergency Procedures.* 1st ed. Philadelphia, PA: Lippincott Williams & Wilkins, 2012, pp. 14–21.

Roman AM. Noninvasive airway management. In: Tintinalli JE, Stapczynski JS, Ma OJ, Clince DM, Cydulka, RK, Meckler GD. *Tintinalli's Emergency Medicine: A Comprehensive Study Guide.* 7th ed. New York, NY: McGraw-Hill, 2011, pp. 183–190.

Vissers RJ, Danzl DF. Tracheal intubation and mechanical ventilation. In: Tintinalli JE, Stapczynski JS, Ma OJ, Clince DM, Cydulka, RK, Meckler GD. *Tintinalli's Emergency Medicine: A Comprehensive Study Guide.* 7th ed. New York, NY: McGraw-Hill, 2011, pp. 198–215.

Shock

Lauren M. Smith, MD

Nihja O. Gordon, MD

Key Points

- Do not wait for hypotension to diagnose shock.
- Early identification and initiation of aggressive therapy can significantly improve patient survival.
- Initiate early goal-directed therapy in patients with septic shock.
- Early revascularization is key to improving outcome in patients with cardiogenic shock.

INTRODUCTION

More than 1 million patients present to U.S. emergency departments annually with shock, and despite continued advances in critical care, mortality rates remain very high. Shock occurs when the circulatory system is no longer able to deliver enough O_2 and vital nutrients to adequately meet the metabolic demands of the patient. Although initially reversible, prolonged hypoperfusion will eventually result in cellular hypoxia and the derangement of critical biochemical processes. From a clinical standpoint, shock can be divided into the following subtypes: **hypovolemic, cardiogenic, obstructive**, and **distributive**. Hypovolemic shock results from an inadequate circulating blood volume owing to either profound dehydration or significant hemorrhage. Traumatic hypovolemia is the most common type of shock encountered in patients <40 years of age. Cardiogenic shock occurs when the heart is unable to provide adequate forward blood flow secondary to impaired pump function or significant dysrhythmia. Myocardial infarction is the leading cause of cardiogenic shock and typically occurs once ~40% of the myocardium is dysfunctional. Obstructive shock results from an extracardiac blockage of adequate venous return of blood to the heart (eg, pericardial tamponade, tension pneumothorax, and massive pulmonary embolism [PE]). Finally, distributive shock occurs secondary to an uncontrolled loss of vascular tone (eg, sepsis, anaphylaxis, neurogenic shock, and adrenal crisis). Neurogenic shock most commonly occurs in trauma patients with high cervical cord injuries and a secondary loss of sympathetic tone and should always be considered a diagnosis of exclusion. Classically these patients will present with hypotension and a paradoxical bradycardia. Suspect septic shock in elderly, immunocompromised, and debilitated patients who are toxic appearing despite only vague symptoms. The prognosis for patients with cardiogenic and septic shock remains grave, with mortality rates between 30% and 90%.

The pathophysiology of shock can be divided into 3 basic categories: a systemic autonomic response, end-organ cellular hypoxia, and the secretion of proinflammatory mediators. The autonomic system initially responds to widespread tissue hypoperfusion by globally increasing the overall cardiac output. As tissue perfusion continues to decline, the body shunts circulating blood away from less vital structures including the skin, muscles, kidneys, and splanchnic beds. Reflexively, the kidneys activate the renin-angiotensin axis, prompting the release of various vasoactive substances, with the net effect to preserve perfusion to the most critical organs, namely the brain and the heart.

When the preceding response is inadequate despite maximal tissue O_2 extraction, cellular hypoxia forces a conversion from aerobic to anaerobic metabolism. By nature, anaerobic metabolism cannot produce enough adenosine triphosphate to maintain regular cellular function. Tissue lactate accumulates, resulting in systemic acidosis, and eventually this breakdown in cellular metabolism leads to widespread tissue death. Injured and dying cells prompt the production and secretion of harmful inflammatory mediators, resulting in the development of the systemic inflammatory response syndrome, defined by the presence of fever, tachycardia, tachypnea, and leukocytosis.

CLINICAL PRESENTATION

▶ History

Vague complaints such as fatigue and malaise may be the only presenting symptoms, especially in elderly patients. Friends, family, and emergency medical service personnel will be vital in obtaining a history in patients with altered mental status. The past medical history including a list of active medications might reveal risk factors such as immunosuppression, underlying cardiac disease, and potential allergic reactions.

▶ Physical Examination

Although hypotension and tachycardia are the cardinal features of shock, many patients will presents with normal vital signs owing to physiologic compensation. Because of the unmet metabolic demands of the central nervous system, altered mental status is not uncommon. Jugular venous distention, cardiac murmurs, and pulmonary rales often accompany cardiogenic shock. A careful skin examination can be invaluable, as patients in distributive shock frequently exhibit warm hyperemic extremities, whereas those in cardiogenic, hypovolemic, and obstructive shock will present with cool mottled extremities secondary to profound systemic vasoconstriction. Furthermore, abnormal findings such as diffuse urticaria, pronounced erythema, or widespread purpura may help identify the type and source of shock. The abdominal exam should focus on careful palpation and looking for signs of peritonitis or a pulsatile mass. Measure urine output, as low volumes indicate an absolute or relative volume deficiency and may help guide resuscitation.

DIAGNOSTIC STUDIES

▶ Laboratory

No single laboratory test is diagnostic of shock. Complete blood count testing may reveal an elevated, normal, or low white blood cell (WBC) count. No matter the absolute WBC count, a bandemia >10% suggests an ongoing infectious process. Comprehensive metabolic panel analysis will assess both kidney and liver function and acid–base status. An elevated anion gap may indicate underlying lactic acidosis, uremia, or toxic ingestion. Blood gas analysis is useful to determine the serum pH, lactate level, and base deficit. Serum lactate is a highly sensitive marker for tissue hypoperfusion and predictive of overall mortality in septic shock. Lactate levels >4 mmol/L are significant and indicate ongoing cellular hypoxia. Other tests useful in the appropriate clinical scenario include cardiac markers, urinalyses, coagulation profiles, toxicologic screens, and pregnancy testing. Obtain blood and urine cultures (and possibly cerebrospinal fluid) if sepsis is a concern.

▶ Imaging

No single radiologic test is diagnostic of shock. Chest x-ray may reveal evidence of an infiltrate (sepsis), enlarged cardiac silhouette (cardiac tamponade), subdiaphragmatic free air (sepsis), pulmonary edema (cardiogenic shock) or pneumothorax. Bedside ultrasound can guide the work-up, treatment, and disposition of patients in shock in multiple clinical situations including sepsis, blunt abdominal trauma, pregnancy, abdominal aortic aneurysm, and pericardial tamponade. Furthermore, ultrasonographic inferior vena cava measurement can help guide appropriate fluid resuscitation. Computed tomography imaging has become the modality of choice for diagnosing PE, aortic dissection, and intra-abdominal pathology.

PROCEDURES

Endotracheal intubation may be required in patients with profound shock to reduce the work of breathing and systemic metabolic demands. Central venous line placement can expedite fluid or blood product infusion, vasopressor administration, and central venous pressure (CVP) analysis.

MEDICAL DECISION MAKING

Once shock is recognized, rapidly attempt to identify both the subtype and inciting factor to determine the appropriate therapy (Table 12-1). Time is truly of the essence in these patients, and any delay will significantly impact patient outcome. Concurrently address the patient airway, breathing, and circulation (ABCs) and stabilize all severely ill patients. Use the ancillary laboratory and imaging studies mentioned previously to guide the diagnosis and treatment (Figure 12-1).

Table 12-1. SHOCK: differential diagnosis.

Shock Mnemonic	
S	Septic, spinal (neurogenic)
H	Hypovolemic, hemorrhagic
O	Obstructive (pulmonary embolism, tamponade)
C	Cardiogenic
K	Kortisol (adrenal crisis), AnaphylaKtic

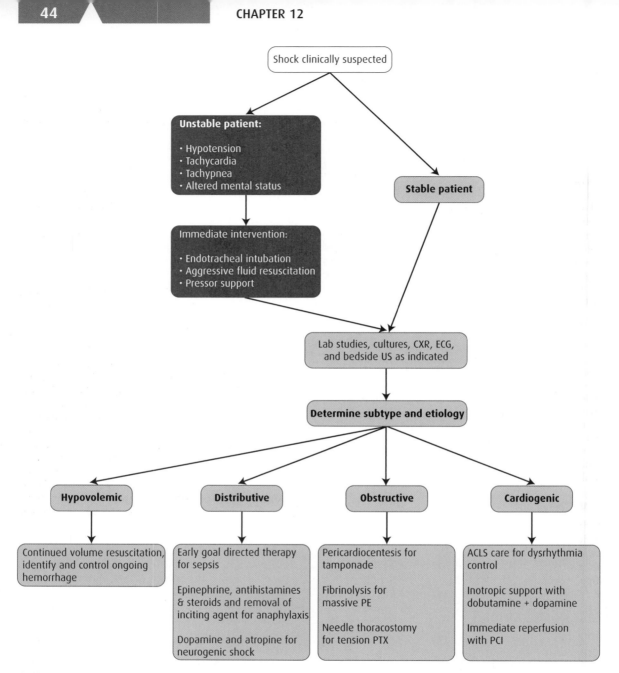

▲ **Figure 12-1.** Shock diagnostic algorithm. ACLS, advanced cardiac life support; PCI, percutaneous coronary intervention PE, pulmonary embolism; PTX, pneumothorax.

TREATMENT

The goal of treatment is 2-fold, namely to restore normal cellular function and reverse the inciting factor. Place all patients on supplemental O₂ and consider early mechanical ventilation in those with markedly elevated metabolic demands, as hyperactive respiratory muscles can steal away up to 50% of normal cerebral blood flow. Place a minimum of 2 large-bore peripheral IV lines in all patients and consider central line placement in those who will require multiple infusions, vasopressor support, or CVP monitoring. Administer boluses of normal saline to replenish an absolute or relative vascular depletion. Transfuse red blood cells as needed to augment circulating O_2 delivery. Initiate vasopressor support in patients who either fail to respond or have a contraindication (eg, cardiogenic shock) to repeated fluid boluses. Place a Foley catheter to accurately measure urine output. The management of specific types of shock is discussed next.

Hypovolemic Shock

Restore adequate tissue perfusion by rapidly expanding the intravascular volume. Infuse several liters of normal saline followed by several units of packed red blood cells in hemorrhagic patients who fail to respond. Patients with simple dehydration will improve rapidly. Of note, avoid overly aggressive volume expansion in trauma patients, as this may trigger recurrent hemorrhage at previously clotted sites. Titrate therapy in these patients to a goal mean arterial pressure (MAP) of 60 mmHg and restoration of normal mental status.

Distributive Shock

Sepsis

Begin early goal-directed therapy in all patients with septic shock. Monitor the CVP to guide fluid resuscitation in these patients. Begin treatment by aggressively bolusing several liters of normal saline to achieve a goal CVP between 8 and 12 mmHg. Initiate vasopressor support with a norepinephrine infusion in patients who remain hypotensive and titrate to a goal MAP >65 mmHg. Start broad-spectrum antibiotics targeted at the proposed source and pursue surgical drainage/debridement when indicated.

Neurogenic Shock

Address all other potential causes of shock first, as neurogenic shock is a diagnosis of exclusion. Aggressively expand the circulating blood volume by bolusing several liters of normal saline. Initiate a dopamine infusion for vasopressor support in all patients who fail to respond. Use small doses of IV atropine (eg, 0.5 mg) to treat symptomatic bradycardia refractory to the previously mentioned measures.

Anaphylaxis

Anaphylactic shock can be rapidly fatal and requires immediate treatment. Administer normal saline boluses, IV antihistamines, and IV corticosteroids to all patients. Give intramuscular epinephrine (1:1,000 solution) in 0.3- to 0.5-mg doses as needed to maintain systemic perfusion. In patients refractory to the preceding, administer 0.3- to 0.5-mg doses of IV epinephrine (1:10,000 solution) over a 2- to 3-minute duration. Actively search for and remove any ongoing allergen exposure (eg, retained soft tissue bee stinger).

Obstructive Shock

Cardiac Tamponade

Administer 1–2 L of normal saline followed by emergent bedside pericardiocentesis. Perform an emergency department thoracotomy in patients with penetrating thoracic trauma who fail to respond.

Pulmonary Embolism

Administer small boluses of normal saline (250–500 mL) followed by vasopressor support in unstable patients. Fibrinolysis is the treatment of choice for massive PE presenting with profound hypotension (MAP <60), severe refractory hypoxemia (SpO_2 <90 despite supplemental O_2), or cardiac arrest.

Tension Pneumothorax

Administer 1–2 L of normal saline while performing emergent needle thoracostomy followed by chest tube placement.

Cardiogenic Shock

The goal of treatment is to improve cardiac output while at the same time reducing myocardial workload. Administer IV fluids judiciously to avoid undesired elevations in the left ventricular preload and secondary pulmonary edema. Begin inotropic and vasopressor support in patients who remain hypotensive despite IV fluids. First-line therapy is often a combination of dopamine and dobutamine (as dobutamine monotherapy will exacerbate hypotension), with norepinephrine reserved for patients who fail to respond. Of note, all of the aforementioned modalities are temporizing measures pending definitive revascularization (ie, percutaneous coronary intervention or fibrinolysis).

DISPOSITION

Admit all patients in shock to a critical care bed.

SUGGESTED READING

Cherkas D. Traumatic hemorrhagic shock: Advances in fluid management. *Emerg Med Pract.* 2011;13:1–20.

Dellinger, RP, Levy, MM, et al. Surviving Sepsis Campaign: International guidelines for management of severe sepsis and septic shock: 2008. *Crit Care Med.* 2008;36:296–327.

Otero RM, Nguyen HB, Rivers EP. Approach to the patient in shock. In: Tintinalli JE, Stapczynski JS, Cline DM, Ma OJ, Cydulka RK, Meckler GD, eds. *Tintinalli's Emergency Medicine: A Comprehensive Study Guide.* 7th ed. New York, NY: McGraw-Hill, 2011.

Reynolds HR, Hochman JS. Cardiogenic shock: Current concepts and improving outcomes. *Circulation.* 2008;117: 686–697.

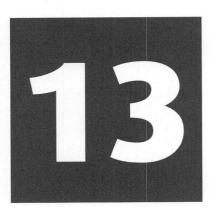

Chest Pain

Jonathon D. Palmer, MD

Key Points

- Chest pain is a very common complaint in emergency department patients.
- A rapid electrocardiogram and chest x-ray will help distinguish between multiple emergent causes of chest pain.
- The exclusion of life-threatening sources of chest pain should be the emergency physician's chief diagnostic concern.

INTRODUCTION

Chest pain is one of the most common presenting complaints in the emergency department (ED). As several fatal conditions present with chest pain, it is imperative to rapidly and thoroughly evaluate these patients to distinguish between emergent and nonemergent causes. Approach chest pain with a broad differential diagnosis and utilize your history, physical exam, and ancillary testing to narrow down the etiology.

The pathophysiology of chest pain will vary tremendously depending on the specific etiology. Regardless of the source, pain sensation ultimately occurs owing to stimulation of either visceral or somatic nerve fibers. Somatic nerve fibers innervate the skin and parietal pleura. Patients will typically complain of a pain that is sharp in nature and easily localized. Potential etiologies include pulmonary embolism, pneumothorax, musculoskeletal injury, herpes zoster infection, pneumonia, and pleurisy. Conversely, visceral nerve pain is often vague in quality, poorly localized, and will frequently radiate to nearby structures. Patients may deny the actual sensation of "pain" and rather describe their condition as a heaviness, pressure, or simple discomfort. Potential etiologies include acute coronary syndrome (ACS), aortic dissection, gastroesophageal reflux, and pericarditis.

CLINICAL PRESENTATION

History

A detailed history is essential when evaluating patients with chest pain, as no single element in isolation is sensitive or specific enough to determine either the etiology or the severity of the complaint. Ascertain the character of the pain to help determine a somatic or visceral source. For example, a sharp and stabbing pain is less likely in patients with ACS, but rather common in patients with pulmonary embolism. Identify the exact location of the pain and whether there is any associated radiation. Prototypical ischemic chest pain presents either just beneath the sternum or on the left side and radiates to either the left arm or jaw, whereas a mid-thoracic "tearing type" pain radiating straight through to the back is classically associated with aortic dissection. Determine the severity and duration of the pain. A mild, sharp pain lasting only seconds in duration is rarely associated with a serious pathology, whereas pain lasting greater than 10 minutes *may* suggest a more serious etiology. Recurrent pain that lasts for many hours or days per episode is unlikely to be cardiac.

In patients with a known history of heart disease, ascertain whether or not their symptoms mirror prior presentations. Patients with pain that is either similar to or more severe than a previous myocardial infarction (MI) have a markedly increased likelihood of ACS. Identify exacerbating or relieving factors, as this can quickly impact management. Patients with potential cardiac presentations frequently complain of pain that is worse with exertion and improved with rest. Pain that is worse with cough or deep inspiration (pleuritic pain) is typically associated with either pleurisy, a musculoskeletal etiology, or pulmonary embolism. Epigastric pain that is worse with meals usually signifies a gastrointestinal etiology. Pain that is aggravated by emotional stress may point to an underlying psychiatric etiology. Finally, inquire about any associated symptoms. For example, nausea and diaphoresis have been associated with a higher likelihood for ACS.

Unfortunately, the long-term risk factors for underlying heart disease (high cholesterol, smoking, hypertension, diabetes, family history) have not been shown to help in the differentiation of acute chest pain patients in the ED. Nonetheless, this history should be taken. A history of an underlying hypercoagulable state (eg, pregnancy, malignancy) should alert you to a possible pulmonary embolism (PE), whereas a history of an underlying connective tissue disorder (eg, Marfan syndrome) should prompt an evaluation for aortic dissection. Ask about any illicit drug habits, as cocaine use has been associated with accelerated atherosclerosis, acute MI, and aortic dissection.

▶ Physical Examination

Note the general appearance of the patient. Those with ACS or other serious etiologies may be clutching their chest and frequently appear anxious, pale, and diaphoretic. This "sick vs not sick" mentality will guide the rapidity of your examination. As with all emergency patients, assess the vital signs and ensure adequate airway, breathing, and circulation (ABCs). Note abnormal vital signs to help guide your differential diagnosis. A detailed examination of the heart, lungs, abdomen, extremities, and neurologic systems will ensure that no emergent causes of chest pain are overlooked. Listed next are some emergent presentations matched with potential physical exam findings.

ACS. Vital signs will vary widely depending on the region of ischemia or infarction. For example, an inferior wall MI may present with bradycardia and hypotension owing to increased vagal tone. Murmurs and abnormal heart sounds such as an S3 or S4 may be present. Inspiratory crackles on lung exam are consistent with secondary pulmonary edema.

Tension pneumothorax. Look for the classic signs of decreased breath sounds, tracheal deviation, and respiratory distress. Consider spontaneous pneumothorax in young, thin patients with an acute onset of chest pain and shortness of breath.

Pericardial tamponade. Although usually limited to patients in extremis, patients may exhibit the classic signs of Beck's triad (hypotension, diminished heart sounds, and jugular venous distension). Pulsus paradoxus >10 mmHg has shown a high sensitivity but low specificity for tamponade, as any condition causing increased intrathoracic pressure may demonstrate this.

Pulmonary embolism. Dyspnea is the most common complaint of patients with PE. They may also describe a pleuritic-type chest pain, especially those with segmental PEs that cause secondary infarction of the parietal pleura. Patients with significantly large (massive or submassive) PE are generally ill-appearing and hemodynamically unstable owing to the sudden severe increase in pulmonary vascular resistance. A detailed examination of the heart and lungs may reveal rales, gallops, or a prominent P2. Lower extremity exam may reveal unilateral swelling consistent with a deep venous thrombosis.

Aortic dissection. The pain is often most severe at onset and typically extends above and below the diaphragm. These patients are often hypertensive and may have a pulse deficit in either the radial and/or femoral arteries. A marked discrepancy in blood pressure compared between each arm (>20 mmHg) is highly suggestive.

DIAGNOSTIC STUDIES

Perform an electrocardiogram (ECG) within 10 minutes of presentation for all patients who complain of chest pain or have signs and symptoms concerning for ACS. Obtain cardiac markers including a troponin assay ± CK-MB analysis in all patients with suspected ACS. D-dimer can aid the evaluation of low-risk patients in whom PE is a diagnostic possibility.

CXR should be ordered on most patients in the ED with chest pain. Posteroanterior and lateral views are ideal, but a portable anteroposterior view is sufficient for patients who require continuous cardiac monitoring. Acute aortic dissection may present with a widened mediastinum or abnormal aortic contour. Pneumothoraces and subcutaneous air are readily identified. Pneumomediastinum ± a left-sided pleural effusion (owing to the relative thinness of the left esophageal wall) is seen with esophageal rupture (Boerhaave syndrome).

Newer generation CT angiography is the modality of choice to diagnose pulmonary embolism and aortic dissection and may have an evolving role in the evaluation of patients with potential coronary artery disease.

Transthoracic echo is often readily available and clinically useful to evaluate for possible pericardial effusions and tamponade physiology, ventricular hypokinesis in patients with ACS, and right ventricular strain in patients with massive PE. A bedside transesophageal echo is very sensitive for diagnosing acute aortic dissection in patients who are not candidates for CT angiography.

MEDICAL DECISION MAKING

A detailed history and physical exam in combination with an ECG and/or chest radiograph may provide sufficient evidence to exclude a myriad of emergent conditions.

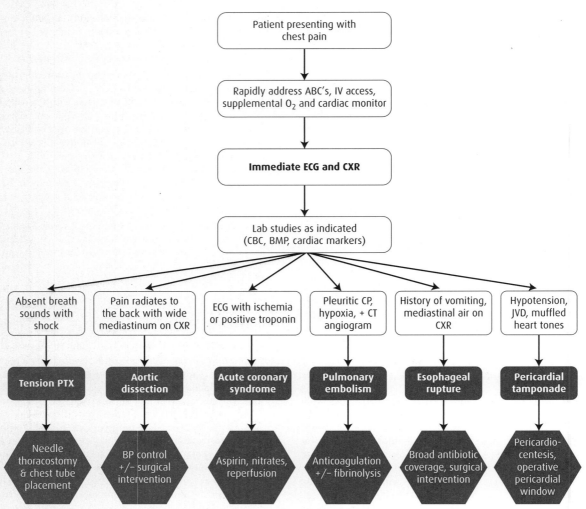

▲ **Figure 13-1.** Chest pain diagnostic algorithm. BMP, basic metabolic panel; BP, blood pressure; CBC, complete blood count; CP, chest pain; CT, computed tomography; CXR, chest x-ray; ECG, electrocardiogram; JVD, jugular venous distention.

When this is not adequate, a thoughtful use of laboratory studies combined with the pretest probability of disease will guide decision making (Figure 13-1).

TREATMENT

▶ Acute Coronary Syndrome

Provide supplemental O_2, administer a loading dose aspirin (162–365 mg), and begin sublingual nitroglycerin (0.4 mg every 5 minutes) on all ACS patients without known contraindications (eg, allergy, hypotension). Further antithrombotic (eg, clopidogrel) and anticoagulation (eg, low-molecular-weight heparin) therapy will differ by institution and cardiologist. Of note, the preceding interventions are often only temporizing measures, as early revascularization is definitive, especially in those patients presenting with an ST-elevation MI.

▶ Aortic Dissection

Patients with an aortic dissection require an immediate and aggressive reduction in both heart rate and blood pressure. The goal of treatment is to maintain a heart rate <60 bpm and systolic blood pressure <100 mmHg. There are multiple medication options for this purpose, and often concurrent infusions are required to meet the preceding targets. When utilizing dual therapy, it is of utmost importance to control the heart rate before dropping the blood pressure to avoid a "reflex tachycardia" and consequent expansion of the underlying dissection.

▶ Pulmonary Embolism

Treatment will vary based on the hemodynamic impact of the embolism. Anticoagulate stable patients with either low-molecular-weight or unfractionated heparin. Hemodynamic instability may necessitate the use of thrombolytic therapy.

Boerhaave Syndrome

Esophageal rupture is uncommon and classically presents with the sudden onset of chest pain after vomiting. Initiate broad-spectrum antibiotic coverage while arranging for definitive surgical repair.

Pneumothorax

Place all patients with a pneumothorax on supplemental O_2 via a nonrebreather mask. Those with a tension pneumothorax require immediate needle decompression followed by chest tube thoracostomy. Simple pneumothoraces can be treated with tube thoracostomy or simple observation.

Pericardial Tamponade

The recognition of tamponade is much easier in the age of bedside ultrasonography. Perform immediate pericardiocentesis in unstable patients while arranging for an operative pericardial window via cardiothoracic surgery.

DISPOSITION

Admission

Admit all patients with concerning presentations to a monitored bed. The following chapters discuss the disposition of patients with specific conditions in greater detail.

Discharge

Many patients with chest pain can be discharged with close primary care follow-up and a list of strict indications for reevaluation. Take care to exclude emergent causes and discharge only those cases with a clear nonemergent etiology (eg, chest wall pain, zoster, dyspepsia). If clinical doubt exists, it is certainly prudent to err on the side of caution and admit for inpatient observation.

SUGGESTED READING

Anderson JL, Adams CD, Antman EM, et al. ACC/AHA 2007 Guidelines for the management of patients with unstable angina/non ST-elevation MI: A report of the ACC/AHA task force of practice guidelines. *Circulation.* 2007;116: e148.

Fesmire FM, Brown MD, Espinosa JA, et al. Critical issues in the evaluation and management of adult patients presenting to the emergency department with suspected pulmonary embolism. *Ann Emerg Med.* 2011;57:628–652.

Green GB, Hill PM. Chest pain: Cardiac or not. In: Tintinalli JE, Stapczynski JS, Ma OJ, Cline DM, Cydulka RK, Meckler GD. *Tintinalli's Emergency Medicine: A Comprehensive Study Guide.* 7th ed. New York, NY: McGraw-Hill, 2011, pp. 361–367.

Swap CJ, Nagurney JT. Value and limitations of chest pain history in the evaluation of patients with acute coronary syndromes. *JAMA.* 2005;294:2623–2639.

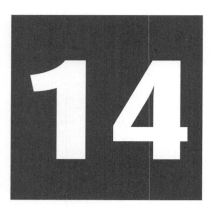

Acute Coronary Syndromes

Christopher Ross, MD

Key Points

- Consider acute coronary syndrome (ACS) in the initial assessment of all patients presenting with chest pain and/or difficulty breathing.
- Atypical presentations are common, especially in women, the elderly, and diabetics.
- Obtain an emergent electrocardiogram in all patients with concern for ACS to rapidly identify ST-segment elevation myocardial infarctions (STEMI).
- Patients with STEMI require immediate reperfusion therapy with either thrombolytics or percutaneous coronary intervention to salvage the maximum amount of viable myocardium.

INTRODUCTION

Acute coronary syndrome (ACS) encompasses a spectrum of disease that includes unstable angina (UA), non–ST-segment elevation myocardial infarctions (NSTEMI), and ST-segment elevation myocardial infarctions (STEMI). The distinction between the 3 is based on historical factors, electrocardiogram (ECG) analysis, and cardiac biomarker measurements. ACS is the leading cause of mortality in the industrialized world and accounts for more than 25% of all deaths in the United States. More than 5 million patients per year present to U.S. emergency departments with symptoms concerning for ACS, although fewer than 10% will be diagnosed with acute myocardial infarctions (AMI). That said, between 2% and 4% of all patients with ACS are initially misdiagnosed and improperly discharged from the ED, resulting in significant morbidity and mortality and accounting for the leading source of malpractice payouts in the United States.

The pathophysiology of myocardial ischemia can be broken down into a simple imbalance in the supply and demand of coronary perfusion. Atherosclerosis is responsible for almost all cases of ACS. This insidious process begins with the deposition of fatty streaks in the coronary arteries of adolescent patients and progresses by early adulthood to the formation of organized fibro-fatty plaques. As plaques enlarge throughout adulthood, they progressively limit coronary blood flow and may eventually induce the development of anginal symptoms with exertion. In time, plaques can rupture, causing secondary intraluminal thrombus formation and a sudden reduction in coronary perfusion (ie, AMI).

UA is a clinical diagnosis that has no pathognomonic ECG findings or confirmatory elevations in cardiac biomarkers. Patients with classic anginal symptoms that are either new, accelerating in frequency or severity, or that occur without exertion are considered to have UA. UA and NSTEMI are very similar from a pathophysiologic standpoint with the latter being distinguished by the presence of elevated cardiac biomarkers. Both conditions arise from the non-complete occlusion of coronary blood flow with the secondary development of ischemia and infarction, respectively. Complete occlusions of the coronary arteries typically result in transmural infarctions of the myocardium with associated ST segment elevation (STEMI) on the ECG and increased biomarker levels. Of note, the mortality rates of patients with NSTEMI and STEMI are identical at the 6-month follow-up point.

It is very important to understand the basic anatomy of the coronary arteries to identify concerning ECG patterns and predict clinical complications. The left coronary artery (ie, left mainstem artery) arises from the aortic root and branches almost immediately into the left anterior descending artery (LAD) and left circumflex artery (LCX). The LAD runs down the anterior aspect of the heart and provides the main blood supply to the anterior left ventricle and ventricular septum, whereas the LCX runs in the atrioventricular (AV) sulcus between the left atrium and left ventricle and provides blood to the lateral and posterior regions of the heart. The right coronary artery (RCA) also arises directly from the aortic root. It runs in the AV sulcus between the right atrium and right ventricle and provides blood to the right side of the heart and inferior portion of the left ventricle. The sinoatrial node is perfused by the RCA, whereas the AV node is perfused by a combination of the RCA and LAD in most patients.

Risk factors predictive of underlying coronary artery disease (CAD) have been identified and include age >40 years, male patients or postmenopausal females, hypertension, dyslipidemia, diabetes mellitus, smoking, family history of CAD, truncal obesity, and a sedentary lifestyle. It is important to remember that these risk factors are based on large demographic analyses and cannot be used to predict the presence or absence of CAD in a given patient. Approximately half of all patients presenting with ACS have no identifiable risk factors outside of age and sex.

CLINICAL PRESENTATION

History

A thorough history is the most sensitive tool for the detection of ACS, and an experienced clinician will always be wary of its variable presentation. Chest pain is the most common presenting complaint. Myocardial ischemia is classically described as pressure-like or squeezing sensation located in the retrosternal area or left side of the chest. Inquire about the quality, duration, frequency, and intensity of the pain. Determine whether there is radiation of pain, associated symptoms, and provoking and palliating factors. Symptoms commonly associated with myocardial ischemia include nausea, diaphoresis, shortness of breath, and palpitations. Anginal pain can radiate in almost any direction depending on the individual patient and the affected region of the heart, but radiation to the shoulder, arm, neck, and jaw is most common. It should be noted that the intensity of pain is not predictive of the overall severity of the myocardial insult, and even minimal symptoms can correlate with significant mortality.

Up to a third of patients with ACS will present with symptoms other than chest pain. Also known as "anginal equivalents," these presentations further complicate the accurate diagnosis of ACS. Possible complaints include dyspnea, vomiting, altered mental status, abdominal pain, and syncope. Patients at an increased risk of atypical presentations include the elderly, women, diabetics, polysubstance abusers, psychiatric patients, and nonwhite minorities. These patients have a near 4-fold increase in mortality owing to inherent delays in their diagnosis, treatment, and disposition. Always obtain a detailed social history and inquire about any recent and chronic substance abuse. Habitual tobacco use has been proven to be an independent risk factor for CAD, whereas cocaine use can not only induce significant coronary spasm in the acute setting, but also accelerate the atherosclerotic process when chronically abused.

Physical Examination

There are no physical findings specific for ACS, and the exam is frequently normal. Obtain a complete set of vital signs and closely monitor unstable patients. Bradycardia is common with inferior wall ischemia owing to an increase in vagal tone, whereas tachycardia may represent compensation for a reduction in stroke volume. Concurrent hypertension increases the myocardial O_2 demand and may exacerbate the underlying ischemia, whereas acute cardiogenic shock has an extremely poor prognosis.

Carefully auscultate the heart for any abnormal sounds. Acute changes in ventricular compliance may result in an S3, S4, or paradoxically split S2. The presence of a new systolic murmur may signify either papillary muscle infarction with secondary mitral valve insufficiency or ventricular septal infarction with secondary perforation. Look for signs of acute congestive heart failure (CHF), including jugular venous distension, hepatojugular reflux, and inspiratory crackles. Perform a rectal exam to look for evidence of gastrointestinal bleeding, and document a thorough neurologic exam in patients who may require treatment with anticoagulant or thrombolytic medications.

DIAGNOSTIC STUDIES

Electrocardiogram

Obtain a 12-lead ECG immediately on presentation for patients with symptoms concerning for ACS. The emergent identification of a STEMI ensures that definitive therapy can be arranged as quickly as possible to limit further myocardial loss. The use of prehospital ECG analysis has further reduced any delays in appropriate therapy. Keep in mind that a single ECG provides only an isolated snapshot of myocardial electrical activity, and as such, any changes in clinical status should prompt repeat testing. In addition, fewer than half of all AMIs are of the STEMI variety, and ECG interpretation may be completely normal in the setting of NSTEMI or UA. ST-segment elevations suggest the presence of an acute transmural infarction, whereas ST-segment depressions suggest active myocardial ischemia. The morphology of the ST-segment elevations

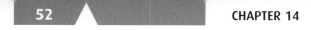

Table 14-1. Anatomical regions of the heart by ECG analysis.

Anatomic Location	Occluded Artery	Ischemic Leads	Reciprocal Leads
Anterior wall	LAD	V2, V3, V4	II, III, aVF
Lateral wall	LCX	I, aVL, V5, V6	V1, V2
Inferior wall	RCA, LCX	II, III, aVF	Variable
Posterior	RCA, LCX	V8, V9	V1, V2
Right ventricle	RCA	V1, V4R	Variable

with AMI is typically straight or convex upward ("tombstone") in appearance, whereas concave ST-segment elevations generally indicate a more benign etiology (left ventricular hypertrophy, benign early repolarization, pericarditis). Concerning ST-segment changes with ACS, whether elevations or depressions, should be seen in a distinct anatomical region with corresponding reciprocal changes (Table 14-1). Additional findings concerning for

cardiac ischemia include inverted and hyperacute T-waves (wide-based asymmetric high-amplitude T-waves). Q waves indicative of myocardial necrosis generally appear late in the course of patients with ACS and cannot be relied on in the acute decision-making process.

The ECG analysis for ACS should always occur in a standard fashion based on the anatomic distribution of the coronary arteries (Figures 14-1 and 14-2). Of particular interest, inferior wall AMIs generally represent occlusion of the RCA. ST-segment elevation that is more pronounced in lead III versus lead II is a subtle clue for involvement of the right ventricle (RV). Obtain a right-sided ECG (lead V4r, analogous to lead V4 but placed on the right side of the sternum) in these patients to better evaluate the RV, and use nitroglycerin very carefully to avoid precipitating hemodynamic collapse. Furthermore, as the posterior descending arteries (PDA) of most patients arise directly from the RCA, acute occlusion of the RCA should raise concern for a concurrent posterior wall infarction. Findings on the ECG suggestive of a posterior wall infarction include an R-wave amplitude > S-wave amplitude in leads V1 and V2 along with corresponding ST-segment depressions and tall upright T-waves

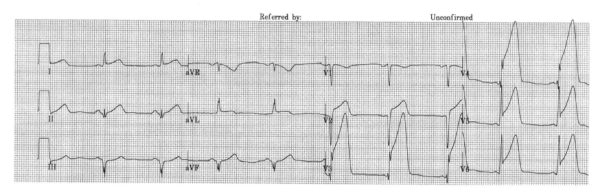

▲ **Figure 14-1.** Anterior wall myocardial infarction. This patient had a 100% occlusion of the left anterior descending artery.

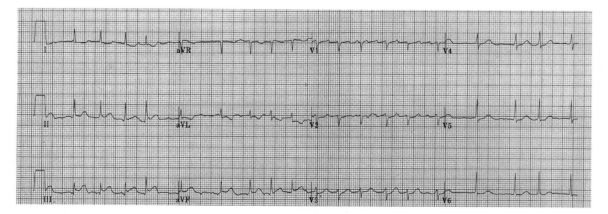

▲ **Figure 14-2.** Inferior wall myocardial infarction. Note the ST segment elevations in leads II, III, and aVF. Elevation in lead III is more pronounced than lead II, suggesting right ventricular wall involvement.

in leads V1-V4. Obtain a posterior ECG (leads V8 and V9) in these patients.

Observe patients closely for the development of any form of irritability, dysrhythmia, conduction delay, or heart block (See Chapter 15 for further details). High-degree AV block (second or third degree) is present in 6% of patients with AMI. The incidence is higher in patients with inferior wall infarctions (15%) owing to the secondary increase in vagal tone or ischemia of the AV node. Anterior wall infarctions can also produce AV blocks as a result of ischemia of either the bundle of His or bilateral bundle branches, resulting in a wide QRS complex brady-dysrhythmia. The presence of a new left bundle branch block in the appropriate clinical context should be considered and treated analogous to a STEMI.

▶ Laboratory

Injury to myocardial tissue results in the release of unique cardiac enzymes into the vascular space, which can be readily measured via serum analysis. Keep in mind that patients with ECG findings consistent with STEMI do not require confirmatory testing with serum markers but rather warrant immediate reperfusion therapy. That said, serum markers are very useful in patients with nondiagnostic ECGs to diagnose the presence of a NSTEMI. Of note, there is no single cardiac marker analysis that has sufficient accuracy to reliably identify or exclude AMI within the first 6 hours of symptoms onset. Furthermore, elevations can and do occur secondary to non-ACS-related conditions, including myocarditis, decompensated CHF, and acute pulmonary embolism.

The usual laboratory studies used for the diagnosis of AMI are the troponins (both T and I subtypes). Troponin (Tn) levels are the most specific marker for myocardial necrosis and have become the gold standard for diagnosis. Elevated levels can be detected within 3 hours of injury, peak at 12 hours, and remain elevated for a period of 3–10 days. The degree of myocardial damage and mortality is correlated with the degree of troponin elevation.

Creatinine kinase is found in all forms of muscle tissue, but the MB subunit is far more specific for myocardial injury. CK-MB elevations can usually be detected within 4–6 hours after symptom onset, peak at 24 hours, and typically return to normal within 2–3 days. Myoglobin assays are also in common use for the evaluation of AMI. Although attractive in theory as significant elevations can be detected within 1–2 hours of symptom onset, a poor specificity limits the clinical utility of serum myoglobin analysis.

▶ Imaging

Obtain an emergent chest x-ray in all patients who present with a chief complaint of chest pain or shortness of breath. That said, there are no radiographic findings specific for the diagnosis of ACS, and its role in this setting is primarily for excluding alternative diagnoses.

Acute CHF secondary to ACS may present with classic radiographic findings.

MEDICAL DECISION MAKING

Order an ECG immediately on presentation to identify patients with STEMI, as they require immediate and aggressive reperfusion. Patients with cardiogenic shock, acutely decompensated CHF, ventricular dysrhythmias, and severe symptoms refractory to aggressive medical therapy also typically warrant emergent percutaneous coronary intervention (PCI). In patients with nondiagnostic ECGs, proceed with cardiac marker testing. Patients with elevated cardiac markers should be treated as having a NSTEMI. Those whose initial set of cardiac markers are negative require serial ECG and biomarker testing. These patients should be stratified to identify those who are at high risk for adverse cardiovascular outcomes. Concerning factors that may identify high-risk patients include patients ≥65 years of age, the presence of at least 3 risk factors for CAD, known prior coronary stenosis of ≥50%, ST-segment deviations on ECG, elevated cardiac markers, the use of aspirin within the prior 7 days, and at least 2 anginal episodes within the past 24 hours. Further treatment should be dictated by the patient's category of risk (Figure 14-3).

TREATMENT

The proper management of ACS demands rapid and aggressive care. These patients require treatment in an area with ready access to resuscitation equipment including advanced airways and defibrillators. Address the patient's airway and circulatory status and place the patient on the cardiac monitor. Obtain IV access and administer supplemental oxygen to maintain an SpO_2 ≥94%. The immediate goals of therapy are to limit the supply-demand mismatch by improving coronary perfusion while reducing myocardial oxygen demand. Further treatment is dictated by condition into either STEMI or UA/NSTEMI pathways.

▶ Nitroglycerin

Nitroglycerin is widely used in patients with ACS and provides benefit via several different actions. It decreases myocardial oxygen demand by reducing the ventricular preload, improves myocardial perfusion by dilating the coronary vascular bed, and exhibits some mild antiplatelet properties. Start with sublingual doses of 0.4 mg in a disintegrating tablet or spray. This can be repeated every 3–5 minutes as necessary for refractory pain provided that the patient maintains a systolic blood pressure >100 mmHg. Chest pain that persists after 3–5 doses warrants the initiation of IV therapy. Start an infusion at 10–20 mcg/min and rapidly titrate upward in 10–20 mcg/min increments to achieve adequate pain control. Immediately stop

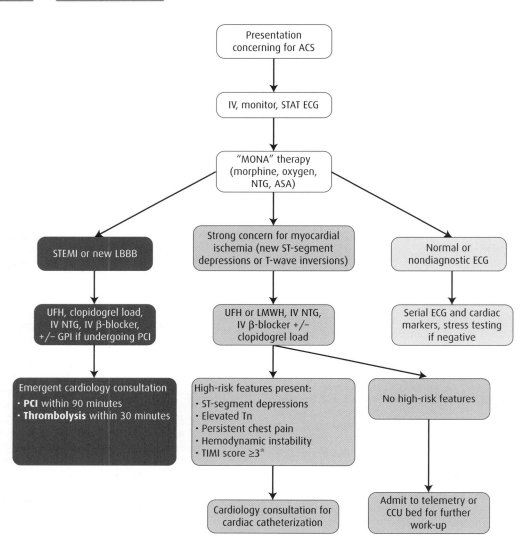

* TIMI risk score for UA/NSTEMI equals the number of the following 7 risk factors that are present: Age ≥ 65, ≥3 CAD risk factors, known CAD, ASA use within the past week, recent angina, elevated cardiac markers, and ST-segment deviations ≥ 0.5mm. A score of 3 carries a 13% risk of an adverse cardiac event (AMI, death, revascularization) within the next 14 days.

 Figure 14-3. ACS diagnostic algorithm. ACS, acute coronary syndrome; AMI, acute myocardial infarction; ASA, aspirin; CAD, coronary artery disease; CCU, critical care unit; ECG, electrocardiogram; GPI, glycoprotein IIb/IIIa inhibitors; LBBB, left bundle branch block; LMWH, low-molecular-weight heparin; NTG, nitroglycerin; NSTEMI, non–ST-segment elevation myocardial infarction; PCI, percutaneous coronary intervention; STEMI, ST-segment elevation myocardial infarction; TIMI, Thrombolysis In Myocardial Infarction; Tn, troponin; UA, unstable angina; UFH, unfractionated heparin.

the infusion and administer IV fluid boluses to any patients with signs of secondary hypotension. Patients with infarctions that involve the right ventricle are particularly prone to hypotension given their preload dependent condition.

▶ **Morphine**

Administer IV morphine to all patients with persistent pain despite treatment with nitroglycerin. Morphine reduces myocardial O_2 demand by decreasing vascular tone (preload) and limiting the catecholamine surge that typically accompanies ACS. Avoid the use of morphine in hypotensive patients.

Antiplatelet Therapy

Begin immediate treatment with aspirin (ASA) in all patients with presentations concerning for ACS. Give ≥162 mg of a non–enteric-coated version. The first dose should be crushed or chewed to improve absorption and more quickly reach therapeutic blood levels. Aspirin alone reduces mortality by 23% in STEMI patients. Minor contraindications (remote history of peptic ulcer disease, vague allergy, etc) should not preclude its use.

Clopidogrel, prasugrel, and ticagrelor all function to inhibit platelet activation via blockade of the adenosine diphosphate (ADP) receptors and therefore work in harmony with aspirin therapy. Clopidogrel has been the most extensively researched of the 3 and, therefore, is the most commonly used. A loading dose of 600 mg is recommended for patients with STEMI undergoing emergent PCI, whereas a 300-mg load is recommended for patients undergoing reperfusion with thrombolytics and those with UA/NSTEMI. No loading dose is recommended in patients older than 75 years because of a concern for increased bleeding complications. Both prasugrel and ticagrelor produce a more intense platelet inhibition, but do so at the expense of an increase in major bleeding complications. Although there is a legitimate concern for excessive bleeding in patients given ADP-receptor antagonists who subsequently undergo coronary artery bypass grafting (CABG), the definite benefit of platelet inhibition in patients with ACS far outweighs the potential concern for bleeding in the very low number of patients who actually require emergent CABG.

Glycoprotein IIb/IIIa inhibitors represent the third class of antiplatelet medications and function by inhibiting platelet aggregation via blockade of the surface binding sites for activated fibrin. There are currently 3 available agents in this class (abciximab, eptifibatide, and tirofiban), and their use in patients with ACS has been extensively researched. These agents have been associated with an increase in major bleeding complications, and current guidelines recommend their use only for patients with ACS undergoing PCI.

Anticoagulation

Administer either unfractionated heparin (UFH) or low-molecular-weight heparin (LMWH) in all patients with ACS and no known contraindications. LMWH (enoxaparin) is generally preferred given its more predictable weight-based onset of activity, reduced tendency for immune-mediated thrombocytopenia, and lack of requirement for laboratory monitoring. That said, the longer half-life and lack of easy reversibility of LMWH is problematic in patients for whom invasive interventions are planned. UFH is typically recommended for patients undergoing PCI, whereas LMWH is preferred for patients with UA/NSTEMI who are not undergoing emergent reperfusion.

Fondaparinux and bivalirudin (a direct thrombin inhibitor) are two of the newer anticoagulant agents available for the management of patients with ACS and will likely have an expanding role in the near future. Both have been shown to be equally effective with fewer bleeding complications as compared with standard treatment with UFH or LMWH in select patient populations.

Beta-Blockers

Beta-blockers exhibit antiarrhythmic, anti-ischemic, and antihypertensive properties. They reduce myocardial O_2 demand via decreasing the heart rate, cardiac afterload, and ventricular contractility. Current guidelines recommend the initiation of treatment in all ACS patients with no contraindications (decompensated CHF, hypotension, heart blocks, and reactive airway disease). Metoprolol can be given in 5-mg IV doses every 5 minutes for a total of 3 doses or as a single 50-mg oral dose if IV treatment is not required.

Reperfusion Therapy

Patients with STEMI require immediate reperfusion therapy with either PCI or thrombolysis. The American College of Cardiology guidelines recommend a duration of no more than 90 minutes between patient presentation and balloon inflation in those undergoing PCI and a duration of no more than 30 minutes between presentation and treatment in those undergoing thrombolysis. PCI is the preferred modality owing to a decreased risk of bleeding complications, lower incidence of recurrent ischemia and infarction, and improved rates of survivability. For patients with UA or NSTEMI, an early invasive approach (within 24–48 hours) utilizing PCI reduces the risk of death, AMI, and recurrent ACS. Thrombolysis is not recommended for patients with either UA or NSTEMI.

DISPOSITION

Admission

Admit all patients with suspected ACS to a monitored bed for serial ECG testing and cardiac marker analysis. High-risk patients including those with elevated cardiac markers, ischemic ECG changes, and refractive symptoms warrant admission to a critical care setting for early PCI. STEMI patients require admission to a critical care setting after appropriate reperfusion therapy (PCI or thrombolysis).

Discharge

Patients at a very low risk for ACS (young healthy patient, atypical history, normal ECG, and negative serial cardiac markers) who remain symptom free during an emergency department observation period of several hours can be safely discharged home with early stress testing arranged in the outpatient setting.

▼ SUGGESTED READING

Green G, Hill P. Chest pain: Cardiac or not. In: Tintinalli JE, Stapczynski JS, Ma OJ, Cline DM, Cydulka RK, Meckler GD. *Tintinalli's Emergency Medicine: A Comprehensive Study Guide.* 7th ed. New York, NY: McGraw-Hill, 2011, pp. 361–367.

Hollander J, Dierks D. Acute coronary syndromes: Acute myocardial infarction. In: Tintinalli JE, Stapczynski JS, Ma OJ, Cline DM, Cydulka RK, Meckler GD. *Tintinalli's Emergency Medicine: A Comprehensive Study Guide.* 7th ed. New York, NY: McGraw-Hill, 2011, pp. 367–385.

Congestive Heart Failure

Tarlan Hedayati, MD
Negean Afifi, DO

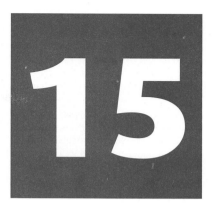

Key Points

- A normal ejection fraction does not exclude congestive heart failure (CHF), as CHF can occur secondary to either systolic or diastolic dysfunction.
- Nitroglycerin is the initial treatment of choice because it reduces both preload and afterload and rapidly improves patient symptoms.
- Consider acute coronary syndrome as the primary precipitant of CHF.
- CHF associated with cardiogenic shock maintains a very high mortality rate despite appropriate medical management.

INTRODUCTION

Congestive heart failure (CHF) is the leading cause of hospitalizations in the United States in patients older than 65 years. Once symptomatic, up to 35% of patients will die within 2 years of the diagnosis, and more than 60% will succumb within 6 years. The annual costs of treatment are more than $27 billion and will only increase given the aging population.

Heart failure occurs when the myocardium is unable to provide sufficient cardiac output to meet the metabolic demands of the body. As the myocardium can no longer keep up with the return of venous blood, pulmonary and systemic vascular congestion occurs. Common causes of CHF include myocardial infarction, valvulopathies, cardiomyopathies, and chronic uncontrolled hypertension.

Based on the underlying pathophysiology, heart failure can be divided into systolic and diastolic subtypes. Systolic heart failure develops when a direct myocardial injury impairs normal cardiac contractility causing a secondary decline in ejection fraction (eg, myocardial infarction). Diastolic heart failure develops when impaired cardiac compliance limits ventricular filling (preload) causing a consequent drop in overall cardiac output (eg, left ventricular hypertrophy).

In acute decompensated CHF, the global decrease in cardiac output forces a compensatory increase in systemic vascular resistance (SVR) to maintain vital organ perfusion. This increase in SVR is actually counterproductive and causes a further reduction in cardiac output as the already compromised myocardium now faces an ever higher afterload. The downward spiral continues as myocardial oxygen demand increases because of the increased ventricular workload, resulting in further compromise of the myocardium. Consequent elevations in left atrial and ventricular pressures eventually beget pulmonary edema and respiratory distress.

Decompensated CHF is commonly precipitated by acute coronary syndrome (ACS), rapid atrial fibrillation, acute renal failure, or medication and dietary noncompliance. Other important precipitants to consider are pulmonary embolus, uncontrolled hypertension, profound anemia, thyroid dysfunction, and states of increased metabolic demand such as infection. Cardiotoxic drugs including alcohol, cocaine, and some chemotherapeutic agents should also be considered.

CLINICAL PRESENTATION

▶ History

Patients most commonly present with shortness of breath with exertion or at rest with severe exacerbations.

Orthopnea, or dyspnea while lying flat, is common as a result of the redistribution of fluid from the lower extremities to the central circulation when the legs are elevated. The increase in central circulation produces a higher pulmonary capillary wedge pressure and secondary pulmonary edema. Attempt to quantify the severity of the orthopnea by asking on how many pillows the patient sleeps and note any changes from baseline. Paroxysmal nocturnal dyspnea occurs when sleeping patients awake suddenly with marked shortness of breath with the need to sit up and hang the legs over the side of the bed or go to a window for air. In certain patients, pulmonary congestion presents rather occultly with a persistent mild nocturnal cough as the only symptom.

Patients may complain of peripheral edema, but this is neither sensitive nor specific for CHF and should prompt an investigation for alternative etiologies. Right upper quadrant pain may occur in patients with hepatic congestion and can be confused with biliary colic.

Always obtain a detailed review of systems to try to identify any possible precipitants of CHF. Specifically, ask patients about antecedent or ongoing chest pain, palpitations, recent illnesses or infections, and medication or dietary changes or noncompliance.

▶ Physical Examination

Quickly evaluate patient stability with a careful assessment of vital signs and a focused physical exam. Check the respiratory rate, obtain a pulse oximetry, look for accessory muscle use, and determine whether the patient can speak in complete sentences to assess the severity of respiratory distress. Decreased stroke volume and impaired cardiac output may manifest as tachycardia, a narrowed pulse pressure, or marked peripheral vasoconstriction. Recognize hypotension and/or signs of hypoperfusion immediately and treat as cardiogenic shock.

After the initial assessment, focus on signs of total body volume overload. Patients with left ventricular failure typically present with pulmonary signs, including inspiratory crackles, a persistent cough, or a "cardiac wheeze." Patients with right ventricular failure show signs of systemic congestion. Check for peripheral edema, jugular venous distention, and hepatojugular reflux (an increase in jugular venous pressure with deep palpation of the right upper quadrant) (Figure 15-1). Auscultate the heart for murmurs or gallops. Although often difficult to appreciate in the emergency department (ED), an S3 gallop is highly specific for decompensated heart failure.

DIAGNOSTIC STUDIES
▶ Laboratory

Obtain a complete blood count to look for signs of anemia and a serum chemistry to evaluate renal function and rule out any electrolyte abnormalities (eg, hyperkalemia) that

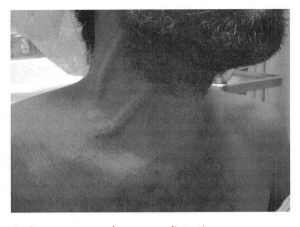

▲ **Figure 15-1.** Jugular venous distention.

may lead to cardiac irritability and impaired function. Order cardiac enzymes to rule out ACS as the precipitating event, although patients in decompensated CHF may exhibit mild elevations in the absence of ACS because of the excessive strain placed on the myocardium. Regardless of etiology, patients in CHF with elevated cardiac enzymes have a worse prognosis. Check thyroid function tests if either hypothyroidism or thyrotoxicosis is thought to be the source of heart failure.

Brain natriuretic peptide (BNP) is released from the ventricular myocytes in the presence of ventricular wall distention. Measurement of serum BNP is especially helpful in differentiating CHF from underlying pulmonary conditions such as chronic obstructive pulmonary disease (COPD) or pneumonia. Levels <100 ng/dL have a high negative predictive value, whereas those >400 ng/dL are consistent with decompensated CHF. Levels between 100 and 400 ng/dL are neither sensitive nor specific for CHF and may be indicative of pulmonary embolism, cor pulmonale, cirrhosis, or renal failure. Remember that heart failure is a clinical diagnosis, and BNP measurement is most helpful in clinically indeterminate cases.

▶ Electrocardiogram

Obtain an emergent electrocardiogram (ECG) on all patients with suspected CHF to look for evidence of new or old myocardial injury, as well any precipitating arrhythmias. Signs of atrial or ventricular hypertrophy may also be seen.

▶ Imaging

Obtain a chest x-ray (CXR) in all patients. Findings consistent with CHF include cardiomegaly, bilateral pleural effusions, perihilar congestion, Kerley B lines (transverse radio-opaque lines seen at the lung periphery), and vascular cephalization (Figure 15-2). CXR may reveal alternative sources for the patient's dyspnea, including pneumonia,

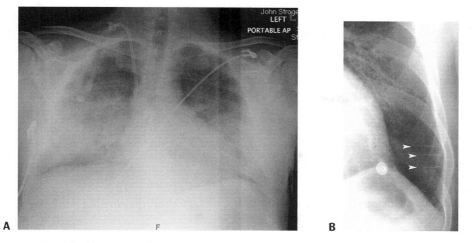

▲ **Figure 15-2. A.** Bilateral infiltrates, cardiomegaly and cephalization can be seen in this patient with pulmonary edema. **B.** Kerley B Lines in patient with pulmonary edema (white arrowheads). (B: Reprinted with permission from Schwartz DT. Chapter 1–7. Congestive Heart Failure—Interstitial Lung Markings. In: Schwartz DT, ed. *Emergency Radiology: Case Studies.* New York: McGraw-Hill, 2008.)

pneumothorax, or malignancy. Importantly, a normal CXR does not exclude CHF, as radiographic findings can lag the onset of clinical symptoms by up to 6 hours.

Echocardiography is often performed on an inpatient basis to assess ventricular size and function and rule out underlying valvular disease. Emergency practitioners skilled in ultrasonography may use bedside echocardiography to assess global cardiac function in the critically ill or clinically indeterminate cases.

MEDICAL DECISION MAKING

Rapidly address any signs of respiratory distress. Mildly symptomatic patients require supplemental oxygen, whereas patients in moderate to severe respiratory distress often require some form of ventilatory assistance. After respiratory stabilization, address the patient's hemodynamic status. A hypotensive patient with signs of shock requires vasopressor/inotropic support, whereas a hypertensive patient will benefit from vasodilator and diuretic therapy. The differential diagnosis of CHF is broad and includes many of its precipitants such as ACS, cardiac dysrhythmias, pulmonary embolus, and valvular disease. Bronchospastic disease and chronic pulmonary conditions (eg, COPD) may be difficult to distinguish from acute CHF. A good history combined with ancillary studies, including a BNP or CXR, may help with diagnosis (Figure 15-3).

TREATMENT

The goals of treatment include symptom management, hemodynamic stabilization, and reversal of precipitating factors. Place all dyspneic and hypoxic patients on supplemental oxygen via a nonrebreather mask and rapidly escalate to noninvasive positive pressure ventilation (NIPPV) (eg, bilevel positive airway pressure) in patients who fail to respond. When initiated early, NIPPV will reduce the need for endotracheal tube placement and mechanical ventilation in patients with decompensated CHF. The higher intrathoracic pressure improves oxygenation by recruiting additional alveoli and decreasing cardiac preload, thereby curtailing further pulmonary edema. Contraindications to NIPPV include patients who are at risk for aspiration, unable or too confused to cooperate, or those with significant facial trauma. Endotracheally intubate and initiate mechanical ventilation in patients who do not qualify for or fail NIPPV.

Patients with hypotension and/or signs of systemic hypoperfusion are by definition in cardiogenic shock and require immediate hemodynamic support. Initiate a dobutamine infusion for inotropic (cardiac pump) support, but beware of worsening hypotension because of its vasodilatory properties. Most patients will require concurrent dopamine or norepinephrine infusions to maintain an adequate blood pressure. Aggressively seek the precipitating factor, keeping in mind that acute myocardial infarction is the most likely culprit. Obtain early cardiology consultation to facilitate emergent bedside echocardiography and admission to an intensive care unit/critical care unit setting for further management.

The majority of patients in acute CHF present with marked hypertension. In these patients, vasodilators are the initial therapy of choice. Nitroglycerin is the preferred agent as it rapidly decreases the ventricular preload and at higher doses reduces the cardiac afterload, thereby improving overall cardiac output. Start with sublingual doses of

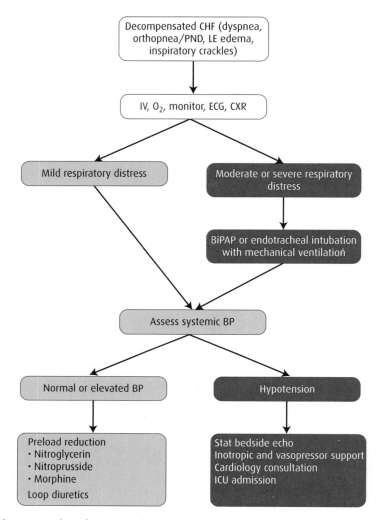

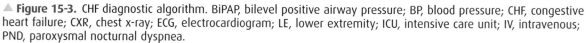

▲ **Figure 15-3.** CHF diagnostic algorithm. BiPAP, bilevel positive airway pressure; BP, blood pressure; CHF, congestive heart failure; CXR, chest x-ray; ECG, electrocardiogram; LE, lower extremity; ICU, intensive care unit; IV, intravenous; PND, paroxysmal nocturnal dyspnea.

0.4 mg every 5 minutes. Severe exacerbations warrant IV nitroglycerin infusions. Start at a rate between 20 and 50 mcg/min and rapidly increase in increments of 20–40 mcg/min every 5–10 minutes. Titrate the infusion to symptomatic relief or systemic hypotension. Consider nitroprusside in patients who don't adequately respond, as it is a more potent arterial vasodilator. It is important to ask any patient requiring vasodilator therapy about the current use of phosphodiesterase-5 inhibitors (eg, sildenafil, used in erectile dysfunction and pulmonary hypertension), as the combination of agents may lead to life-threatening drops in systemic blood pressure. Avoid overaggressive vasodilation in patients with right ventricular infarction, aortic stenosis, and hypertrophic cardiomyopathy, as all are preload dependent conditions.

Initiate IV loop diuretics (eg, furosemide) in all patients with signs of volume overload. Furosemide is not only a potent diuretic but also an effective venodilator, often producing symptomatic improvement long before the onset of diuresis. Start the dosing at 40 mg IV in patients naïve to the drug, whereas those who take the agent chronically should have their home dose doubled. Evaluate patients who fail to diurese within 30 minutes for any evidence of urinary obstruction and re-dose as necessary. Bumetanide, torsemide, and ethacrynic acid are alternative loop diuretics, with ethacrynic acid being the agent of choice in patients with a history of severe sulfa allergy.

A summary of medications used to treat acute CHF exacerbations is listed in Table 15-1.

Table 15-1. Medications used in CHF.

	Dosing	Titration	Mechanism of Action	Adverse Effects	Notes
Vasodilators					
Nitroglycerin sublingual	0.4 mg SL	Repeat q 3–5 min to symptoms	Preload reduction	Hypotension, tachycardia, headache	Assess BP between doses.
Nitroglycerin IV	25–50 mcg/min	Titrate by 10–20 mcg/min q 3–5 min to symptoms. Max: 400 mcg/min	Preload reduction; some afterload reduction at higher doses	Hypotension, tachycardia, headache	Should not be used longer than 24 hours as tachyphylaxis/ tolerance develops.
Nitroprusside IV	10–20 mcg/min	Titrate by 5–10 mcg/min q 5 min Max: 400 mcg/min	Marked afterload reduction	Hypotension, cyanide & thiocyanate toxicity	Risk of toxicity increases with prolonged use and larger doses. Rebound vasoconstric- tion may occur.
Loop Diuretics					
Furosemide	40–80 mg IV	May re-dose at 30 min if no diuresis, then q 12 hour dosing Max: 200 mg/dose	Sodium and water excretion + initial venodilatory effects Onset: 15–30 min	Electrolyte abnormalities Sulfa allergy Ototoxicity	Patients on chronic home therapy or with renal insufficiency will require higher dosing.
Bumetanide	1 mg IV	May re-dose at 2 hours	Same Onset 10 min	Same	May be used with furosemide allergy
Torsemide	10 mg IV	May re-dose at 2 hours	Same Onset 10 min	Same	
Ethacrynic acid	50 mg IV	May be re-dosed at 8 hours	Same Onset 5 min	Same	May be used with sulfa allergy
Inotropes/Pressors					
Dobutamine	2–5 mcg/kg/min	Titrate to effect, Max: 20 mcg/kg/min	Primarily Beta 1, some Beta 2 & alpha	Vasodilator potential may decrease BP	Primarily inotropic, limited by vasodilation
Dopamine	3–5 mcg/kg/min	Titrate to effect, Max: 20 mcg/kg/min	Low dose: dopamine intermed: Beta 1 & 2 High dose: alpha	Variability in dose-related effects	May be used with dobutamine as second agent in cardiogenic shock
Norepinephrine	2–5 mcg/min	Titrate to effect, Max: 30 mcg/min	Alpha, Beta 1	Vasoconstriction	May be used with dobutamine as second agent in cardiogenic shock

The outpatient management of CHF includes treatment with angiotensin-converting enzyme inhibitors and beta-blockers, as both have been shown to reduce patient mortality. Of note, both of these agents are contraindicated in patients with acute decompensation. Oral furosemide is typically used for symptomatic relief, but no mortality benefits have ever been demonstrated.

DISPOSITION

▶ Admission

The vast majority of patients with acute CHF exacerbations require admission to a monitored unit. Previously undiagnosed cases require an inpatient work-up including echocardiography and medication titration. All admitted patients require education regarding medication compliance, as more than half will be readmitted for the same within the next 6 months.

▶ Discharge

Asymptomatic patients with stable vital signs and a negative ED work-up may be safely discharged provided the precipitant for their presentation has been identified and adequately addressed. Counsel these patients on the disease process and the importance of medication and dietary compliance. Provide appropriate discharge instructions, including return precautions, and arrange close outpatient follow-up.

SUGGESTED READING

Collins S, Storrow AB, Kirk JD, et al. Beyond pulmonary edema: Diagnostic, risk stratification, and treatment challenges of acute heart failure management in the emergency department. *Ann Emerg Med.* 2008;51:45.

Heart Failure Society of America, Lindenfeld J, Albert NM, et al. HFSA 2010 Comprehensive Heart Failure Practice Guideline. *J Card Fail.* 2010;16:e1.

Peacock WF. Congestive heart failure and acute pulmonary edema. In: Tintinalli JE, Stapczynski JS, Ma OJ, Cline DM, Cydulka RK, Meckler GD. *Tintinalli's Emergency Medicine: A Comprehensive Study Guide.* 7th ed. New York, NY: McGraw-Hill, 2011, pp. 405–414.

Silvers SM, Howell JM, Kosowsky JM, et al. Clinical policy: Critical issues in the evaluation and management of adult patients presenting to the emergency department with acute heart failure syndromes. *Ann Emerg Med.* 2007;49:627.

Dysrhythmias

Marianne Haughey, MD

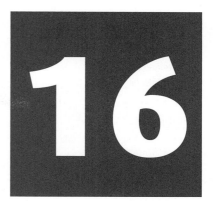

Key Points

- Quickly address airway, breathing, and circulation (the ABCs), provide supplemental O₂, secure intravenous access, and initiate continuous cardiac monitoring.
- Rapidly distinguish between stable versus unstable presentations, as unstable patients require immediate intervention.

- Order a 12-lead electrocardiogram on stable patients and address potential etiologies, including acute coronary syndrome, electrolyte abnormalities, toxic ingestions, and medication side effects.

INTRODUCTION

The recognition of dysrhythmia is an essential skill for all emergency physicians, as patients presenting with dysrhythmias are relatively common and have the potential for rapid hemodynamic deterioration. Clinically, dysrhythmias are classified as stable or unstable based on the presence or absence of adequate end-organ perfusion (ie, systemic hypotension, cardiac ischemia, pulmonary edema, or mental status changes). Dysrhythmias are further divided by their rate into either bradydysrhythmias (heart rate [HR] <60) or tachydysrhythmias (HR >100). An additional subset of dysrhythmia, atrioventricular blocks, can present with any HR and represent a malfunction in electrical conduction between the sinoatrial (SA) node, atrioventricular (AV) node, and bilateral ventricles.

A thorough understanding of the origins of normal cardiac rhythm and electrical conduction is essential to properly comprehend cardiac dysrhythmia. Normal cardiac conduction originates in the SA node and conducts through the atria to the AV node. In the majority of patients, the AV node is the only site where electrical signals can transmit between the atria and ventricles and therefore functions as the ultimate "gatekeeper" to the ventricles. Impulses then travel sequentially from the AV node to the bundle of His, the right and left bundle branches, the Purkinje fibers, and ultimately the ventricular myocardium.

The normal electrocardiogram (ECG) waveform contains a P wave, QRS complex, and T wave. The P wave represents atrial depolarization. It is immediately followed by the PR interval, which normally lasts between 120 and 200 msec in duration. The QRS complex represents ventricular depolarization and is normally <100 msec in duration. Delays in intraventricular conduction result in a widened (>100 msec) QRS complex. The ST segment represents the plateau of ventricular depolarization and is normally isoelectric in appearance. Finally, the T wave represents ventricular repolarization. Of note, the segment extending from the end of a T wave to the beginning of the next P wave, known as the TP segment, should be used as the isoelectric baseline when performing any type of ECG analysis.

Bradydysrhythmias occur either because of depressed sinus node activity or inhibited electrical signal conduction. These are common in patients with structural heart damage, excessive vagal tone, taking certain cardioactive medications, or with specific electrolyte abnormalities (eg, hyperkalemia). Tachydysrhythmias occur because of enhanced automaticity from either the SA node or an ectopic focus and can originate from both atrial and ventricular sources. Supraventricular tachycardia (SVT) occurs when re-entry loops are present in the AV node or accessory conduction pathways.

Rhythms with a wide QRS complex represent ventricular depolarization that occurs outside of the normal

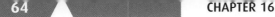

Table 16-1. PIRATES: Causes of atrial fibrillation.

P	PE, pneumonia, pericarditis
I	Ischemia (coronary artery disease and myocardial infarction)
R	Rheumatic heart disease, respiratory failure
A	Alcohol ("holiday heart")
T	Thyrotoxicosis
E	Endocrine (Ca), enlarged atria (mitral valve disease, cardiomyopathy)
S	Sepsis, stress (fever)

conduction system, whereas those with normal QRS durations originate from a focus either superior to or within the AV node that then travel through standard conduction pathways.

Cardiac dysrhythmias vary by etiology, severity, and treatment. Atrial fibrillation (AF), for example, is common and has multiple causes (Table 16-1). Although occasionally symptomatic and/or requiring emergent intervention, many patients are typically unaware when they are in AF. Asymptomatic bradycardia is also a very common rhythm, especially in young, athletic patients. It can be a normal finding in some people or result from medication use at therapeutic levels. Other bradydysrhythmias, such as third-degree heart block, always elicit emergent concern. Tachydysrhythmias vary in a similar manner, from an isolated asymptomatic atrial tachycardia to an emergently life-threatening ventricular fibrillation, the initial dysrhythmia for the majority of patients in cardiac arrest.

There are several important questions that need to be answered when attempting to identify a pathologic rhythm. First, determine the hemodynamic stability of the patient. Look for any signs of hypoperfusion, including systemic hypotension, cardiac chest pain, pronounced diaphoresis, altered mental status (AMS), or congestive heart failure. Second, quantify the rate of the dysrhythmia and classify as normal, slow, or fast. Third, identify the morphology of the rhythm (eg, narrow vs wide complex QRS). Next, determine whether the observed dysrhythmia is irregular or regular in cadence. Finally, assess for any evidence of an AV conduction block. AV blocks are divided into first, second, and third degrees based on the PR interval and the cardiac rhythm.

Narrow rhythms:

- Fast: Atrial fibrillation, atrial flutter, SVT
- Slow: Sinus bradycardia, junctional escape rhythm

Wide rhythms:

- Fast: Ventricular tachycardia (VT), AF, or flutter with aberrant conduction
- Slow: Hyperkalemia, third-degree (complete) heart block

CLINICAL PRESENTATION

▶ History

Unstable patients may be too altered to offer any meaningful history. Employ any available friends, family, and emergency medical service personal for possible critical details. Unstable patients require immediate intervention, and time should not be wasted on an excessively detailed history. In stable patients, ask about any previous episodes, current medications, illicit drug use, and the timing of symptom onset. Inquire about a history of any underlying structural anomalies (eg, Wolf-Parkinson-White syndrome [WPW]), as this will help guide therapy (Figure 16-1).

Finally, ascertain about past medical history. Although sinus bradycardia is a common finding in healthy adults, older patients with underlying coronary artery disease (CAD) and slow heart rates often have a pathologic source for their bradydysrhythmia (eg, inferior wall ischemia, electrolyte abnormalities, or pharmacologic side effects). Similarly, although sinus tachycardia often accompanies conditions with increased sympathetic tone (eg, exercise, fever, cocaine use), older patients with a history of CAD, valvulopathy, or underlying pulmonary disease often have a pathologic source for their tachydysrhythmia.

▶ Physical Examination

Evaluate the patient's hemodynamic stability. Always note the triage vital signs and repeat frequently. Carefully palpate peripheral pulses to determine whether they correspond with the dysrhythmia displayed on the cardiac monitor. Assess for signs of end-organ hypoperfusion, including detailed cardiovascular (weak peripheral pulses), pulmonary (rales), and neurologic (AMS) examinations.

Check for additional findings that may help identify the source of the dysrhythmia. Patients with thyrotoxicosis may have a goiter, peripheral tremor, and ocular proptosis. Discovering a dialysis catheter or palpable AV fistula should prompt concern for hyperkalemia. A sternotomy scar should prompt concern for either acute coronary syndrome (ACS) or valvular disease as the precipitating source.

DIAGNOSTIC STUDIES

▶ Electrocardiogram

The initial evaluation of all patients with suspected dysrhythmia includes continuous cardiac monitoring and an immediate 12-lead ECG unless patient instability necessitates either immediate cardioversion or electrical pacing. Measure the rate, determine whether the rhythm is regular or irregular (may need an additional rhythm strip), and classify the QRS complex as narrow (normal) or wide (>100 msec).

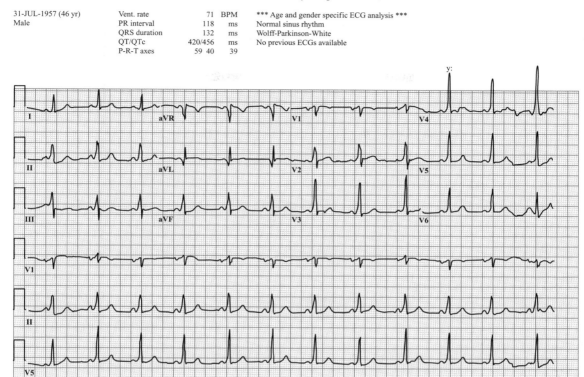

Cook County Hospital

31-JUL-1957 (46 yr)	Vent. rate	71	BPM	*** Age and gender specific ECG analysis ***
Male	PR interval	118	ms	Normal sinus rhythm
	QRS duration	132	ms	Wolff-Parkinson-White
	QT/QTc	420/456	ms	No previous ECGs available
	P-R-T axes	59 40 39		

▲ **Figure 16-1.** Wolf-Parkinson-White syndrome. Note the short PR interval and slurred upstroke of the QRS complex (delta wave) due to abnormal atrioventricular signal conduction through the Bundle of Kent.

▶ Laboratory

Obtain a complete blood count to exclude anemia and a metabolic panel to rule out electrolyte anomalies as the source of the dysrhythmia. Check cardiac enzymes when underlying cardiac ischemia is suspected and a serum digoxin level in any patient taking it. Consider a d-dimer and thyroid function tests in select patients with tachycardia at risk for either pulmonary embolism (PE) or thyroid disease, respectively.

▶ Imaging

Imaging studies should include a chest x-ray looking for signs of congestive heart failure or valvulopathy.

MEDICAL DECISION MAKING

The evaluation of dysrhythmia is very algorithmic. Rapidly assess the hemodynamic stability of the patient and intervene in unstable patients. In stable patients, obtain a 12-lead ECG with or without rhythm strip to identify the rhythm. Treatments will vary depending on the rhythm and inciting event and range from vagal maneuvers to antidysrhythmic medications to DC electricity (defibrillation, cardioversion, or cardiac pacing) (Figure 16-2).

▶ Bradydysrhythmias

In stable patients, examine the rhythm to ensure that a P wave precedes each QRS complex and that the PR interval remains constant throughout. A slow regular rhythm with a constant PR interval is either sinus bradycardia or sinus bradycardia with a first-degree AV block (PR interval >200 msec) and requires no urgent intervention. Search for and address any predisposing conditions. Bradycardic rhythms that feature more P waves than QRS complexes typically represent second- or third-degree AV blocks. Second-degree AV block is divided in Mobitz types I (Wenckebach) and II. Type I presents with a PR interval that progressively elongates until an impulse is not conducted to the ventricles, resulting in a dropped QRS on the ECG. A progressively decreasing interval between consecutive R waves is classic for this dysrhythmia. In second-degree AV block type II, although the PR interval remains constant, occasional P waves will not be conducted to the ventricles, resulting in a dropped QRS. Type II is more

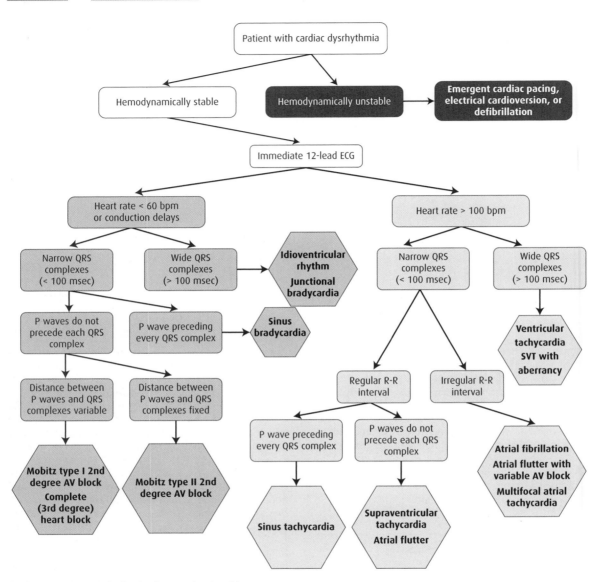

▲ **Figure 16-2.** Dysrhythmia diagnostic algorithm.

serious than type I and typically represents a conduction blockade distal to the AV node. Complete disruption of signal conduction between the atria (P waves) and ventricles (QRS complexes) represents third-degree or complete heart block. The P waves and QRS complexes march independently of one another with no consistency between the two. The QRS complexes are referred to as escape beats and can be either narrow (junctional) or wide (ventricular) depending on their site of origin (Figure 16-3).

Two additional bradycardias warrant mention. Junctional bradycardia is a slow regular rhythm with a narrow QRS complex and absent or abnormal P waves owing to its origin within the AV node. As this condition typically occurs because

of medication side effects (eg, beta-blockers), carefully elicit a medical history to help identify the etiology. Idioventricular rhythms (ventricular escape rhythms) originate in the ventricles and appear as regular wide QRS complex rhythms at a rate of 20–40 bpm with no discernible P waves.

▶ Tachydysrhythmias

In stable patients, assess for the regularity of the rhythm and distinguish between a supraventricular (narrow QRS) versus ventricular etiology (QRS >100 msec) (Figure 16-4). A rhythm that is fast, narrow, and regular is typically either sinus tachycardia, atrial flutter, or SVT. Slowing the heart

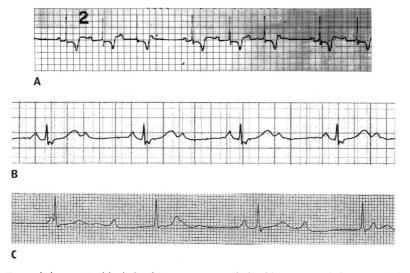

▲ **Figure 16-3. A.** Second-degree AV block (Mobitz type I; Wenckebach). **B.** Second-degree AV block (Mobitz type II). **C.** Third-degree AV block. (Reproduced with permission from Tintinalli JE, Kelen GD, Stapczynski JS. *Emergency Medicine: A Comprehensive Study Guide.* 6th ed. New York: McGraw-Hill, 2004.)

rate with vagal maneuvers or adenosine aids in identifying the underlying rhythm and may treat SVT. Although appropriate concern should arise when using adenosine in patients with either known or ECG findings concerning for pre-excitation (eg, WPW), it is generally safe provided that the QRS complexes are narrow. Of note, SVT with aberrancy (conduction through an accessory pathway or bundle branch block) is typically difficult to distinguish from VT. Always assume VT until proven otherwise, especially in elderly patients with underlying cardiac disease.

Sinus tachycardia will appear with a P wave preceding each QRS and regular R-R intervals. Sinus tachycardia is often secondary to noncardiac issues, including pain, fever, anxiety, PE, illicit drug use (cocaine), alcohol withdrawal, thyrotoxicosis, volume depletion, and anemia. Focus on identifying and treating the underlying cause of the tachycardia.

SVT can be subdivided into AV nodal re-entry tachycardias (AVNRT) and atrioventricular re-entry tachycardias (AVRT) depending on the anatomy of the re-entry circuit. AVNRT has a re-entry loop contained within the AV node itself, whereas AVRT requires the presence of an accessory pathway (eg, WPW) to complete the re-entry loop. With AVRT, signals that travel downward through the AV node and re-enter the atria through the accessory pathway (orthodromic) will exhibit narrow QRS complexes. The reverse situation is known as antidromic conduction and will exhibit wide QRS complexes. Wide QRS complexes are also present in patients with underlying bundle branch blocks (SVT with aberrancy). Regardless of SVT subtype, discernible P waves preceding the QRS complexes will be absent and the R-R intervals will be regular.

Atrial flutter has a classic "saw tooth" appearance from the multiple flutter waves that precede the QRS complexes.

The R-R intervals are usually regular unless there is variable conduction through the AV node. The most common presenting rate is ~150 bpm and occurs when the flutter waves are conducted through the AV node in a 2:1 ratio.

In addition to atrial flutter with a variable block, atrial fibrillation (AF) and multifocal atrial tachycardia (MAT) represent the irregular narrow QRS complex tachycardias. AF can be identified by irregular R-R intervals without discernible P waves. Although MAT is often confused with AF, the distinction is critical, as the treatment varies markedly. MAT will have varying P wave morphologies and irregular P-R and R-R intervals, but unlike AF, P waves will precede each QRS. MAT is most common in patients with underlying pulmonary disease, and as there is no specific cardiac treatment. Focus on addressing the underlying lung pathology.

Wide complex tachycardias typically require more emergent intervention than their narrow complex counterparts and are often encountered in the unstable or "coding" patient. Besides the aforementioned SVT with aberrancy, VT and ventricular fibrillation (VF) are the remaining possibilities. VT presents with a rate >120 bpm, QRS intervals >120 msec, and no discernible P waves.

Torsade de pointes is a unique subset of polymorphic VT that features a beat to beat variation in QRS morphology with a progressive twist in QRS axis. This condition usually arises from abnormal ventricular repolarization.

TREATMENT

Address patient airway, breathing, and circulation (ABCs), provide supplemental O_2, ensure adequate peripheral IV access, and initiate continuous cardiac monitoring. Tailor

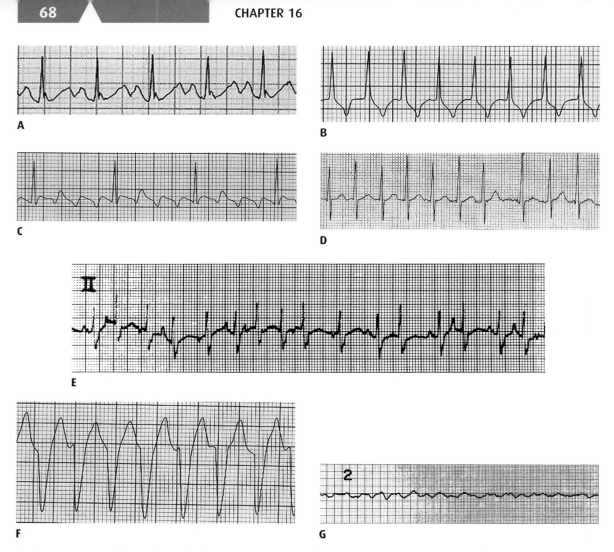

▲ **Figure 16-4. A.** Sinus tachycardia. **B.** Supraventricular tachycardia. **C.** Atrial flutter. **D.** Atrial fibrillation. **E.** Multifocal atrial tachycardia. **F.** Ventricular tachycardia. **G.** Ventricular fibrillation. (B., F. Reproduced with permission from Ferry DR. *Basic Electrocardiography in Ten Days*. New York: McGraw-Hill, 2001. E., G. Reproduced with permission from Tintinalli JE, Kelen GD, Stapczynski JS. *Emergency Medicine: A comprehensive study guide*. 6th ed. New York: McGraw-Hill, 2004.)

the remaining treatment to the patient's underlying rhythm.

▶ Bradydysrhythmias

Unstable patients require immediate intervention. Treat those who are unstable with IV doses of atropine (0.5–1.0 mg) and epinephrine (0.3–0.5 mg over 2–3 minutes) if refractory. Initiate transcutaneous pacing and consider placement of an introducer catheter into the internal jugular or subclavian vein for transvenous pacing in all patients who fail to respond. Catecholamine infusions (eg, dopamine) may be necessary to maintain an adequate HR and blood pressure.

Whereas second-degree AV block Mobitz type I typically requires no specific treatment, Mobitz type II and third-degree heart block require emergent intervention. Place transcutaneous pacer pads on the chest and initiate pacing in those that become unstable. To do so, set your defibrillator to the pacing mode with a rate of ~80 bpm and gradually increase the voltage until a normal ventricular rate is captured. Most patients will require IV analgesia and sedation while pacing. When transcutaneous pacing fails, the placement of a temporary transvenous pacer will be necessary. Obtain emergent cardiology consultation in all Mobitz type II and third-degree patients, as most will require intensive care/critical care unit admission and definitive pacemaker placement.

Treat both junctional bradycardia and idioventricular rhythms analogous to other bradyrhythmias if symptomatic. Accelerated idioventricular rhythms (rates >40 bpm) often accompany myocardial infarction and reperfusion and are typically well tolerated by the patient. Avoid treatment with typical antidysrhythmics and aggressively search for the inciting event.

▶ Tachydysrhythmias

Tachydysrhythmias vary widely with regard to etiology, severity, and treatment. Proper identification is essential to ensure appropriate intervention. Rapidly determine patient stability, as unstable patients require immediate electrical cardioversion or defibrillation. For cardioversion, ensure that the defibrillator is set to the SYNC mode before delivering the shock to avoid precipitating VF. Defibrillate patients in pulseless VT and VF in the unsynchronized (default) mode.

Treat AF and atrial flutter similarly by controlling the ventricular response and evaluating for the source of the tachycardia. Useful agents for slowing AV nodal conduction include beta-blockers, nondihydropyridine calcium channel blockers (ie, diltiazem) and digoxin. Diltiazem is an excellent first-line agent in the emergency department (ED) and can be given as an initial bolus of 0.25 mg/kg bolus followed by an infusion of 5–15 mg/hr. Carefully monitor for signs of hypotension and administer a second bolus (0.35 mg/kg) in 15 minutes as necessary for adequate rate control. Additional agents used to treat AF with a rapid ventricular rate include procainamide and amiodarone.

Treat SVT with vagal maneuvers and adenosine. Vagal maneuvers such as carotid massage, ice-water immersion of the face, and patient-induced Valsalva are sometimes successful. If unsuccessful, administer escalating doses of IV adenosine in doses of 6 mg, and then 12 mg. Administer the medication rapidly, followed by a saline flush, as adenosine is quickly cleared from the circulation.

Clinically, VT can present as a stable perfusing rhythm, a hemodynamically unstable patient, or a patient in cardiac arrest. Treat such patients with antiarrhythmic agents (eg, amiodarone, procainamide), synchronized cardioversion, or defibrillation, respectively.

Treatment of torsade de pointes should focus on removing the inciting agent and narrowing the QT interval. IV magnesium sulfate (2 g slow IV push) is the first-line agent for treatment.

VF is never a stable rhythm. The rhythm tracing will demonstrate no discernible P waves or QRS complexes. This rhythm requires immediate defibrillation as it very quickly deteriorates.

DISPOSITION

▶ Admission

Admit all patients with dysrhythmia accompanied by signs of end-organ hypoperfusion or cardiac ischemia to an intensive care setting. Patients at risk for recurrent dysrhythmia or in need of medication titration should be admitted to a monitored setting.

▶ Discharge

Patients with known AVNRT who are successfully treated in the ED or patients with AF/atrial flutter and adequate rate control can be safely discharged provided they remain asymptomatic and have access to appropriate follow up.

▼ SUGGESTED READING

Knight J Sarko J. Ventricular dysrhythmias. In: Peacock WF, Tiffany BR, eds. *Cardiac Emergencies.* New York, NY: McGraw Hill, 2006, pp. 219–236.

Moffa DA. Cardiac conduction blocks. In: Peacock WF, Tiffany BR, eds. *Cardiac Emergencies.* New York, NY: McGraw-Hill, 2006, pp. 250–268.

Piktel JS. Cardiac rhythm disturbances. In: Tintinalli JE, Stapczynski JS, Ma OJ, Clince DM, Cydulka RK, Meckler GD, eds. *Tintinalli's Emergency Medicine: A Comprehensive Study Guide.* 7th ed. New York, NY: McGraw-Hill, 2011, pp. 129–154.

Walters DJ, Dunbar LM. Atrial arrhythmias. In: Peacock WF, Tiffany BR, eds. *Cardiac Emergencies.* New York, NY: McGraw-Hill, 2006, pp. 237–249.

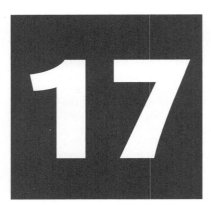

Aortic Dissection

David A. Wald, DO

Key Points

- Always consider aortic dissection in patients presenting with the acute onset of chest or thoracic back pain.
- Initiate a rapid reduction in heart rate and blood pressure in all patients with a high clinical suspicion for aortic dissection before obtaining confirmatory diagnostic imaging.

- Stanford type A (proximal) dissections typically require surgical intervention, whereas Stanford type B (distal) dissections are managed medically.
- Complications of acute dissection include myocardial infarction, cardiac tamponade, aortic valve insufficiency, stroke, renal failure, paralysis, limb ischemia, and death.

INTRODUCTION

Acute aortic dissection is a rare but potentially life-threatening condition. Although the true incidence is unknown, it is estimated that there are between 6,000 and 10,000 new cases annually in the United States. Aortic dissection is more prevalent in men and in patients with advanced age, with approximately 75% occurring in patients between 40 and 70 years of age. Younger patients with aortic dissection usually have a history of an underlying connective tissue disease. Of note, about half of all aortic dissections in women under the age of 40 years occur in the third trimester or early postpartum period.

Risk factors for acute aortic dissection include chronic hypertension, a bicuspid aortic value, coarctation of the aorta, or inherited connective tissue disorders such as Ehlers-Danlos and Marfan syndromes. Vascular inflammatory disorders such as giant cell arteritis or Takayasu arteritis are additional risk factors for dissection.

Aortic dissection results from a tear in the intimal layer of the vessel wall. Common inciting factors include the chronic conditions listed previously, as well as illicit drug use or blunt thoracic trauma. High-pressure pulsatile blood will travel through this tear into the media layer of the aorta, thereby separating the intima from the adventitia. This creates a false lumen for aortic blood flow that can extend distally (antegrade), proximally (retrograde), or in both directions. Rarely, the false lumen will rupture through the adventitia, resulting in immediate hemodynamic collapse. The majority of aortic dissections originate in the ascending aorta (65%), the aortic arch (10%), or just distal to the ligamentum arteriosum (20%). The Stanford classification system divides aortic dissections clinically into types A and B. Type A dissections involve the ascending aorta, whereas type B dissections involve only the distal aorta (origin of the intimal tear is distal to the left subclavian artery) (Figure 17-1).

CLINICAL PRESENTATION

▶ History

The classic presentation of an acute thoracic aortic dissection is that of a 55- to 65-year-old male with chronic hypertension who develops a sudden onset of severe sharp or tearing chest pain radiating to the intrascapular area. Keep in mind that this is a fairly rare condition that often presents in an atypical manner. When obtaining the history, identify relevant risk factors and inquire about the quality, radiation, and intensity at onset of the pain. Type A dissections present most commonly with anterior chest pain (71%) and less commonly with either back (47%) or abdominal pain (21%).

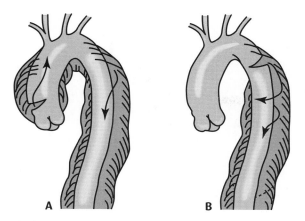

▲ **Figure 17-1.** Stanford classification of aortic dissections **A.** Type A. **B.** Type B. (Reproduced with permission from Brunicardi FC, Andersen D, Billiar T, et al. *Schwartz's Principles of Surgery*. 8th ed. New York: McGraw-Hill Education, 2005.)

Additional presenting complaints include syncope (13%) and stroke-like symptoms (6%). Type B dissections present most often with acute back (64%) and chest (63%) pain with increasing rates of abdominal pain (43%). Atypical presentations include patients with intermittent symptoms, pleuritic or positional pain, and isolated syncope. Painless aortic dissections have also been reported. Corresponding visceral symptoms including diaphoresis, nausea, vomiting, and pallor are often present.

▶ Physical Examination

The physical examination should initially focus on the general appearance of the patient and an assessment of his or her vital signs. Patients with acute dissections are typically very uncomfortable and ill-appearing. Palpate peripheral pulses in all 4 extremities and measure the blood pressure in both arms, taking note of any discrepancies. The presenting blood pressure cannot be used to either diagnose or exclude this condition, as roughly half of patients will have an elevated blood pressure, whereas an equal proportion will be either normotensive or hypotensive. Although a small percentage of the normal population will exhibit a blood pressure differential between the upper extremities, a blood pressure differential ≥20 mmHg in this clinical context should be considered highly suspicious. That said, the absence of a blood pressure differential does not exclude aortic dissection.

The cardiac examination should focus on any abnormal heart sounds. Consider pericardial tamponade in patients with distant heart tones and associated hypotension, jugular venous distention, and tachycardia. The presence of a diastolic murmur suggests secondary aortic regurgitation. Perform a focused neurologic examination, looking for signs of hemiplegia or paraplegia.

Some of the more rare clinical findings associated with aortic dissection include Horner's syndrome, superior vena cava syndrome, acute arterial occlusion with limb ischemia, lower cranial nerve palsies, and bilateral testicular tenderness. It is important to realize that many of the classic physical examination findings are frequently absent, and therefore the history of present illness is often more significant than the physical exam. Always maintain a high index of suspicion for aortic dissection in the patient presenting with an acute coronary syndrome associated with neurologic or vascular signs and symptoms.

DIAGNOSTIC STUDIES

▶ Laboratory

There are no laboratory studies that can reliably rule out the diagnosis of acute aortic dissection. A screening d-dimer assay has been shown to be highly sensitive (94–99%), but it should not be used in isolation to rule out acute dissection. Other laboratory studies (complete blood count, basic metabolic profile, troponin I, etc.) are often used to exclude or confirm an alternative diagnosis or complication of aortic dissection.

▶ Electrocardiogram

The electrocardiogram (ECG) has no primary role in the diagnosis of acute aortic dissection. It is often normal (31%) or may show nonspecific abnormalities such as left ventricular hypertrophy (26%). As proximal aortic dissections can frequently involve the coronary arteries (right > left), the ECG can be useful for detecting secondary cardiac ischemia.

▶ Imaging

Plain chest radiography is the most common initial imaging test. Approximately 80–90% of patients with aortic dissection will have an abnormal chest radiograph. An abnormal aortic contour (71%) and widened mediastinum (64%) are the most commonly encountered findings. Additional findings include a left-sided pleural effusion or apical cap, a widened space (>5 mm) between the external vessel wall and calcified intima (egg-shell sign), rightward deviation of the trachea or a nasogastric tube, and downward deviation of the left mainstem bronchus (Figure 17-2). Comparison with a prior chest radiograph is often useful. Of note, the classic radiographic findings are not reliably present, and a normal chest x-ray (CXR) cannot be used to rule out acute aortic dissection.

Reliably excluding or confirming the presence of acute aortic dissection requires one or more advanced imaging techniques. Computed tomography (CT) angiography is the most commonly employed modality. Newer generation helical CT imaging is readily available in most emergency departments (EDs) and is both highly sensitive (100%) and specific (98%) for dissection. Furthermore, it can

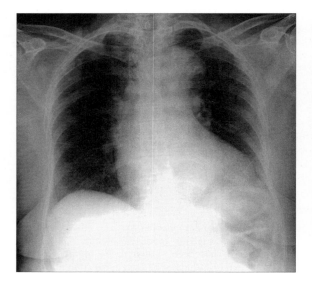

▲ **Figure 17-2.** Chest radiograph of a 74-year-old female with an aortic dissection. Note the widened mediastinum and rightward tracheal deviation.

clearly delineate the vascular anatomy to distinguish between ascending and descending pathology and can identify potential alternative diagnoses for the patient's presentation (Figure 17-3 and 17-4). The limitations of CT angiography include the need to transfer the patient out of the acute care setting, exposure to ionizing radiation, and the administration of radiocontrast media.

   Bedside echocardiography is a reasonable alternative for patients deemed too unstable for CT. Although relatively easy and quick to perform, transthoracic echocardiography is only 59.3% sensitive for the detection of acute dissection. Transesophageal echocardiography (TEE), however, is 98%

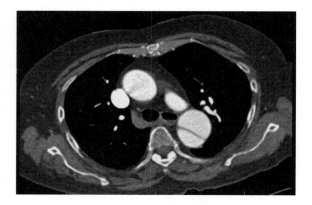

▲ **Figure 17-3.** Computed tomography angiography of the patient from Figure 17-2. Note the intimal flap in the descending aorta consistent with a Stanford type B dissection.

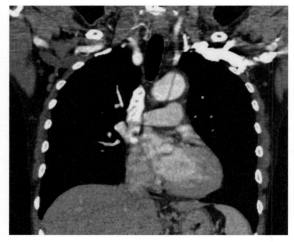

▲ **Figure 17-4.** Coronal computed tomography angiogram of a 49-year-old male with a Stanford type A aortic dissection.

sensitive for dissection. Furthermore, TEE can identify concurrent pericardial effusion and valvular pathology.

   Magnetic resonance imaging (MRI) is also a highly sensitive modality for diagnosing acute aortic dissection. However, the variable availability of MRI combined with the prolonged time required outside of the ED severely limits its utility in this context.

MEDICAL DECISION MAKING

In cases of a suspected aortic dissection, an accurate patient history will likely provide the most valuable information to guide your work up. Always consider alternative life-threatening conditions in your differential diagnoses, including acute myocardial infarction, pulmonary embolism, abdominal aortic aneurysm, and tension pneumothorax. Use the patient's description of the pain, a history of relevant risk factors, and the results of rapid bedside imaging techniques (eg, portable CXR, bedside ultrasound) to drive the formation of your differential diagnosis. Rapidly determine patient stability, as this will dictate how urgently consulting physicians should be called to the bedside and whether the patient will be able to leave the department for advanced diagnostic imaging (Figure 17-5).

TREATMENT

The initial management of acute aortic dissection should focus on a rapid reduction in heart rate and blood pressure to decrease the shear forces on the aorta wall and limit further propagation of the false lumen. Numerous medications are available for this purpose, and regardless of the specific agent(s) employed, the target heart rate is <60 bpm and target systolic blood pressure is 90–120 mmHg. Ensure

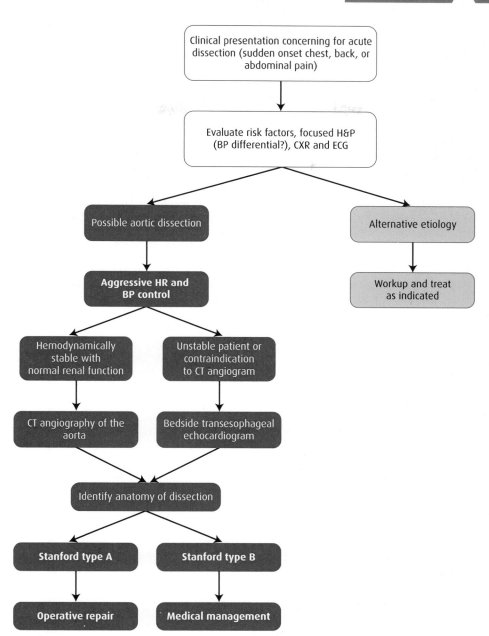

▲ **Figure 17-5.** Aortic dissection diagnostic algorithm. BP, blood pressure; CT, computed tomography; CXR, chest x-ray; ECG, electrocardiogram; H&P, history and physical examination; HR, heart rate.

adequate pain control with the use of opiates to limit excessive sympathetic stimulation. Initiate treatment in all patients with a high clinical suspicion before a confirmatory diagnosis is made.

Beta-blockers are generally considered the first-line therapy for acute dissection given their ability to reduce both blood pressure and heart rate. Because of its short duration of action and rapid onset, esmolol is an excellent first-line agent. Start with a loading dose of 500 mcg/kg given over 1 minute followed by a continuous infusion at 50 mcg/kg/min. If the desired ventricular response has not been achieved within 5 minutes, repeat the loading dose and increase the infusion to 100 mcg/kg/min. If the desired ventricular response has not been achieved within another

5 minute span, give a third and final loading dose of 500 mcg/kg and increase the infusion up to a max rate of 200 mcg/kg/min.

Patients frequently remain hypertensive despite achieving the ideal heart rate. In such situations, begin a continuous infusion of an arterial vasodilator such as nitroprusside (0.3-3.0 mg/kg/min). Alternative vasodilators including nicardipine or clevidipine are acceptable. Regardless of which medication is used, never initiate vasodilator therapy until the heart rate is adequately suppressed with beta-blockers to avoid reflex tachycardia and propagation of the dissection.

As an alternative, labetalol is a reasonable single agent due to its selective α_1 and nonselective beta-blocking properties. Give an initial dose of 10–20 mg as a slow IV bolus over 2 minutes. If the desired blood pressure and heart rate are not achieved within 10 minutes, administer escalating doses (ie, 20 mg, 40 mg, 80 mg, 160 mg) at 10-minute intervals to a cumulative maximum dose of 300 mg. Labetalol can also be given as a continuous infusion. Start the infusion at 0.5 mg/min and increase by 0.5 mg/min every 15 minutes to a max dose of 2.0 mg/min as necessary. If necessary, additional boluses of IV labetalol can be given while concurrently titrating the infusion to more rapidly achieve the goal heart rate and blood pressure. Stanford type A dissections require prompt cardiothoracic consultation for operative repair, whereas type B dissections are typically managed medically.

DISPOSITION

▶ Admission

All patients with an acute aortic dissection require hospital admission to an intensive care unit setting.

▶ Discharge

A patient in whom aortic dissection has been ruled out should be discharged only when there was an initial low clinical suspicion and all other concerning etiologies for the presenting complaints have been excluded. Patients with known chronic aortic dissections can be safely discharged provided their blood pressure is adequately controlled and their presenting complaint is unrelated to the underlying dissection. At times subspecialty consultation may be necessary to assist with disposition.

SUGGESTED READING

Klompas M. Does this patient have an acute thoracic aortic dissection? *J Am Med Assoc.* 2002;287:2262–2272.

Upadhye S, Schiff K. Acute aortic dissection in the emergency department: Diagnostic challenges and evidence-based management. *Emerg Med Clin N Am.* 2012;30:307–327.

Wittels K. Aortic emergencies. *Emerg Med Clin N Am.* 2011; 29:789–800.

Hypertensive Emergencies

Erik K. Nordquist, MD

Key Points

- Hypertension is a very common finding in emergency department patients. Evidence of acute end-organ dysfunction in the setting of hypertension is rare but requires emergent diagnosis and treatment.

- Depend on the history and physical to guide the clinical evaluation of patients with severe hypertension.

- Emergent blood pressure control is contraindicated in asymptomatically hypertensive patients without evidence of end-organ dysfunction.

INTRODUCTION

Hypertension affects up to 30% of the total adult population and is one of the most common medical conditions in the United States. Of these individuals, nearly 75% have inadequately controlled blood pressure (BP) (beyond normotensive limits of 140/90 mmHg), and only half are taking their medications correctly as prescribed. That said, fewer than 1% of all patients with hypertension will ever develop a hypertensive emergency.

Patients presenting with a systolic BP ≥180 mmHg or a diastolic BP ≥110 mmHg are classified as having severe hypertension. Evaluating a patient with severe hypertension should focus on the rapid distinction between hypertensive emergency or hypertensive urgency, as the treatment and disposition differ dramatically. Hypertensive emergency is defined as an acute elevation in BP (≥180/110 mmHg) associated with active end-organ damage, specifically ongoing injury to the brain, heart, aorta, kidneys, and/or eyes. Hypertensive urgency is less clearly defined, but can be thought of as a severe elevation in blood pressure without evidence of acute end-organ dysfunction.

The suggested mechanism behind hypertensive emergency requires a sudden increase in systemic vascular resistance due to an unregulated surge in circulating vasoconstrictors. This spike in BP causes undo stress on the vascular wall with consequent endothelial injury. The injured endothelium produces pathologic increases in vascular permeability, activation of the platelets and coagulation cascade, and the localized deposition of intraluminal fibrin. Secondary fibrinoid necrosis of the arteriolar end-organ circulation results in significant tissue hypoperfusion and consequent organ system dysfunction.

Most individuals presenting with hypertensive emergency will carry a previous diagnosis of hypertension. When determining the goals for BP treatment, it is important to understand the effects of longstanding hypertension on the cerebral circulation. Chronic hypertension forces a shift in cerebral autoregulation, allowing patients to tolerate significant elevations in blood pressure without any signs of cerebral end-organ damage. Consequently, the overaggressive reduction of systemic BP in this setting, even if only decreased to normotensive limits, may lead to secondary hypoperfusion and ischemia of the central nervous system (CNS). Always remember that treating blood pressure based on numbers alone, without considering the clinical context, can be altogether quite harmful for the patient.

CLINICAL PRESENTATION

▶ History

Patients with severe hypertension require a rapid evaluation for evidence of end-organ damage. Start with a focused history and comprehensive review of systems, inquiring about the presence of chest pain, back pain, shortness of breath, hematuria or decreased urine output, and neurologic complaints including numbness, weakness, headache, confusion, and visual disturbances. A more detailed history related to specific diagnoses follows.

Hypertensive encephalopathy. Patients with hypertensive encephalopathy present with neurologic complaints including altered mental status, severe headache, seizures, vomiting, and visual disturbances. The mental status changes range from drowsiness to confusion to outright coma.

Intracranial hemorrhage. Patients with intracranial hemorrhage present with severe headache (often sudden onset), focal neurologic deficits, and/or altered mental status.

Acute pulmonary edema. Patients with flash pulmonary edema present with acute shortness of breath. Variable associated symptoms include orthopnea, hemoptysis, and chest pain or pressure.

Acute coronary syndrome. Patients with acute coronary syndrome usually present with chest pain, although subtle signs of congestive heart failure may be the only presenting complaint.

Aortic dissection. Patients with aortic dissection present with severe chest and/or back pain, often of a tearing quality. Associated symptoms include neurologic deficits, syncope, and abdominal pain, as well as constitutional symptoms such as nausea, vomiting, or diaphoresis.

Acute renal failure. Patients with acute renal failure often present with relatively subtle symptoms. A carful history will often elicit hematuria, oliguria, or anuria. Patients may also present with swelling of the lower extremities or shortness of breath due to significant fluid retention.

▶ Physical Examination

Begin by verifying that the elevated BP reading was obtained with a cuff appropriately sized for the patient. Cuffs that are too small will lead to spuriously high BP readings. The width of the cuff bladder (inflatable portion of the cuff) should equal approximately 40% of the arm circumference. The length of the cuff bladder should equal ~80% of the arm circumference. Perform a detailed physical exam, focusing on the neurologic, cardiac, pulmonary, and abdominal examinations. A more detailed description of expected findings related to specific diagnoses follows.

Hypertensive encephalopathy. Check for any signs of altered mental status. Of note, this can present as only a subtle confusion. Focal neurologic findings may also be present and do not always follow the normal vascular distributions associated with stroke syndromes due to the global breakdown of the entire cerebral autoregulatory system. Careful funduscopic examination may reveal retinal hemorrhages and papilledema.

Intracranial hemorrhage. Focal neurologic deficits or coma may be noted. Meningeal irritation (eg, nuchal rigidity) may be present in a patient with hemorrhage in the subarachnoid space.

Acute pulmonary edema. Patients are typically in significant distress. Inspiratory crackles will be present. Lower extremity edema, jugular venous distention, and an accessory gallop (S3 or S4) may be noted.

Acute coronary syndrome. Patients will often be diaphoretic and may have evidence of heart failure on exam.

Aortic dissection. A blood pressure differential of >20 mmHg between arms or a new aortic insufficiency murmur suggests the presence of an aortic dissection.

Acute renal failure. Physical exam may reveal evidence of fluid overload but is often rather unremarkable.

DIAGNOSTIC STUDIES

▶ Electrocardiogram

Perform an electrocardiogram with any suspicion for acute cardiac ischemia.

▶ Laboratory

Laboratory studies are most useful to identify end-organ injury. Obtain a urinalysis (specifically looking for hematuria or proteinuria) and serum blood urea nitrogen and creatinine to evaluate for acute kidney injury. Check a urine pregnancy test on all females of reproductive age to rule out evolving eclampsia. Order cardiac enzymes in patients complaining of chest pain, back pain, or shortness of breath.

▶ Imaging

Obtain a head computed tomography (CT), searching for signs of hypertensive encephalopathy or intracranial hemorrhage in patients presenting with altered mental status, papilledema, focal neurologic deficits, or seizure. Order a chest x-ray (CXR) to look for signs of flash pulmonary edema or aortic dissection in patients with chest pain, back pain, or shortness of breath. Pursue CT angiography of the chest and abdomen in patients with suspicion of aortic dissection.

MEDICAL DECISION MAKING

Rapidly evaluate all patients with severe hypertension for the presence of hypertensive emergency (hypertensive encephalopathy, intracranial hemorrhage, flash pulmonary edema, acute coronary syndrome, aortic dissection, and

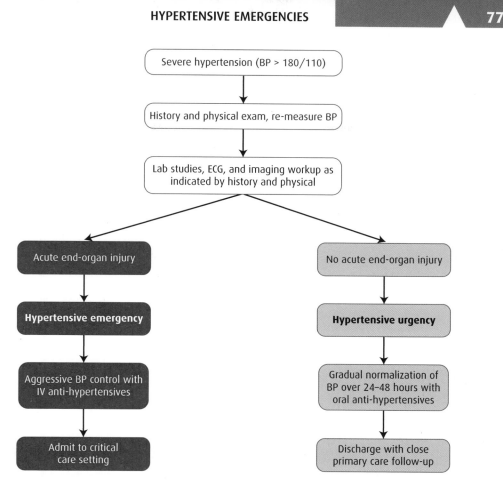

▲ **Figure 18-1.** Hypertensive emergency diagnostic algorithm. BP, blood pressure; ECG, electrocardiogram.

acute kidney injury). Utilize the history and physical exam to help narrow the differential diagnosis and obtain the appropriate laboratory and imaging studies to both confirm end-organ injury and guide further therapy (Figure 18-1 and Table 18-1).

TREATMENT

Hypertensive emergency requires immediate BP reduction to limit continuing end-organ damage. The goal is not to normalize the BP (<140/90 mmHg), but rather to

Table 18-1. Hypertensive emergency diagnoses with findings.

Diagnosis	Findings on H&P, Labs, and Imaging
Hypertensive encephalopathy	AMS, headache, vomiting and papilledema; labs and CT head frequently normal
Intracranial hemorrhage	Headache, coma and focal neurologic deficits; CT head with hemorrhage
Acute pulmonary edema	SOB, chest pain and inspiratory crackles on lung exam; elevated BNP; CXR with cardiomegaly and pulmonary edema
Acute coronary syndrome	Chest pain, SOB; elevated troponin; ECG with ischemic changes
Aortic dissection	Severe chest/back pain; unequal pulses; CXR with wide mediastinum, CT chest with dissection
Acute renal failure	Decreased urine output, hematuria; peripheral edema; urinalysis positive for protein and RBCs ± casts, acutely elevated BUN and creatinine

AMS, altered mental status; BNP, B-type natriuretic peptide; BUN, blood urea nitrogen; CT, computed tomography; CXR, chest x-ray; ECG, electrocardiogram; RBCs, red blood cells; SOB, shortness of breath.

Table 18-2. IV antihypertensive medications used in treatment of hypertensive emergency.

Drug	Mechanism	Onset	Duration	Contraindications	Adverse Effects
Esmolol (500 mcg/kg load, then 50 mcg/kg/min)	Cardio-selective beta-blocker	60 sec	10–20 min	Bradycardia, heart block, decompensated CHF, cocaine toxicity	Bradycardia
Labetalol (20–40 mg every 10 min up to 300 mg)	alpha and beta-blocker	2–5 min	2–4 hr	Active asthma or COPD, bradycardia, heart block, decompensated CHF	Bradycardia, bronchoconstriction
Nicardipine (5–15 mg/hr)	Calcium channel blocker (vascular selectivity)	5–10 min	1–4 hr	Advanced aortic stenosis	Headache, reflex tachycardia
Nitroglycerin (10–200 mcg/min)	Venodilator (arterial vasodilator at higher doses)	2 min	1 hr	Right ventricular infarction, concurrent use of phosphodi-esterase 5 inhibitors	Headache, reflex tachycardia
Nitroprusside (0.3–2 mcg/kg/min)	Arterial and venous vasodilator	seconds	1–2 min	Hepatic or renal dysfunction	Cyanide toxicity with prolonged use (>48 h); recommended usually as second-line treatment when other agents fail
Fenoldopam (0.1–1.6 mcg/kg/min)	Dopamine 1 receptor agonist	5 min	30–60 min	(Limited availability in clinical practice)	Reflex tachycardia at higher doses, headache, flushing, nausea

CHF, congestive heart failure; COPD, chronic obstructive pulmonary disease.

reduce the mean arterial pressure (MAP = 1/3 systolic BP + 2/3 diastolic BP) by ~20% in the first half-hour. This is accomplished with the use of easily titratable IV medications (Table 18-2). Always tailor your choice of agent to its mechanism of action to ensure the optimal management of individual hypertensive emergencies (Table 18-3).

Aortic dissection is the exception to this rule and requires a rapid reduction in systolic BP to <100 mmHg and heart rate to <60 bpm. Regarding the treatment of intracranial hemorrhage, ideal BP goals remain controversial. A cautious reduction of systolic BP <200 mmHg or diastolic BP <110 mmHg is recommended, and immediate consultation with a neurosurgeon is advised. Immediate aggressive BP reduction is contraindicated in hypertensive urgency, as overzealous treatment can lead to secondary cerebral hypoperfusion and CNS ischemia. Gradually reduce the BP to normotensive limits over a period of 24–48 hours with the use of oral antihypertensive medicines.

DISPOSITION

▶ Admission

Admit all patients with hypertensive emergency to an intensive care setting for careful titration of IV antihypertensives and close hemodynamic monitoring.

Table 18-3. Recommended agents for specific hypertensive emergencies.

Diagnosis	Suggested Agents
Hypertensive encephalopathy	Nitroprusside Fenoldopam Labetalol
Intracranial hemorrhage	Nicardipine Labetalol
Acute pulmonary edema	Nitroglycerin loop diuretic Nitroprusside
Acute coronary syndrome	Nitroglycerin Labetalol
Aortic dissection	Esmolol AND nicardipine OR nitroprusside Labetalol
Acute renal failure	Fenoldopam Nicardipine

▶ Discharge

Severely hypertensive patients without evidence of acute end-organ damage (ie, hypertensive urgency) can be safely discharged with oral antihypertensive medications and close outpatient follow-up.

SUGGESTED READING

Cline DM, Machado AJ. Systemic and pulmonary hypertension. In: Tintinalli JE, Stapczynski JS, Ma OJ, Cline DM, Cydulka RK, Meckler GD. *Tintinalli's Emergency Medicine: A Comprehensive Study Guide*. 7th ed. New York, NY: McGraw-Hill, 2011, pp. 441-448.

Marik PE, Rivera R. Hypertensive emergencies: an update. *Curr Opin Crit Care*. 2011;17:569.

Marik PE, Varon J. Hypertensive crisis: challenges and management. *Chest*. 2007;131:1949.

19

Syncope

Trevor J. Lewis, MD

Key Points

- Place all patients with syncope on a cardiac monitor, obtain a STAT bedside glucose level, and check continuous pulse oximetry.

- Obtain a detailed history of the events surrounding the episode, including pertinent data from any available bystanders such as family and emergency medical service personnel.

- All patients with a syncopal episode require an electrocardiogram.

- Admit all patients with risk factors for a cardiac etiology or alternative life-threatening conditions.

INTRODUCTION

Syncope is defined as a transient loss of consciousness with an inability to maintain postural tone. The event is classically followed by a spontaneous recovery to normal mentation. Between 12% and 48% of the U.S. population will experience a syncopal episode at some point in their lifetime. It is the presenting complaint in 1–3% of emergency department (ED) visits and accounts for 1–6% of hospital admissions. The etiology of syncope encompasses a wide variety of disorders ranging from the benign to the acutely life-threatening. Often the cause of syncope remains elusive within the ED. That said, a careful history and physical exam combined with the appropriate ancillary testing will help identify high-risk individuals who require hospital admission for further work-up and management.

Syncope occurs secondary to impaired blood flow to either the reticular activating system or the bilateral cerebral hemispheres. Potential etiologies include transient systemic hypotension or isolated central nervous system (CNS) hypoperfusion (eg, subarachnoid hemorrhage). The reduction in cerebral perfusion produces unconsciousness and a loss of postural tone. A reflexive sympathetic response combined with the recumbent positioning of the patient results in restored cerebral perfusion and a return to a normal level of consciousness. Patients who experience the sensation of nearly "passing out" without an overt loss of consciousness are termed near-syncope or presyncope. From a clinical standpoint, both near-syncope and syncope are approached in the same manner.

For clinical purposes, syncope is classified by etiology. Examples include neural mediated (reflex), orthostatic, cerebrovascular, and cardiac.

Neurally mediated (reflex) syncope. Also referred to as "vasovagal syncope," this occurs because of an excessive parasympathetic output in response to a stressful event. The resulting combination of bradycardia and vasodilation reduces the overall cardiac output and thereby inhibits adequate cerebral perfusion. Prodromal symptoms are common and include subjective feelings such as dizziness, warmth, or lightheadedness. Certain situations involving increased vagal tone such as forceful coughing, micturition, and defecation can also initiate this reflex.

Orthostatic syncope. This occurs because of transient arterial hypotension after a positional change to either sitting upright or standing. The underlying mechanism depends on either significant volume depletion (bleeding, dehydration) or intrinsic autonomic dysfunction. Elderly patients tend to be the most prone to autonomic dysfunction secondary to blunted sympathetic responses and medication side effects.

Cerebrovascular syncope. Cerebrovascular disorders are rarely the cause of syncope. That said, loss of consciousness can occur after a subarachnoid hemorrhage when the intracranial pressure rises suddenly and the cerebral perfusion is transiently lowered. Patients typically have a prolonged post-event recovery, which helps to differentiate cerebrovascular syncope from alternative etiologies.

Cardiac syncope. This occurs when either structural heart defects or cardiac dysrhythmias transiently impair cardiac output. These events frequently occur without warning, which helps to distinguish cardiac syncope from alternative etiologies. In cases of structural heart disease, the syncopal event typically occurs during or immediately following exercise. Classic examples include hypertrophic cardiomyopathy and aortic stenosis. Very rarely, aortic dissection and massive pulmonary embolism (PE) can present as isolated syncope. Of note, cardiac syncope tends to have the worst prognosis, with 1-year mortality rates of 18–33%.

CLINICAL PRESENTATION

▶ History

A comprehensive history is critical and may identify the etiology in up to 40% of cases. It is very important to clarify all of the events immediately preceding, during, and after the episode. Interview all family members and emergency medical service personnel present during the event. Inquire about any concerning prodromal symptoms including headache (ie, subarachnoid hemorrhage [SAH]), chest pain (ie, myocardial infarction [MI], aortic dissection, PE), and abdominal or back pain (ie, ruptured abdominal aortic aneurysm [AAA] or ectopic pregnancy). Obtain a detailed past medical history and review all current medications. Patients with significant cardiac histories are at higher risk of arrhythmia, whereas elderly patients on multiple medications are predisposed to orthostatic syncope.

Antecedent dizziness, nausea, and diaphoresis or symptoms occurring after moving from a recumbent or sitting to upright position suggest a benign vasovagal or orthostatic episode respectively. Syncope that occurs either suddenly without prodrome or with physical exertion suggests arrhythmia or structural heart disease (aortic stenosis, hypertrophic cardiomyopathy). A prolonged recovery period after syncope indicates a cerebrovascular etiology (stroke, seizure, SAH), as classically all patients should regain consciousness within several seconds of the event.

▶ Physical Examination

Always obtain triage vital signs and repeat when abnormal. Obtain blood pressure (BP) measurements in both arms, looking for unequal pressures suggestive of aortic dissection. Consider orthostatic vitals, comparing recumbent and standing vital signs. Significant BP findings include a drop in systolic BP by ≥20 mmHg or an absolute value ≤90 mmHg when standing. Orthostasis suggests volume depletion or medication side effects. The cardiovascular exam should include a detailed auscultation of the heart, listening for arrhythmias or any murmurs suggestive of underlying structural heart disease. A detailed neurologic exam should identify any focal neurologic deficits. Perform a rectal exam with stool guaiac analysis to assess for gastrointestinal (GI) blood loss.

DIAGNOSTIC STUDIES

▶ Laboratory

Routine laboratory evaluation is useful only when indicated by the history and physical exam. Obtain a rapid bedside glucose in all patients with an altered sensorium. Beside urine pregnancy testing is important for all females of reproductive age. Check a complete blood count in all patients with a history of bleeding or a positive stool guaiac. Order a basic metabolic panel with any concern for cardiac dysrhythmia secondary to significant electrolyte abnormalities. Finally, check cardiac markers in patients with antecedent chest pain or shortness of breath.

▶ Electrocardiogram

Although the yield is relatively low (<5%) for discerning the source of a syncopal event, obtain an electrocardiogram (ECG) in all patients to rapidly identify any emergent life threats. Concerning abnormalities on ECG include the following:

1. Signs of ischemia or strain (Q waves, T wave, and ST-segment changes, right bundle branch block)
2. Signs of conduction anomalies (prolonged QRS or QT intervals, atrioventricular blocks, sinus pauses/arrest)
3. Signs of ectopy or arrhythmia (frequent premature ventricular contractions, pre-excitation, Brugada criteria, significant bradycardia <50 bpm) (Figure 19-1)
4. Signs of cardiomyopathy (left ventricular hypertrophy with or without strain pattern)

▶ Imaging

Routine computed tomography (CT) imaging of the head is not warranted unless directed by the history and physical. Indications include signs and symptoms suggestive of a cerebrovascular etiology such as an antecedent headache, focal neurologic deficits on physical exam, or a prolonged recovery phase after the syncopal event. Chest radiographs may be helpful to evaluate for signs of cardiomegaly, aortic dissection, or congestive heart failure (CHF). Indications include syncope that occurs without prodrome or is preceded by chest pain or shortness of breath.

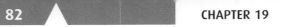

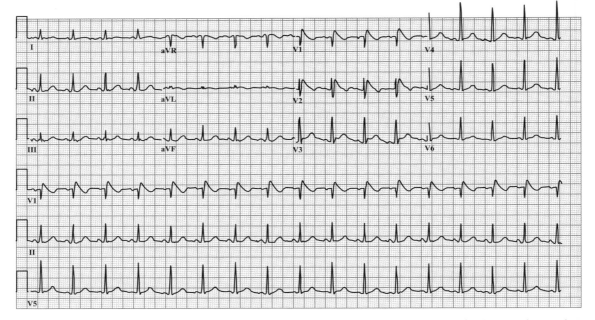

▲ **Figure 19-1.** ECG demonstrating Brugada syndrome. Note the classic rSR appearance in leads v1 and v2 with a downsloping ST-segment elevation.

MEDICAL DECISION MAKING

Manage all syncopal patients in a standardized stepwise fashion. Start with a broad differential focusing on life-threatening causes of syncope. Review the patient's initial vital signs and obtain a bedside capillary glucose. Obtain a STAT ECG and place the patient on the cardiac monitor. Take a careful and detailed history including any bystander accounts. Review the patient's past medical history and note all current medications. Focus the physical exam on the cardiovascular and neurologic systems. Tailor any ensuing laboratory and imaging studies to abnormalities discovered during the history and physical exam. After excluding any acute life threats, focus on the more benign causes, keeping in mind that often times the exact etiology is not identified in the ED (Figure 19-2).

TREATMENT

Rapidly determine hemodynamic stability and initially focus on supportive care. Obtain IV access, start supplemental oxygen in hypoxic or dyspneic patients, and initiate continuous cardiac monitoring. Check a bedside glucose and give supplemental dextrose as indicated. The remainder of treatment should focus on the inciting event.

Cardiac syncope. Follow standard advanced cardiac life support guidelines for any cardiac rhythm disturbances.

Avoid agents that primarily reduce the cardiac preload (eg, nitroglycerin) in patients with hypertrophic cardiomyopathy or aortic stenosis. With concern for PE or aortic dissection, obtain appropriate imaging and tailor treatment to the results.

Cerebrovascular syncope. If SAH is suspected, obtain an emergent head CT and dictate further management accordingly.

Orthostatic syncope. Initiate volume resuscitation with isotonic saline as tolerated. If internal hemorrhage is suspected (eg, ruptured ectopic, AAA, GI bleed), begin aggressive fluid resuscitation and proceed with the appropriate confirmatory studies. Identify and avoid any potentially contributing medications that the patient might be taking (eg, beta-blockers, nitrates).

Reflexive/vasovagal syncope. Often no additional treatment is necessary. Attempt to identify the precipitating event to limit further occurrences.

DISPOSITION

▶ Admission

Admit all patients with either clinical findings or risk factors concerning for cardiac syncope to a monitored setting. Although there is no consensus regarding which items should prompt serious concern, patients with any of the following generally warrant admission: age >45 years, abnormal vital signs including hypoxia or a systolic BP <90 mmHg, ECG abnormalities, an underlying history of CHF or coronary

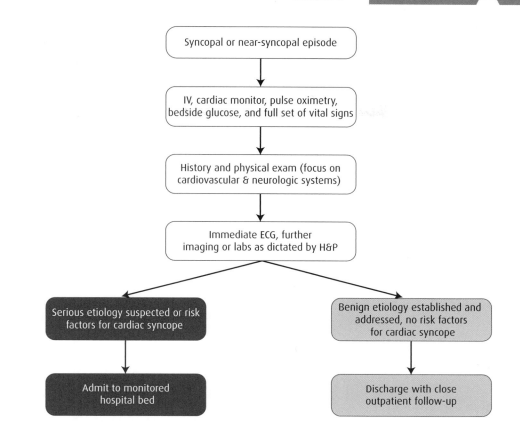

▲ **Figure 19-2.** Syncope diagnostic algorithm. ECG, electrocardiogram; H&P, history and physical examination.

artery disease (CAD), a laboratory hematocrit <30%, an abnormal physical exam, a positive stool guaiac test, syncope that occurs either with exertion or without prodrome, and syncopal episodes that were accompanied by shortness of breath.

▷ **Discharge**

Patients with a low risk for a cardiac etiology (normal physical exam, no history of CAD or CHF, normal ECG, age <45 years) can be safely discharged home. This assumes the exclusion of all other noncardiac life threats. Further work-up including Holter monitoring or tilt-table testing can be arranged in the primary care setting.

▼ **SUGGESTED READING**

Chen L, Benditt D, et al. Management of syncope in adults: An update. *Mayo Clin Proc.* 2008;83:1280–1293.

Huff J, Decker W, et al. Clinical policy: Critical issues in the evaluation and management of patients presenting to the ED with syncope. *Ann Emerg Med.* 2007;49:431–444.

Quinn J. Syncope. In: Tintinalli JE, Stapczynski JS, Ma OJ, Cline DM, Cydulka RK, Meckler GD. *Tintinalli's Emergency Medicine: A Comprehensive Study Guide.* 7th ed. New York, NY: McGraw-Hill, 2011, pp. 399–405.

Quinn J, McDermott M, et al: Prospective validation of the San Francisco rule to predict patients with serious outcomes. *Ann Emerg Med.* 2006;47:448–454.

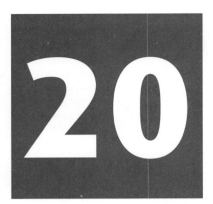

Dyspnea

Shari Schabowski, MD

Chuang-yuan Lin, MD

Key Points

- Determine whether an immediate life threat is present.
- Answer 3 key questions when approaching patients in moderate to severe respiratory distress.
- Diagnose causes of dyspnea by using a structured step-by-step anatomic approach.
- Do not hesitate. Initiate treatment in cases of respiratory distress immediately, even if the diagnostic work-up is incomplete.

INTRODUCTION

Dyspnea, from the patient's perspective, is known as "shortness of breath." This is a sensation of breathlessness or "air hunger" manifested by signs of difficult or labored breathing, often owing to a physiologic aberration. Tachypnea is rapid breathing. Dyspnea may or may not involve tachypnea. Hyperventilation is ventilation that exceeds metabolic demands, such as can be caused by a psychological stressor (eg, anxiety attack).

From the physician's perspective, dyspnea is caused by impaired oxygen delivery to tissues. This can begin at the mechanical level, with any possible cause of airway obstruction, and can end at the cellular level, with any chemical inability to offload oxygen to tissues. If time permits, a systematic walk-through from airway to tissue can help elucidate the more difficult diagnoses. However, treatment for life-threatening severe respiratory distress must be initiated during, or even before, the diagnostic work-up.

CLINICAL PRESENTATION

Start your initial assessment of the severity of the presentation with these 3 questions:

1. **Does the patient need to be intubated immediately?**

This may be demonstrated by the patient's:

a. Failure to oxygenate

b. Failure to ventilate

c. Failure to protect the airway

If "yes" to any of the above, intubate immediately. If the patient cannot oxygenate, there will be anoxic injury, especially brain injury, within seconds to minutes. The inability to perform the act of breathing (failure to ventilate) leads to carbon dioxide buildup, and the ensuing acidosis can lead to cardiac dysfunction. Finally, if the patient cannot maintain an open airway (due to brain injury, mechanical occlusion, etc.), there will be threat to both oxygenation and ventilation, warranting immediate intubation.

2. **Is the respiratory distress rapidly reversible?**

Recognizing and promptly intervening on the rapidly reversible causes of severe respiratory distress can prevent the need for intubation. Delays in therapy may cause the patient to quickly decompensate. Some of these reversible causes (and their solutions) are as follows:

Hypoxia (administer oxygen)

Bronchospasm (beta-agonists/steroids/epinephrine)

Hypertensive pulmonary edema (nitrates/diuresis)

Pneumothorax (needle decompression/chest tube)

Allergic reaction (steroids/epinephrine/antihistamine)

3. Can he run?

Imagine the patient had to run for his or her life (in many ways, this is what the patient is doing). How long could the patient go before he or she collapsed? What is the patient's physiologic reserve? For example, is the patient young and healthy or elderly with comorbidities? Consider all of the following in this assessment: airway, chest wall/musculature, diaphragmatic excursion, posture, age, body mass index, cardiopulmonary status, and baseline exercise tolerance. The decision to intubate or to wait is based on the patient's ability to maintain the work of breathing. If the patient is stable, set time limits and reassess response to therapy frequently. If the patient has poor reserve or already has respiratory fatigue, it may be wiser to intubate *electively* rather than during a crashing situation.

History

Relevant questions to answer during history taking include the following: What makes the dyspnea worse? Is it exertional? Is it positional? When does the dyspnea occur? Has the patient felt this dyspnea, or similar dyspnea, before? What are the circumstances surrounding the dyspnea? What is the patient's medical condition; any predispositions toward dyspnea? While asking those questions, consider the following factors.

Positional dyspnea. In an upright position, fluid is dependent and aeration is maximized at the apices. The upright tripod position is the optimal position for effective respirations: The diaphragm is able to reach full excursion; there is no restriction of chest wall movement; the airway is maximally patent. A history of dyspnea when lying down suggests congestive heart failure (CHF) or pericardial effusions.

Exertional dyspnea. If oxygen delivery is compromised, any increase in cardiac work and oxygen demand will exacerbate the problem. This applies to every cause of dyspnea, from primary pulmonary disease to cardiac disease to anemia. Determine whether there are recent changes to how easily a patient starts feeling dyspneic. Be especially concerned if there is new dyspnea at rest.

Transient dyspnea. If defined events of dyspnea are described that resolve without intervention, this suggests a reversible or transient cause (ie, dysrhythmia, pulmonary embolism [PE], perceived dyspnea with panic attacks).

Recurrent dyspnea. The past predicts the future. "The last time I had these symptoms it was my _____". Fill in the blank: asthma, PE, CHF, dysrhythmia.

Past medical history. A baseline pulmonary disease, cardiac disease, history of bleeding, or bleeding disorder may manifest unexpectedly as a patient complaint of dyspnea.

Exposures. Several exposures can provoke dyspnea, including cleaning products, angiotensin-converting enzyme inhibitors, allergens, irritants, carbon monoxide.

In these cases, there is a temporal relationship between exposure and onset of dyspnea.

Activities of daily living. Baseline exercise tolerance is important historic information that helps you to judge the severity of the acute process in addition to providing information regarding cardiac status. Ask about whether the patient can do day-to-day chores. A patient who reports trouble changing clothes or doing dishes tells much about their baseline—and how quickly they may decompensate in the emergency department.

Physical Examination

A patient's visual appearance reveals much about their degree of respiratory distress. This assessment can be done concurrently with the history. Patients sit in the tripod position (hands on knees with chest propped forward, neck extended) to open their airways while in severe distress. Look for retractions, intercostal tugging, or even paradoxical breathing (sucking in the abdomen when breathing), which indicates mechanical breathing insufficiency. Patients in extremis can look groggy or lethargic due to respiratory fatigue/collapse.

Next guide your physical exam by mentally walking down the anatomy required for oxygenation and ventilation. The radiographic studies mentioned in this section are adjuncts meant to confirm the findings on your physical exam.

Upper airway. Dyspnea caused by partial upper airway obstruction is typically associated with sonorous respirations if it originates in the oropharynx (ie, the tongue), or stridor and voice change if anatomically related to the trachea or vocal cords. Causes of dyspnea in the upper airway are typically visible on exam or by nasopharyngeal scope. Use radiographs or a contrast computed tomography (CT) of the neck to evaluate soft tissue swellings near the pharynx.

Bronchi. When dyspnea is caused by bronchial pathology—whether by foreign body, inflammation, infection, or bronchospasm—it is typically associated with wheezing (most commonly expiratory, but may be inspiratory, or both). Chest x-ray (CXR) may reveal bronchial cuffing.

Alveolar. Alveoli function by maximizing contact between air pockets and capillary beds. Dyspnea occurs if alveoli are filled with fluid (ie, blood, pus, or water), collapsed (ie, atelectasis), or destroyed (eg, emphysema). Alveolar pathology is typically associated with crackles or rales on exam and CXR will show "socked in" solid consolidations.

Interstitial space. Fluid or inflammation in the interstitial space inhibits oxygen transfer to blood cells. This unusual and potentially illusive cause of dyspnea will manifest with dry crackles on exam and be seen on CXR as a "hazy but spongy" density.

Diaphragm. The diaphragm is responsible for active inspiration. If the diaphragm is restricted (ie, increased intra-abdominal pressure from mass, pregnancy, or ascites or paresis/paralysis of the musculature), full tidal volume may not be achieved. On the physical exam, gross asymmetric chest wall expansion or abdominal distention/ascites can be clues of diaphragmatic dysfunction or impairment. Look for asymmetric diaphragmatic excursion on a good inspiratory CXR.

Chest wall. Chest wall expansion is important for unimpeded respiration. Any disorder that restricts wall motion may cause dyspnea (ie, paresis/paralysis, neuromuscular junction or muscular dysfunction, pain from contusion or rib fractures). Do not underestimate splinting from chest wall pain—even from apparently minor injuries. Inspection of the chest wall during respiration will help you to assess this aspect of breathing. Use CXR to look for rib fractures and/or pulmonary contusion (haziness at site of trauma).

Pleural space. The pleural space is a potential space present to facilitate movement of the lungs within the chest wall. If the space is filled with fluid (ie, effusion, pus, blood) or air, dyspnea can occur. If the pleural space is occupied, it will typically cause decreased breath sounds on the effected side. Fluid causes decreased resonance, whereas air causes increased resonance. Abnormalities will typically be seen on CXR; the addition of a lateral decubitus radiograph of the chest may be helpful. Look for extra-lucent edges that indicate a pneumothorax and lenticular, dependent, or meniscal opacifications consistent with an effusion.

Cardiac. The heart pumps deoxygenated blood to the lungs and oxygenated blood to the tissues. Any impairment of pump function (ie, ischemia, dysrhythmia, valvular dysfunction, septal defects, pericardial fluid) can cause dyspnea. Do not hesitate to initiate relevant cardiac work-ups when a patient presents with dyspnea. On the physical exam, assess for cardiac murmurs, gallops, and rhythm aberrations. These are important clues to expand the differential to cardiac problems.

Hemoglobin. There must be enough healthy red blood cells to carry the oxygen to the tissues (ie, no significant anemia), and the hemoglobin must be unadulterated so that oxygen can bind in the lungs and release at the tissues (ie, no CO or CN poisoning). A lack or impairment of hemoglobin can also manifest as dyspnea. Consider a stool guaiac exam if there is any clinical or historical signs of anemia (eg, pallor, cachexia). Replete with a blood transfusion as necessary.

Blood volume. Adequate circulating volume is necessary to deliver red blood cells to the lungs and then distribute them throughout the body. Determine the volume status by assessing vital signs, pulses, mucus membranes, skin turgor, amount of secretions, etc.

Blood vessels. Blood must be able to flow freely to all parts of the lungs to pick up oxygen. A PE may obstruct blood flow to lung tissue and effect gas exchange, resulting in dyspnea. Unfortunately, the physical exam may not reliably assist with this diagnosis, although wheezing

may occur. Be especially suspicious if there are signs of unilateral leg swelling. Entertain the thought of pulmonary embolism in any patient who is short of breath, especially if the cause of dyspnea is unclear.

DIAGNOSTIC STUDIES

Diagnostic studies will vary based on the clinical presentation and physical exam.

▶ Laboratory

Pulse oximetry is a rapid, noninvasive test that is useful to screen for hypoxia. An SaO_2 >98% predicts a PaO_2 >80 mmHg. An SaO_2 >90% predicts a PaO_2 >60 mmHg. This is important because an SaO_2 of 90% is at the precipitous edge of the oxygen dissociation curve; the patient may drop from 90% to 70% far quicker than from 95% to 90%. An arterial blood gas is the only way to directly measure the PaO_2 and the pCO_2. The pCO_2 is useful in the management of patients with chronic obstructive pulmonary disease, asthma, or sleep apnea. The complete blood count can help in assessing whether anemia is a cause of dyspnea. A metabolic panel can elucidate the patient's renal status as well as give further information about the patient's acid–base status (bicarbonate). Blood cultures are important in cases of pneumonia. Remember to obtain before starting antibiotics.

▶ Electrocardiogram

ECG is useful to assess for cardiac ischemia, arrhythmias, and even pericarditis or pericardial effusion.

▶ Imaging

CXR can help to assess the bronchial tree, alveoli, and interstitium. It is also useful for evaluating bony structures, the mediastinum, heart silhouette, and even aberrations of the pleural space. Chest CT can be useful to assess mass lesions, consolidations, effusions/exudates or pulmonary emboli. Soft tissue plain radiograph or CT of the neck can be used in stable patients to determine the presence of epiglottitis, foreign body, or neck abscesses.

MEDICAL DECISION MAKING

As stated previously, the first goal of a dyspnea work-up is to determine whether the patient is in extreme respiratory distress. If the patient is unable to oxygenate, ventilate, or preserve the airway, the patient must be intubated immediately (question 1). Next, if the patient has signs of a reversible cause of dyspnea, such as asthma, CHF, anaphylaxis, or tension pneumothorax, initiate treatment as soon as possible (question 2). Finally, once the patient is stable, begin the diagnostic work-up (question 3, begin walking down respiratory system anatomically) (Figure 20-1).

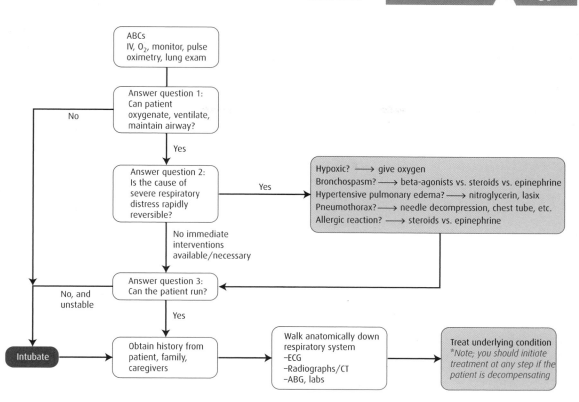

▲ **Figure 20-1.** Dyspnea diagnostic algorithm. ABCs, airway, breathing, and circulation; ABG, arterial blood gas; CT, computed tomography; ECG, electrocardiogram.

TREATMENT

Establish IV access, cardiac monitor, and a pulse oximeter. Think of monitors as a therapeutic intervention; being aware of the patient's airway and gas exchange status is just as important as intervening.

Supplemental O_2 can come in multiple forms. Nasal cannula can accommodate 2–6 L/min of O_2 comfortably. This can increase FiO_2 by 2–4% for each liter increase. A nonrebreather mask (NBM) can and should go up to 15 L/min of flow; any less leads to drawing back environmental air through the mask, defeating the purpose. NBM can supply up to 60–70% FiO2 at 15 L/min (Figure 20–2). Bag-valve-mask (BVM) provides 90–100% of FiO_2 with 15 L/min of flow. Proper 2-handed technique is highly recommended with BMV use when there is an assistant available. Endotracheal intubation is performed if respiratory arrest is imminent.

DISPOSITION

▶ Admission

Patients who are intubated, unstable, or have the potential to become unstable should be admitted to the intensive care unit. Patients who were initially unstable but improved after therapy may be observed on a telemetry unit.

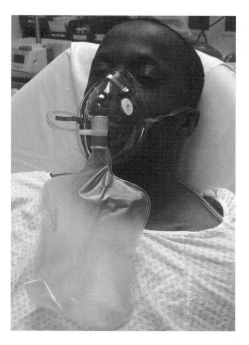

▲ **Figure 20-2.** Patient with nonrebreather mask.

▶ Discharge

Patients who are stable with improvement in symptoms, an identified nonemergent condition, and good medical follow-up may be discharged.

▼ SUGGESTED READING

Sarko J, Stapzynski S. Respiratory distress. In: Tintinalli JE, Stapczynski JS, Ma OJ, Cline DM, Cydulka RK, Meckler GD. *Tintinalli's Emergency Medicine: A Comprehensive Study Guide.* 7th ed. New York, NY: McGraw-Hill, 2011, pp. 465–473.

Asthma

Matthew C. Tews, DO

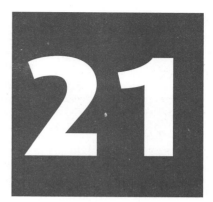

Key Points

- Patients with severe asthma exacerbations may have such severe restriction of airflow that they do not exhibit wheezing on examination.
- Beta-2 agonists are the mainstay of treatment for acute asthma exacerbations.
- Corticosteroids should be given to patients who do not respond initially to beta-2 agonists and in those with moderate to severe exacerbations.

- Peak expiratory flow rate and forced expiratory volume in 1 second are objective measures of the severity of a patient's asthma exacerbation and should be followed serially to measure improvement.

INTRODUCTION

Asthma is a chronic disorder of the airways that is associated with inflammation, bronchial hyperreactivity, and intermittent airflow obstruction. The most common chronic disease in childhood, it is also common in the adult population. Presentations of acute asthma account for more than 2 million emergency department (ED) visits annually. The causes are multifactorial, but the pathophysiology is characterized by the release of inflammatory cell mediators that lead to airway smooth muscle constriction, pulmonary vasculature leakage, and mucous gland secretion.

Asthma is characterized by progressive shortness of breath, variable airflow obstruction, and wheezing. Symptoms fluctuate over time, and patients with worsening symptoms due to a trigger are considered to have an "exacerbation" and require prompt treatment to reverse the airflow obstruction.

CLINICAL PRESENTATION

An acute asthma presentation is due to a decrease in expiratory airflow and is characterized by progressive symptoms of shortness of breath, a nonproductive cough, and wheezing in all lung fields. Symptoms may develop over a period of hours, days, or weeks, but often there is an acute worsening that prompts the patient to seek medical care. The most common trigger of acute asthma is an upper respiratory tract infection, but other factors may lead to sudden worsening of symptoms (Table 21-1).

► History

Obtaining a thorough history may not be possible in an acute asthma exacerbation. A focused history should be obtained in parallel with initiation of therapy to reverse

Table 21-1. Acute asthma triggers.

Environmental allergens
Exercise-induced
Gastroesophageal reflux disease
Tobacco smoke
Occupational exposures
Inhaled irritants
Stress-induced
Environmental changes (weather)
Air pollutants

Table 21-2. Risk factors for mortality in asthma.

Chronic steroid usage
>2 canisters of short acting beta-2 agonists per month
≥2 hospitalizations in the past year
≥3 emergency department visits in the past year
History of intensive care unit admissions
Previous intubations for asthma
Cardiopulmonary comorbidities
Illicit drug use
Low socioeconomic status or inner-city residence

airflow obstruction, regardless of the trigger. Once the patient has improved and is able to provide more history, an attempt should be made to characterize the triggering event, rapidity of symptom onset, and the severity of the exacerbation, which will help guide further treatment and disposition. Characterization of the severity of the patient's underlying asthma may help predict mortality (Table 21-2).

Attempting to define the patient's underlying long-term asthma control does not aid in the management of an acute exacerbation, but will be important to understand when prescribing outpatient therapeutic regimen and follow-up. Patients should be asked about the frequency and duration of their current asthma symptoms and recent beta-agonist usage.

Numerous medical conditions can present in a similar fashion to asthma, including pulmonary embolism (PE), pneumonia, congestive heart failure (CHF), acute myocardial infarction (AMI), or chronic obstructive pulmonary disease (COPD). The initial history should focus on differentiating asthma from other life-threatening causes of shortness of breath and wheezing.

▶ Physical Examination

Patients may present with a wide spectrum of severity, from an increase in coughing to obvious respiratory distress with tachypnea and accessory muscle use. Mental status should be assessed initially because alterations in consciousness may affect the patient's ability to protect their airway. A diminished level of consciousness is an indicator of impending respiratory arrest. The neck should be palpated for tracheal deviation and crepitus, as might occur with spontaneous pneumothorax. The lung exam is variable and demonstrates prolonged expiration with wheezing. However, the severity of the airflow obstruction cannot be gauged by the loudness of the wheezing. The patient who is audibly wheezing may still have good air movement on auscultation, whereas the quiet sounding chest with little air movement is a sign of severe disease because there is not enough airflow to produce a wheeze. Percussion of the thorax reveals hyperresonance due to air trapping. Evaluation of extremity edema will help differentiate asthma from other causes of difficulty breathing.

DIAGNOSTIC STUDIES

The use of diagnostic studies is limited in the evaluation of a patient with an asthma exacerbation. However, certain diagnostic modalities may be indicated, depending on the clinical situation.

▶ Laboratory

An arterial blood gas (ABG) may demonstrate an increased pCO_2 level, indicating ventilatory failure and need for admission to the intensive care unit (ICU). However, the patient's clinical condition is more important than an ABG to predict outcome or the need for intubation. Electrolytes and renal function may be helpful if the patient has comorbidities that make metabolic derangements more likely. An elevated white blood cell count may aid in the diagnosis of concomitant pulmonary infection.

▶ Imaging

Hyperinflation of the lungs is seen in moderate to severe exacerbations and may be reflected on the chest x-ray (CXR) as an increased anterior-posterior diameter and flattening of the diaphragm muscles. A CXR should be considered in patients not responding to treatment, those with fevers, and those requiring hospitalization or intubation. About 15% of these patients have unsuspected pneumonia, CHF, pneumothorax, or pneumomediastinum.

▶ Electrocardiogram

The electrocardiogram (ECG) is not routinely useful and often demonstrates sinus tachycardia. In severe asthma exacerbations, a right ventricular strain pattern that normalizes with improvement of airflow may be seen. Dysrhythmias and ischemia may occur in older patients with coexistent heart disease.

PROCEDURES

▶ Peak Expiratory Flow Rate

Forced expiratory volume in 1 second (FEV1) and peak expiratory flow rate (PEFR) are objective measurements of the degree of airway obstruction that can be performed at the bedside (Figures 21-1 and 21-2). These aid the physician in monitoring the progression of treatment and determination of patient disposition. Predicted values for FEV1 and PEFR are based on the patient's age, sex, and height and compared with a standardized chart or by using the percent of the patient's personal best peak flow. PEFRs <25% predicted indicate a life-threatening exacerbation and require aggressive management. The severity of asthma can be determined by the percentage PEFR and categorized as mild (>70%), moderate (40–69%), or severe (<40%) and will guide further therapy. PEFR values at 1 hour from presentation and beyond are useful to determine need for hospitalization. Either FEV1 or PEFR can be used in acute exacerbations.

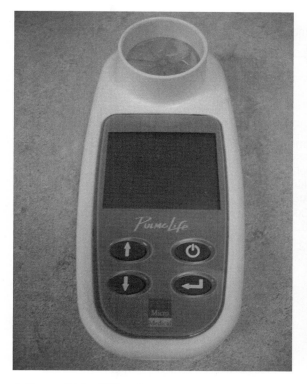

▲ **Figure 21-1.** FEV1 meter.

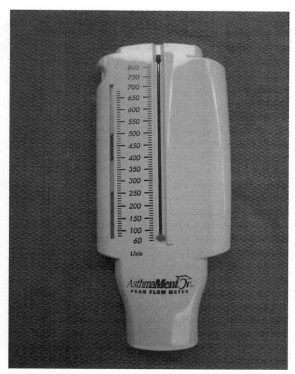

▲ **Figure 21-2.** Peak flow meter.

▶ Nebulizer

The components of a nebulizer treatment include the mouthpiece, medication reservoir, O_2 tubing, and "accordion" extension tube. The albuterol is placed within the reservoir, and the components are fastened together. The extension tube provides a reservoir of "trapped" O_2 and nebulized albuterol that can be inhaled with each breath. The O_2 tubing is hooked up to the green wall O_2 port and turned to 6 L/min because the yellow wall port only delivers air (21% FiO_2). The patient holds the nebulizer during the treatment (Figure 21-3). If the patient is unable to hold the treatment, a facemask is used instead.

MEDICAL DECISION MAKING

The diagnosis of an asthma exacerbation in the ED is relatively straightforward. Any patient who has a history of asthma and presents with wheezing, cough, and dyspnea likely has asthma as the underlying cause. However, there are several situations in which wheezing may not be asthma. Anaphylaxis may present with wheezing, but the patient will often have urticaria and sometimes gastrointestinal symptoms. CHF may present with "cardiac wheezing," but the patient will often have "wet" lungs sounds with rales in the bases, an enlarged heart on CXR, peripheral edema, and jugular venous distention. CHF can have many underlying causes, but often these individuals will have underlying heart disease and other comorbidities. The presence of wheezing is common in COPD, but unless the patient has a history of α_1-antitrypsin deficiency, this type of presentation is found in patients with smoking history and who are

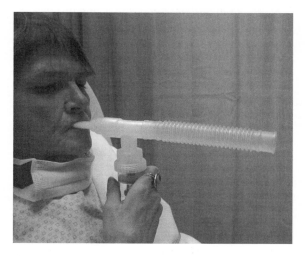

▲ **Figure 21-3.** Handheld nebulizer treatment.

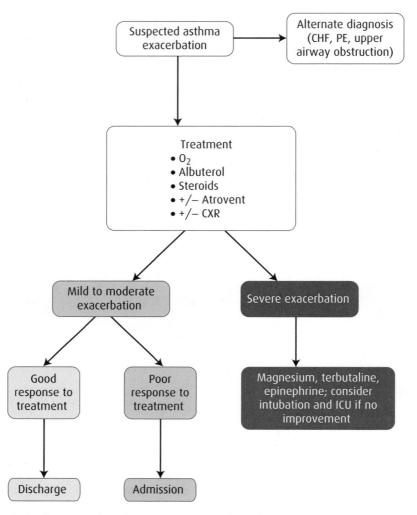

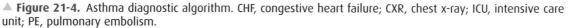

▲ **Figure 21-4.** Asthma diagnostic algorithm. CHF, congestive heart failure; CXR, chest x-ray; ICU, intensive care unit; PE, pulmonary embolism.

typically over the age of 40 years. Patients with pneumonia may have underlying wheezing, but typically have a fever and an infiltrate of CXR. Other diagnoses such as foreign body aspiration, PE, and upper airway obstruction should also be considered. Stridor is an indicator of upper airway swelling and should be differentiated from wheezing in the lung fields.

Once the diagnosis of asthma has been made, the treatment decisions are based on the severity of illness (Figure 21-4). Mild exacerbations can be treated with beta-1 agonists and other supporting medications, and the patient can be discharged. Moderate disease may require further treatments with beta-2 agonists, and the disposition will depend on the response to treatment. Severe presentations will require aggressive management with serial or continuous beta-agonist

treatments and can require other medications such as magnesium and epinephrine.

TREATMENT

Patients who present with difficulty breathing should have oxygen applied via nasal cannula or facemask and titrated to keep the level of oxygenation >94%. Cardiac monitoring and IV access should be used in moderate to severe asthmatics. In conjunction with these, beta-2 agonist therapy should be instituted as the first-line therapy. Patients who are started on beta-2 agonists will still receive oxygen though the nebulized treatment. There are several other therapies that should be considered during an exacerbation, depending on the severity. All medications discussed here are safe to use during pregnancy except epinephrine, which is associated with congenital malformations and premature labor.

Beta Agonists. Albuterol is the most commonly used beta-2 agonist agent and is considered first-line therapy. It causes bronchodilation by increasing cyclic adenosine monophosphate and relaxing airway smooth muscles. Its onset of action is <5 minutes. The nebulized form consists of albuterol 2.5 mg in 3 mL of saline given every 20 minutes × 3, or as a continuous nebulizer for severe asthmatics using albuterol 10 mg over a period of 1 hour. A metered dose inhaler (MDI) delivers albuterol using 2 puffs with a spacer every 20–30 minutes and requires active participation. A spacer is a chamber that keeps the nebulized drug in suspension to allow a more reliable delivery of the bea agonist to the lungs. Bronchodilation from MDI beta-2 agonists is equivalent to that achieved by nebulization.

Parenteral beta agonists include terbutaline 0.25 mg or epinephrine 0.3 mg subcutaneously and can be useful in a life-threatening exacerbation. Avoid in patients with a history of ischemic heart disease.

Corticosteroids. Steroids suppress inflammation, increase the responsiveness of beta-2 adrenergic receptors in the airway smooth muscle, and decrease the recruitment and activation of inflammatory cells. They are indicated in moderate to severe exacerbations, patients who fail to respond to initial beta-2 agonist therapy, patients who are on chronic steroids, and for patients who meet the criteria for hospitalization. The clinical effect of corticosteroids is not seen immediately, as the peak effect occurs within 6 to 12 hours. Oral or IV routes may be used as both have equal bioavailability. Prednisone 60 mg orally or methylprednisolone (Solu-Medrol) 125 mg IV are equivalent doses. Aerosolized corticosteroids are important in chronic treatment and prevention of relapse in asthmatic patients, but they do not play a role in the treatment of acute exacerbations.

Anticholinergic agents. Ipratropium bromide 0.5 mg via nebulizer can be used in conjunction with beta-2 agonist therapy for moderate to severe asthma exacerbations. It competitively antagonizes acetylcholine and subsequently decreases cyclic guanosine monophosphate, causing bronchodilation. The onset of action is 20 minutes, with a peak effect within 1–6 hours.

Other treatments. Magnesium sulfate ($MgSO_4$) 2 g IV over 20 minutes is given for severe asthma exacerbations and works by causing relaxation of smooth muscle. Antibiotics should be given for evidence of pneumonia. Methylxanthines (Theophylline) is not recommended in the emergency setting. Heliox is a helium-oxygen (80:20 or 70:30) mixture that has a lower density compared with room air, which allows it to travel through narrow air passages in a more laminar fashion instead of causing turbulence. This allows increased delivery of oxygen or bronchodilator medications to the alveoli, thereby decreasing the work of breathing.

Noninvasive positive pressure ventilation (NPPV) may be used in patients with significant work of breathing and early fatigue. Although its use in COPD and CHF patients has been well established, the use of NPPV in acute asthma needs further evidence to determine the optimal recommendations.

Intubation with mechanical ventilation may be required for severe acute asthma due to fatigue, persistent hypoxia, worsening hypercarbia, or altered mentation. Ketamine (2 mg/kg) should be used as the induction agent because it causes bronchodilation. The goal is to maintain adequate oxygenation until the patient responds to therapies and mechanical ventilation can be withdrawn. However, during mechanical ventilation patients can develop high lung pressures because they are unable to expire a full breathe. This can lead to barotrauma, pneumothorax, or hypotension. Several strategies can be used to prevent these complications. Using the largest endotracheal tube possible will decrease airway resistance, and ventilator settings should be set to allow for increases in the expiration time to prevent air trapping. This is done by using a low respiratory rate (permissive hypercarbia) and low tidal volumes (5–7 mL/kg). However, if all other therapies fail, intubation is necessary.

DISPOSITION

▶ Admission

The decision to admit is based on the combination of patient symptoms, physical examination findings, responses to treatment, O_2 saturation, PEFR/FEV1 measurements, and the patient's social limitations to medical care. ICU admission should be considered in patients with severe exacerbations and poor response to treatment judged by altered mentation or continued respiratory distress. Patients who require continuous albuterol, noninvasive ventilation, or intubation should be admitted to the ICU. Floor admission is considered for patients with continued symptoms and a PEFR/FEV1 that remains <70% of predicted despite treatment.

▶ Discharge

It is acceptable to discharge patients without respiratory distress or hypoxia, who have good aeration and diminished wheezing, with a sustained response after the final albuterol treatment. The goal of the FEV1 or PEFR should be >70% predicted before discharge. Discharged patients should be sent home with an inhaler and spacer and should be instructed on their proper use. Proper technique for use of the MDI is to remove the cap and shake; exhale completely; place mouth on end of spacer; depress inhaler so that 1 puff is delivered into the spacer; start inspiration of medicine from spacer; continue slow, deep inspiration; hold breath 5–10 seconds; and wait 20 seconds between each puff.

A steroid burst should also be used in patients who had a moderate to severe exacerbation, but who improved enough to go home. This includes a 5- to 10-day course of prednisone at 40–60 mg per day to keep the inflammatory effects of asthma under control. Patients should also have peak flow meters with instructions on a home asthma action plan detailing when to return to the ED based on their symptoms and PEFR. In addition, patients should be given instructions to avoid asthma triggers (eg, smoking) and be provided with appropriate follow-up information.

SUGGESTED READING

Cydulka RK. Acute asthma in adults. In: Tintinalli JE, Stapczynski JS, Ma OJ, Clince DM, Cydulka, RK, Meckler GD. *Tintinalli's Emergency Medicine: A Comprehensive Study Guide*. 7th ed. New York, NY: McGraw-Hill, 2011, pp. 504–511.

National Heart Lung and Blood Institute. Expert Panel Report 3: Guidelines for the Diagnosis and Management of Asthma: Managing Exacerbations of Asthma. http://www.nhlbi.nih.gov/guidelines/asthma/, Accessed April 16, 2007, pp. 373–405.

Pollart SM, Compton RM, Elward KS. Management of acute asthma exacerbations. *Am Fam Phys*. 2007;84:40–47.

Chronic Obstructive Pulmonary Disease

David H. Rosenbaum, MD

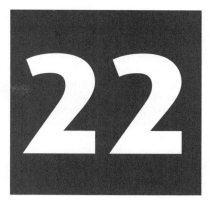

Key Points

- Respiratory infections are responsible for most acute exacerbations of chronic obstructive pulmonary disease (COPD).
- Beta-adrenergic agonists and anticholinergic drugs remain the primary bronchodilators and are most effective when used together.
- Steroids should be given to nearly all patients presenting to the emergency department (ED) with COPD exacerbations, and ongoing therapy should be prescribed for those patients who are discharged.
- Antibiotics are an important adjunct to therapy, although their use should be guided by the patient's signs and symptoms.
- Noninvasive ventilation is a critical component of therapy that is best used early in the ED course to avoid the need for intubation.

INTRODUCTION

Chronic obstructive pulmonary disease (COPD) is defined as an illness characterized by irreversible, progressive airway obstruction that is associated with inflammatory pulmonary changes. It is extraordinarily common, and patients with exacerbations of COPD will continue to inundate emergency departments (EDs) in search of respiratory relief. In the United States, COPD is the fourth most common cause of death.

The use of the term COPD encompasses patients with chronic bronchitis and emphysema, as well as those patients with asthma who have a component of *irreversible* airflow obstruction. Airflow obstruction is the end result of a process that begins with particulate air pollution exposure (usually from tobacco smoke). Particulate exposure initiates a cascade of events, including airway inflammation and narrowing of the small airways, as well as airway destruction and remodeling in the setting of diminished repair mechanisms and fibrosis, resulting in fixed airflow obstruction and air trapping. Although there are clearly pathophysiologic differences between these groups, their evaluation and treatment is largely the same.

A COPD exacerbation is an event characterized by a worsening of the patient's respiratory symptoms beyond the normal day-to-day variation. Typically, this involves one or all of the following: worsening dyspnea, increased sputum as well as a change in the character of sputum, and an increase in the frequency and severity of cough.

CLINICAL PRESENTATION

▶ History

The critical aspects of the history in evaluating patients with dyspnea due to a presumed COPD exacerbation are to establish the patient's baseline function, assess the severity of the exacerbation, determine a cause, and rule out disorders that may mimic a COPD exacerbation. Most patients experiencing a COPD exacerbation present with complaints of increased dyspnea in the setting of a recent onset respiratory infection (ie, upper respiratory infection). As a result, they may complain of a productive or sometimes a nonproductive cough that differs from their baseline cough, rhinorrhea and nasal congestion, and fevers and chills, as well as the constitutional symptoms that frequently accompany systemic illness. Most such patients are chronically ill and often quite frail, so the key to determining the severity of the exacerbation is establishing their baseline health. To do this, it helps to ascertain their oxygen use, their current treatment regimen, their level of function and ability to perform activities of daily living, the frequency of hospitalizations and the timing of their most recent hospitalization, their history of mechanical ventilation, and any comorbid illnesses (eg, ischemic heart disease and congestive heart failure [CHF]).

Patients who present with symptoms that seem to develop over a long period of time may actually have underlying CHF, whereas patients with abrupt onset symptoms may have a pneumothorax (from a ruptured bleb) or a pulmonary embolus (PE). Although acute coronary syndrome should also be considered among patients presenting with dyspnea, chest tightness is a common complaint among patients with relatively uncomplicated COPD or asthma exacerbations. One helpful historical detail is to discern whether chest tightness is a common feature of past COPD exacerbations.

▶ Physical Examination

Patients with COPD exacerbations frequently present with tachypnea, tachycardia, and hypoxia. Because the majority of patients have an underlying respiratory infection, they may also have a fever. Most of what the clinician needs to make a quick assessment can be gathered from vital signs and a quick glance at the patient on entering the room. Patients with severe exacerbations may be sitting upright or leaning forward in the "tripod" position with both of their hands planted on their knees. Such patients may be confused and diaphoretic, unable to converse comfortably, and use accessory muscles in the neck and chest wall to help them breathe. Cyanosis is an ominous, but uncommon finding. Patients with less severe exacerbations speak in complete sentences, and the chest exam reveals diffusely diminished breath sounds with wheezing or a prolonged expiratory phase. Patients with emphysema pathology are often thin and frail appearing with a barrel chest. Some patients with prolonged COPD will have evidence of right heart failure including jugular venous distension and lower extremity edema. Finally, although bedside spirometry in the form of a peak expiratory flow rate (PEFR) assessment is more useful in asthma, it can be a helpful adjunct to the physical exam of COPD patients because several patients with COPD have a reversible component to their disease. In patients with a known baseline, an easy comparison can be made to determine the severity of airflow obstruction. Most patients do not recall past PEFR values, but a PEFR <200 L/min suggests a significant component of airflow obstruction.

DIAGNOSTIC STUDIES

▶ Laboratory

Given that patients with COPD often have several comorbidities, routine laboratory studies including a complete blood count, electrolytes, and an assessment of renal function should be ordered in most patients. Brain natriuretic peptide (BNP) appears to be tailor made to help differentiate patients with COPD from those with CHF. BNP levels less than 100 pg/mL have a very high negative predictive value for CHF, whereas most patients with CHF have levels >400 pg/mL. However, many patients have values that fall somewhere in between, and discordance between BNP values and patient symptoms occurs often enough that single measurements need to be interpreted carefully. If available, the patient's prior records should be sought out to compare current and past values to determine trends and to establish a baseline. Furthermore, some patients may have a mixture of presenting problems contributing to their dyspnea, so an elevated BNP does not exclude a concomitant COPD exacerbation.

Cardiac markers such as troponin are frequently ordered, but usually unnecessary. Because patients with severe COPD exacerbations often suffer from hypoxia and tachycardia, myocardial oxygen demand is increased, and many patients will have small troponin elevations owing to "demand ischemia." In these patients, serial troponin measurements should be used to help exclude an acute coronary syndrome.

D-dimer levels may also be useful in patients with a presumed COPD exacerbation to help exclude PE. Given their comorbidities (CHF, a low flow state), sedentary lifestyle, history of smoking, and increased risk for an underlying malignancy, many patients with COPD are at increased risk for PE. Because d-dimer levels are also likely to be falsely elevated in this population, it is wise to limit d-dimer testing to those patients in whom there is a reasonable clinical suspicion of PE (abrupt onset, unilateral leg swelling).

Finally, arterial blood gases (ABG) have long been part of the routine evaluation of patients with severe COPD exacerbations. ABGs provide information about oxygenation (PaO_2), ventilation ($PaCO_2$), and overall acid–base status (pH). Blood gas readings in patients with significant COPD exacerbations will reveal a primary respiratory acidosis, with elevated CO_2 levels (>40 mmHg) resulting in a decreased pH (<7.30).

▶ Imaging

The chest x-ray (CXR) primarily helps to diagnose pneumonia and to exclude alternative conditions such as CHF, a pneumothorax, or significant atelectasis or lobar collapse. The classic findings are hyperinflation and bullous changes (Figure 22-1). Vascular markings and heart size are often decreased in patients with emphysema pathology and increased in patients with chronic bronchitis.

▶ Electrocardiogram

As with the CXR, electrocardiograms are primarily useful to exclude alternative diagnoses, such as cardiac ischemia. In patients with pulmonary hypertension, peaked P waves

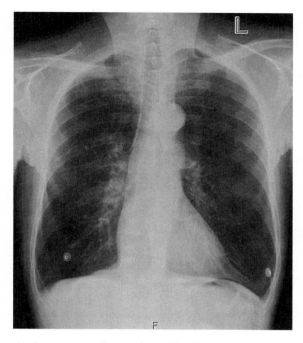

▲ **Figure 22-1.** Chest radiograph of a patient with chronic obstructive pulmonary disease.

in lead II may be present (p pulmonale), reflecting right atrial enlargement, whereas other patients may have signs of right ventricular hypertrophy (large R wave in v1 and v2 with prominent S waves in v5 and v6), a right bundle branch block, or right axis deviation. Multifocal atrial tachycardia (MAT) is the classic arrhythmia associated with COPD patients. MAT is an irregularly irregular rhythm, like atrial fibrillation (AF), but there are P waves of differing morphologies before every QRS complex, and it tends to be slower than AF.

MEDICAL DECISION MAKING

The fundamental challenge in evaluating patients with a presumed COPD exacerbation is to exclude alternative diagnoses that may mimic COPD, such as pneumonia, CHF, PE, pneumothorax, or an acute coronary syndrome. In concert with a CXR, the history and physical is ordinarily sufficient to establish the diagnosis and initiate treatment. Some patients may require more extensive testing, including BNP or d-dimer levels, as well as cardiac markers. However, most patients present with a self-diagnosis, and there is little ambiguity to the underlying process (Figure 22-2).

TREATMENT

Patients should receive an IV line, monitor, and oxygen. If a patient appears clinically unstable, with significant tachypnea,

accessory muscle use, diaphoresis, and hypoxia, then he or she should be intubated using rapid sequence intubation. In such cases, there is no indication for delaying intubation to obtain a blood gas or CXR or to do any other diagnostic studies.

In somewhat more stable patients, a trial of bilevel positive airway pressure (BPAP) is appropriate. BPAP (often referred to as BiPap, which is a brand name of a specific ventilator) is particularly useful because it actually assists in ventilating patients by delivering a higher inspiratory positive airway pressure (IPAP) in concert with a lower expiratory positive airway pressure (EPAP). The pressure difference between these numbers is what drives ventilation. Typical initial settings are 10/5 (IPAP =10, EPAP = 5). BPAP is most effective when used early in the ED course as a means to avoid intubation, as opposed to being deployed on the verge of intubation as a "rescue therapy." However, the only absolute contraindications to its use are respiratory arrest, inability to fit the mask, and patient noncompliance. When used appropriately, BPAP use in patients with COPD exacerbations has been shown to decrease intubation, mortality, hospital length of stay, and number of days patients spend in intensive care unit settings.

Most patients presenting with a COPD exacerbation do not present *in extremis* but with moderate to severe respiratory distress and hypoxia. Hypoxemia is the critical life threat in this group of patients and should never be left untreated. Although it's true that $PaCO_2$ levels rise in COPD patients to whom oxygen is administered, only a very small fraction of patients experience enough of a rise to cause CNS depression and a depressed respiratory effort (called "CO_2 narcosis"). However, oxygen should be limited to only what is needed, with a target oxygen saturation (SaO_2) of 90–94% (PaO_2 of 60–65 mmHg). Venturi masks provide a convenient means of titrating oxygen delivery more accurately.

Despite the prevalence of COPD, there are few evidence-based guidelines regarding pharmacologic therapy. However, the conventional triad of short-acting bronchodilators, steroids, and antibiotics remains unchanged. In COPD patients, beta-adrenergic agonists (albuterol 2.5 mg in 3 mL of saline) are used in concert with anticholinergic agents (ipratropium bromide 0.5 mg in 3 mL saline) via a nebulizer.

Steroids should be given to all patients presenting to the ED with a COPD exacerbation. Although steroids are not as effective in COPD patients as in patients with asthma, steroids reduce treatment failures and obstructive symptoms, as well as hospital length of stay with an uncertain effect on mortality. In the ED, methylprednisolone is the preferred parenteral agent (Solu-Medrol 125 mg IV), although patients with mild exacerbations can be given 80 mg of prednisone orally. All patients should receive a prescription for 40–60 mg of prednisone to be taken daily for at least 1 week after discharge. Steroid prescriptions do not need to be tapered when prescribed for less than 3 weeks.

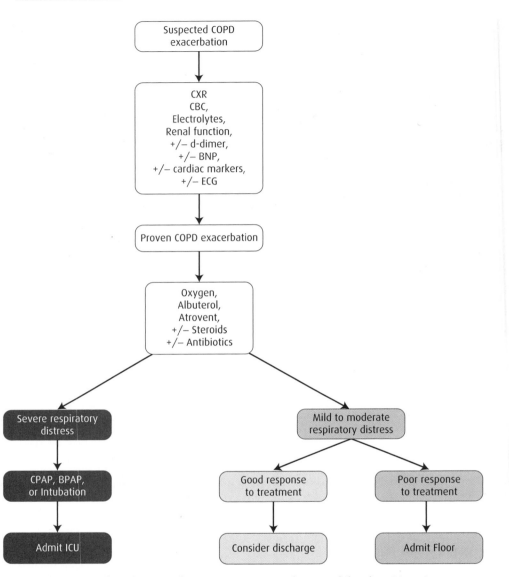

▲ **Figure 22-2.** COPD diagnostic algorithm. BNP, brain natriuretic peptide; BPAP, bilevel positive airway pressure; CBC, complete blood count; COPD, chronic obstructive pulmonary disease; CPAP, continuous positive airway pressure; CXR, chest x-ray; ECG, electrocardiogram; ICU, intensive care unit.

Antibiotics are frequently given to patients with COPD exacerbations and are indicated for patients with signs of infection such as fever and an increase in sputum production or a change in sputum purulence or color. Because most COPD exacerbations are caused by respiratory infections, most patients receive antibiotics. Although only a subset of patients have bacterial infections, it is effectively impossible to differentiate these patients clinically. Admitted patients should be given ceftriaxone or a respiratory fluoroquinolone such as levofloxacin. Discharged patients are candidates for azithromycin (or other macrolides), doxycycline, or levofloxacin.

DISPOSITION

▶ Admission

Patients with COPD have very little reserve capacity, are slow to recover from exacerbations, and often have multiple comorbidities. As a result, most patients presenting to the ED with a COPD exacerbation should be admitted to the hospital, including all patients presenting with a respiratory acidosis.

▶ Discharge

Patients with mild symptoms that respond rapidly to minimal therapy may be amenable to discharge. In such cases, it is helpful to incorporate the patient into the decision-making process, as they often have a sense of whether they can safely manage their disease as an outpatient.

▼ SUGGESTED READING

Bates CG, Cydulka RK. Chronic obstructive pulmonary disease. In: Tintinalli JE, Stapczynski JS, Ma OJ, Clince DM, Cydulka, RK, Meckler GD. *Tintinalli's Emergency Medicine: A Comprehensive Study Guide.* 7th ed. New York, NY: McGraw-Hill, 2011;511–517.

Gruber P, Swadron S. The acute presentation of chronic obstructive pulmonary disease in the emergency department: A challenging oxymoron. *Emerg Med Pract.* 2008;10:1–28.

Brulotte CA. Acute exacerbations of chronic obstructive pulmonary disease in the emergency department. *Emerg Med Clin North Am.* 2012;30:223–247.

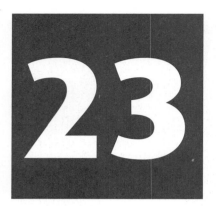

Pneumonia

Brandon C. Tudor, MD

Key Points

- Focus on diagnosing pneumonia early.
- Identify risk factors that influence treatment decisions (eg, antibiotic choice and disposition).
- Blood cultures and empiric antibiotics should be started in the emergency department for patients admitted with pneumonia.
- Tuberculosis should be considered for patients with human immunodeficiency virus or other significant risk factors to avoid further spread.

INTRODUCTION

Pneumonia is the sixth leading cause of death and the leading cause of death from an infectious disease in the United States. The annual incidence of community-acquired pneumonia (CAP) in the United States is 4 million cases, and it results in about 1 million hospitalizations. Most deaths occur in the elderly or immunocompromised.

Pneumonia is an infection of the pulmonary alveoli caused by aspiration, inhalation, or hematogenous seeding of pathogens. An inflammatory response in the alveoli leads to sputum production and a cough, although atypical organisms may produce other findings such as mental status changes or weakness.

Pneumonia can be divided into 4 categories based on where it is acquired. CAP occurs in patients who have not been recently in a nursing home or hospitalized. Hospital-acquired pneumonia (HAP) occurs more than 2 days after hospital admission. Ventilator-associated pneumonia (VAP) occurs 2–3 days after endotracheal intubation. Health care–associated pneumonia (HCAP) occurs within 90 days of a 2-day hospital stay; in a nursing home resident; within 30 days of receiving IV antibiotics, chemotherapy, or wound care, or after a hospital or hemodialysis clinic visit; or in any patient in contact with a multidrug-resistant pathogen.

In about half of cases of pneumonia, the etiology will not be determined. In those whose cause can be determined, "typical" pathogens (*Streptococcus pneumoniae*, *Haemophilus influenzae*, and *Klebsiella pneumoniae*) account for about 25%, with *S. pneumoniae* being the most common bacterial pathogen identified. "Atypical" pathogens (*Mycoplasma pneumoniae*, *Chlamydia pneumoniae*, and Legionella) account for 15%. Viral pathogens (influenza, parainfluenza, and adenovirus) account for about 17%. HCAP may also be due to other agents, including *Pseudomonas aeruginosa*, *Staphylococcus aureus*, and *Enterobacter* species. In patients with diminished mental status, aspiration of a foreign substance (eg, gastric contents) into the lungs leads to a pneumonitis and a polymicrobial infection. Determining risk factors, such as comorbidities, alcohol abuse, and the patient's environment, can help guide therapies and disposition decisions.

CLINICAL PRESENTATION

▶ History

In most adults and adolescents, the diagnosis of pneumonia can be made by history and physical examination alone. Patients will typically complain of a cough productive of purulent sputum, fevers, shortness of breath, fatigue, and pleuritic chest pain. Patients at the extremes of age (children and the elderly) and immunocompromised patients often present with atypical symptoms. In many cases, they present with mental status changes or deterioration of baseline function alone.

Be sure to ask about risk factors for pulmonary tuberculosis (TB) (history of TB, exposure to TB, persistent weight loss, night sweats, hemoptysis, incarceration, human immunodeficiency virus [HIV]/acquired immune deficiency syndrome [AIDS], homelessness, alcohol abuse, immigration from a high-risk area).

▶ Physical Examination

Vital sign changes can include tachycardia, hypotension, increased respiratory rate, or decreased pulse oximetry. These can be late findings and may not be present. On examination, patients may have coarse rales or rhonchi in the involved segments. Other evidence of pulmonary consolidation includes decreased breath sounds, dullness to percussion, egophony, and tactile fremitus. Test for egophony by asking the patient to say "ee" while you are auscultating. Normally, a muffled long *E* sound is heard. When "ee" is heard as "ay," egophony is present and indicates an underlying consolidation. Tactile fremitus refers to an increase in the palpable vibration transmitted through the bronchopulmonary system to the chest wall when a patient speaks. Increased tactile fremitus suggests an underlying consolidation.

DIAGNOSTIC STUDIES

▶ Laboratory

In ambulatory, mildly symptomatic patients who are otherwise healthy, no testing may be indicated. The diagnosis of pneumonia is often clinical, but laboratory studies may aid in the diagnosis or treatment decisions. There is often an elevated white blood cell count in patients with bacterial pneumonia. Obtain a chemistry panel in ill-appearing patients to rule out metabolic derangements. For patients who are hospitalized with pneumonia, obtain blood cultures before initiating antibiotics (if possible). Do not delay antibiotics for critically ill patients. More than 25% of hospitalized patients with pneumonia have bacteremia. Sputum Gram stain and cultures are rarely obtained in the emergency department (ED), but can help determine the bacterial pathogen and narrow specific antimicrobial therapy.

▶ Imaging

Chest x-ray (CXR) may demonstrate evidence of pneumonia, but cannot be relied on to completely exclude pneumonia (especially in immunocompromised patients). Typical findings on CXR include lobar consolidation, segmental or subsegmental infiltrates, or an interstitial pattern (Figure 23-1). Cavitation is seen with anaerobic, aerobic gram-negative bacilli, *S. aureus*, and mycobacterial or fungal infections (Figure 23-2). Radiologic findings are nonspecific for

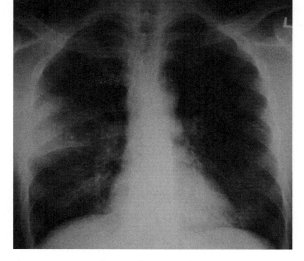

▲ **Figure 23-1.** Chest radiograph showing pneumonia in the right middle lobe.

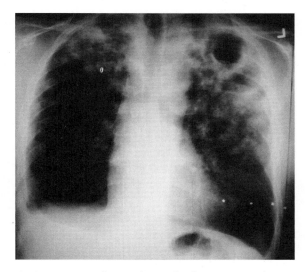

▲ **Figure 23-2.** Chest radiograph of a patient with tuberculosis. Note the bilateral apical infiltrates and the cavitary lesion in the left upper lobe.

predicting a particular infectious etiology and can lag behind clinical findings. Also, radiographic signs of pneumonia can persist well after clinical resolution.

MEDICAL DECISION MAKING

The differential diagnosis of patients with a cough and CXR abnormality includes pulmonary embolism, congestive heart failure, lung cancer, connective tissue disorders,

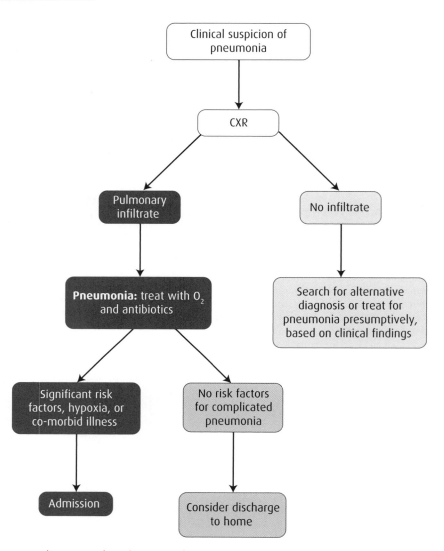

▲ **Figure 23-3.** Pneumonia diagnostic algorithm. CXR, chest x-ray.

granulomatous disease, fungal infections, and chemical or hypersensitivity pneumonitis. The radiographic signs of pneumonia vary, so it is difficult to predict the causative organisms by the radiographic appearance alone. The clinical presentation, in conjunction with CXR findings, will aid in treatment decisions (Figure 23-3).

TREATMENT

Start with supplemental oxygen by nasal cannula or face mask if the patient is short of breath or hypoxic. For patients with severe respiratory distress or shock, mechanical ventilation can decrease the work of breathing and can be lifesaving.

Empiric antibiotics can be started based on the likely pathogens and overall clinical picture. Timely administration of antibiotics (<6 hours from presentation) is associated with improved outcomes for patients requiring hospital admission. The antibiotic recommendations listed are representative of recommended treatments, but are not comprehensive (Table 23-1). Other antibiotic regimens may also be effective, and the clinician should consider local resistance patterns and allergies.

Consider whether or not your patient requires measures to prevent transmission of disease. These include droplet and airborne precautions. When the pathogen has not been identified, err on the side of caution and apply the precaution based on the suspected pathogen. These measures

Table 23-1. Recommended antibiotic regimens to treat pneumonia.

Outpatients age <60 years and otherwise healthy	Consider azithromycin (500 mg PO for 1 day, then 250 mg PO for 4 days) or levofloxacin (750 mg PO daily for 14 days) or doxycycline (100 mg PO bid for 14 days)
Outpatients age >60 years or with comorbidities (without HCAP)	Consider amoxicillin-clavulanate (2 g PO bid for 14 days) plus azithromycin or levofloxacin (750 mg PO daily for 14 days)
Admitted with CAP	Third-generation cephalosporin (ceftriaxone 1 g IV daily) and a macrolide (azithromycin 500 mg IV daily)
Aspiration pneumonia	Clindamycin (600 mg IV every 8 hours) or ampicillin-sulbactam (3 g IV every 12 hours) or moxifloxacin (400 mg IV daily)
HAP, HCAP, or neutropenia	Antipseudomonal beta-lactam (eg, Zosyn 4.5 g IV every 6 hours), an anti-MRSA antibiotic (vancomycin 15 mg/kg IV every 12 hours) and a fluoroquinolone (levofloxacin 750 mg IV every 8 hours)
HIV/AIDS suspected of PCP pneumonia	Add trimethoprim/sulfamethoxazole (5 mg/kg of the trimethoprim component IV every 8 hours) and prednisone 40 mg PO 30 minutes before antibiotics when the pO_2 is <70 mmHg

AIDS, acquired immune deficiency syndrome; CAP, community-acquired pneumonia; HAP, hospital-acquired pneumonia; HCAP, health care–acquired pneumonia; HIV, human immunodeficiency virus; MRSA, methicillin-resistant *Staphylococcus aureus*; PO, per os (by mouth); PCP, *Pneumocystis carinii* pneumonia.

should be performed early in the ED visit (preferably from triage) and continue when the patient is admitted.

Droplet Precautions

Droplets are particles >5 microns that travel in the air but only remain floating for a very limited time. Transmission occurs usually within 3 feet of the patient. Common pathogens transmitted by the droplet route include respiratory viruses (eg, influenza, parainfluenza, and adenovirus), *Bordetella pertussis*, *Neisseria meningitides* (in the first 24 hours of treatment), *Mycoplasma pneumoniae*, rubella, and severe acute respiratory syndrome (SARS).

In addition to standard precautions, healthcare workers should wear a mask when working within 6 feet of the patient. Respirator masks and air handling systems are not necessary. The door to the patient's room doesn't have to be closed (as transmission is limited to 3 feet), but doing so can help remind health care workers they are entering a room with droplet precautions. If a single patient room is not available, the patient should be more than 3 feet away from other patients and a curtain drawn between them.

Airborne Precautions

Airborne droplets are <5 microns and can remain suspended in the air for extended periods of time. Human to human transmission usually occurs via inhalation. The most common pathogen transmitted via the airborne route is TB. Other common pathogens include measles, varicella (until lesions are crusted over), disseminated herpes, and SARS (though predominantly transmitted via droplet).

Health care workers should place patients in airborne infection isolation rooms (AIIR). These are negative pressure rooms with a minimum of 6–12 air changes per hour

and a door that can be closed. When entering the room, health care workers need to wear respirator masks for which the efficacy of the seal formed is evaluated. These N-95 respirator masks remove 95% of droplets. Once the patient vacates the room, the room will need to be open for 1 hour for enough air exchanges to occur to remove any offending organism.

DISPOSITION

Admission

There are several clinical guidelines (Pneumonia Severity Index or CURB-65) to help risk-stratify patients and aid in the disposition. These guidelines consider risk factors associated with increased morbidity and mortality. Risk factors include elderly or nursing home residents, the presence of comorbid disease (congestive heart failure, cancer, liver disease, stroke, chronic renal disease), altered mental status, respiratory rate >30 breaths/min, systolic blood pressure <90 mmHg, temperature <35°C (95°F) or >40°C (104°F), pulse >125 bpm, pH <7.35, blood urea nitrogen >30 mg/dL, Na <130 mEq/L, glucose >250 mg/dL, hematocrit <30%, arterial pO_2 <60 mmHg, and pleural effusion. Although these risk factors and clinical guidelines should be considered in deciding to admit a patient, other factors such as the social situation, ability to follow-up, and other medical conditions may also play a role in the decision to admit the patient. Consider infection control measures, as outlined previously, on all admitted patients.

Discharge

Patients without a complicated course or risk factors and who have a good social situation may be discharged home with appropriate follow-up.

SUGGESTED READING

Emerman CL, Anderson E, Cline DM. Community-acquired pneumonia, aspiration pneumonia, and noninfectious pulmonary infiltrates. In: Tintinalli JE, Stapczynski JS, Ma OJ, Cline DM, Cydulka RK, Meckler GD. *Tintinalli's Emergency Medicine: A Comprehensive Study Guide.* 7th ed. New York, NY: McGraw-Hill, 2011, pp. 479–491.

Mandell, LA, Wunderink, RG, Anzueto A, et al. Infectious Diseases Society of America/American Thoracic Society Consensus guidelines on the management of community-acquired pneumonia in adults. *Clin Infect Dis.* 2007;44:S27–72.

Nazarian DJ, Eddy OL, Lukens TW, et al. Clinical policy: Critical issues in the management of adult patients presenting to the emergency department with community-acquired pneumonia. *Ann Emerg Med.* 2009;54:704–731.

Pneumothorax

Michelle Sergel, MD

Brian Krieger, MD

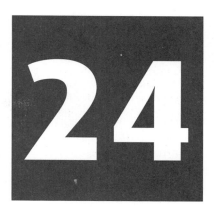

Key Points

- Tension pneumothorax is a clinical diagnosis that should be considered in any patient with shock and respiratory distress. Treatment should not be delayed for radiologic confirmation.

- Appropriate treatment of a tension pneumothorax is a needle thoracostomy, followed by tube thoracostomy.

- Unless a pneumothorax is spontaneous, small (<20%), minimally symptomatic, and primary, definitive treatment is tube thoracostomy.

INTRODUCTION

Pneumothorax is an accumulation of air within the pleural space. Spontaneous pneumothorax is acquired in the absence of trauma. A primary spontaneous pneumothorax is found in patients without underlying pulmonary pathology. A secondary spontaneous pneumothorax is found in patients with underlying lung disease and damage to the alveolar-pleural barrier (most commonly seen with chronic obstructive pulmonary disease [COPD] or asthma).

Spontaneous primary pneumothoraces have the greatest incidence of occurrence in young adults. They are more common in males than females (6:1), greater height-weight ratios, and smokers. Smoking is the most important modifiable risk factor, with a lifetime risk of 12% compared with 0.1% in nonsmokers. Spontaneous secondary pneumothoraces are most common in patients older than 40 years with COPD. Recurrence rates range from 30–45%.

The parietal pleura lines the thoracic cavity and closely adheres to the visceral pleura, which surrounds the lungs. The potential area between these 2 layers is known as the pleural space. If air accumulates within this potential space, the pressure causes the thoracic cavity to expand and the lung to collapse, creating a pneumothorax.

Secondary spontaneous pneumothoraces are the result of a damaged alveolar-pleural barrier or underlying lung problems that cause an increase in intrabronchial pressures. Tension pneumothoraces occur when air enters the pleural space on inspiration but cannot escape on expiration (known as ball-valve effect). There is progressive accumulation of air in the pleural space, resulting in collapse of the affected lung and shift of the mediastinal structures to the opposite side. This ultimately causes compression of the contralateral lung, impairment of venous return, decreased cardiac output, and signs of cardiovascular collapse requiring immediate intervention with a needle thoracostomy.

CLINICAL PRESENTATION

▶ History

Symptoms can vary, but are predicated on the pneumothorax size, rate of formation, and cardiorespiratory reserve. A typical history includes a sudden onset of ipsilateral pleuritic chest pain and/or dyspnea with a nonproductive cough. Patients, however, range from clinically silent to agitated, restless, altered mental status, and/or cardiac arrest if severe respiratory compromise is present.

CHAPTER 24

▶ Physical Examination

The physical examination can range from unremarkable to a patient in shock. Vital signs typically include a mild tachycardia and tachypnea, although only 5% of patients have a respiratory rate greater than 24. Findings on the lung examination may be subtle if there is a small pneumothorax. Decreased breath sounds occur in 85%, whereas hyperresonance to percussion occurs in less than 33%. Patients with tension pneumothorax present in extremis with hypotension, cyanosis, severe respiratory distress, and tracheal deviation to the contralateral side.

DIAGNOSTIC STUDIES

▶ Laboratory

Laboratory studies do not assist in making the diagnosis of pneumothorax, but may be helpful in evaluating other causes of the patient's symptoms.

▶ Imaging

A standard inspiratory posteroanterior chest x-ray (CXR) is obtained initially. The edge of the collapsed lung runs parallel to the chest wall, and lung markings cannot be identified beyond that border (Figure 24-1). The size of the pneumothorax can be roughly estimated as a percentage with each centimeter equal to approximately 10% decreased lung volume. Pneumothoraces >2 cm are considered large. If a pneumothorax is not seen on the film, but still highly suspected, an expiratory, lateral, and/or decubitus film may help. The intrapulmonary pressure is decreased during expiration, causing decreased lung volumes and a relative increase in the size of the pneumothorax. Computed

tomography (CT) has higher sensitivity for the detection of pneumothoraces, especially in the supine patient. CT also has high specificity in differentiating bullae from pneumothoraces. Patients with pneumothoraces identified solely on a CT, however, uncommonly require treatment. Ultrasonography is another modality to detect a pneumothorax that capitalizes on changes in artifact when comparing normal lung with collapsed lung. The utility of ultrasound, however, is vastly tied to the ability of the operator.

PROCEDURES

Needle decompression is performed if a tension pneumothorax is suspected. Using a long 14- or 16-gauge angiocatheter, puncture the second intercostal space at the mid-clavicular line on the affected side. A gush of air will be heard, as the hemodynamics improve. Ultimately, a tube thoracostomy must be placed. Tube thoracostomy is discussed in detail in Chapter 7.

Complications include re-expansion pulmonary edema, extrapleural placement, intraparenchymal placement, empyema, and penetration of solid organs.

MEDICAL DECISION MAKING

Suspicion for a pneumothorax begins with the history and physical examination. If a pneumothorax is suspected, the vital signs are critical in the medical decision making. Stable vital signs allow time for chest radiographs, confirming the diagnosis. Pneumothorax with hypotension equates to a tension pneumothorax requiring needle thoracostomy followed immediately by tube thoracostomy (Figure 24-2).

TREATMENT

Oxygen is a mainstay of treatment. Reabsorption, normally occurring at a rate of 1–2% per day, is hastened with O_2 (3–4 L/min increases the rate 4-fold). Tube thoracostomy is indicated in patients with secondary spontaneous pneumothoraces; those greater than 20% in size or expanding pneumothoraces; bilateral or tension pneumothoraces; those associated with significant symptoms; or in patients requiring positive pressure ventilation or air transport.

Small (<20%) pneumothoraces can be observed and the patient can be discharged if there is no progression seen on a CXR repeated after 6 hours. Failure rates, defined by the eventual need for tube thoracostomy, with observation alone are as high as 40%.

Catheter aspiration reduces a moderate to large pneumothorax to a small one that will resolve on its own. A CXR is needed immediately after aspiration and again 6 hours later to verify successful aspiration and to ensure that there is no reaccumulation of air. Catheter aspiration decreases length of stay without affecting mortality or complications.

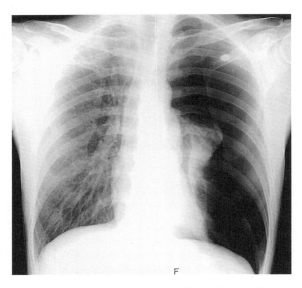

▲ **Figure 24-1.** Complete pneumothorax of the left lung.

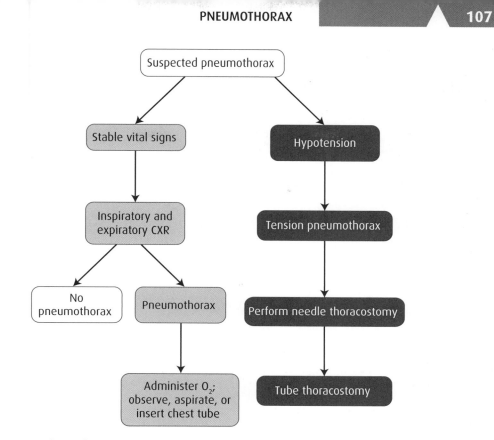

▲ Figure 24-2. Pneumothorax diagnostic algorithm. CXR, chest x-ray.

A trend toward discharging patients after insertion of a small-bore catheter with a small 1-way valve attached (ie, Heimlich valve) has emerged. After consultation with a specialist (cardiothoracic surgeon or pulmonologist), discharge is either completed after an observation period or immediately with a next-day follow-up appointment.

DISPOSITION

▶ Admission

If a chest tube is inserted, patients are admitted to the hospital. The chest tube must be attached to a water seal and vacuum device (Pleur-Evac). Patient with small (<20%) traumatic pneumothoraces that are managed conservatively are usually admitted for observation.

▶ Discharge

If the pneumothorax is small (<20%) and patients are healthy, reliable, and minimally symptomatic, they may be observed. A second CXR 6 hours later should be performed to ensure that there has been no change in the size of the pneumothorax before discharge. Close follow-up with a specialist should be arranged. Patients must avoid air travel until the pneumothorax shows complete resolution.

SUGGESTED READING

Humphries RL, Young WF. Spontaneous and iatrogenic pneumothorax. In: Tintinalli JE, Stapczynski JS, Ma OJ, Cline DM, Cydulka RK, Meckler GD. *Tintinalli's Emergency Medicine: A Comprehensive Study Guide.* 7th ed. New York, NY: McGraw-Hill, 2011, pp. 500–504.

Henry M, Arnold T, Harvey J. BTS guidelines for the management of spontaneous pneumothorax. *Thorax.* 2003;58:ii39–ii52.

Kulvatunyou N, Vigayasekaran A, et al. Two-year experience of using pigtail catheters to treat traumatic pneumothorax: A changing trend. *J Trauma Injury Infect Crit Care.* 2011;71:1104–1107.

Sahn SA, Heffner JE. Spontaneous pneumothorax. *N Engl J Med.* 2000;342:868–874.

Wakai A, O'Sullivan R, McCabe G. Simple aspiration versus intercostals tube drainage for primary spontaneous pneumothorax in adults. *Cochrane Database Syst Rev.* 2011;1:CD004479.

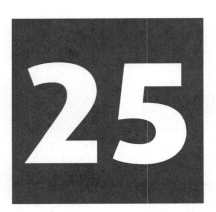

Pulmonary Embolism

Harsh Sule, MD

Key Points

- Consider pulmonary embolism (PE) in patients with complaints of dyspnea, chest pain, hemoptysis, or syncope.
- Dyspnea, pleuritic chest pain, or tachypnea is present in 92% of patients with PE.

- If PE is considered in the differential, use clinical decision rules (PERC, Wells, Geneva) to help guide decisions regarding the patient work-up.
- Consider thrombolytics in hemodynamically unstable patients with confirmed PE.

INTRODUCTION

Pulmonary embolism (PE) is a potentially life-threatening condition associated with a partial or complete obstruction of the pulmonary artery caused by a thrombus that breaks off from a peripheral vein, migrates via the right side of the heart, and lodges in the pulmonary artery circulation. About 90% of emboli originate from venous thrombi in the lower extremities and pelvis. The presence of emboli in the pulmonary vasculature blocks normal blood flow to the lung and increases pulmonary resistance. This, in turn, increases pulmonary artery pressure and right ventricular pressure. When greater than 50% of the vasculature is occluded, the patient experiences significant pulmonary hypertension and acute cor pulmonale. Undetected, this leads to long-term morbidity and death.

PE is the third most common cause of death from cardiovascular disease, with approximately 650,000 cases of PE occurring per year in the United States. The diagnosis is frequently missed, with 30% of cases diagnosed antemortem. Massive PE occurs in only 5% of cases, but has an associated mortality rate of 40%. Overall, mortality is 3–10% if treated and 15–30% if untreated.

CLINICAL PRESENTATION

History

The classic triad of chest pain, dyspnea, and hemoptysis is present in fewer than 20% of patients. Dyspnea is the most common symptom associated with PE, occurring in up to 80% of confirmed cases, with 67% experiencing rapid onset of shortness of breath. Pleuritic chest pain is present in 52% of patients, but substernal chest pain is present in <20%. Other symptoms include fainting, cough, palpitations, hemoptysis, and calf/thigh pain or swelling.

Risk factors for deep vein thrombosis (DVT) and PE are inherited or acquired and continue to follow Virchow's triad described in 1856: venous stasis (eg, bed rest >48 hours, long-distance auto or air travel, recent hospitalization), alterations in coagulation (eg, malignancy, previous PE/DVT, pregnancy, or protein C deficiency), and vascular injury (eg, trauma, recent surgery, central lines, IV drug use). Ninety-four percent of all patients with PE have one or more risk factors.

Physical Examination

Tachypnea (≥ 20/min) is one of the most sensitive clinical findings, with a prevalence of 70% in PE confirmed cases.

Tachycardia (≥100/min) has a prevalence of 26%. Pulse oximetry is frequently normal in patients with a PE and cannot be used to exclude the diagnosis. Lung examination may be clear or may reveal rales, whereas extremity examination is useful only if signs of a DVT are present. Rectal examination for blood is useful to assess bleeding risk if anticoagulation becomes necessary.

DIAGNOSTIC STUDIES

▶ Laboratory

Although many patients with PE are hypoxic ($PaO_2 < 80$ mmHg), this is not universally true. The A-a gradient can be used as an indirect measure of ventilation-perfusion V/Q abnormalities, although 15% of patients with PE have a normal A-a gradient.

D-dimer is a fibrin degradation product that circulates in a patient with a dissolving fibrin thrombus. It is found in the serum within 1 hour and stops circulating after 7 days. Multiple d-dimer tests exist with varying sensitivities and specificities, but a negative d-dimer test (enzyme-linked immunosorbent assay or turbidimetric) in patients with a low pretest probability implies a risk for PE of less than 1%.

Troponin and brain natriuretic peptide have been studied in the context of PE, and at this time their value may be limited to risk stratification only.

▶ Electrocardiogram

An electrocardiogram (ECG) is useful to rule out a primary cardiac etiology and is neither specific nor sensitive for PE. Approximately 30% of patients with PE have a normal ECG. Sinus tachycardia is present in up to 36% of patients with PE. The classic S1Q3T3 combination of findings (S wave in lead I, Q wave in lead III, and T wave inversion in lead III) is present in <20% of patient with confirmed PE. Right-sided heart strain seen as T-wave inversions in the anterior leads (v1–v4) may be present in massive PE.

▶ Imaging

A chest x-ray (CXR) is useful in evaluating other causes of the symptoms. In PE, CXR is nonspecific and nondiagnostic, with a normal radiograph reported in up to 24% of patients. Common abnormalities seen in patients with PE include atelectasis, parenchymal abnormalities, elevated hemidiaphragm, or pleural effusions. Hampton's hump is a triangular pleural-based infiltrate, representing a pulmonary infarct (sensitivity 22% and specificity 82%). Westermarck's sign is dilatation of pulmonary vessels proximal to the PE with collapse of distal vessels (sensitivity 12% and specificity 97%).

Chest CT angiography (CTA) is the accepted diagnostic modality of choice (Figure 25-1). It is rapid and sensitive for detecting proximal PEs. The clinical outcome after a negative CTA is favorable, and the likelihood for subsequent

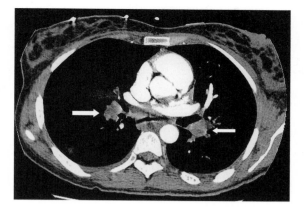

▲ **Figure 25-1.** Computed tomography angiography with pulmonary embolism.

thromboembolic events is extremely low. CTA is also useful to identify alternate diagnoses.

V/Q lung scan results are interpreted as normal, low, intermediate, or high probability for PE. A normal scan effectively rules out PE with a negative predictive value of 97%. However, this test is infrequently used today except when specific contraindications to a CTA exist. Although previously favored for pregnant patients, guidelines now typically recommend CTA in pregnant patients too.

Lower extremity duplex ultrasound may be used to diagnose DVT in a patient with a high clinical suspicion of PE and a negative CTA.

MEDICAL DECISION MAKING

The diagnosis of PE can be elusive, and with growing concerns of excessive testing and resultant radiation, the clinician must determine not only how to work up the patient, but also which patients need to be worked up. Although experience and clinical gestalt may reproduce the output of some decision rules, it is felt that the use of clinical prediction rules is warranted.

The Pulmonary Embolism Rule-Out Criteria (PERC rule) was prospectively derived and validated to identify very low-risk patients who do not require diagnostic testing (Table 25-1). When there is a low clinical gestalt for PE and all 8 criteria are met (with no contraindications for use of the rule), then patients are determined to be very low risk for PE with a 45–day incidence of venous thromboembolism or death of less than 2%. In these patients, no further work-up for PE is recommended.

If the PERC rule does not apply, a patient's pretest probability for PE should be calculated using 1 of 2 rules (Geneva or Wells) that utilize findings from the history and physical examination (Box 25-1 and Table 25-2). The results risk-stratify the patient into two groups—PE unlikely or PE likely. Both simplified revised Geneva and

Table 25-1. The Pulmonary Embolism Rule Out Criteria (PERC) for excluding PE without testing.

Age <50 years
Pulse <100 bpm
Pulse oximetry >94%
No unilateral leg swelling
No hemoptysis
No recent surgery/trauma
No oral hormone use
No prior venous thromboembolism

If there is a low clinical gestalt pretest probability for PE AND all 8 criteria are fulfilled, sensitivity is 97.4%.

PERC rule may not be applied if concurrent beta-blocker use, transient tachycardia, thrombophilia, strong family history of thrombosis, patient with an amputation, massively obese (leg swelling cannot be reliably assessed), or baseline hypoxemia (<95% long-term).

Based on data from: Kline JA, Mitchell AM, Kabrhel C, Richman PB, & Courtney, DM. Clinical criteria to prevent unnecessary diagnostic testing in emergency department patients with suspected pulmonary embolism. *Journal of thrombosis and haemostasis.* 2004;2(8):1247–55.

Wells rules have been shown to be comparable. In patients with an "unlikely" pretest probability of PE, a d-dimer should be ordered. If the d-dimer is negative, no further testing is required. If the d-dimer is positive, the clinician proceeds to chest CTA to adequately exclude PE. In

Box 25-1. Geneva Score (Revised and Simplified).

The Geneva score is predictive for PE. It was developed in 2001, revised in 2006, and simplified in 2008. The items below are scored and summed in patients with suspected PE to give a total score.
PE unlikely if score 0–2
PE likely if score ≥ 3

RISK FACTORS

Give 1 point for each:
1. Older than 65 years
2. Previous DVT or PE
3. Surgery requiring general anesthesia OR fracture of the lower limb in the last month
4. Active malignancy (tumor or blood) within the last year

SYMPTOMS

Give 1 point for each:
1. Pain in a unilateral lower extremity
2. Hemoptysis

CLINICAL SIGNS

Give 1 point each:
1. Heart rate 75–94 bpm
2. Deep venous palpation elicits pain and unilateral edema

Give 2 points for:
3. Heart rate greater than 95 bpm

Table 25-2. Well's criteria for determining the pretest probability of pulmonary embolism.

Variable	Points
Hemoptysis	1.0
Heart rate >100 bpm	1.5
Immobilization (bedrest, except for use of bathroom, for >3 days or surgery within 4 weeks)	1.5
Previous diagnosis of DVT or PE	1.5
Malignancy (currently receiving treatment, treatment within 6 months, or palliative care)	1.0
Clinical signs and symptoms of DVT (objectively measured leg swelling and pain with palpation in the deep vein region)	3.0
PE as likely as or more likely than an alternate diagnosis	3.0
PE unlikely	**0–4**
PE likely	**>4**

Adapted from: Wells PS, Anderson DR, Rodger M, et al. Derivation of a simple clinical model to categorize patient's probability of pulmonary embolism: increasing the models utility with the SimpliRED D-dimer. *Thrombosis and Haemostasis.* 2000; Mar;83(3):416–420.

patients with "likely" pretest probability of PE, CTA is obtained (Figure 25-2).

TREATMENT

Oxygen should be administered as needed. Endotracheal intubation may be necessary for cases of refractory hypoxia. Vasopressors such as norepinephrine (10 mcg/min) are indicated in patients with hypotension. Large IV fluid boluses should be avoided. Fluids can exacerbate already elevated right ventricular pressures, leading to further compromise of left ventricular outflow and shock.

Anticoagulation is the mainstay of treatment and prevents additional thrombi from forming, but does not dissolve existing clot. Endogenous fibrinolysis and clot resolution typically occurs over weeks to months, but may be incomplete. Short-term therapy with unfractionated heparin (5,000 unit or 80 IU/kg bolus, followed by a nomogram-adjusted infusion), low-molecular-weight heparins (enoxaparin, dalteparin, etc.), or fondaparinux is used as a bridge to long-term therapy with a vitamin K antagonist such as warfarin. The target international normalized ratio for warfarin administration is 2.0–3.0. Length of treatment may be limited to 3 months if a clear precipitant (transient or reversible) is identified, but otherwise long-term treatment is recommended as long as the benefits outweigh the risks. Newer medications such as direct thrombin inhibitors are promising alternatives to warfarin, but are still being studied. An inferior vena cava filter is indicated in patients with contraindications to anticoagulation (eg, active gastrointestinal bleeding) or who have failed anticoagulant therapy.

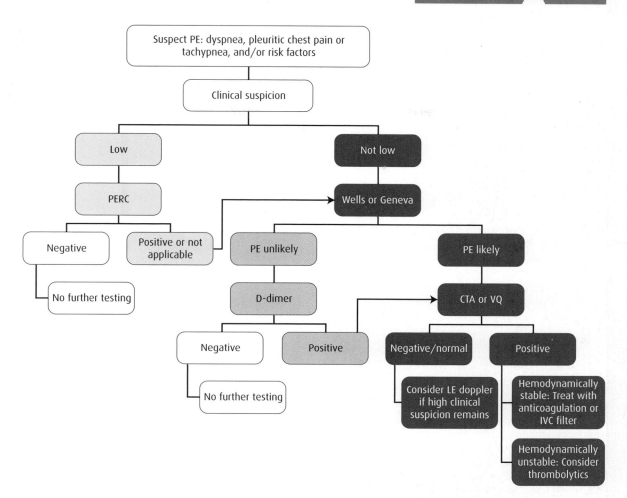

▲ **Figure 25-2.** Pulmonary embolism diagnostic algorithm. CTA, computed tomography angiography; IVC, intravenous catheter; LE, lower extremity; PE, pulmonary embolism; VQ, ventilation/perfusion.

Thrombolytic agents that directly lyse the clot are indicated in hemodynamically unstable patients with confirmed PE, when the benefits of treatment outweigh the risks of life-threatening bleeding complications (13% risk of major hemorrhage).

DISPOSITION

▶ Admission

Recent studies seem to indicate that it may be possible to manage patients with confirmed PE and low-risk findings as outpatients. However, pending further data, the current standard remains admission for all patients with newly diagnosed PE. Patients with refractory hypoxia or cardiovascular dysfunction should be admitted to an intensive care setting.

▶ Discharge

Patients with a clear alternative diagnosis may be discharged based on the severity and appropriate management of the alternate diagnosis.

▼ SUGGESTED READING

ACEP Clinical Policy. Critical issues in the evaluation and management of adult patients presenting to the emergency department with suspected pulmonary embolism. *Ann Emerg Med.* 2011;57:628–652.e75.

Goldhaber SZ, Bounameaux H. Pulmonary embolism and deep vein thrombosis. *Lancet.* 2012;6736:1–12.

Kline JA. Thromboembolism. In: Tintinalli JE, Stapczynski JS, Ma OJ, Cline DM, Cydulka RK, Meckler GD. *Tintinalli's Emergency Medicine: A Comprehensive Study Guide.* 7th ed. New York, NY: McGraw-Hill, 2011, pp. 430–440.

Ouellette DW, Patocka C. Pulmonary embolism. *Emerg Med Clin North Am.* 2012;30:329–375.

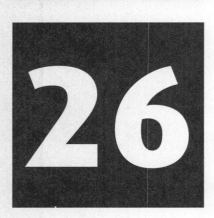

Acute Abdominal Pain

David C. Gordon, MD

Key Points

- A primary survey should be conducted to rapidly screen for vascular catastrophes, abdominal sepsis, or perforated viscus.
- Appendicitis should always be on the differential diagnosis for acute abdominal pain.
- Females of childbearing age with abdominal pain are presumed to have an ectopic pregnancy until proven otherwise.

- Older and immunocompromised patients may have an atypical presentation of disease.
- The white blood cell count is an unreliable predictor of disease and should not be used in isolation to confirm or exclude a critical diagnosis.

INTRODUCTION

Abdominal pain is a common presenting complaint and represents up to 10% of all emergency department (ED) visits. Although the etiology of abdominal pain frequently goes undiagnosed, the role of the emergency physician is to first identify and treat any immediate life- or organ-threatening conditions. Imminent causes of abdominal pain that need to be promptly diagnosed are those driven by a vascular event, infectious process, or perforated viscous (eg, ruptured abdominal aortic aneurysm [AAA], cholangitis, perforated gastric ulcer). Other disease processes may not pose an immediate threat to the patient but should be diagnosed before discharge, as delays in treatment can result in patient morbidity (eg, appendicitis, pelvic inflammatory disease).

Abdominal pain can be classified as visceral, parietal, or referred in origin. Depending on the disease process, pain may begin as visceral and become parietal, as in the stretching and subsequent rupture of a hollow viscus. Visceral pain occurs with the stretching of nerve fibers in the walls of hollow organs or the capsules of solid organs. The location of pain is not well localized, but often has an embryologic basis that aids in determining the diagnosis. Epigastric pain occurs in patients with stretching of foregut organs (stomach to duodenum, including biliary tree

and pancreas). Periumbilical pain represents pathology of midgut organs (distal duodenum to transverse colon). Suprapubic pain is due to problems of the hindgut organs (distal transverse colon, rectum, and urogenital tract). Parietal pain is due to irritation of the parietal peritoneum. The patient is more readily able to localize the pain (eg, left lower quadrant pain in diverticulitis), but when the entire peritoneal cavity is involved, the pain is diffuse. Referred pain is defined as pain experienced at a site distant from its source. Its anatomic basis lies in afferent nerves from different locations sharing the same spinal cord segment. Abdominal pain may be referred from organs above the diaphragm (eg, myocardial infarction causing epigastric pain). Alternatively, abdominal pathology may refer pain to sites above the diaphragm (eg, splenic rupture causing shoulder pain).

Older and immunocompromised patients warrant special consideration as higher risk groups. Older patients have a greater incidence of vascular catastrophes and surgical disease, with as high as 40% of patients older than 65 years requiring operative intervention (Table 26-1). Compared with younger counterparts, older patients are more likely to have atypical presentations, have nonspecific symptoms, and present later in the disease course. In addition to being vulnerable to opportunistic pathogens, immunocompromised patients may not develop peritoneal

Table 26-1. Causes of abdominal pain in patients <50 and >50 years of age.

Age <50	%	Age >50	%
Nonspecific abdominal pain	40	Nonspecific abdominal pain	20
Appendicitis	32	Cholecystitis	16
Cholecystitis	6	Appendicitis	15
Obstruction	3	Obstruction	12
Pancreatitis	2	Pancreatitis	7
Diverticulitis	< 0.1	Diverticulitis	6
Hernia	< 0.1	Cancer	4
Vascular	< 0.1	Hernia	3
Cancer	< 0.1	Vascular	2

findings despite a serious underlying infection owing to their blunted immune response. For both these populations, a low threshold must be maintained to pursue critical diagnoses.

CLINICAL PRESENTATION

History

A thoughtful history is important in obtaining an accurate diagnosis, but some specific historical elements can lead to the rapid development of a targeted differential. While keeping in mind that patients may have an atypical presentation of disease, the location of the pain, the nature of the pain at onset, and how the pain behaves since onset can help efficiently discriminate between different diagnostic considerations (Figure 26-1). Pain that is sudden and severe at onset is often associated with the rupture of a blood vessel or hollow viscus (eg, ruptured AAA, perforated peptic ulcer), occlusion of a blood vessel or hollow viscus (eg, acute mesenteric ischemia, ureteral colic), or gonadal torsion. In contrast, inflammatory conditions tend to have a more insidious onset, as is seen with appendicitis. Pain whose progression is colicky in nature is suggestive of peristaltic activity in the setting of an obstructed lumen (eg, ureteral, biliary, intestinal colic).

The manner in which the pain radiates can suggest a specific disease. Pain radiating to the back is often seen with pancreatitis. Pain radiating to the right infrascapular region is associated with biliary tract disorders. Pain that radiates to the groin may indicate a ruptured aortic aneurysm or nephrolithiasis.

Associated symptoms involving the gastrointestinal, genitourinary, and cardiopulmonary systems should be obtained. The clinician, however, must keep a broad differential as the same symptom can be seen across many disease processes. Nausea and vomiting are nonspecific

symptoms, although it is worthwhile noting the temporal relationship between them. Surgical causes of abdominal pain classically present with pain preceding vomiting, whereas the reverse is often seen with medical etiologies. The clinician must be cautious in using diarrhea as conclusive evidence of gastroenteritis, as it can also be seen with appendicitis, diverticulitis, and partial small bowel obstruction. Irritative voiding symptoms such as dysuria and frequency are suggestive of a urinary tract infection; however, they can also be caused by appendicitis or pelvic abscess. Hematuria should raise concern for nephrolithiasis or a malignancy in the genitourinary tract. Vaginal bleeding and discharge are important to elicit in assessing for ectopic pregnancy and pelvic inflammatory disease. As pneumonia, pulmonary embolism, and acute coronary syndrome can all present with abdominal pain, the presence of cough, chest pain, and shortness of breath should be ascertained.

A thorough past medical/surgical history, medications, allergies, and social history should also be obtained. The existence of known coronary artery or cerebrovascular disease should raise suspicion for vascular disease of the abdomen. Corticosteroids and immunosuppressants should alert the clinician that the patient may not present with typical symptoms or exam findings. Knowledge of anticoagulants is critical in constructing the differential diagnosis as well as making sure reversal is not needed before any operative intervention. Heavy alcohol use raises the possibility of hepatitis or pancreatitis.

Physical Examination

Vital signs should be readily noted, with tachycardia and/or hypotension raising immediate concern for the presence of shock. Hemodynamic instability, in conjunction with fever and warm skin, points toward septic shock; the presence of cold and clammy skin suggests hypovolemic shock.

The general appearance of the patient can provide important diagnostic information. The inability to lie still or find a position of comfort is seen with ureteral colic, ovarian torsion, and mesenteric ischemia. Patients with peritonitis—whose pain is worsened with movement—prefer to lie still.

A thorough abdominal examination should be performed, starting with visual inspection, followed by auscultation, and then palpation. Inspection may reveal abdominal distention or surgical scars from surgeries not initially volunteered by the patient. The presence of hyperactive high-pitched bowel sounds may signify a small bowel obstruction. Palpation should begin with a nontender location followed by the tender quadrants. One should look for the presence of guarding (contraction of the abdominal wall musculature) as well as facial grimacing. Rebound tenderness lacks sensitivity or specificity as a finding of peritonitis. A more specific marker is "cough pain." The patient is asked to cough, and the examiner looks for signs of pain such as flinching, grimacing, or

Right Upper Quadrant	Epigastric	Left Upper Quadrant
Biliary: colic, cholecystitis, cholangitis Hepatic: hepatitis, abscess Pancreatitis Renal: nephrolithiasis, pyelonephritis Intestinal: retrocecal appendicitis Pulmonary: pneumonia, embolus	Biliary disease: colic, cholecystitis, cholangitis Gastric: PUD, gastritis Pancreatitis Cardiac: ACS Vascular: AAA, aortic dissection	Gastric: PUD, gastritis Splenic: infarct, rupture Pancreatitis Renal: nephrolithiasis, pyelonephritis Pulmonary: pneumonia, embolus Cardiac: ACS

Periumbilical
Intestinal: early appendicitis, small bowel obstruction
Vascular: AAA, aortic dissection, mesenteric ischemia

Right Lower Quadrant	Suprapubic	Left Lower Quadrant
Intestinal: appendicitis, colitis, IBD, hernia OB-GYN: ectopic pregnancy, PID, TOA, ovarian torsion GU: testicular torsion Renal: nephrolithiasis, pyelonephritis	Intestinal: appendicitis, diverticulitis, colitis, IBD, hernia OB-GYN: ectopic pregnancy, PID, TOA, ovarian torsion GU: testicular torsion Renal: nephrolithiasis, pyelonephritis	Intestinal: diverticulitis, colitis, IBD, hernia OB-GYN: ectopic pregnancy, PID, TOA, ovarian torsion GU: testicular torsion Renal: nephrolithiasis, pyelonephritis

Diffuse
Intestinal: bowel obstruction, early appendicitis, perforation
Vascular: aortic dissection, AAA, mesenteric ischemia
Peritonitis
Sickle cell crisis
Diabetic ketoacidosis
Black widow spider bite

AAA = abdominal aortic aneurysm; ACS = acute coronary syndrome; IBD = inflammatory bowel disease; PID = pelvic inflammatory disease; PUD = peptic ulcer disease; TOA= tubo-ovarian abscess

Figure 26-1. Causes of abdominal pain based on location.

grabbing the abdomen. Children can be asked to jump up and down as an indirect means of inciting peritoneal irritation. In addition to signs of peritonitis, the physician should examine for the presence of a pulsatile mass consistent with an aortic aneurysm.

A pelvic exam should be performed in women with lower or undifferentiated abdominal pain to help separate a pelvic from abdominal source. Cervical motion tenderness can be found with appendicitis, but the presence of a cervical mucopurulent discharge supports the diagnosis of pelvic inflammatory disease. A genitourinary exam (GU) in males should be performed to evaluate for testicular disease, prostatitis, and hernias. Adolescents with testicular torsion may only complain of abdominal pain making a systematic GU exam paramount to timely diagnosis.

DIAGNOSTIC STUDIES

Laboratory

Complete blood count. Although leukocytosis may alert the physician that the patient is sicker than initially perceived, the white blood cell count (WBC) must be used with caution. A normal WBC does not exclude serious infection, and an elevated WBC can be seen in many benign conditions. Overall, the WBC is a poor predictor of disease and should not replace clinical judgment.

Electrolytes and glucose. It is important to correct any electrolyte derangement that can occur in the setting of fluid losses from excessive vomiting or diarrhea. Conversely, electrolyte or glucose derangement may be the cause of abdominal pain, as seen in hypercalcemia and diabetic ketoacidosis.

Blood urea nitrogen and creatinine. Renal function tests should be obtained in patients for whom there is concern for dehydration or severe sepsis. They are also necessary before intravenous contrast is given for a computed tomography (CT) scan to prevent patients with renal insufficiency incurring contrast nephropathy.

Urinalysis. A urinary tract infection (UTI) is suggested by the presence of leukocyte esterase, nitrates, pyuria, and bacteria. Careful interpretation of this test is necessary, as inflammatory processes (eg, appendicitis, diverticulitis) near the ureter may produce pyuria in the absence of a UTI.

Pregnancy test. All females of childbearing age should be tested for pregnancy. This is routinely accomplished through qualitative testing of the urine. If positive, this is followed by a quantitative serum beta human chorionic gonadotropin level in conjunction with pelvic ultrasound to exclude an ectopic pregnancy.

Liver function tests (LFTs). LFT abnormalities can be seen in both hepatic and biliary tract disorders. A hepatic picture involves increases in aspartate aminotransferase (AST) and alanine aminotransferase (ALT) greater than alkaline phosphatase (ALP). An obstructive (cholestatic) picture is seen when the increase in ALP is greater than that of AST/ALT, along with the presence of hyperbilirubinemia. Marked transaminitis (>1,000 IU/L) is typically only seen in toxin/drug-induced hepatitis, acute viral hepatitis, or ischemic hepatitis (shock liver).

Lipase. A value 2 times normal is 94% sensitive and 95% specific for pancreatitis. An elevated lipase in conjunction with cholestatic LFT abnormalities should raise concern for gallstone pancreatitis.

Coagulation tests. Patients on warfarin should have their international normalized ratio checked for both diagnostic and treatment purposes. Being subtherapeutic in the setting of atrial fibrillation could raise concern for mesenteric ischemia. Supra-therapeutic levels can raise suspicion for hemorrhagic diseases such as a rectus sheath hematoma. Patients on warfarin going to the operating room may require reversal beforehand.

Type and screen (T&S). T&S should be obtained in patients presenting with hemorrhage or going to the operating room. It is also necessary in determining the Rh status of females being evaluated for ectopic pregnancy.

▶ Electrocardiogram

An electrocardiogram should be obtained as an initial screening tool in patients with unexplained epigastric pain or older patients with poorly localized pain. Cardiac markers can be ordered for additional risk stratification.

▶ Imaging

Plain radiographs offer little diagnostic value in evaluating nonspecific abdominal pain, but can serve as an initial imaging study for perforated viscus, small bowel obstruction, volvulus, or foreign bodies. Radiographs offer the advantage of being quick and portable, but owing to their poor sensitivity, cannot be used to definitively rule out disease. Upright chest x-ray can be used to screen for free air under the diaphragm (Figure 26-2). When a patient is unable to sit upright, a lateral decubitus may alternatively be used.

Ultrasound plays a central role in evaluating patients for disorders of the biliary tract, reproductive system, or abdominal aorta. It is the primary radiologic modality in investigating for cholecystitis, gonadal torsion, ectopic pregnancy, and tubo-ovarian abscess. In children and

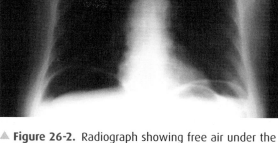

▲ **Figure 26-2.** Radiograph showing free air under the diaphragm in a patient with a perforated viscus.

pregnant women, it can serve as the initial imaging study of choice in evaluating for appendicitis. In hemodynamically unstable patients, bedside ultrasound enables the emergency physician to rapidly assess for the presence of an abdominal aortic aneurysm, intrauterine pregnancy, or free intraperitoneal fluid suggestive of hemorrhage.

Computed tomography (CT) is widely employed in the diagnosis of abdominal diseases including infections (appendicitis, diverticulitis, abscess), vascular events (aortic dissection, mesenteric ischemia), bowel obstruction, perforated viscus, and nephrolithiasis. It is the radiologic study of choice when imaging is being pursued for undifferentiated abdominal pain. Its use is limited by contrast nephropathy, contrast allergies, and exposure to ionizing radiation.

The use of contrast agents is dictated by the study indication. Noncontrasted CT is obtained when confirming nephrolithiasis. IV contrast is utilized in investigating neoplastic, infectious, and inflammatory diseases. IV contrast accentuates areas of high blood flow (eg, appendicitis). IV contrast is furthermore utilized in detecting vascular lesions such as intimal flaps (aortic dissection), occlusion (mesenteric ischemia), and leakage (AAA). Oral contrast allows for visualization of the bowel lumen. Variation in opinion exists over its use. Conditions in which it can facilitate diagnosis include bowel perforation, fistulas, and partial bowel obstruction. Both abscesses and loops of bowel appear as fluid-filled structures on CT, so oral contrast will help discriminate between them, as only bowel should fill with contrast.

MEDICAL DECISION MAKING

A primary survey guided by vital signs, general appearance, and a focused abdominal exam should be conducted to screen for a life- or organ-threatening disease

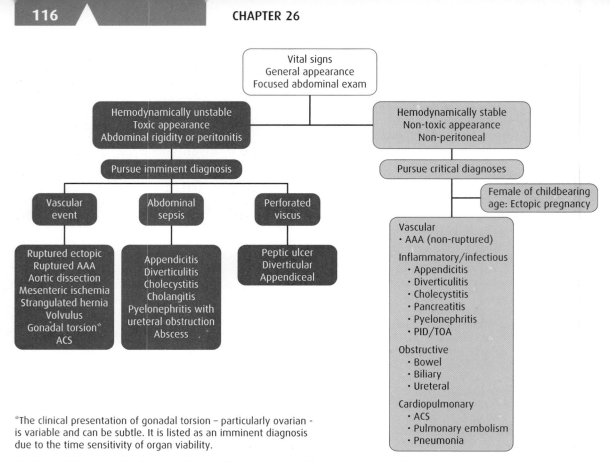

*The clinical presentation of gonadal torsion – particularly ovarian - is variable and can be subtle. It is listed as an imminent diagnosis due to the time sensitivity of organ viability.

▲ **Figure 26-3.** Acute abdominal pain diagnostic algorithm. AAA, abdominal aortic aneurysm; ACS, acute coronary syndrome; PID, pelvic inflammatory disease; TOA, tubo-ovarian abscess.

processes (imminent diagnoses). If not found, a secondary search should begin for disease states requiring identification before discharge (critical diagnoses). Certain diagnoses should be automatically considered in different age groups: AAA in the older adult, testicular torsion in the adolescent male, and ectopic pregnancy in females of reproductive age. As the most common surgical disease of the abdomen, appendicitis should always be placed on the differential diagnosis regardless of age (Figure 26-3).

TREATMENT

Resuscitation should be initiated in patients with hemodynamic instability without delay. Volume repletion should begin with rapid infusion of isotonic crystalloid. In the setting of massive hemorrhage, emergency release blood (type O) can be transfused until typed and crossed blood is available. In septic shock, a vasopressor should be employed for persistent hypotension (mean arterial pressure [MAP] <65) after volume status has been optimized

or during volume resuscitation in the setting of severe hemodynamic compromise (MAP <40–50 mmHg).

Antibiotics should be promptly administered in patients with abdominal sepsis, peritonitis, or perforated viscus. Specific diseases requiring antibiotic treatment include appendicitis, cholecystitis, diverticulitis, pyelonephritis, and pelvic inflammatory disease.

Pain control can be tailored to the suspected disease process. When gastritis/peptic ulcer disease (PUD) is suspected, a "GI cocktail" (typically a combination of Maalox, viscous lidocaine, and Donnatal) may provide relief. Ketorolac is useful in the setting of biliary colic and nephrolithiasis, but should be avoided in patients with PUD or chronic kidney disease. Multiple randomized studies have shown that narcotic pain medications do not interfere with diagnostic ability. These agents should not be withheld in patients with significant pain.

Consultation with the appropriate surgical service should be emergently obtained for hemodynamic instability, suspected vascular catastrophe (ruptured AAA, ruptured ectopic, acute mesenteric occlusion), or abdominal rigidity (ie, perforation). For patients with severe sepsis secondary to an intra-abdominal abscess or obstruction of the biliary tract, consultation with interventional radiology can be pursued for percutaneous drainage.

DISPOSITION

▶ Admission

Patients found to have a surgical disease, abdominal sepsis, or intractable pain or vomiting regardless of the etiology should be admitted to the hospital.

▶ Discharge

Patients with resolution of symptoms without suspicion of serious underlying pathology may be discharged. Follow-up with a primary physician should be ensured, and the patient should be instructed to return if there is progression of symptoms. Patients with acute abdominal pain of unclear etiology who are discharged should be instructed to be re-examined within 12–24 hours by a health care provider if still having active pain.

▼ SUGGESTED READING

Cartwright SL, Knudson MP. Evaluation of acute abdominal pain in adults. *Am Fam Physician.* 2008;77:971–978.

Graff LG, Robinson D. Abdominal pain and emergency department evaluation. *Emerg Med Clin North Am.* 2001;19: 123–136.

O'Brien MC. Acute abdominal pain. In: Tintinalli JE, Stapczynski JS, Ma OJ, Cline DM, Cydulka, RK, Meckler GD. *Tintinalli's Emergency Medicine: A Comprehensive Study Guide.* 7th ed. New York, NY: McGraw-Hill, 2011, pp. 519–527.

Ragsdale L, Southerland L. Acute abdominal pain in the older adult. *Emerg Med Clin North Am.* 2011;29:429–448.

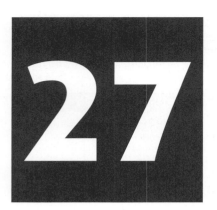

Appendicitis

Anitha E. Mathew, MD

Key Points

- The absence of leukocytosis or the presence of diarrhea does not rule out appendicitis.
- Appendicitis is a clinical diagnosis, with imaging aiding in atypical presentations or cases of diagnostic uncertainty.
- Rapid diagnosis and early surgical intervention help to avoid complications associated with rupture.
- Intravenous antibiotics should be administered if perforation is likely or has occurred.

INTRODUCTION

The lifetime risk of developing acute appendicitis in the United States is 12% for males and 25% for females. Appendicitis is caused by luminal obstruction of the appendix, typically by a fecalith, and less frequently by lymphatic tissue, gallstones, tumors, or parasites. Continued luminal secretion results in increased intraluminal pressure and vascular insufficiency, leading to bacterial proliferation, inflammation, and ultimately perforation.

CLINICAL PRESENTATION

▶ History

One half of patients present to the emergency department within 24 hours of symptom onset, and another one third present within the following 24 hours. Early on, patients complain of general malaise, indigestion, anorexia, or bowel irregularity. The presence of diarrhea should not be used to exclude appendicitis. The classic patient presentation begins with periumbilical abdominal pain followed by nausea, with or without emesis, and low-grade fever, after which the pain migrates to the right lower quadrant (RLQ) (Table 27-1). Atypical presentations of appendicitis are common. Perforation often results in sudden resolution of pain and should be suspected in patients who present more than 48 hours after symptom onset.

Table 27-1. Frequency of historical features of appendicitis.

Feature	Frequency
Abdominal pain	100%
Anorexia	92%
Nausea	78%
Vomiting	54%
Migration of pain	50%
Fever	20%
Diarrhea	15%

▶ Physical Examination

Patients should receive a complete physical examination, including a pelvic exam for any women of childbearing age. Vague periumbilical abdominal tenderness is observed early in the disease and then migrates to the McBurney point, located one-third of the distance between the right anterior superior iliac spine and the umbilicus. Rebound tenderness and involuntary guarding suggest peritonitis. Rovsing sign, or pain in the RLQ with palpation of the left lower quadrant (LLQ), can also be present. The psoas sign is elicited if abdominal pain is produced with extension of the right leg at the hip while the patient lies on the left side. The obturator test elicits pain with internal and external rotation of the hip. Perforation should be suspected in patients with generalized tenderness, rigidity, or a palpable mass in the RLQ.

Up to one third of patients have atypical presentations of acute appendicitis, often owing to anatomic variations. A retrocecal appendix can produce right flank or pelvic pain, whereas malrotation of the colon results in appendiceal transposition with LUQ pain. Although pregnant women with appendicitis most commonly complain of RLQ pain, they can have RUQ tenderness owing to gravid uterine displacement of the abdominal organs.

DIAGNOSTIC STUDIES

▶ Laboratory

Individuals with acute appendicitis commonly have a mild leukocytosis with a left shift, but a normal white blood cell count (WBC) is not uncommon. An elevated WBC and/or C-reactive protein can have a combined sensitivity up to 98%, and normal values of both make appendicitis very unlikely. Although hematuria or sterile pyuria can be present in acute appendicitis, isolated microscopic hematuria may support a diagnosis of renal colic, and pyuria can suggest pyelonephritis. A negative pregnancy test should be documented in females of childbearing age to rule out ectopic or heterotopic pregnancy.

▶ Imaging

Early surgical consultation should be obtained before imaging in straightforward cases of suspected appendicitis (ie, male with classic presentation and onset of pain <48 hours). Plain radiography is not helpful. Abdominal computed tomography (CT) should be obtained in nonpregnant females and males for whom the diagnosis is unclear. CT has a sensitivity of >94% and a positive predictive value of >95%. Many centers recommend CT imaging with both IV and oral contrast, although noncontrast CT imaging is increasingly being used. Typical findings include a dilated appendix >6 mm with a thickened wall, periappendiceal stranding, and visualization of an appendicolith or abscess (Figure 27-1). Luminal obstruction may be relieved with perforation, leading to disappearance of imaging hallmarks and difficulty visualizing the appendix. Patients with abdominal pain for >48 hours usually require a CT scan to diagnose abscess formation that is treated with percutaneous drainage rather than surgery. Ultrasonography is the imaging modality of choice in both pregnant females and

▲ **Figure 27-1.** CT scan showing appendicitis. Note the increased uptake of intravenous contrast in the wall of the appendix and the absence of oral contrast in the lumen (arrow).

children. Typical findings include a thickened, noncompressible appendix >6 mm in diameter. Magnetic resonance imaging is increasingly being used to diagnose appendicitis when ionizing radiation needs to be avoided, although IV gadolinium should be avoided in pregnancy and cannot be given to patients with renal insufficiency.

MEDICAL DECISION MAKING

Acute appendicitis is largely a clinical diagnosis and should be considered in any patient with atraumatic right-sided abdominal, periumbilical, or flank pain who has not had an appendectomy. The differential diagnosis of such a patient is broad and includes diverticulitis, volvulus, colitis, ileitis, bowel obstruction, irritable bowel disease, incarcerated hernia, intra-abdominal abscess, intussusception, malrotation, mesenteric lymphadenitis, ectopic pregnancy, ovarian torsion, ovarian vein thrombosis, pyelonephritis, referred testicular pain, renal colic, tubo-ovarian abscess, abdominal wall hematoma, and psoas abscess (Figure 27-2).

TREATMENT

Patients with acute appendicitis typically require appendectomy, so surgical consult should be obtained promptly. Patients should be kept NPO (nothing by mouth) to avoid operative delays and be given IV hydration, antiemetics, and analgesics, including narcotics, as needed. Perioperative antibiotics should be given once the diagnosis has been made or if the patient exhibits signs of peritonitis. Appropriate choices should include broad coverage of aerobic and anaerobic gram-negative organisms, such as ciprofloxacin and metronidazole.

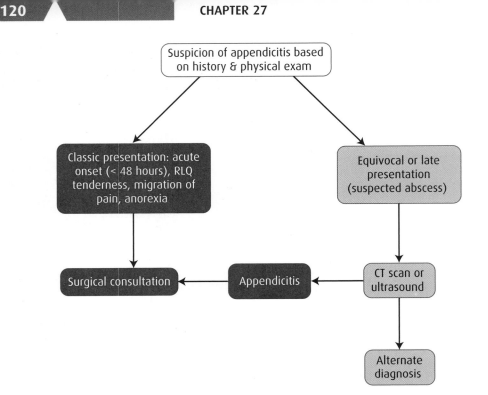

Figure 27-2. Appendicitis diagnostic algorithm. CT, computed tomography; RLQ, right lower quadrant.

DISPOSITION

▶ Admission

All patients with appendicitis should be admitted to the hospital after consultation with a general surgeon. Patients with equivocal diagnoses can be observed with serial examinations.

▶ Discharge

Stable, nontoxic patients with adequate pain control, toleration of oral fluids, and no significant comorbidities who have been ruled out for appendicitis and other surgical conditions may be considered for discharge with timely follow-up. Discharged patients should be given written instructions that identify signs or symptoms needing earlier return.

▼ SUGGESTED READING

Andersson RE. Meta-analysis of the clinical and laboratory diagnosis of appendicitis. *Br J Surg.* 2004;91:28–37.

DeKoning EP. Acute appendicitis. In: Tintinalli JE, Stapczynski JS, Ma OJ, Cline DM, Cydulka RK, Meckler GD. *Tintinalli's Emergency Medicine: A Comprehensive Study Guide.* 7th ed. New York, NY: McGraw-Hill, 2011, pp. 574–578.

Humes DJ, Simpson J. Acute appendicitis. *Br Med J.* 2006;333: 530–534.

Pittman-Waller VA, Myers JG, Stewart RM, et al. Appendicitis: why so complicated? Analysis of 5755 consecutive appendectomies. *Am Surg.* 2000;66:548–554.

Vissers RJ, Lennarz WB. Pitfalls in appendicitis. *Emerg Med Clin North Am.* 2010;28:103–118.

Acute Cholecystitis

Casey Glass, MD

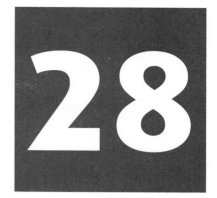

Key Points

- Biliary colic frequently presents with epigastric or right upper quadrant pain that resolves in a few hours and is not associated with fever or leukocytosis.
- Acute cholecystitis cannot be established or excluded based on history and examination alone.
- Antibiotics should be administered early in ill-appearing patients when acute cholecystitis is suspected.

INTRODUCTION

Acute cholecystitis can be a challenging diagnosis because the spectrum of disease ranges from biliary colic, a self-limited condition, to emphysematous cholecystitis or gallbladder perforation with sepsis. Additionally, no single historical feature, exam finding, or test result is adequate to exclude the disease in its early stages.

When a gallstone moves into the gallbladder neck, cystic duct, or common bile duct, it causes obstruction. Obstruction in turn causes an increase in luminal pressure in the gallbladder or common bile duct. In biliary colic, the obstruction is intermittent, and symptoms resolve when the blockage is relieved. If obstruction is persistent, there is a resulting increase in mucosal inflammation and irritation. Ultimately this leads to ischemia of the gallbladder wall and bacterial invasion.

Biliary colic is pain due to transient gallbladder neck blockage with a gallstone. Acute cholecystitis is inflammation of the gallbladder due to persistent obstruction from gallstones and is sometimes associated with infection. Acalculous cholecystitis accounts for 2–15% of cases of acute cholecystitis and occurs in the absence of gallstones. Acalculous cholecystitis is believed to be secondary to gallbladder ischemia and is more common in diabetics, the elderly, and the critically ill and carries a higher mortality rate. Emphysematous cholecystitis is acute cholecystitis with superinfection by gas-forming bacteria and has a more severe course and poorer prognosis. When gallstones become lodged in the common bile duct, the condition is referred to as choledocholithiasis. Choledocholithiasis is associated with ascending cholangitis and pancreatitis.

Gallstones are present in 10–15% of the population in the United States, but only 10–20% of persons with asymptomatic stones will develop complications over a 20-year period, and only 1–3% will develop acute cholecystitis each year. When patients do develop acute cholecystitis, the mortality rate is approximately 4%. The mortality rate for emphysematous cholecystitis is approximately 20%.

CLINICAL PRESENTATION

▶ History

Patients with biliary colic present with acute onset of constant crampy pain in the right upper quadrant or epigastrium that may radiate to the back. Pain persisting for more than 6 hours is unusual and should raise concern for early cholecystitis. Nausea and vomiting are present to varying degrees, and fever is usually absent.

Acute cholecystitis presents in much the same way as biliary colic, but symptoms are persistent and localize to the right upper quadrant. The pain may radiate to the right or left shoulder owing to irritation of the diaphragm. Fever

Table 28-1. Test characteristics of common historical, exam, and laboratory findings in acute cholecystitis.

Findings	Sensitivity (%)	Specificity (%)
Fever	35	80
Nausea	77	36
Emesis	71	53
RUQ pain	81	67
RUQ tenderness	77	54
Murphy sign	65	87
Leukocytosis (>12,000/mL)	63	57

RUQ, right upper quadrant.

Reproduced with permission from Roe J: Clinical assessment of acute cholecystitis in adults. *Ann Emerg Med* Jul; 48(1):101–103, 2006.

may develop but it is often absent, especially in elderly or immunosuppressed patients.

No historical or exam finding is adequately sensitive or specific to exclude or confirm the diagnosis of cholecystitis (Table 28-1). The history should focus on previous episodes of similar symptoms and previous surgery. Patients may describe exacerbations of pain related to food or late at night. Although uncommon, patients who have had a cholecystectomy can retain stones in the common bile duct after surgery or develop them later. It is important to ask about respiratory or cardiac symptoms to help exclude a thoracic cause for the pain. Family history of gallstones, female sex, parity, rapid weight loss, and hemolytic disorders are several important risk factors for gallstones.

Physical Examination

The physical examination should focus on excluding other abdominal or thoracic causes of pain and determining the degree of pain in the right upper quadrant. In biliary colic, tenderness on examination may be mild. The Murphy sign is the most specific physical exam finding for cholecystitis and is described as the patient halting inspiration when the examiner is palpating deeply in the right upper quadrant. The examiner should also assess for costovertebral angle tenderness and right lower quadrant tenderness.

DIAGNOSTIC STUDIES

Laboratory Studies

It is hard to discriminate biliary colic from early cholecystitis, and laboratory evaluation is almost always indicated. A complete blood count (CBC) may help in determining the presence of infection, especially because fever may be absent. However, the CBC may be normal in acute

cholecystitis. Liver function tests may help identify biliary obstruction or hepatic inflammation. Serum lipase is helpful when there is a concern for choledocholithiasis and associated gallstone pancreatitis.

Imaging

Ultrasound evaluation of the gallbladder and common bile duct remains the best test for identifying cholecystitis. The sensitivity (88–94%) and specificity (80–90%) vary depending on what criteria are used to establish the diagnosis. On ultrasound examination, gallstones appear as hyperechoic intraluminal structures, and larger stones will cast an ultrasound shadow (Figure 28-1). Findings suggestive of cholecystitis include gallbladder wall thickness greater than 3–5 mm and pericholecystic fluid. A common bile duct diameter greater than 5–8 mm is abnormal. The sonographic Murphy sign is positive when maximal pain is produced with transducer pressure over the gallbladder. When combined with the presence of gallstones, the sonographic Murphy sign has a positive predictive value of 92%. The sonographic Murphy sign can be masked by

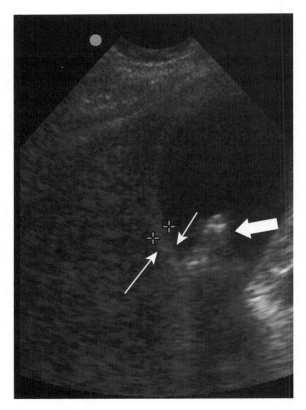

▲ **Figure 28-1.** Short axis view of the gallbladder demonstrating a gallbladder neck stone (large arrow) and gallbladder wall thickening (small arrows).
© Casey Glass, MD.

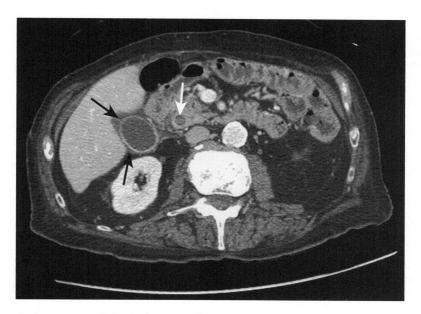

▲ **Figure 28-2.** Abdominal CT scan showing an enlarged gallbladder with pericholecystic fluid (black arrows) and a dilated common bile duct (white arrow). © Casey Glass, MD.

prior pain medication and can be absent in diabetics or gangrenous cholecystitis.

Abdominal computed tomography (CT) scan is helpful when other diagnoses are also being considered. CT scanning is less sensitive for acute cholecystitis than ultrasound (50–90%), but is as sensitive for choledocholithiasis and can identify complications such as perforation or abscess formation. CT findings include wall thickening, pericholecystic fluid, and biliary tree dilation (Figure 28–2). Notably, only 20% of gallstones are radio-opaque, which limits the utility of CT in early cases of cholecystitis or for patients with biliary colic.

MEDICAL DECISION MAKING

The patient with classic symptoms of biliary colic or acute cholecystitis is easy to identify, but many patients present with atypical symptoms (Figure 28-3). It is important to consider other conditions that may masquerade as gallbladder pain. This may include pyelonephritis of the right kidney or retrocecal appendicitis. Right lower lobe pneumonia can also present with right upper quadrant pain and vomiting. Patients with choledocholithiasis are often misdiagnosed as having pancreatitis or gastritis. In elderly patients or those with coronary disease, it is important to consider the possibility of an inferior myocardial infarction. Patients who appear septic or with peritoneal signs may have perforation or ascending cholangitis. Other gastrointestinal (GI) conditions such as pancreatitis, peptic ulcer disease, or hepatitis should also be considered.

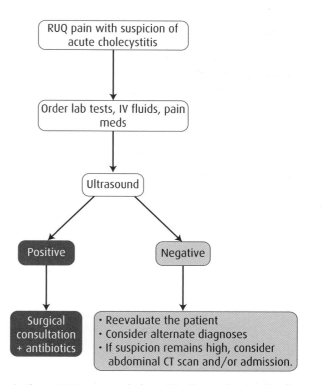

▲ **Figure 28-3.** Acute cholecystitis diagnostic algorithm. CT, computed tomography; IV, intravenous; RUQ, right upper quadrant.

TREATMENT

All patients are likely to need pain control. Morphine (0.1 mg/kg) IV or hydromorphone (0.0125 mg/ kg IV) are common choices. Antiemetics are also helpful, with common regimens being ondansetron 4–8 mg IV, promethazine 12.5–25 mg IV or intramuscularly, or metoclopramide 10 mg IV. If vomiting has been prolonged, then fluid resuscitation at 10–20 mL/kg is indicated, unless there is a concern for volume overload (history of congestive heart failure, end-stage renal disease). Patients should be made NPO (nothing by mouth) until it is clear they will not need surgery.

Surgical consultation is necessary when the diagnosis of acute cholecystitis is established. Cholecystectomy is usually performed within 48–72 hours. If testing is equivocal, then admission for further work-up is appropriate. Consultation with a GI specialist is necessary for choledocholithiasis to facilitate timely endoscopic retrograde cholangiopancreatography and sphincterotomy.

There is no clear role for antibiotics in uncomplicated cholecystitis. If there are signs of infection (leukocytosis, fever), then antimicrobial coverage with a second-generation cephalosporin or quinolone with metronidazole is appropriate. If the patient presents with sepsis or is at risk to develop sepsis (elderly, immune system compromise, high-risk presentation such as ascending cholangitis, emphysematous cholecystitis), then broad-spectrum antibiotics should be started promptly. The antibiotic regimen should cover both gram-positive and gram-negative organisms. Antibiotic choices include piperacillin-tazobactam 3.375 g IV and vancomycin 1 g IV, or in penicillin allergic patients, ciprofloxacin 400 mg IV, metronidazole 500 mg IV, and vancomycin 1 g IV.

DISPOSITION

▶ Admission

Patients with acute cholecystitis should be admitted to a surgical service. Patients with sepsis or severe disease should be admitted to an intensive care unit setting. Admission should also be strongly considered for patients with persistent symptoms but without definitive evidence of acute cholecystitis, as testing can be normal early in the course of the disease.

▶ Discharge

Patients with biliary colic can be discharged home if their pain has resolved, testing is normal, and they can tolerate oral fluids. They should be told to return for persistent symptoms, more severe pain, or fever. Outpatient follow up should include referral to a general surgeon.

▼ SUGGESTED READING

Atilla R, Oktay C. Pancreatitis and cholecystitis. In: Tintinalli JE, Stapczynski JS, Ma OJ, Cline DM, Cydulka RK, Meckler GD. *Tintinalli's Emergency Medicine: A Comprehensive Study Guide.* 7th ed. New York, NY: McGraw-Hill, 2011, pp. 558–566.

Barie PS, Eachempati SR. Acute acalculous cholecystitis. *Gastroenterol Clin North Am.* 2010;39:343–357.

Fox JC, Scruggs WP. Ultrasound Guide for Emergency Physicians: An Introduction. 2008. http://sonoguide.com/biliary.html

O'Connor OJ, Maher MM. Imaging of cholecystitis. *AJR Am J Roentgenol* 2011;196:W367–W374.

Strasberg SM. Clinical practice. Acute calculous cholecystitis. *N Engl J Med* 2008;358:2804S–2811S.

Abdominal Aortic Aneurysm

Alex de la Fuente, MD

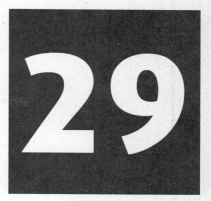

Key Points

- Diagnosis of ruptured abdominal aortic aneurysm (AAA) is frequently missed or delayed. The most common misdiagnosis is renal colic.
- AAA must be considered in any elderly patient with back, flank, or groin pain.
- Suspected ruptured AAA requires emergent consultation, with the goal of immediate open or endovascular repair.
- Patients with incidentally discovered AAAs must be referred for surveillance or elective repair.

INTRODUCTION

Abdominal aortic aneurysm (AAA) is an increase in the diameter of the aorta of more than 50%, or an infrarenal aortic diameter greater than 3 cm. The etiology and pathogenesis of AAA is unclear, although atherosclerosis, connective tissue disorders, genetic factors, and smoking have all been implicated. A family of enzymes known as matrix metalloproteinases may be largely responsible for the inflammatory destruction of elastin and collagen fibers in the medial and adventitial layers of the aortic wall that can ultimately lead to AAA formation, enlargement, and rupture.

The rate of expansion and risk of rupture are related to tension on the wall of the aneurysm, which in turn is related to the diameter of the aneurysm and to the underlying pressure. Rupture of aneurysms smaller than 4 cm is rare, whereas the annual risk of rupture for aneurysms larger than 8 cm has been estimated at 30–50%.

AAA causes 15,000 deaths in the United States a year. It is a common cause of sudden death and is responsible for 1–2% of all deaths in men older than 65 years. The overall mortality rate of a patient with a ruptured AAA is 90%, and 50% of patients with ruptured AAA do not survive to reach the hospital. In patients who arrive at the hospital, the mortality rate improves to 60%. The mortality rate for elective open operative repair is 2–7%; recent advances in endovascular technique have mitigated early morbidity and mortality.

The incidence of AAA begins to increase in men older than 55 years. By age 80 years, 5% of men have an AAA, and 5% of women age 90 years have AAA. There is an increased incidence in smokers, whites, and those with a family history of AAA. First-degree relatives of patients with AAA have up to an 8-fold increase in the chance of developing AAA.

CLINICAL PRESENTATION

▶ History

The emergency department (ED) presentation of AAA is varied, with symptoms due to expansion and rupture, distal thromboembolic complications, local mass effects, or erosion into adjacent structures. Most AAAs are asymptomatic and discovered incidentally while evaluating patients for unrelated conditions. These patients require little more than referral. At the other end of the spectrum, AAA rupture can constitute one of the most acutely life-threatening emergencies in medicine.

The classic triad of abdominal/back pain, hypotension, and a pulsatile abdominal mass is present in substantially less than one half of patients with a ruptured AAA. The vast majority of patients with ruptured AAA will have pain, typically in the abdomen, back, flank, or groin, depending on the extent and direction of rupture. Rarely, patients with rupture can present with syncope alone or with nonspecific symptoms such as vomiting, diarrhea, or dizziness.

Physical Examination

Patients with ruptured AAA may present with evidence of hemorrhagic shock: hypotension, tachycardia, and exam findings of poor perfusion. However, the patient may be normotensive or even hypertensive. Transient hypotension may also occur and can be erroneously attributed to a vasovagal etiology. Abdominal examination may detect a pulsatile mass, but this can be difficult with small aneurysms or obese patients and is subject to significant interobserver variability. Absence of a pulsatile mass on exam does not exclude the diagnosis of AAA. Lower extremity pulses should be assessed, as lower limb ischemia is present in 5% of cases.

DIAGNOSTIC STUDIES

Laboratory

Any patient with a possible ruptured AAA should have blood sent for type and crossmatch, although often uncrossmatched blood will be required emergently. Anemia can be seen in ruptured AAA, with hematocrit less than 38 in 40% of patients. D-dimer assays have been investigated as a possible screen for patients deemed to be at low risk for AAA, but their use for this indication has not yet been validated.

Imaging

Ultrasound has a sensitivity approaching 100% and can be obtained at the bedside even in unstable patients. In addition to the aneurysm, ultrasound may reveal intraperitoneal free fluid in cases of rupture. However, because many AAAs rupture into the retroperitoneum, ultrasound is insensitive in detecting this complication, and a lack of free fluid should not be reassuring. Ultrasound can also be limited by obesity and by overlying bowel gas.

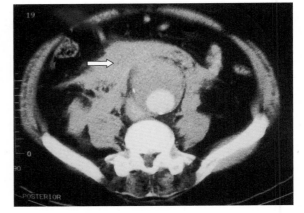

▲ **Figure 29-1.** CT scan showing a ruptured AAA. This AAA is rupturing into the peritoneal cavity (arrow). The majority of ruptured AAAs are retroperitoneal (70%).

Abdominal computed tomography (CT) is helpful for preoperative planning, is better at detecting suprarenal aneurysms, and shows retroperitoneal bleeding not visible on ultrasound. CT can also reveal alternative etiologies for abdominal pain and can be considered a first-line diagnostic modality in stable patients (Figure 29-1).

PROCEDURES

Bedside ultrasound allows for rapid detection of an aortic aneurysm. Place the abdominal probe in the epigastric area in the transverse plane (Figure 29-2). The aorta is located anterior and just to the left of the vertebral bodies. Move the probe inferiorly until the aorta bifurcates at the umbilicus. Next, rotate the probe 90 degrees to obtain a longitudinal view.

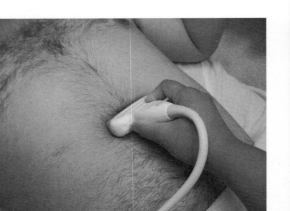

A

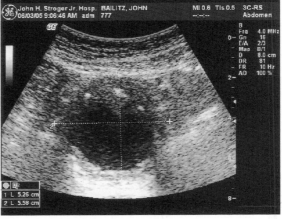

B

▲ **Figure 29-2.** Ultrasound of an AAA. **A.** Transverse position of probe. **B.** Transverse view of AAA.

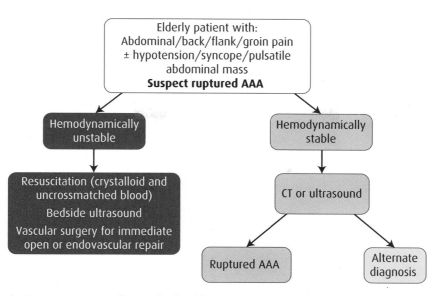

Figure 29-3. AAA diagnostic algorithm.

MEDICAL DECISION MAKING

AAA must be ruled out in any elderly patient who presents with abdominal, back, flank, or groin pain. Hemodynamically stable patients can be evaluated with CT, whereas unstable patients are better assessed with a bedside ultrasound (Figure 29-3). Other emergent causes of abdominal, back, and flank pain should be considered and evaluated concurrently. Consider ruptured AAA in elderly patients "found down" or with otherwise unexplained hypotension. Any patient with abdominal pain and previous repair of AAA, either open or endovascular, merits consultation with the patient's surgeon.

TREATMENT

Patients with ruptured AAA require immediate treatment in the ED with 2 large-bore (16-gauge) IV lines in the antecubital veins or a large-bore (8F) central line and subsequent resuscitation with IV crystalloid and uncrossmatched blood. The ideal goal blood pressure is not known, and many practitioners will allow relative hypotension pending definitive operative repair. A vascular surgeon should be consulted immediately, and the patient should be taken to the operating room or angiography suite as soon as possible to repair the AAA.

Unruptured, symptomatic AAAs require evaluation by a vascular surgeon. These patients may benefit from early elective repair, depending on the size of the aneurysm. Patients with incidentally discovered asymptomatic aneurysms should be referred for surveillance or elective repair. Consider smoking cessation counseling, beta-blockers, antihyperlipid agents, and low-dose aspirin, as appropriate.

DISPOSITION

▶ Admission

All patients with symptomatic AAAs should be admitted for observation, further investigation, or surgery, in consultation with a vascular surgeon. If vascular surgery consultation is not available, consider transfer. Both open and endovascular outcomes are superior in centers that perform a high volume of AAA repair. Ruptured AAA mandates immediate surgery or endovascular repair if the patient is to have any reasonable chance of survival.

▶ Discharge

Patients with an asymptomatic AAA (i.e., incidental finding) and an alternate benign cause for their symptoms may be discharged after follow-up with a vascular surgeon has been arranged and appropriate risk factor modification has been initiated.

SUGGESTED READING

Aggarwal S, Qamar A, Sharma V, et al. Abdominal aortic aneurysm: A comprehensive review. *Exp Clin Cardiol.* 2011;16:11–15.

Lewiss RE, Egan DJ, Shreves A. Vascular abdominal emergencies. *Emerg Med Clin North Am.* 2011;29:253–272.

Metcalfe D, Holt PJE, Thompson MM. The management of abdominal aortic aneurysms. *BMJ.* 2011;342:d1384.

Prince LA, Johnson GA. Aneurysms of the aorta and major arteries. In: Tintinalli JE, Stapczynski JS, Ma OJ, Cline DM, Cydulka RK, Meckler GD. *Tintinalli's Emergency Medicine: A Comprehensive Study Guide.* 7th ed. New York, NY: McGraw-Hill, 2011, pp. 453–458.

Wittels K. Aortic emergencies. *Emerg Med Clin North Am* 2011;29:789–800.

30

Gastrointestinal Bleeding

Jeffery A. Baker, MD

Key Points

- Aggressive resuscitative measures (intravenous access, crystalloid bolus, and blood products) are necessary in unstable patients with gastrointestinal (GI) bleeding.
- A negative nasogastric lavage does not completely exclude an upper GI bleed.
- A brisk upper GI bleed should be considered in the differential of patients who present with hematochezia.
- Octreotide should be administered in patients with liver disease and significant upper GI bleeding, even when the diagnosis of esophageal varices has not been confirmed.
- Emergent endoscopy should be arranged when active upper GI bleeding is present.

INTRODUCTION

Gastrointestinal (GI) bleeding accounts for 5% of admissions from the emergency department (ED). An intervention is required to stop ongoing hemorrhage in 10% of patients. Bleeding can occur anywhere along the GI tract and can be grossly divided into upper and lower sources. Upper GI bleeding is defined as occurring proximal to the ligament of Treitz (the suspensory ligament of the duodenum). Lower GI bleeding is defined as occurring distal to the ligament of Treitz. Upper GI bleeding is 4–8 times more common than lower GI bleeding.

It is not always possible to clinically distinguish between upper and lower GI bleeding in the ED, but appearance of the gastric contents and stool can provide clues to the source of the hemorrhage. Hematemesis is the vomiting of blood and indicates an upper GI bleed. "Coffee ground" emesis suggests that the blood has partially digested and that bleeding is either slow or has stopped. A nasogastric (NG) tube aspirate positive for blood also indicates an upper GI source of bleeding. NG lavage can be negative in 25% of patients with an upper GI source of bleeding because the nasogastric tube does not reliably pass the pylorus.

Melena is black, tarry stool that reflects the presence of blood in the GI tract for more than 8 hours. At least 300 mL of blood must be present to produce melena. Melena is 4 times more likely to be from an upper GI source of bleeding and almost always reflects bleeding proximal to the right side of the colon. Hematochezia is bright red or maroon-colored blood per rectum. It is 6 times more likely to be from a lower GI source. An exception is a rapid upper GI source of bleeding. Hematochezia is present in 10% of upper GI bleeds.

The three most common causes of upper GI bleeding are peptic ulcer disease, gastritis, and varices (Table 30-1). Lower GI bleeding may be due to multiple causes, but

Table 30-1. Causes of upper GI bleeding.

Cause	Percentage
Peptic ulcer (duodenal 2/3)	40%
Erosive gastritis	25%
Varices (esophageal and gastric)	20%
Mallory-Weiss tear	5%
Other (epistaxis, aortoenteric fistula, carcinoma, caustic ingestion)	10%

Table 30-2. Causes of lower GI bleeding.

Cause	Percentage
Diverticulosis	60%
Inflammatory bowel disease	13%
Hemorrhoids, anal fissure	11%
Neoplasia	9%
Coagulopathy	4%
Arteriovenous malformation	3%

diverticulosis is most common (Table 30-2). Less common causes include pseudomembranous colitis, infectious diarrhea, aortoenteric fistula, radiation colitis, mesenteric ischemia, and Meckel diverticulum.

CLINICAL PRESENTATION

▶ History

In most cases, patients will report hematemesis, coffee-ground emesis, hematochezia, or melena. The duration and frequency of these symptoms should be elicited. For hematemesis, it is important to determine whether blood was present initially or appeared after several episodes of vomiting. The latter history suggests a Mallory-Weiss tear. A history compatible with cirrhosis (chronic alcohol use, hepatitis, IV drug use) suggests varices. These patients may also have a coagulopathy, making control of hemorrhage more difficult. When bleeding has been slow but chronic, the patient may present with lightheadedness, fatigue, chest pain, or shortness of breath owing to anemia without any knowledge of GI bleeding. Patients with peptic ulcer disease may report epigastric abdominal pain related to eating. Agents that increase the risk of peptic ulcer disease include nonsteroidal anti-inflammatory drugs (NSAIDs), aspirin, and cigarettes. Elderly patients with acute hemorrhage may initially present with syncope or near-syncope.

▶ Physical Examination

Vital signs should be obtained immediately. When abnormalities are present, treatment is frequently necessary before obtaining a thorough history. Tachycardia and hypotension indicate hypovolemic shock and require immediate resuscitation. Cool, pale, and clammy skin is evidence of anemia or shock. The abdomen should be thoroughly examined, noting areas of tenderness or peritonitis. Rectal examination should be performed with Hemoccult testing. The presence of hemorrhoids should be documented. They may or may not be the source of lower GI bleeding. Examination should also elicit any evidence of the stigmata of cirrhosis including ascites, spider angioma, jaundice, or palmar erythema.

DIAGNOSTIC STUDIES

▶ Laboratory

Complete blood count, electrolytes, renal function, and coagulation studies should be obtained. It is important to remember that a normal hemoglobin value does not rule out a massive acute hemorrhage. Compensatory hemodilution may not occur for 2–3 hours. Blood bank should be contacted for immediate type and screen. Blood products should be ordered for patients with unstable vital signs or significant blood loss. Upper GI bleeding may elevate blood urea nitrogen because of the digestion and absorption of hemoglobin.

▶ Imaging

Upright chest x-ray is indicated in patients with suspicion of perforation or aspiration. The presence of free air under the diaphragm is diagnostic of perforation and is a surgical emergency. Routine imaging otherwise offers little clinical value in GI bleeding.

▶ Electrocardiogram

An electrocardiogram should be obtained on patients with risk factors for coronary artery disease, patient with known heart disease, or patients with symptoms concerning for coronary ischemia. Silent ischemia can occur as a result of decreased oxygen delivery related to blood loss.

PROCEDURES

Nasogastric aspiration should be performed on patients suspected of having an upper GI bleed. Aspirate appearing like gross blood or "coffee grounds" is evidence of an upper GI source. The stomach may then be lavaged with 200–300 mL saline to see if the aspirate clears. Note that false negatives may occur with bleeding distal to the pylorus, and false positives may occur from nasal trauma. NG aspiration is an especially uncomfortable and anxiety-provoking procedure for the patient, and the use of topical anesthetic is advised. Although NG aspiration in GI bleeding is routinely performed, it will only yield a useful diagnostic result in a minority of cases.

MEDICAL DECISION MAKING

The exact location of GI bleeding is usually not determined in the initial ED evaluation. Examination of any emesis, stool, or NG aspirate may help to determine the general location of the hemorrhage and direct further diagnostic and treatment strategies (Figure 30-1).

TREATMENT

Patients with active GI bleeding should be placed on a cardiac monitor with supplemental oxygen. Large peripheral IV catheters should be inserted in unstable patients. If these

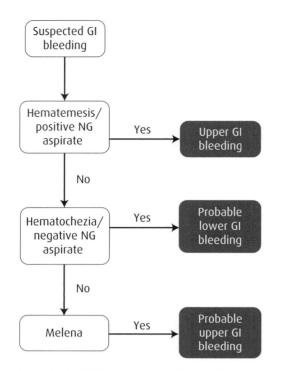

▲ **Figure 30-1.** GI bleeding diagnostic algorithm.
GI, gastrointestinal; NG, nasogastric.

lines cannot be inserted, a large-bore (8F) central line should be placed to maximize volume resuscitation. IV fluid bolus of 1–2 L of normal saline should be administered. If the patient remains unstable after the fluid bolus, administration of packed red blood cells (RBCs) is indicated. Uncross-matched type O blood is ordered for patients with unstable vital signs and significant blood loss. If a coagulopathy is suspected, fresh-frozen plasma is also ordered.

For upper GI bleeding, histamine-2 antagonists are frequently administered, although they have not been shown to be of any benefit in the acute setting. Proton pump inhibitors decrease the rate of re-bleeding. Pantoprazole 80 mg IV bolus followed by 5 mg/hr infusion is recommended. Octreotide is beneficial in decreasing the rate of bleeding, the incidence of rebleeding, and mortality by decreasing portal hypertension. It is particularly useful in variceal bleeding, but may also reduce bleeding from nonvariceal sources. Administer a 50-mcg IV bolus followed by 50 mcg/hr IV drip. Emergent endoscopy is indicated for patients with fresh blood in the NG aspirate and hematochezia from an upper GI source. Patients with liver disease also benefit from early endoscopic intervention. Surgical intervention may be required in patients with uncontrolled hemorrhage, perforation, or patients with liver disease and portal hypertension.

In the setting of a suspected lower GI source of bleeding, consult gastroenterology and surgical services early in unstable patients. Diagnostic and therapeutic options include

angiography, technetium-labeled RBC scan, colonoscopy, or surgical intervention for partial colectomy. Angiography allows for localization and arterial embolization, whereas a technetium-labeled RBC scan localizes the bleeding site only. In emergent cases, colonoscopy misses the diagnosis in 40% of cases because of poor bowel preparation. When the site of bleeding is identified during colonoscopy, it may allow for therapeutic interventions to stop bleeding, but is unsuccessful in 20% of cases. Surgical intervention is required in cases of massive lower GI bleeding when other therapies fail.

DISPOSITION

▶ Admission

Upper GI bleed. Most patients with an upper GI bleed require admission. Admission to an intensive care unit (ICU) setting should be strongly considered for patients with unstable vital signs, age >75 years, persistent bleeding that does not clear with NG lavage, presence of coagulopathy or severe anemia (hematocrit <20%), evidence of portal hypertension, or unstable comorbid conditions.

Lower GI bleed. Most patients with lower GI bleeding will require admission. ICU admission is appropriate for unstable patients. Mortality is higher in elderly patients with comorbidities, and these features should prompt consideration for admission to an intensive care setting.

▶ Discharge

Upper GI bleed. Discharge with close follow-up can be arranged for reliable patients who meet all of the following criteria: age <65 years, no comorbidities including coagulopathy, no significant liver disease, normal vital signs, negative NG lavage and no melena, and a hemoglobin >10 gm/dL. Recent clinical scoring systems (Glasgow-Blatchford bleeding score) may help predict which patients can be safely discharged from the ED without endoscopy.

Lower GI bleed. Young stable patients with normal hemoglobin, no active bleeding, evidence of hemorrhoids or fissures as a possible source, and no evidence of portal hypertension, coagulopathy, or other significant comorbidities may be discharged with close follow-up.

▼ SUGGESTED READING

Lo BM. Lower gastrointestinal bleeding. In: Tintinalli JE, Stapczynski JS, Ma OJ, Cline DM, Cydulka RK, Meckler GD. *Tintinalli's Emergency Medicine: A Comprehensive Study Guide.* 7th ed. New York, NY: McGraw-Hill, 2011, pp. 545–548.

Overton DT. Upper gastrointestinal bleeding. In: Tintinalli JE, Stapczynski JS, Ma OJ, Cline DM, Cydulka RK, Meckler GD. *Tintinalli's Emergency Medicine: A Comprehensive Study Guide.* 7th ed. New York, NY: McGraw-Hill, 2011, pp. 543–545.

Stanley AJ, Ashley D, Dalton HR, et al. Outpatient management of patients with low-risk upper-gastrointestinal haemorrhage: Multicentre validation and prospective evaluation. *Lancet.* 2009;373:42.

Intestinal Obstruction

Conor D. Schaye, MD
Colleen N. Hickey, MD

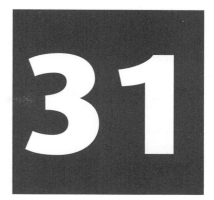

Key Points

- Intestinal obstruction presents with acute abdominal pain, abdominal distension, and vomiting.
- Abdominal radiographs can demonstrate obstruction, but computed tomography is more sensitive.
- Intestinal obstruction is treated with intravenous fluids, nasogastric suctioning, antiemetics, narcotic pain medications, and antibiotics in select cases.
- Strangulation is a complication of obstruction that can lead to bowel ischemia, peritonitis, and sepsis.

INTRODUCTION

Intestinal obstruction refers to failure of intestinal contents to pass through the bowel lumen. Mechanical obstruction refers to physical blockage of luminal contents. This occurs in either small bowel (80% of cases) or large bowel (20% of cases). The most common cause of mechanical obstruction is adhesions from prior abdominal surgery (50%), followed by malignancy (20%), hernias (10%), inflammatory bowel disease (5%), and volvulus (3%).

Intestinal obstructions can be either partial or complete. Partial obstructions are often managed nonoperatively. Complete obstructions carry more risk of morbidity and can result in strangulation. As bowel contents are prevented from forward flow, increased secretions result in overdistention, which causes bowel wall edema and reduced lymphatic and venous outflow. This is referred to as strangulation and can progress to bowel ischemia, necrosis, perforation, and peritonitis. Up to 40% of small bowel obstructions become strangulated, most commonly from volvulus, adhesions, and hernias. A closed-loop obstruction occurs when there is mechanical blockage both proximal and distal to a bowel segment. This results in very high risk of strangulation because bowel contents are prevented from both forward and retrograde flow.

Small bowel obstructions represent 15% of hospital admissions for acute abdominal pain. Approximately 300,000 operations are performed every year in the United States for obstruction. Mortality rate overall is approximately 5%, whereas the mortality rate from strangulated obstructions approaches 30%.

In contrast to mechanical obstruction, functional obstruction (eg, adynamic ileus) occurs when intestinal contents fail to pass because of disturbances in gut motility. It most commonly occurs immediately after surgery, but can also be seen in inflammatory conditions, electrolyte abnormalities, and from certain medications (namely, narcotics). Unless noted otherwise, the remainder of this chapter refers to mechanical obstruction.

CLINICAL PRESENTATION

▶ History

The most common initial complaint is intermittent colicky abdominal pain. If the obstruction is proximal, the patient may also complain of nausea and vomiting. More distal obstructions can result in delayed onset of vomiting. Although obstipation (lack of flatus and bowel movements) can suggest an obstruction, the presence of flatus or bowel movements should not be used as evidence that an obstruction has *not* occurred, as these can be seen early in the course of even complete obstructions. The patient history should include questions about prior surgeries, history of hernias, and history of obstruction in the past, as prior intestinal obstructions have up to 50% recurrence rate.

Physical Examination

Vital signs may be normal or abnormal. Fever, tachycardia, and hypotension are ominous signs and may suggest peritonitis or sepsis. Patients will usually appear uncomfortable regardless of their position. Physical exam is significant for a distended, diffusely tender abdomen, tympany to percussion, and hyperactive bowel sounds. If strangulation has occurred there may be peritonitis on exam. Patients should be examined for evidence of prior abdominal surgeries (eg, incision scars) and examined for hernias.

DIAGNOSTIC STUDIES

Laboratory

Electrolyte abnormalities such as hypokalemia and acid–base disturbances can occur due to vomiting. Third spacing of fluid and dehydration from vomiting may cause elevated blood urea nitrogen or creatinine. Intestinal ischemia can cause an anion gap metabolic acidosis with an elevated lactic acid. Leukocytosis may be present on a complete blood count and also suggests ischemia or peritonitis. Consideration should be given to checking liver function studies, amylase, lipase, and urinalysis to evaluate for other etiologies of the patient's symptoms.

Imaging

Radiographs are 50-66% sensitive in diagnosing an intestinal obstruction. An "obstructive series" classically consists of 3 radiographs: upright chest film, supine abdominal film, and upright abdominal film. A lateral decubitus x-ray may also be included. The upright chest film is used to evaluate for evidence of perforation (free air under the diaphragm). The upright abdominal film will show dilated loops of bowel (>3 cm), air-fluid levels (layering of intestinal contents), and absence of air in the rectum (Figure 31-1A). The "string of pearls" sign is a series of small pockets of gas in a row. It represents a predominance of fluid in the bowel lumen with small amounts of air trapped between the valvulae conniventes of the bowel. In adynamic ileus, radiographs will demonstrate dilation of the bowel without air-fluid levels.

An abdominal CT scan is much more sensitive than radiographs (92-100% sensitive) (Figure 31-1B). CT also has the advantage of being able to determine the location of obstruction, as well as bowel wall edema, and findings suggestive of bowel ischemia. A CT scan may also show the cause of the obstruction (eg, hernia, malignancy). If no cause is identified, adhesions may be the etiology. In patients with fever, localized abdominal pain, or abnormal vital signs, a CT scan should be the initial study of choice owing to its greater sensitivity and the need for timely diagnosis.

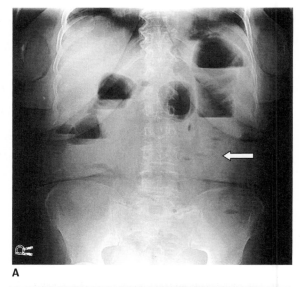

A

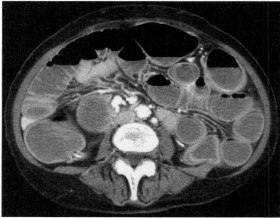

B

▲ **Figure 31-1. A.** Upright abdominal radiograph of small bowel obstruction. Note the multiple air-fluid levels and the "string of pearls" sign (arrow). **B.** Abdominal CT scan demonstrating bowel obstruction.

PROCEDURES

Most intestinal obstructions benefit from decompression with a nasogastric (NG) tube. Placement of an NG tube is uncomfortable for the patient and should be carried out in the following manner to decrease pain and anxiety:

1. Sit the patient upright with the head of the stretcher at 90°. Determine which nostril is less congested by having the patient blow the nose on both sides. Inject viscous lidocaine into the nostril or alternatively spray benzocaine into the nostril and mouth.

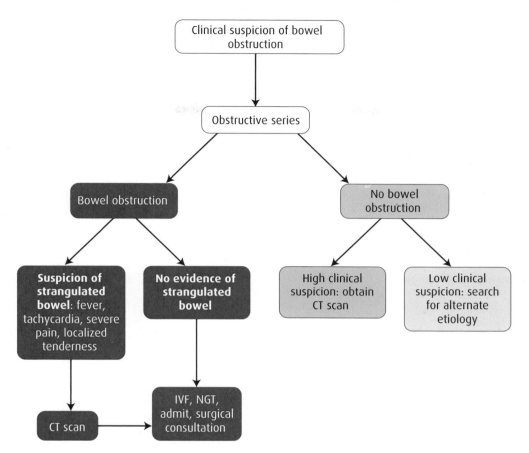

▲ **Figure 31-2.** Intestinal obstruction diagnostic algorithm. CT, computed tomography; IVF, Intravenous fluids; NGT, nasogastric tube.

2. Insert the NG tube straight back until the tip is at the posterior pharynx, and then pause. Give the patient a glass of water with a straw. Instruct the patient that as they begin to swallow the water, you will insert the tube.

3. Insert the tube as the patient swallows. The tube is inserted to approximately 30-40 cm. Coughing after placement suggests inadvertent placement in the lung.

4. *Check the location of the tube by inserting 60 mL of air and listening over the stomach for gurgling.* Aspiration of stomach contents will also indicate that the tube is in the proper location. An abdominal radiograph should be used to confirm the correct location.

5. Tape the tube securely to the nose. Place the tube to low intermittent suction (LIS).

MEDICAL DECISION MAKING

Diagnosis of intestinal obstruction relies on careful patient history, physical exam, and interpretation of imaging studies (Figure 31-2). Obstruction should be considered in any patient with a history of prior surgeries, as adhesions are the leading cause. Do not rule out obstruction based on the presence of flatus or bowel movements or the lack of vomiting, as these findings may develop later. If clinical suspicion is high enough, consider starting with a CT scan instead of radiographs. If the patient appears acutely ill, begin with resuscitation and consult a surgeon immediately even if imaging studies have not been completed.

TREATMENT

Establish intravenous (IV) access promptly and begin administration of fluids. An initial bolus of 1–2 L of 0.9 normal saline is appropriate, but some patients may require more aggressive fluid resuscitation to replace third-spaced volume loss. Antiemetics should be given (ondansetron 4 mg IV, prochlorperazine 10 mg IV, promethazine 25 mg IV). Consider narcotic pain medications (morphine 4 mg IV, hydromorphone 0.5 mg IV) and repeat as needed. An NG tube should be inserted once the diagnosis of obstruction has been made and should be placed to low intermittent suction (LIS). This results in decompression of the bowel lumen, provides symptomatic relief, and may avoid the need for surgery. Broad-spectrum antibiotics that cover gram-negative and anaerobic organisms (eg, piperacillin-tazobactam, ciprofloxacin plus metronidazole) should be given in the presence of fever, peritonitis, or evidence of strangulation. Surgical consultation should be obtained in case the patient requires surgical intervention. For patients with adynamic ileus, treatment involves cessation of any narcotic medications and initiation of motility agents (eg, metoclopramide).

DISPOSITION

▶ Admission

All patients with intestinal obstruction require admission, either to a surgical service or a medicine service with a surgeon on consult. Most patients can be admitted to floor units. Intensive care unit admission is indicated for patients with unstable vital signs (tachycardia, hypotension) or sepsis. Urgent surgery is required in patients with peritonitis, perforation, or strangulation.

▶ Discharge

None.

▼ SUGGESTED READING

Diaz JJ Jr, Bokhari F, Mowery NT. Guidelines for management of small bowel obstruction. *J Trauma.* 2008 Jun;64(6):1651–64.

Markogiannakis H, Messaris E, Dardamanis D. Acute mechanical bowel obstruction: clinical presentation, etiology, management and outcome. *World J Gastroenterol.* 2007 Jan 21;13(3): 432–7.

Miller G, Boman J, Shrier I, Gordan PH. Etiology of small bowel obstruction. *Am J Surg.* 2000 Jul;180(1):33–6

Vicario SJ, Price TG. Bowel obstruction and volvulus. In: Tintinalli JE, Stapczynski JS, Ma OJ, Cline DM, Cydulka RK, Meckler GD. *Tintinalli's Emergency Medicine: A Comprehensive Study Guide.* 7th ed. New York, NY: McGraw-Hill, 2011, pp. 581–583.

Mesenteric Ischemia

Ross A. Heller, MD

Carl M. Kraemer, MD

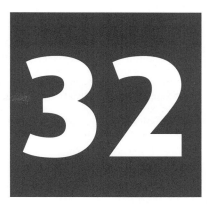

Key Points

- The classic presentation of mesenteric ischemia is acute abdominal pain that is "out of proportion" to exam.
- The majority of patients with mesenteric ischemia have an embolus due to atrial fibrillation.
- Morbidity and mortality remains very high despite advances in care, and survival is dependent on early recognition and treatment.
- Obtain early surgical consultation if mesenteric ischemia is suspected.

INTRODUCTION

Acute mesenteric ischemia is a syndrome characterized by inadequate blood flow to the mesentery with resultant hypoxemia of the tissue. Over time, the hypoxemia results in tissue break down with loss of bowel integrity.

The incidence of mesenteric ischemia is reported to be 0.1% of hospitalized patients, and this number is thought to be increasing as the average age of the population increases. The mortality is more than 60%. Delay in diagnosis is common, but with reports that early intervention increases survival rate, it is important to always have this diagnosis in the differential for elderly patients presenting with abdominal pain.

Four etiologies of mesenteric ischemia are described, and each has different risk factors and variation in presentation. The most common cause of mesenteric ischemia is arterial emboli (50%), usually owing to atrial fibrillation. Arterial thrombosis at the narrowing of mesenteric arteries in patients with atherosclerosis is responsible for 20% of acute presentations. These patients frequently have other forms of atherosclerosis such as coronary artery disease. Mesenteric venous thrombosis, which may be associated with peripheral deep vein thrombosis, accounts for 5–10% of presentations. Nonocclusive mesenteric ischemia is seen in up to 20–25% of presentations. It is due to low flow states typically seen in shock syndromes. It occurs most commonly in hospitalized patients and is difficult to diagnose.

The mesenteric vessel affected is responsible for the presenting symptoms and area of injury. The superior mesenteric artery (SMA) is the most commonly involved site because of the sharp takeoff of this vessel from the aorta. Approximately 80% of mesenteric blood flow supplies the bowel mucosa, making it the most sensitive to ischemia.

CLINICAL PRESENTATION

▶ History

Symptoms are nonspecific and common to many conditions. Abdominal pain, nausea, vomiting, and diarrhea are frequently seen. Any patient older than 50 years with risk factors (eg, atrial fibrillation) who experiences acute onset abdominal pain lasting >2 hours should be suspected of having acute mesenteric ischemia. Pain out of proportion to the physical examination is very concerning for mesenteric ischemia. Late findings include peritonitis (eg, pain with movement), fever, weakness, and altered mental status.

Patients with chronic mesenteric ischemia will give a history of "abdominal angina" or pain after eating. This is due to narrowing of the mesenteric artery usually associated with chronic atherosclerosis. With eating there is increased demand for blood flow, causing a relative ischemia until demand is lowered. These patients go on to have thrombotic occlusion of their narrowed vessels, presenting then with the common acute symptoms.

Physical Examination

Early physical findings may be nonexistent or nonspecific. A patient complaining of extreme pain who has an essentially normal abdominal exam (especially no pain on palpation) should prompt consideration of mesenteric ischemia. If not diagnosed at this stage, the ischemia progresses to necrosis and perforation. The physical examination will then reveal abdominal distension and peritonitis. Hemoccult positive stools are found in only 25% of cases.

DIAGNOSTIC STUDIES

Laboratory

Lab testing is usually nonspecific and therefore of little help ruling in or excluding the diagnosis. The white blood cell count is frequently high, but this is nonspecific. There is a lack of consensus on the role of lactic acid. It has 100% sensitivity if there is bowel infarction; however, it may be normal early. If elevated at presentation, it predicts a higher morbidity and mortality and should prompt an aggressive search for ischemia. An electrocardiogram should be performed to diagnose atrial fibrillation.

Imaging

The classic reported finding on plain radiographs is "thumb-printing," representing bowel wall thickening and edema. However, this is a mid to late finding and is seen in only 40% of patients. Nonspecific findings such as ileus are seen in up to 60% of patients. Pneumatosis intestinalis, portal venous air, and free air are late findings (Figure 32-1A).

Computed tomography (CT) angiography is much more sensitive and frequently shows bowel edema, lack of arterial flow, or venous thrombus with ischemia. It has become the imaging study of choice in suspected acute mesenteric ischemia (Figure 32-1B).

MEDICAL DECISION MAKING

Any patient who is part of the "at risk" population who presents with moderate to severe abdominal pain should be considered at risk for mesenteric ischemia (Figure 32-2). A lactic acid level should be obtained as soon as possible and the stool should be tested for blood. Involve your surgical consultant early. If the diagnosis is in question, a CT angiogram should be performed.

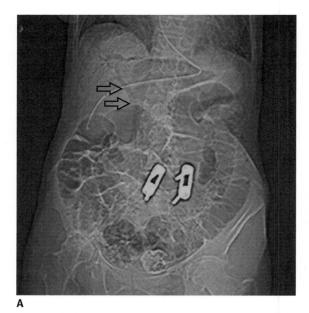

A

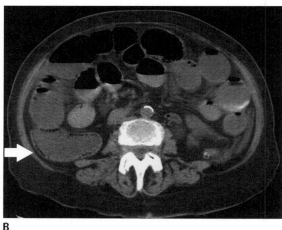

B

▲ **Figure 32-1. A.** Portal venous air, a late finding of mesenteric ischemia, is seen in this patient (arrows). **B.** Pneumatosis intestinalis demonstrated in a loop of bowel on CT scan (arrow).

TREATMENT

In the emergency department, aggressive fluid therapy to correct hypotension and hypovolemia is instituted. Central venous access and monitoring may be necessary. Administer broad-spectrum antibiotics in the setting of suspected perforation.

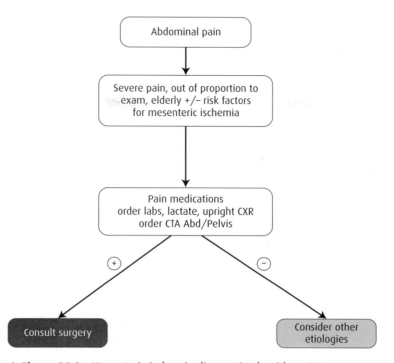

▲ **Figure 32-2.** Mesenteric ischemia diagnostic algorithm. CTA, computed tomography angiogram; CXR, chest x-ray.

Surgery is the mainstay of treatment for mesenteric ischemia due to embolus or thrombosis. Early surgical consultation has been shown to improve outcomes even in patients ultimately treated nonsurgically. Patients with ischemia due to nonocclusive disease or venous thrombosis are not amenable to surgery, but surgery may be necessary to remove necrotic bowel. There are several nonsurgical management options involving angiography. Infusion of papaverine into the SMA for vasodilation has been reported to improve survival rate. Venous thrombosis is treated with anticoagulation.

DISPOSITION

All patients with mesenteric ischemia need rapid surgical consult and admission.

SUGGESTED READINGS

Deehan DJ, Heys SD, Brittenden J. Mesenteric ischemia: prognostic factors and Influence of delay upon outcome. *J R Coll Surg Edinb.* 1995;40:112–115.

Edwards MS, Cherr GS, Craven TE. Acute occlusive mesenteric ischemia: surgical management and outcomes. *Ann Vasc Surg.* 2003;17:72–79.

O'Brien MC. Acute abdominal pain. In: Tintinalli JE, Stapczynski JS, Ma OJ, Cline DM, Cydulka RK, Meckler GD. *Tintinalli's Emergency Medicine: A Comprehensive Study Guide.* 7th ed. New York, NY: McGraw-Hill, 2011, pp. 519–527.

Oldenburg WA, Lau LL, Rodenberg TJ. Acute mesenteric ischemia. *Arch Intern Med.* 2004;164:1054.

Ruotolo RA, Evans SR. Mesenteric ischemia in the elderly. *Clin Geriatr Med.* 1999;15:527–557.

Fever

Krista A. Grandey, DO

Key Points

- Fever is a symptom, not a disease.
- Fever should not be confused with hyperthermia. Temperatures higher than 41°C (105.8°F) are almost always due to hyperthermia and not fever.
- Be thoughtful in your evaluation of fever to avoid misdiagnosing a serious bacterial illness as "just another viral syndrome."
- Provide empiric antibiotics early for moderate to severely ill patients with a possible infectious etiology. Give directed antibiotic treatment in the emergency department to patients with serious focal bacterial infections.

INTRODUCTION

The human body temperature is controlled within a narrow range between 36 and 37.8 °C (96.8 –100.4°F). Fever is defined as a core temperature >38° C (100.4 °F) in infants and >38.3°C (100.9°F) in adults. It is the result of the body resetting the temperature control center, the hypothalamus, in response to infection. Endogenous (cytokines) and exogenous (bacterial and viral) pyrogens trigger production of prostaglandin E2 (PGE2) in the hypothalamus. PGE2 raises the hypothalamic temperature set point. The body then generates and conserves heat to reach this new hypothalamic set point, thereby raising the body temperature. Fever is sustained as long as the levels of pyrogens and PGE2 are elevated. Cyclooxygenase inhibitors decrease fever by blocking the production of PGE2.

Fever is one of the most common presenting complaints in the emergency department (ED). It accounts for 5% of adult visits, 15% of elderly visits and 40% of pediatric visits to the ED. The most important thing to recognize about fever is that it is a symptom, not a disease, and it represents an underlying problem that must be evaluated and treated. The most common sites of infection vary based on age and immune system status. In the elderly and immunosuppressed, respiratory, genitourinary, and bacterial skin infections predominate. In younger patients the cause of fever is often self-limited and benign (eg, upper respiratory infection), but serious focal bacterial infections (eg, meningitis) requiring antibiotics, diagnostic procedures, and admission, must be detected.

CLINICAL PRESENTATION

▶ History

The differential diagnosis for fever is quite broad, but in 85% of cases the cause is identified by a thorough history and physical examination. Important historical information includes the onset, magnitude, duration, pattern, any associated symptoms, travel within the past year, chronic illnesses, recent medication changes, recent hospitalizations, chemotherapy, radiotherapy, or the presence of indwelling vascular access devices or artificial heart valves. The age and overall health of the patient must be taken into account when taking the history and making medical decisions.

▶ Physical Examination

The site of temperature recording should be noted, as rectal temperatures are more accurate and usually 1°C higher than oral temperatures. Rectal temperature should be

Table 33-1. Physical examination in fever.

General	Cachexia or other signs of chronic illness
Neurologic	Perform a brief mental status examination. In the elderly, AMS may be the only sign of an occult infection.
Ear, nose, and throat	Examine the tympanic membranes and pharynx for evidence of otitis media or exudative pharyngitis. Assess the neck for thyroid enlargement, lymphadenopathy, and meningismus.
Chest	Auscultate for evidence of pneumonia (eg, rales or rhonchi), new murmurs suggesting endocarditis, or the rub of pericarditis.
Abdomen	Palpate for signs of focal or generalized peritonitis. Check for costovertebral angle tenderness. Perform a genitourinary examination in males and a pelvic examination in females with abdominal pain.
Skin	Disrobe the patient and examine for rashes (petechiae of meningococcemia) or focal infection (joint inflammation, cellulitis, infected ulcers, or abscess).

taken in infants, children, and adults with significant tachypnea, tachycardia, or altered mental status (AMS). Heart rate (HR) and respiratory rate (RR) increase as fever rises. An increase in temperature of 1°C results in an increase in HR by approximately 10 bpm. The RR may also increase 2-4 breaths/minute per degree Celsius. The elderly and immunosuppressed patients may not mount a febrile response despite serious infection.

In most patients, the examination is directed by the patient's symptoms (Table 33-1). Patients with significant alterations in mental status, respiratory distress, and cardiovascular instability require rapid assessment and stabilization. Once the patient has been stabilized, assess for infectious causes that may be a threat to life (eg, toxic shock, septic shock, meningitis, peritonitis).

DIAGNOSTIC STUDIES

▶ Laboratory

In children and the elderly, the highest yield laboratory test will be the urinalysis. It is highly accurate for urinary tract infection. In most cases, a complete blood count (CBC) will be sent to look for an elevated white blood cell (WBC) count, but this test lacks specificity and sensitivity. The WBC count can be normal in cases of severe infection or falsely elevated when no infection is present. The most helpful component of the CBC is the neutrophil count, as it can provide a measure of response to infection or determine whether a patient is neutropenic and unable to mount a response to infection (eg, immunocompromised chemotherapy patient). Gram stains, blood, urine, and

wound cultures can be obtained in the ED. Although not helpful in the ED management of the patient, these studies direct targeted antibiotic therapy in the future.

▶ Imaging

The chest x-ray is helpful in patients with suspected pneumonia, but may be difficult to interpret in the dehydrated patient or those with underlying pulmonary or cardiovascular disorders. For patients with abdominal pain, a computed tomography (CT) scan of the abdomen can be performed to evaluate for appendicitis, diverticulitis, cholecystitis, and intra-abdominal abscess. A head CT should be performed for patients with focal neurologic findings, seizures, AMS, human immunodeficiency virus (HIV)/acquired immune deficiency syndrome or signs of increased intracranial pressure. The administration of antibiotics should not be delayed in patients with suspected meningitis awaiting CT scan results.

PROCEDURES

For patients with altered mental status or meningismus, a lumbar puncture should be performed to evaluate the cerebrospinal fluid for infectious causes (see Chapter 5).

MEDICAL DECISION MAKING

The differential diagnosis for fever is extensive, and the cause can be infectious or noninfectious. The majority of causes of fever are infectious (Table 33-2). Noninfectious causes include pulmonary embolism, intracranial hemorrhage, cerebrovascular accident, neuroleptic malignant syndrome/serotonin syndrome, malignant hyperthermia, thyroid

Table 33-2. Differential diagnosis of infectious causes of fever.

Neurologic	Meningitis, cavernous sinus thrombosis, encephalitis, or brain abscess
Respiratory/ear, nose, and throat	Epiglottitis, retropharyngeal abscess, pneumonia, peritonsillar abscess, otitis media, pharyngitis, sinusitis, or upper respiratory infection
Cardiovascular	Endocarditis, myocarditis, or pericarditis
Gastrointestinal	Peritonitis, cholangitis, appendicitis, cholecystitis, diverticulitis, intra-abdominal abscess, colitis, or enteritis
Genitourinary	Fournier's gangrene, urinary tract infection (cystitis, pyelonephritis), tubo-ovarian abscess, pelvic inflammatory disease, epididymitis, orchitis, or prostatitis
Skin and soft tissue	Necrotizing fasciitis, cellulitis, or abscess
Bloodborne	Sepsis, bacteremia, human immunodeficiency virus, malaria

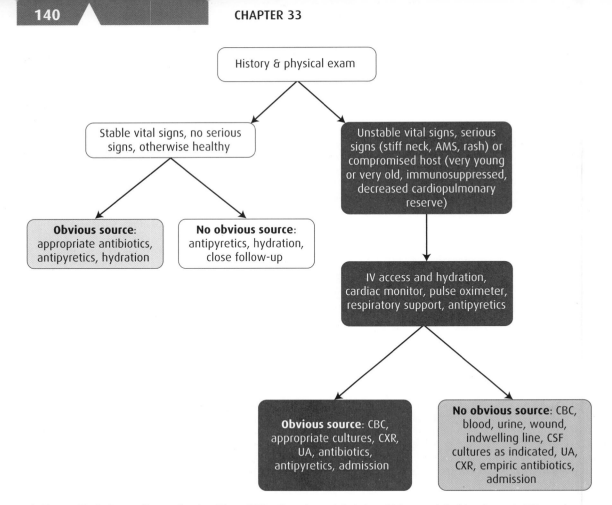

▲ **Figure 33-1.** Fever diagnostic algorithm. AMS, altered mental status; CBC, complete blood count; CSF, cerebrospinal fluid; CXR, chest x-ray; UA, urinalysis.

storm, transfusion reaction, malignancy, autoimmune disorders, or drug fever.

Use the history and physical examination to make decisions about testing and treatment. If the patient is stable and there is an obvious source of infection, antipyretics should be given and antibiotics when appropriate. In the hemodynamically unstable patient, intravenous fluid resuscitation should be initiated along with monitoring, respiratory support, and antipyretics (see Chapter 34). Empiric antibiotic treatment with broad-spectrum antibiotics should be started immediately in the ED for unstable patients if an obvious source cannot be found (Figure 33-1).

TREATMENT

Antipyretics (eg, acetaminophen or ibuprofen) are administered to increase patient comfort and reduce the metabolic demand. Patients who are stable can be treated with hydration and appropriate antibiotics. Patients with signs and symptoms of shock (eg, AMS, hypotension, tachycardia)

require monitoring and aggressive fluid resuscitation. Patients with signs of respiratory compromise or airway obstruction may require intubation. In critically ill or immunocompromised patients, administer antibiotic therapy early. If there is no known source of infection, administer broad-spectrum antibiotic therapy to cover aerobic (gram-positive and gram-negative) and anaerobic organisms. The choice of antibiotic is based on the most likely cause of the fever as well as patient considerations such as neutropenia. Antibiotic dosing may be altered in patients with renal insufficiency or in patients with specific conditions (eg, bacterial meningitis).

DISPOSITION

▶ Admission

Patients who are unstable, immunocompromised (eg, HIV, elderly, neonate), have serious localized infection (eg, meningitis), or have serious comorbidities (eg, pneumonia and congestive heart failure) should be admitted to the hospital for further stabilization and treatment. Admission may also be warranted in patients with no obvious source of infection, but signs of serious illness.

Discharge

Young healthy patients without comorbidities or serious focal infections can usually be discharged home with close follow-up.

SUGGESTED READING

Bentley DW. Practice guideline for evaluation of fever and infection in long-term care facilities. *Clin Infect Dis*. 2000;31:640–653.

Darowski A, Najim Z, Weinberg JR. The febrile response to mild infections in elderly hospital residents. *Age Ageing*. 1991;20:193–198.

Fontanarosa PB, Kaeberlein FJ, Gerson LW, Thomson RB. Difficulty in predicting bacteremia in elderly emergency patients. *Ann Emerg Med*. 1992;21:842–848.

Sepsis

Rakesh S. Engineer, MD

Key Points

- Identification of the septic patient is the important first step. All other critical actions are missed if this does not occur.
- Lactate measurement is critical to determining sepsis severity, response to therapy, and prognosis.

- Early administration of appropriate antimicrobials and early goal-directed therapy are the mainstays of treatment.
- Resuscitation of the critically ill septic patient should occur concurrent or before diagnostic evaluation.

INTRODUCTION

Sepsis is now defined as "infection plus systemic manifestations of infection" (Table 34-1). Systemic inflammatory response syndrome is no longer a strict criteria. There are 3 sepsis syndromes (stages): uncomplicated sepsis, severe sepsis, and septic shock. Sepsis becomes severe sepsis when there is tissue hypoperfusion or organ dysfunction (Table 34-2). Septic shock is defined as a systolic blood pressure (SBP) <90 mmHg or 40 mmHg below one's baseline blood pressure, despite two 20- to 30-mL/kg boluses.

Sepsis affects 751,000 patients per year, with an annual mortality that exceeds that of AIDS and breast cancer and approaches that of myocardial infarction. The lungs, abdomen, and urinary tract are the most frequent source of infection, but sepsis can come from anywhere in the body. In approximately 20% of cases, the etiology cannot be determined. Risk factors for the development of sepsis syndromes are extremes of age, immunosuppression (chemotherapy, organ transplantation, steroid use, HIV, etc.), severe comorbid disease, exposure to multiple drug-resistant organisms, vascular catheters and other indwelling devices, intravenous (IV) drug abuse, trauma, and burns.

CLINICAL PRESENTATION

▶ History

Any patient presenting with an infectious syndrome should be considered for potential sepsis. Those at the extremes of age or the immunosuppressed may not mount a fever. Other patients may have defervesced before triage vital signs. High clinical suspicion will be required in properly identifying these patients. Furthermore, patients with reduced physiologic reserve are at risk for rapid clinical deterioration.

History should elicit the source of infection. Straightforward complaints include cough, purulent phlegm, headache with stiff neck, dysuria, or rashes. More subtle cues include fluctuating mentation suggesting delirium; rigors suggest influenza, pneumonia, and biliary sepsis; and fevers shortly after administration of total parenteral nutrition (TPN) suggest central line infection.

▶ Physical Examination

As with all potentially unstable patients, airway, breathing, and circulation (ABCs) should be assessed on arrival. Vital signs should be assessed next, remembering that lack of fever does not exclude infectious etiology. Tachycardia may be a response to fever, or it may represent a physiologic

Table 34-1. Diagnostic criteria for sepsis.

Infection, documented or suspected, and some of the following:
General variables
Fever (>38.3°C)
Hypothermia (<36°C)
Heart rate >90 beats/min
Tachypnea
Altered mental status (delirium)
Significant edema or positive fluid balance
(>20 mL/kg over 24 hrs)
Hyperglycemia (>140 mg/dL) in the absence of diabetes
Inflammatory variables
Leukocytosis (WBC count >12,000/μL)
Leukopenia (WBC count <4000/μL)
Normal WBC count with >10% immature forms
Plasma C-reactive protein >2 SD above the normal value
Plasma procalcitonin >2 SD above the normal value
Hemodynamic variables
Arterial hypotension (SBP <90 mmHg; MAP <70 mmHg; or an SBP
decrease >40 mmHg in adults or >2 SD below normal for age)
Organ dysfunction variables
Arterial hypoxemia (PaO2/FIO2 <300)
Acute oliguria (urine output <0.5 ml/kg/hr for at least 2 hrs,
despite adequate fluid resuscitation)
Creatinine increase >0.5 mg/dL
Coagulation abnormalities (INR >1.5 or a PTT > 60 secs)
Ileus (absent bowel sounds)
Thrombocytopenia (platelet count, <100,000/μL)
Hyperbilirubinemia (total bilirubin >4 mg/dL)
Tissue perfusion variables
Hyperlactatemia (>4 mmol/L)
Decreased capillary refill or mottling

Diagnostic criteria for sepsis in the pediatric population are signs and symptoms of inflammation plus infection with hyper- or hypothermia (rectal temperature >38.5°C or <35°C), tachycardia (may be absent in hypothermic patients), and at least one of the following indications of altered organ function: altered mental status, hypoxemia, increased serum lactate level, or bounding pulses.

INR, international normalized ratio; MAP, mean arterial pressure; PTT, activated partial thromboplastin time; SBP, systolic blood pressure; SD, standard deviation; WBC, white blood count.

Adapted from Levy MM, Fink MP, Marshall JC, et al: 2001 SCCM/ESICM/ACCP/ATS/SIS International Sepsis Definitions Conference, *Crit Care Med* 2003;31:1250–1256

Table 34-2. Diagnostic criteria for severe sepsis.

Severe sepsis is sepsis with tissue hypoperfusion or organ dysfunction as defined by the following criteria:
Hypotension
Lactate greater than the upper limits of normal laboratory results
Urine output <0.5 ml/kg/hr for >2 hrs, despite adequate fluid resuscitation
ALI with PaO2/FIO2 <250 in the absence of pneumonia
ALI with PaO2/FIO2 <200 in the presence of pneumonia
Creatinine >2.0 mg/dL
Bilirubin >2 mg/dL
Platelet count <100,000/μL
Coagulopathy (INR >1.5)

ALI, acute lung injury; INR, international normalized ratio.
Data from Levy MM, Fink MP, Marshall JC, et al: 2001 SCCM/ESICM/ACCP/ATS/SIS International Sepsis Definitions Conference, Intensive Care Med 2003;29:530–538. ACCP/SCCM Consensus Conference Committee: American College of Chest Physicians/Society of Critical Care Medicine Consensus Conference: Definitions for sepsis and organ failure and guidelines for the use of innovative therapies in sepsis, *Crit Care Med* 1992;20:864–874

baseline blood pressure, despite two 20- to 30-mL/kg boluses. (That's 4-6 L for a 100-kg patient!) Patients, family members, and electronic medical records can be useful in determining baseline blood pressures.

A detailed physical exam starts with general appearance, head and neck, respiratory, cardiovascular, abdominal, genitourinary, integument, and neurologic exam. Particular attention should be paid to mental status. Delirium is characterized by inattention, altered level of consciousness, and change in cognition. These symptoms tend to fluctuate over periods of time.

DIAGNOSTIC STUDIES

The purpose of diagnostic studies is to (1) determine the presence and etiology of sepsis and (2) assess the severity and response to therapy. A patient with focal symptomatology (fever, cough, purulent sputum) may need only focused evaluation (chest x-ray). The discussion that follows assumes the presentation is more nebulous.

▶ Laboratory

A typical diagnostic work-up for the presence and etiology of sepsis involves assessment for leukocytosis or leukopenia (complete blood count), two blood cultures, and urinalysis. Blood cultures should be performed before administration of antimicrobials, with at least one from a peripheral site. Each vascular access device should have one blood culture drawn. Other laboratory assessments, such as wound cultures, synovial fluid, peritoneal fluid, and

attempt to augment cardiac output. Tachypnea may be a sign of hypoxia or may represent respiratory compensation of a metabolic (lactic) acidosis. "Normal" blood pressures should not be used as an indication of stability. Shock is defined as an SBP <90 mmHg or 40 mmHg below one's

cerebrospinal fluid, should be obtained when clinical suspicion indicates.

Because severe sepsis is defined by organ failure, look for evidence of acute kidney injury, shock liver (elevated bilirubin), coagulopathy (elevated prothrombin time/international normalized ratio/partial thromboplastin time), and thrombocytopenia. PaO_2 measurement compared with FiO_2 may be useful in determining the presence of acute lung injury and acute respiratory distress syndrome.

Patients with sepsis should undergo risk stratification. This begins with initial lactate assessment with levels >4 mmol/L diagnostic for severe sepsis. Although arterial and venous samples are nearly equivalent, lactate is ideally measured at the bedside. In the time it takes for blood to travel to the lab, blood cells undergo anaerobic metabolism, causing false elevations. Repeat measurement should occur after treatment or after 6 hours. Clearance of lactate (delta lactate) of 10% or greater indicates a significant reduction in mortality, whereas no change may signify a 60% mortality.

▶ Imaging

Chest radiographs are typically included for most septic patients when the presentation is concerning or the etiology is uncertain. Targeted imaging should be considered based on clinical presentation (eg, computed tomography scan of the abdomen/pelvis in the febrile patient with abdominal pain and recent surgery for Crohn disease to assess for potential abscess).

PROCEDURES

Targeted diagnostic procedures should be considered when indicated, such as lumbar puncture for suspected meningitis or arthrocentesis for suspected septic joint.

Invasive central monitoring such as central line placement, arterial line, and urinary catheterization is indicated when there is evidence of acute end-organ failure, lactate ≥4 mmol/L, or shock.

MEDICAL DECISION MAKING

The initial step is to determine who is at risk for infection. Next, determine the sepsis severity through clinical assessment, point of care lactate, laboratory assessment for end-organ injury, and blood pressure response to fluid resuscitation. Patients with uncomplicated sepsis should have investigation to determine the infectious source and be treated with antimicrobials and fluids.

Patients with severe sepsis and septic shock should receive early aggressive resuscitation, including early antimicrobial therapy and early goal-directed therapy (EGDT). Resuscitation should occur concurrent to the diagnostic evaluation, not after it (Figure 34-1).

TREATMENT

Antibiotics should be administered as early as possible, preferably within 1 hour of recognition of septic shock. Cultures should be obtained before antibiotics, but should not delay their administration when plausible. Every hour delay decreases survival by 7.5% in the hypotensive patient. Initial empiric choice of antibiotics should be against likely pathogens. This can generally be determined by identifying the target organ of infection (eg, lung), setting that the infection was acquired (eg, nursing home), and bacterial susceptibilities within your hospital (the local antibiogram is often available on hospital's internal website).

Patients with severe sepsis or septic shock with a lactate >4 mmol/L or hypotension unresponsive to fluids should receive a bundle of therapies referred to as EGDT. These patients should have a central line and Foley catheter placed for monitoring. An arterial line may also be necessary to accurately measure blood pressure.

The goals of this approach include optimizing preload, afterload, and central venous oxygen saturation ($ScvO_2$) in a stepwise approach. Preload is addressed with fluid resuscitation in the form of 1,000 mL crystalloid boluses administered over 30 minutes and repeated as necessary to achieve a central venous pressure of 8-12 mmHg. Once achieved, afterload is treated with vasopressors (norepinephrine or dopamine) to raise the mean arterial pressure to ≥65 mmHg.

$ScvO_2$ is a measurement of oxygen saturation in blood returning to the superior vena cava. When low, either the body is delivering inadequate oxygen or the tissues need to extract a large amount to correct their oxygen debt. The goal is to achieve a $ScvO_2$ ≥70%. Oxygen delivery (DO_2) can be augmented by administering additional oxygen (maximize the pulse oximetry), increasing oxygen carrying capacity with blood transfusions to a hematocrit of 30%, and increasing oxygen delivery by "whipping" the heart with dobutamine for greater inotropy. If that is unsuccessful, then oxygen utilization (VO_2) can be reduced by sedating, paralyzing, and intubating the patient. A decrease in post-treatment lactate by 10% has been shown to be equivalent to achieving a $ScvO_2$ ≥70%, utilizing the same treatment algorithm.

There are conflicting data on the benefits of steroids in septic shock. Hydrocortisone may be considered in adult patients who are vasopressor refractory or who are steroid dependent.

Lastly, source control involves removal of the nidus of infection when possible (eg, removal of infected central lines or drainage of abscesses).

DISPOSITION

▶ Admission

Most patients with sepsis syndromes will require admission. Patients with persistently elevated lactates,

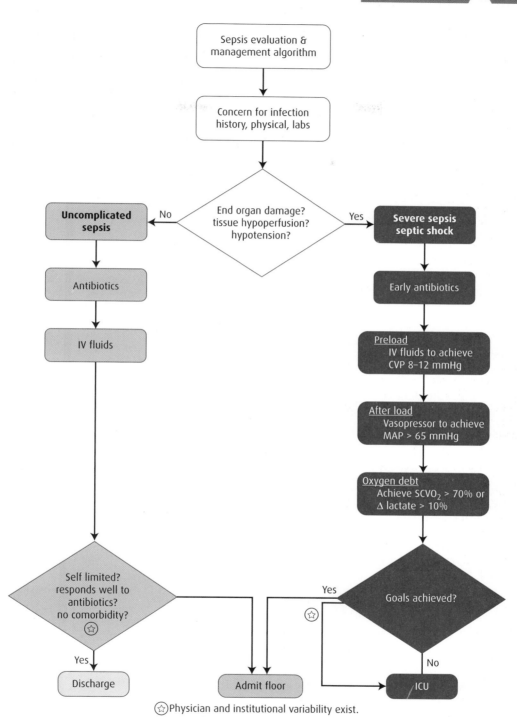

▲ **Figure 34-1.** Sepsis diagnostic algorithm.

hypotension requiring vasopressors, or respiratory failure requiring ventilatory support should be admitted to an intensive care unit. Other patients may be admitted to general medical floor or step down, depending on the nursing ratios and capabilities of that particular unit.

▶ Discharge

A minority of sepsis patients may be discharged. Typically, these are young, healthy patients without tissue hypoperfusion or end-organ failure who have normalized their vital signs and have self-limited infections or infections that are rapidly responsive to antimicrobial therapy. Viral pharyngitis, strep throat, and pyelonephritis are examples of infections that often may enable the patient to be discharged to home.

SUGGESTED READING

Booker E. Sepsis, severe sepsis, and septic shock: Current evidence for Emergency Department management. *Emerg Med Pract*. 2011;13:1-24.

Dellinger RP, Levy MM, Carlet JM, et al. Surviving Sepsis Campaign: International guidelines for management of severe sepsis and septic shock. *Crit Care Med*. 2008;36:296–327 [published correction appears in *Crit Care Med*. 2008;36:1394–1396].

Jones AE, Shapiro NI, Trzeciak S, et al. Lactate clearance vs central venous oxygen saturation as goals of early sepsis therapy: A randomized clinical trial. *JAMA*. 2010;303:739–746.

Jui J. Septic shock. In: Tintinalli JE, Kelen GD, Stapczynski JS, eds. *Tintinalli's Emergency Medicine: A Comprehensive Study Guide*. 7th ed. New York, NY: McGraw-Hill, 2011, pp. 1003–1014.

Kumar A, Roberts D, Woods KE, et al. Duration of hypotension prior to initiation of effective antimicrobial therapy is the critical determinant of survival in human septic shock. *Crit Care Med*. 2006;34:1589–1596.

Rivers E, Nguyen B, Havstad S, et al. Early goal-directed therapy for the treatment of severe sepsis and septic shock. *N Engl J Med*. 2001;345:1368–1377.

Society of Critical Care Medicine. Surviving Sepsis Campaign. www.survivingsepsis.org

Meningitis and Encephalitis

Elizabeth W. Kelly, MD

Michael T. Fitch, MD

Key Points

- The classic triad of meningitis includes fever, neck stiffness, and altered mental status. However, all 3 of these are present less than half of patients with bacterial meningitis.

- Patients who are very young, very old, or immunocompromised may present with atypical signs and symptoms.

- Empiric antibiotics should not be delayed while waiting for a computed tomography (CT) scan before a lumbar puncture (LP) if meningitis is a likely diagnosis. When a CT scan is necessary, draw blood cultures and administer steroids and appropriate antibiotics before the LP.

- Consider the diagnosis of herpes simplex virus encephalitis in patients with focal neurologic findings or altered mental status and add intravenous acyclovir to the empiric antimicrobial regimen.

INTRODUCTION

Bacterial meningitis and viral encephalitis are life-threatening causes of infection and inflammation within the central nervous system (CNS). In the early stages of illness the diagnosis can be very challenging, and evaluation is focused on identifying patients who require urgent diagnostic testing and treatment.

Until antibiotics became available at the beginning of the 20th century, bacterial meningitis was nearly 100% fatal. Morbidity and mortality still remain high even with appropriate treatment. Meningitis affects patients of all ages, but those at the extremes of age or immunosuppressed are at increased risk. Accurate diagnosis, timely administration of antibiotics, and other adjunctive therapies (eg, dexamethasone) are important for patients with suspected bacterial disease.

Meningitis is an inflammatory process of the membranes that surround the brain and spinal cord. The most common causative agents of bacterial meningitis are encapsulated organisms, namely *Streptococcus pneumoniae* and *Neisseria meningitidis*. *Listeria monocytogenes* more commonly infects older patients (>50 years old), infants (<3 months old), and immunocompromised or pregnant individuals. These pathogens often invade the host through the upper airway by infecting the mucosa and bloodstream and ultimately cross the blood–brain barrier, entering the CNS. CNS inoculation can also occur after trauma, surgery, or a contiguous infection such as sinusitis or otitis media.

Changes in epidemiology have mirrored vaccination practices in children and adults against *Haemophilus influenzae, S. pneumoniae,* and *N. meningitidis.* Routine childhood vaccination against *H. influenza* type b has helped decrease this pathogen as a cause of meningitis. Use of the pneumococcal vaccine in adults may be reducing the rate of *S. pneumoniae* disease. Given the success of routine childhood vaccination programs, over the past 25 years, the median age of a patient diagnosed with meningitis has risen from 15 months to 42 years of age.

Aseptic meningitis is due to inflammation from other causes such as drugs, rheumatologic conditions, or nonbacterial infections. Most cases are caused by viral (the most common overall causes of meningitis) or mycobacterial infections. Of the viral etiologies, enteroviruses and echoviruses are the most common, but herpes simplex virus (HSV) is an important pathogen.

Encephalitis is an infection of the brain parenchyma causing inflammation within the CNS. Viral pathogens include HSV, which is the most treatable cause of encephalitis. In the acute care setting, it can be difficult to distinguish encephalitis from severe cases of bacterial meningitis, as patients' signs and symptoms may be similar.

CLINICAL PRESENTATION

History

The classic triad of meningitis includes fever, neck stiffness, and altered mental status, but all of these are present together in less than half of adult patients with bacterial meningitis. Patients may also experience seizure. Many of the symptoms are nonspecific, such as headache, nausea and vomiting, and neck pain, making accurate diagnosis challenging. Patients at the extremes of age and those who are immunocompromised can be further difficult to diagnose, as they can have more subtle presentations or even lack fever. Infants may present with only irritability, lethargy, poor feeding, rash, or a bulging fontanelle. Seizures may be present in up to one third of pediatric patients with bacterial meningitis. Geriatric patients can often present with confusion or altered mental status. The clinical presentation of patients with encephalitis can be similar to patients with meningitis, including fever, headache, or stiff neck, but the diagnosis of encephalitis is characterized by the presence of altered mental status or neurologic symptoms.

Physical Examination

Although not all patients with meningitis will have fever, it is a common physical finding. Classically described meningeal findings include nuchal rigidity (severe neck stiffness due to meningeal irritation), Kernig sign (flexing the hip and extending the knee to elicit pain in the back and the legs) and Brudzinski sign (passive flexion of the neck elicits flexion of the hips). However, these findings cannot be relied on exclusively, as they have relatively poor sensitivities. Neck stiffness may only be present 30% of the time in patients with meningitis. Petechiae and purpura are classically associated with meningococcal meningitis; however, these skin findings can be present with other bacterial causes or may be absent. Altered mental status and focal neurologic findings should raise concern for encephalitis as a possible diagnosis.

DIAGNOSTIC STUDIES

Laboratory

Evaluation of the CSF is most critical. Initial CSF laboratory studies include cell count and differential, protein and glucose levels, and a Gram stain and bacterial culture. Other CSF studies to consider may include HSV or enterovirus polymerase chain reaction, bacterial antigen testing,

or specialized fungal testing. Additional CSF studies may be ordered for immunocompromised patients.

Other studies include a complete blood count, serum glucose and electrolytes, blood urea nitrogen and creatinine, and C-reactive protein. Most laboratory studies are nonspecific for meningitis or encephalitis, although a blood culture drawn before empiric antibiotics when meningitis is likely can be helpful to identify bacterial pathogens.

Imaging and Procedures

A prompt lumbar puncture (LP) is the preferred diagnostic procedure in patients with suspected bacterial meningitis or encephalitis. A computed tomography scan of the brain before LP should be considered under the following circumstances: altered mental status, new-onset seizures, an immunocompromised state, focal neurologic signs, or papilledema. Neuroimaging is intended to identify patients with possible contraindications to LP such as an occult mass from infection, brain tumor, or signs of brain shift or herniation.

MEDICAL DECISION MAKING

The initial history and physical exam are important for guiding diagnostic decisions and initiating emergent therapy when indicated for patients with suspected bacterial meningitis or encephalitis. Elevated numbers of white blood cells in the CSF obtained by LP are diagnostic for meningitis or encephalitis, although it can be a challenge to determine whether the cause is more likely bacterial or nonbacterial in etiology.

CSF findings suggestive of bacterial meningitis include the following:

- Positive Gram stain with identified organism
- Glucose <40 mg/dL or ratio of CSF/blood glucose <0.40
- Protein >200 mg/dL
- WBC >1,000/mL
- >80% polymorphonuclear neutrophils
- Elevated opening pressure of CSF during LP (pressure reading must be obtained with patient in the lateral decubitus position)

See Table 35-1 for classically described CSF findings in bacterial, viral, and fungal meningitis. Although these

Table 35-1. Classically described CSF findings in bacterial, viral, and fungal meningitis.

CSF findings	Bacterial	Viral	Fungal
Opening pressure	High	Normal	High
White blood cell count	1,000–10,000	<300	<500
Neutrophils	>80%	1–50%	1–50%
Glucose	Low	Normal	Low
Protein	High	Normal	High
Gram stain	+	–	–

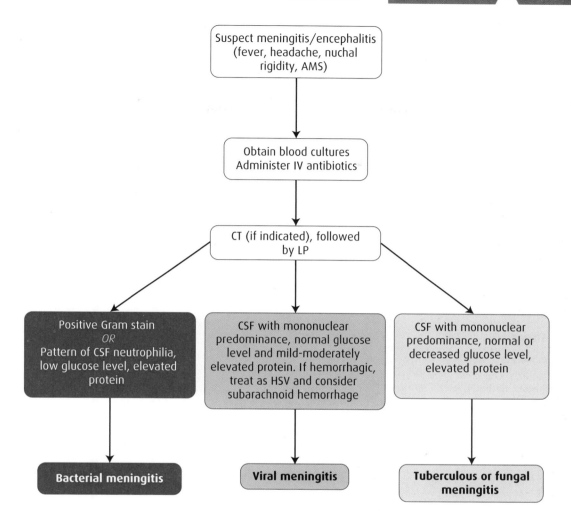

▲ **Figure 35-1.** Meningitis diagnostic algorithm. AMS, altered mental status; CSF, cerebrospinal fluid; IV, intravenous, LP, lumbar puncture.

general guidelines may be helpful to broadly characterize CSF findings in many cases, several studies have demonstrated that no single laboratory finding can accurately categorize the cause of CSF pleocytosis in all patients (Figure 35-1).

CSF studies for patients with encephalitis will lead to similarly abnormal results, with increased numbers of white blood cells in the CSF, generally with a lymphocytic predominance. Results may also reveal increased numbers of red blood cells in the CSF owing to neuronal cell death leading to edema, hemorrhage, and necrosis when encephalitis is present.

TREATMENT

For patients with suspected bacterial meningitis, empiric IV antibiotic therapy and admission to the hospital is recommended (Table 35-2). Recommendations for pediatric

patients are based on patient age. For neonates less than 1 month, empiric IV therapy includes ampicillin and cefotaxime (alternative is ampicillin and gentamicin). Children 1 to 3 months should be given ampicillin and cefotaxime,

Table 35-2. Recommended empiric therapy for adults with suspected bacterial meningitis.*

Patient Age	IV Empiric Therapy*
Adults <50 years	Ceftriaxone or cefotaxime and vancomycin
Adults ≥50 years	Ceftriaxone or cefotaxime and vancomycin and ampicillin

Readers should consult local infectious disease specialists for recommended empiric antibiotic therapy in your local region.
*Remember to add acyclovir in cases of possible HSV encephalitis.

and for those older than 3 months, empiric therapy includes ampicillin or ceftriaxone, and vancomycin. Patients with severe disease may require intensive care unit level care depending on the clinical circumstances.

The role of adjunctive dexamethasone for patients with bacterial meningitis remains somewhat uncertain, as recent work has questioned the value of this treatment that had previously been strongly recommended to reduce mortality and poor neurologic outcomes. For patients in high-income countries, there may be benefit to treatment with IV dexamethasone that is initiated before or at the same time as antibiotic treatment.

In patients with suspected bacterial meningitis who need a CT scan of the brain before LP, blood cultures should be drawn and empiric antimicrobial therapy administered before CT to avoid additional delays to beginning treatment.

The treatment for most cases of encephalitis is supportive care. HSV encephalitis is the only cause of this disease with a specific treatment: IV acyclovir.

DISPOSITION

▶ Admission

Patients who are diagnosed with bacterial meningitis or viral encephalitis should be admitted to the hospital for monitoring, IV antimicrobial agents, and other adjunctive therapies. There may be clinical ambiguity regarding disposition for patients who are clinically well appearing but have mildly elevated white blood cell levels in the CSF suggestive of aseptic meningitis. One option for such patients may include hospital admission for observation with or without empiric antibiotic therapy, pending CSF culture results.

▶ Discharge

In some circumstances, patients with suspected viral meningitis may be appropriate for outpatient management with close follow-up and strict return precautions. When considering discharge home for outpatient management of presumed viral meningitis, it is important to assess the patient's support system, reliability, availability of close follow-up, and mechanisms for contacting the patient if CSF culture results are unexpectedly positive.

▼ SUGGESTED READING

Fitch MT, Abrahamian FM, Moran GJ, Talan DA. Emergency department management of meningitis and encephalitis. *Infect Dis Clin North Am.* 2008;22:33–52, v–vi.

Fitch MT, van de Beek D. Emergency diagnosis and treatment of adult meningitis. *Lancet Infect Dis.* 2007;7:191–200.

Loring KE, Tintinalli JE. Central nervous system and spinal infections. In: Tintinalli JE, Kelen GD, Stapczynski JS, eds. *Tintinalli's Emergency Medicine: A Comprehensive Study Guide.* 7th ed. New York, NY: McGraw-Hill, 2011, pp. 1172–1178.

Quagliarello VJ, Scheld WM. Treatment of bacterial meningitis. *N Engl J Med.* 1997;336:708–716.

Soft Tissue Infections

William Thomas Smith, MD

Nicole M. Deiorio, MD

Key Points

- Most cases of cellulitis can be safely managed as outpatients with oral antibiotics, elevation, and recheck in 24-48 hours.

- All abscesses require drainage. Most patients can be safely discharged without antibiotics, but do need a recheck in 48 hours.

- Patients who are systemically ill or immune compromised require intravenous (IV) antibiotics, laboratory and imaging studies, and admission.

- Patients with pain out of proportion to physical exam findings, crepitus, or rapidly spreading erythema may have a life-threatening necrotizing infection requiring aggressive work-up, broad-spectrum IV antibiotics, and immediate surgical consultation for operative debridement.

INTRODUCTION

Soft tissue infections represent a common complaint in the emergency department (ED). The term "soft tissue infection" refers to an infection of the skin and underlying tissue. It is the emergency physician's objective to distinguish superficial infections (cellulitis, erysipelas, or abscess) from deep infections. If deep infections, such as necrotizing fasciitis, are not emergently diagnosed, they can cause significant morbidity and mortality.

Cellulitis is a progressive bacterial infection of the dermis and subcutaneous fat that is associated with leukocytic infiltration and capillary dilation (seen as erythema). It is caused by bacterial invasion of the skin, most often by *Staphylococcus aureus*, β-hemolytic streptococcus, and gram-negative bacilli such as *Haemophilus influenzae*. Methicillin-resistant *Staphylococcus aureus* (MRSA) is quickly becoming a common infecting agent in many community-acquired cases of cellulitis and abscesses.

Erysipelas is a skin infection that involves the lymphatic drainage system. Primarily, it is caused by invasion of the skin by *Staphylococcus pyogenes* in areas with impaired lymphatic drainage. It is common in infants, children, and older adults. It is usually found on the lower extremities (70%) or face (20%). The characteristic presentation is painful erythematous raised lesions, which may look like an orange peel. Red streaking representing inflammation of the underlying lymphatics may also be present.

Abscesses are localized pyogenic infections that can occur in any part of the body. Approximately 2% of all adult visits to the ED are for the treatment of cutaneous abscesses. Bacteria that normally colonize the skin are often the cause, with *S. aureus* being the most common organism involved. Mixed infections (aerobes and anaerobes) usually occur in the perineal areas.

Necrotizing infections are life and limb-threatening infections that involve the skin, subcutaneous tissue, fascia, and muscle. They usually occur in the setting of skin trauma, surgical procedures, decubitus ulcers, and immune compromise. These deadly infections are caused by a mixture of aerobic and anaerobic bacteria in most cases. Commonly isolated bacteria include *S. aureus*, *S. pyogenes* (ie, "flesh-eating bacteria"), enterococci, and anaerobes such as *Bacteroides* and *Clostridium perfringens* (ie, "gas gangrene").

CLINICAL PRESENTATION

▶ History

Ask about the time course and presence of systemic symptoms. Rapidly progressive infections with systemic symptoms require aggressive care in the ED. Patients should be asked about trauma (including bites, scratches, and possible foreign bodies), as it is the most common risk factor for developing a soft tissue infection. Other risk factors include obesity, malnutrition, immune compromise, intravenous (IV) drug use, vascular or lymphatic insufficiency, surgical procedures, and decubitus ulcers. The past medical history can be relevant, as anything that depresses the immune system (eg, steroids, diabetes, immunosuppressive drugs, elderly) predisposes the patient to soft tissue infections and may mask the severity of illness. Also, the status of tetanus immunization and previous antibiotic allergies should be ascertained.

▶ Physical Examination

Vitals signs provide rapid clues to the severity of infection. Tachycardia and hypotension may indicate sepsis. Fever is not reliable, as it occurs in <10% of patients with simple cellulitis or abscess.

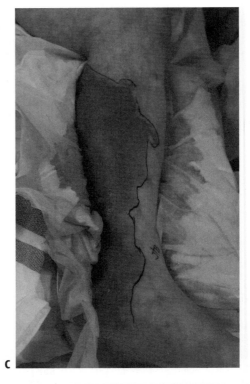

C

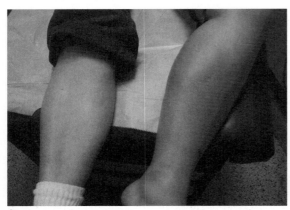

A

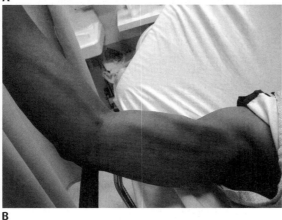

B

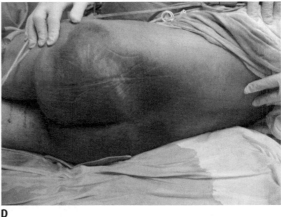

D

▲ **Figure 36-1. A.** Cellulitis of the left leg. **B.** Lymphangitis of the arm in a patient with a hand infection. **C.** Necrotizing fasciitis of the lower extremity. This patient required amputation of the leg to treat his infection. Courtesy of Kevin Jones, MD. **D.** Fournier's gangrene extending up the back of a patient.

The skin examination is crucial, and it is important to completely undress the patient to examine the involved body part. Assess the involved area for erythema, warmth, edema, and tenderness (Figure 36-1A). Lack of tenderness helps differentiate infections from other causes of skin erythema and warmth, such as venous stasis. Evidence of lymphatic spread in the form of red lines tracking proximally from the wound, called lymphangitis, further suggests an infectious etiology (Figure 36-1B). Focal areas of fluctuance and induration may indicate abscess formation.

Marking the extent of erythema on the patient with a pen will allow for comparison on repeat examinations. Rapid extension is concerning for a necrotizing infection (Figures 36-1C and D). Crepitus suggests gas formation in the tissues and is a sign of a more serious necrotizing infection. It is important to remember that necrotizing soft tissue infections often present with severe pain but may have few findings on physical exam. The absence of crepitus does not rule out a deep space infection.

Distal pulses should be examined to assess for arterial insufficiency.

DIAGNOSTIC STUDIES

▶ Laboratory

The diagnosis of simple cellulitis, erysipelas, or an abscess is clinical. Basic laboratory studies, such as a complete blood count or basic metabolic panel, are of little benefit. However, they should be considered if there is a suspicion of necrotizing infection, immune compromise, a history suggestive of hyperglycemia/metabolic abnormalities, or systemic symptoms. A C-reactive protein may also be useful when considering a necrotizing infection, as it will be significantly elevated. Gram stain and wound culture should be obtained in patients with suspected MRSA abscess and necrotizing infections, as it will guide future antibiotic therapy. Routine blood cultures add little to the diagnosis and treatment of soft tissue infections.

▶ Imaging

Ultrasound is becoming more frequently utilized in the ED for the diagnosis of cutaneous abscesses. It is fast, readily available at the bedside, and can easily localize an abscess for incision and drainage (Figure 36-2A). Ultrasound is also more sensitive than plain radiographs for soft tissue

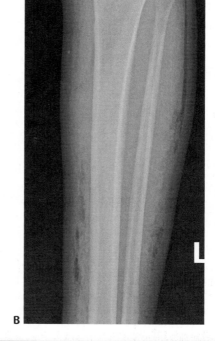

B

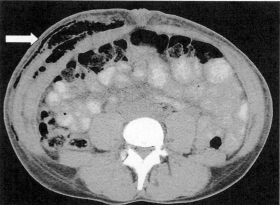

C

▲ **Figure 36-2. A.** Ultrasound of a cutaneous abscess. The abscess cavity is hypoechoic with mixed internal echogenicity. The surrounding skin is hyperechoic because of adjacent tissue edema and possibly cellulitis. **B.** Plain radiograph of the leg demonstrating subcutaneous air. **C.** CT scan in a patient with necrotizing fasciitis of the abdominal wall (arrow).

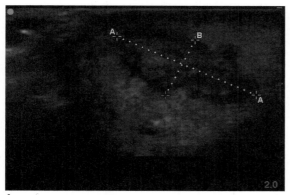

A

air. Plain radiographs are helpful to evaluate for traumatic injury, osteomyelitis, and the presence of gas formation (Figure 36-2B). However, radiographs are insensitive for small amounts of air. Computed tomography scan remains the most sensitive for soft tissue air, deep space abscesses, and foreign bodies (Figure 36-2C).

PROCEDURES

For a description of abscess incision and drainage, see Chapter 1.

MEDICAL DECISION MAKING

Most of the time, a good history and physical examination are all that is needed to make the diagnosis of a soft tissue infection. A patient with cellulitis will likely present with a history of an injury to the skin who then develops superficial erythema, warmth, swelling, and pain. A thorough history and physical will allow differentiation of cellulitis from other diagnoses such as thrombophlebitis, viral and drug exanthems, dermatitis, allergic reactions, insect bites, lymphedema, or fungal infections.

Sometimes a cutaneous abscess can be present along with superficial cellulitis. In these cases, bedside ultrasound becomes useful in determining whether a pus collection has developed underneath the skin. The differential diagnosis for abscess includes cutaneous cysts, tumors, foreign body granulomas, or vascular malformations (especially in the axilla and groin). Knowing the features of an abscess (erythema, induration, fluctuance, and a focal area of pain) becomes important, as only an abscess will have all of those features.

If a necrotizing infection (presence of pain out of proportion to exam, crepitus, bullae formation, skin sloughing, or systemic toxicity) is suspected, it becomes vital that an urgent CT scan is ordered to assess for gas and the extent of infectious involvement. A necrotizing infection requires prompt identification, consultation, and treatment (Figure 36-3).

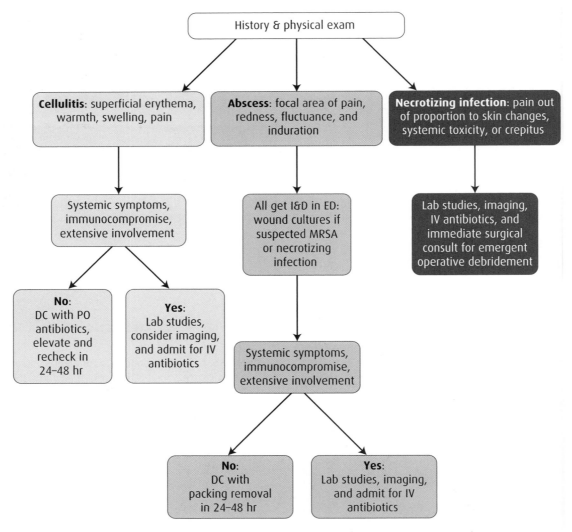

▲ **Figure 36-3.** Soft tissue infections diagnostic algorithm. DC, discharge; ED, emergency department; I&D, incision and drainage; IV, intravenous; MRSA, methicillin-resistant *Staphylococcus aureus*.

TREATMENT

Cellulitis is treated with antibiotics. If there is systemic toxicity, immune compromise, or involvement of high-risk areas (hands, face, perineum, or circumferential extremity) the patient should receive IV antibiotics and admission. If none of the above is present, the patient can be discharged with oral antibiotics (7- to 10-day course) and instructions to be rechecked in 2 days.

Incision and drainage (I&D) is the treatment of choice for an abscess, most of which do not require antibiotics after I&D. The abscess should be packed and a recheck scheduled in 1-2 days. Indications for the addition of antibiotics include systemic symptoms, extensive surrounding cellulitis, or immune compromise.

Treatment of a necrotizing infection involves prompt fluid resuscitation and IV antibiotics. Consultation with a general surgeon should be performed for emergent debridement to stop the advancement of the infection. Empiric broad-spectrum antibiotic coverage should be initiated. Piperacillin/tazobactam with vancomycin and ciprofloxacin is the initial treatment of choice, as it covers mixed aerobic and anaerobic bacteria that are often involved. Vancomycin is being used because high rates of MRSA resistance to clindamycin have been found. However, clindamycin is often added to the preceding regimen, as it has been shown to have bacterial toxin suppressive properties.

DISPOSITION

▶ Admission

Patients with cellulitis or abscesses should be admitted if there is an extensive area of involvement or if they are systemically ill, have significant comorbid illness, or are immune-compromised. All patients with necrotizing infections should be admitted to an intensive care unit for broad-spectrum antibiotic therapy after surgical debridement.

▶ Discharge

Patients with cellulitis or a drained abscess with limited area of involvement, no or minimal systemic symptoms, and no significant comorbidities may be discharged.

▼ SUGGESTED READING

Chambers HF, Moellering RC Jr, Kamitska P. Clincal decisions. Management of skin and soft-tissue infection. *N Engl J Med.* 2008;359:1063.

Dewitz F. Soft tissue. In: Ma OJ, Mateer JR, Blaivas M. *Emergency Ultrasound.* 2nd ed. New York, NY: McGraw-Hill, 2008, pp. 441–444.

Infectious Diseases Society of America. Practice Guidelines for the Diagnosis and Management of Skin and Soft-Tissue Infections. http://www.idsociety.org/uploadedFiles/IDSA/Guidelines-Patient_Care/PDF_Library/Skin%20and%20Soft%20Tissue.pdf. CID 2005:41.

Kelly EW, Magliner D. Soft tissue infections. In: Tintinalli JE, Stapczynski JS, Ma OJ, Cline DM, Cydulka RK, Meckler GD. *Tintinalli's Emergency Medicine: A Comprehensive Study Guide.* 7th ed. New York, NY: McGraw-Hill, 2011, pp. 1014–1024.

Wang CH, Khin LW, Heng KS, Tan KC, Low CO. The LRINEC (Laboratory Risk Indicator for Necrotizing Fasciitis) score: A tool for distinguishing necrotizing fasciitis from other soft tissue infections. *Crit Care Med.* 2004;32:1535–1541.

Human Immunodeficiency Virus

Sorabh Khandelwal, MD

John Davis, MD

Key Points

- A high index of suspicion is needed for the initial diagnosis of human immunodeficiency virus (HIV), particularly in the context of atypical presenting symptoms. Consider acute HIV in the patient who presents with a mononucleosis-like infection, but with negative monospot testing.

- CD4 T-cell count is correlated with risk for opportunistic infection.

- All patients with HIV and respiratory complaints, especially those with CD4 <200 cells/μL should be placed in negative pressure/airborne isolation until the diagnosis of tuberculosis can be excluded.

- With appropriate care and proper management, people living with HIV can live a normal lifespan.

INTRODUCTION

Human immunodeficiency virus (HIV) is a cytopathic retrovirus that attacks the CD4 T-lymphocytes in the immune system. Acquired immunodeficiency syndrome (AIDS) occurs when HIV-induced loss of CD4 cells and the resulting immunosuppression permit infection from opportunistic pathogens. AIDS is defined as a CD4 count <200/μL, a CD4 percentage <14%, or the presence of an AIDS-defining illness. AIDS-defining illnesses include *Pneumocystis jiroveci* pneumonia (PCP), Mycobacterium tuberculosis (TB), toxoplasmosis, cryptococcosis, cryptosporidiosis, esophageal candidiasis, disseminated Mycobacterium avium complex (dMAC), and cytomegalovirus (CMV), among others.

In the United States, approximately 1.2 million persons are infected with HIV, with up to 50,000 new cases every year. The estimated prevalence of HIV-positive patients seen in urban emergency departments (EDs) may be as high as 11.4%. Up to 20% of all HIV-positive persons in the United States are unaware of their HIV status.

Risk factors for HIV acquisition include sexual activity, injection drug use, blood transfusion (particularly before screening of the donor pool commenced in 1985), intrapartum/neonatal exposure to a mother with HIV, and occupational exposure (break of skin with contaminated sharps or blood/body fluid splashes onto mucous membranes/non-intact skin).

Acute retroviral syndrome (ARS) occurs in approximately 50% of acutely infected patients, approximately 2–4 weeks after exposure to HIV, and may clinically manifest as a flu-like or mononucleosis-like illness. Regardless of the presence or absence of ARS, most patients have a high viral load (>10^6 copies/cm³) during this period, and *negative* serologic tests. Seroconversion typically occurs 2–6 weeks (though sometimes up to 6 months) after exposure. An immune response to the virus is then generated, and the viral load falls to a setpoint with a relatively stable CD4 count. This leads to a period of clinical latency (usually 2–10 years) during which CD4 T-cells are continually destroyed and regenerated, and viral replication continues. Ultimately, immune control is ineffective, and the CD4 count falls, leading to increased susceptibility to opportunistic (as well as other) infection. Some CD4 cutoffs are associated with increased risk of certain infections (<200 with PCP, <100 with histoplasmosis, <50 with dMAC and CMV retinitis), but the clinician should be aware that infections may occur at a higher than anticipated CD4 levels.

CLINICAL PRESENTATION

History

All patients presenting to the ED with complaints of infections should be asked about their HIV status, if they have been tested, and about pertinent risk factors. Patients with unknown HIV status, significant risk factors, and symptoms consistent with an opportunistic infection should be assumed to be immunosuppressed. Patients with known HIV should be asked about their latest CD4 count, viral load, medications (including prophylaxis), and history of any opportunistic infections or recent hospitalizations. Patients with counts >500/μL are at lower risk for opportunistic infections.

Some aspects of the history are particularly important for specific, symptomatic presentations in those who are infected with HIV.

Fever. Pulmonary and CNS infections are the chief causes of fever, but infections at these sites may occasionally present without localizing symptoms.

Respiratory complaints. Any pulmonary complaint should raise suspicion for pneumonia or TB. Patients should be asked about prior episodes of PCP or TB. They should also be questioned about the use of prophylactic medications (eg, trimethoprim-sulfamethoxazole) for PCP. The presence of oral candidiasis in a patient with shortness of breath suggests PCP.

Neurologic complaints. New or worsening headache with CD4 count <200/μL suggests central nervous system (CNS) infection (toxoplasmosis or cryptococcal meningitis) or primary CNS lymphoma. Painless visual loss occurs with CMV retinitis.

Gastrointestinal complaints. Difficulty swallowing occurs with candidal esophagitis, and failure to improve with fluconazole (Diflucan) suggests CMV or herpes esophagitis. Acute diarrhea may be caused by bacteria (eg, *Salmonella*), whereas chronic diarrhea may represent a parasitic (eg, *Giardia, Cryptosporidium*) or viral (eg, CMV) cause. Pancreatitis and kidney stones most often occur as a result of antiretroviral therapy.

Physical Examination

A comprehensive physical examination may not only help provide a general picture of the overall health of the patient, it can also help identify the source for any acute presenting complaint. Some key systems to examine include:

Vital signs. History of fever at home requires a workup, even if the patient is afebrile in the ED. Tachypnea and hypoxia suggest PCP.

General appearance. Assess for respiratory distress. Wasting, dehydration, and parietal hair loss are common in patients with advanced AIDS.

Head and neck. Assess visual acuity and perform funduscopic examination for possible CMV retinitis ("ketchup and mayo" retinal findings). Perform oral examination for

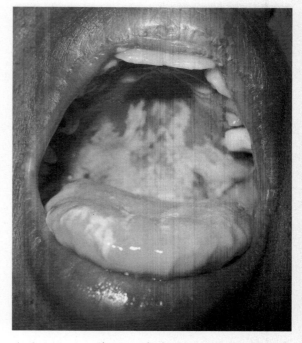

▲ **Figure 37-1.** Photograph showing patient with oral candidiasis.

candidiasis (thrush) and oral hairy leukoplakia (Figure 37-1). Assess the neck for lymphadenopathy or meningismus.

Pulmonary. Auscultate for rales, rhonchi, or wheezes; however, many patients with PCP will have normal breath sounds.

Cardiovascular. Listen for new murmurs, suggesting endocarditis, especially in the IV drug user.

Gastrointestinal. Examine for evidence of peritonitis, pancreatitis, or hepatobiliary disease, which may occur secondary to acute infection or antiretroviral medications.

Neurologic. Assess mental status and any focal deficits (present in up to 60% of patients with toxoplasmosis, though absent in many cases of cryptococcal meningitis).

Skin. Examine for Kaposi sarcoma, cellulitis, abscesses, evidence of disseminated infection (endocarditis, fungal disease, dMAC), or drug reactions.

DIAGNOSTIC STUDIES

Laboratory

Complete Blood Count. Use the absolute lymphocyte count as a correlation for the CD4 count. If the CD4 count is unknown, an absolute lymphocyte count (ALC) can be used to predict the CD4 count. The ALC is equal to the total white blood cell count multiplied by the percentage of lymphocytes. An ALC of <1,000/μL predicts a CD4 count <200/μL. An ALC of >2,000/μL predicts a CD4 count >200/μL.

Chemistry. Useful in patients with prolonged diarrhea, dehydration, or wasting to assess glucose level, electrolytes, and renal function. Can be helpful in patients presenting with abdominal pain to check for lactic acidosis.

Liver profile, lipase, lactate dehydrogenase. In patients with abdominal pain and jaundice. Lactate dehydrogenase (LDH) is also useful in patients with suspected PCP. Elevation >220 IU/L in patients with shortness of breath suggests PCP (94% sensitive), and a normal LDH level suggests an alternative diagnosis.

Blood cultures. In patients with a fever without a source and for suspected serious bacterial (including mycobacterial), viral, or fungal infections.

Urine. Obtain a urinalysis and urine culture in all febrile patients without a source. Many AIDS patients have urinary tract infections without localizing symptoms. The urinary histoplasma antigen can be useful in detecting disseminated histoplasmosis.

Stool. Check for leukocytes, bacterial culture, ova, and parasites (including microsporidia, *Cryptosporidium*, *Isospora*, and *Cyclospora*) in patients with diarrhea or bloody stools. Some causes of diarrhea may require biopsy for diagnosis.

Blood gas. An arterial blood gas should be performed for patients with pulmonary complaints. Patients with PCP and an elevated A-a gradient (>35 mmHg) or low PaO2 (<70 mmHg on room air) are candidates for adjunctive steroid therapy.

Viral load. Rarely used emergently to establish risk of opportunistic infection.

▶ Imaging

Chest x-ray. All HIV-positive patients with pulmonary symptoms or fever without a source. PCP classically shows diffuse bilateral interstitial infiltrates, but findings vary widely and can be normal (39%) or indistinguishable from bacterial pneumonia (Figure 37-2).

Head computed tomography (CT) scan with contrast. All patients with neurologic symptoms (Figure 37-3).

Brain magnetic resonance imaging (MRI) with contrast. Consider for patients with focal neurologic findings but minimal or only subtle changes on head CT. Some lesions of progressive multifocal leukoencephalopathy (PML) or toxoplasmosis are seen only on MRI.

Abdominal CT scan and ultrasound. Immuno suppression masks normal inflammatory responses to serious intra-abdominal pathology such as appendicitis and biliary disease. Maintain a low threshold for imaging patients with abdominal pain.

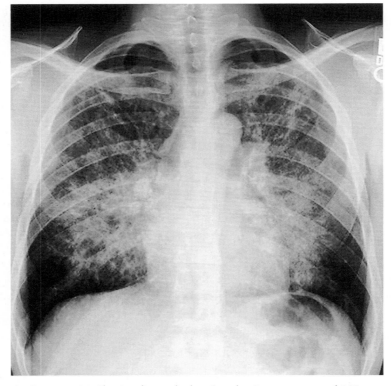

▲ **Figure 37-2.** Chest radiograph showing classic appearance of PCP pneumonia (bilateral interstitial infiltrates).

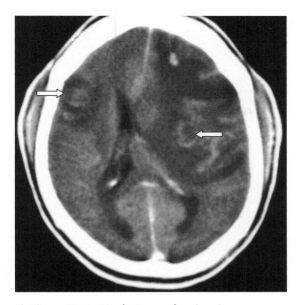

▲ **Figure 37-3.** Head CT scan showing ring-enhancing lesions of CNS toxoplasmosis in a patient with AIDS.

PROCEDURES

Lumbar puncture. In patients with new headache or fever, especially in patients with CD4 count <200/mL. CT before lumbar puncture (LP) is recommended in all patients with HIV to rule out mass lesion and increased intracranial pressure. Check opening pressure (particularly important for cryptococcal meningitis). Routine studies (cell count with differential, total protein, glucose) should be sent. Additional cerebrospinal fluid studies performed in HIV patients include India ink (*Cryptococcus*), viral and fungal culture, toxoplasmosis, cryptococcal titers or antigens, and VDRL for neurosyphilis.

MEDICAL DECISION MAKING

The medical decision-making process is especially dependent on the presenting symptoms in a patient with HIV.

Fever. Although fever in the HIV-positive patient with preserved CD4 count (>500) may be benign, the likelihood that fever represents opportunistic infection goes up markedly with lower CD4 count and should be treated as such. Fever alone in the immunocompromised patient is sufficient grounds for admission/observation. Differential diagnosis includes pneumonia (PCP, bacterial), histoplasmosis (especially for those living in, or recently traveling to, the Ohio/Mississippi river valley areas), toxoplasmosis (disseminated or encephalitis), cryptococcal meningitis, bacterial meningitis and sepsis, TB (anywhere), salmonellosis, sinusitis, lymphoma, CMV, dMAC, or drug reaction.

Respiratory symptoms. Most standard prognosis/decision algorithms do not apply to the immunocompromised. Therefore, admission and empiric treatment are appropriate for the HIV-positive patient with low CD4 count and possible pneumonia. Differential diagnosis includes PCP, community-acquired pneumonia, TB, fungal pneumonia (histoplasmosis, coccidioidomycosis), Kaposi sarcoma, or lymphoma. As a special note, patients with HIV, cough, and fevers are at risk for pulmonary TB. They should be masked and placed in a respiratory isolation room directly from triage. Up to 12% of HIV-infected patients with TB may have a normal chest x-ray.

Neurologic symptoms. Neurologic symptoms in the HIV-positive patient, particularly with low CD4 count, should be treated as a medical emergency. The evaluation is as above, and empiric treatment, when warranted, should not be delayed. Differential diagnosis includes toxoplasmosis, cryptococcal meningitis, bacterial or viral meningitis, encephalitis (JC virus–PML, primary HIV encephalitis, herpes simplex virus, CMV, varicella zoster virus), primary CNS lymphoma, or drug reactions.

Gastrointestinal symptoms. Diarrhea is the most common gastrointestinal (GI) complaint in the HIV-positive population, and this may be due to many factors, including acute retroviral therapy (ART) or opportunistic infection (OI), in addition to usual causes of diarrhea in the non–HIV-infected population. Many GI complaints can be managed successfully without requiring admission, although certain diagnoses (eg, pancreatitis, lactic acidosis) merit close monitoring, usually in an inpatient setting. Differential diagnosis is dependent on the particular GI symptom(s) and includes esophagitis (candida, CMV, herpes), pancreatitis (ART, viral), cholangiopathy (microsporidia), nephrolithiasis (ART), enteritis (CMV, bacterial, parasitic), lactic acidosis (ART).

See Figure 37-4 for a diagnostic algorithm for a patient with HIV presenting with fever, respiratory, or neurologic complaints.

TREATMENT

The treatment and management of HIV itself is rarely an emergency. Data have shown that initiation of ART earlier in the course of HIV infection benefits both those with OI (eg, TB), and those without OI. Current Department of Health and Human Services guidelines recommend treatment for all persons diagnosed with HIV. However, given the complexities associated with initiation of an antiretroviral regimen, the decision about what to start should be made in conjunction with an expert in the management of HIV.

▶ **Fever (Undifferentiated)**

Well-appearing patients with CD4 counts >500/μL without an obvious source of infection do not need specific antimicrobial therapy and are treated as an immunocompetent

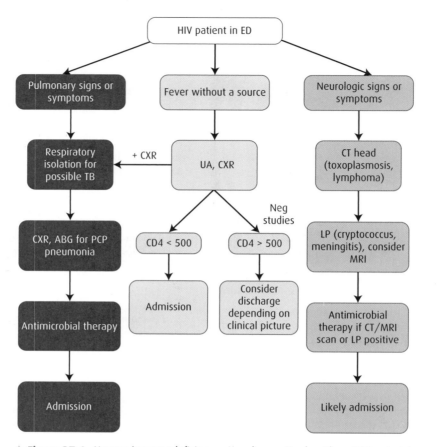

▲ **Figure 37-4.** Human immunodeficiency virus diagnostic algorithm. ABG, arterial blood gas; CT, computed tomography; CXR, chest x-ray; ED, emergency department; HIV, human immunodeficiency syndrome; LB, lumbar puncture; MRI, magnetic resonance imaging; PCP, *Pneumocystis carinii* pneumonia; TB, tuberculosis; UA, urinalysis.

host. Patients who appear ill and have CD4 counts <200/μL should be treated with broad-spectrum antibiotic coverage (piperacillin-tazobactam plus aminoglycoside, consider addition of vancomycin when concerned for methicillin-resistant *Staphylococcus aureus* as etiologic agent).

▶ Pulmonary Complaints

Patients with suspected PCP should be treated with trimethoprim-sulfamethoxazole. If PaO2 is <70 mmHg or A-a gradient is >35 mmHg, adjunctive steroids should be given (usually a prednisone taper). Because PCP is often indistinguishable from community-acquired pneumonia, a third-generation cephalosporin (eg, ceftriaxone) with macrolide (eg, azithromycin), or monotherapy with a respiratory fluoroquinolone (eg, levofloxacin, moxifloxacin) should be added. All patients should be isolated until TB has been ruled out.

▶ CNS Complaints

Patients with CT/MRI findings consistent with toxoplasmosis and mass effect from the CNS lesion require neurosurgical consultation and steroids (dexamethasone 10 mg intravenously [IV]). Cryptococcal meningitis is treated with IV amphotericin B (often with 5-fluorocytosine) after consultation with an infectious disease specialist. Suspected bacterial meningitis should be treated immediately (see Chapter 35) and not delayed for imaging or LP. Retinal lesions consistent with possible CMV retinitis should be treated with ganciclovir (IV) in conjunction with consultation with an ophthalmologist and infectious disease specialist. There is currently no effective treatment for PML, although immune reconstitution can help slow or halt progression of the disease.

▶ GI Complaints

Suspected candidal esophagitis should be treated with oral fluconazole. Failure to improve suggests drug-resistant *Candida*, CMV, or herpes as the cause. Acute diarrhea that is negative for ova and parasites is treated symptomatically (eg, loperamide) in the ED, with outpatient referral.

DISPOSITION

▶ Admission

- Fever without a source if the patient is ill-appearing or the CD4 count is <500/μL.
- Any ill-appearing or dehydrated patient.
- All patients with pulmonary infections should be admitted to an isolation bed until the possibility of TB is excluded.
- Admit all patients with focal neurologic findings or abnormal CT scan or LP findings; with CMV retinitis; and with severe drug reactions.

▶ Discharge

- Fever without a source if the CD4 count is >500/μL and the patient appears well (outpatient follow-up).
- Patient with a headache who appears well with normal CT and LP. Outpatient follow-up should be arranged to check CSF cryptococcal antigen test.

▾ SUGGESTED READING

Marco CA, Rothman RE. HIV infection and complications in emergency medicine. *Emerg Med Clin North Am.* 2008;26:367–387.

Rothman RE, Marco CA, Yang S. Human immunodeficiency virus infection and acquired immunodeficiency syndrome: Introduction. In: Tintinalli JE, Stapczynski JS, Ma OJ, Cline DM, Cydulka RK, Meckler GD. *Tintinalli's Emergency Medicine: A Comprehensive Study Guide.* 7th ed. New York, NY: McGraw-Hill, 2011, pp. 1031–1042.

Torres M, Chin RL. HIV in the Emergency Department. *Emerg Med Clin North Am.* 2010;28:xii–429.

38 Blood and Body Fluid Exposure

Rahul G. Patwari, MD

Key Points

- A blood or body fluid exposure refers to contact with potentially infected fluids through non-intact skin, mucous membranes, or skin penetrated by a sharp object.
- Prevention is the cornerstone to reducing infectious exposures.
- Administering postexposure prophylaxis for human immunodeficiency virus is a time-sensitive decision,

necessitating that the exposed patient visit the emergency department when the employee health office is closed.
- Hepatitis B vaccination greatly reduces the seroconversion rate when a health care worker is exposed to blood and body fluid.

INTRODUCTION

The Centers for Disease Control and Prevention define an exposure to blood and body fluids as contact with potentially infectious fluids that put health care workers at risk of infectious disease. This may come from a break in the skin by a sharp object (eg, a needle or scalpel) or contact with mucous membranes or already present breaks in the skin. The infectious diseases for which a health care worker is at risk include human immune deficiency syndrome (HIV), hepatitis B virus (HBV), and hepatitis C virus (HCV).

Not surprisingly, most needlestick injuries come from teaching hospitals, usually within operating rooms or the emergency department (ED) where sharp instruments are used routinely. Syringe and suture needles are the most common offending devices. The risk of seroconversion after needlestick exposures varies depending on the pathogen. For hepatitis B, the risk of transmission is up to 30% if the source patient is e-antigen positive. If the source patient is e-antigen negative, the risk drops to 1–6%. The risk of transmission of hepatitis B substantially decreases in those who have received the hepatitis B vaccine. The risk of transmission of hepatitis C is 1.8%, whereas the risk of HIV risk is 0.3%. Postexposure prophylactic medications

are administered to decrease the seroconversion rate for HIV and HBV.

Blood or any specimen visibly contaminated with blood is the most common vector for transmission; however, other potentially infectious fluids include semen, vaginal secretions, and cerebrospinal, synovial, pleural, peritoneal, pericardial, and amniotic fluids. The risk of transmission of disease in these fluids is unknown. Fluids that are not considered infectious include feces, nasal secretions, saliva, sputum, sweat, tears, urine, and vomitus, unless of course they contain blood.

The best defense against a blood and body fluid exposure is prevention. Standard precautions should be used when caring for all patients. Standard precautions include proper hand washing; the use of gloves, masks, and gowns; and proper disposal of medical waste and safe needle usage. Health care workers should wash hands before and after contact with every patient, even if gloves were worn. The use of soap and water (or an alcohol-based gel or foam) is the most important factor in decreasing the transmission of disease.

Personal protective equipment (PPE), namely gloves, masks, gowns, and eye shields, is an important part of preventing the transmission of organisms; however, it is not perfect. Microperforations in gloves can allow contamination of the hands. Infection can also occur when removing gloves. Hence hand washing is recommended after removing gloves. Sharp instruments should always be disposed of in proper sharps bins and blood and body fluid contaminated objects in proper biohazard bags.

CLINICAL PRESENTATION

▶ History

An exposure consists of a break in the skin by a sharp object (eg, a needle or scalpel) or contact with mucous membranes or non-intact skin by blood or other body fluids. If a needle is involved, determine whether it was a "less severe" (solid bore, superficial scratch) or "more severe" (large bore hollow needle, deep puncture, visible blood on the device, or the needle was used in the source patient's artery or vein) exposure. For mucous membrane or percutaneous exposures of non-intact skin, the volume and duration of exposure should be noted. Determine information about the source individual (unless this is not possible or prohibited), specifically their HBV, HCV, and HIV infectivity. Lastly, document the patient's tetanus status.

▶ Physical Examination

Examine the patient's skin for any breaks or visible blood. Make sure that the patient has cleaned the area. If not, immediately cleanse the area with copious soap and water. Small wounds can be cleaned with an antiseptic such as an alcohol-based hand hygiene agent (alcohol is virucidal to HIV, HBV, and HCV). Mucosal surfaces and eyes should be flushed with saline or water. There is no evidence that squeezing blood out of the wound reduces the risk of transmission.

DIAGNOSTIC STUDIES

If it is unknown whether the source patient is infected with hepatitis B, hepatitis C, or HIV, then the source patient's blood should be tested after obtaining consent. This will require contacting personnel in the location where the patient is located (eg, operating room). In some regions, consent for such testing is not required. All source patients should be tested for HBsAg, HCV, and HIV, unless they are known to be infectious. Obtaining a rapid HIV test of the source patient's blood is valuable in making decisions about whether to start postexposure prophylaxis from the ED.

The exposed patient's blood may be collected in the ED or the employee health clinic. Many EDs will have a specific protocol to follow regarding what laboratory tests should be drawn on the exposed health care worker. For the person exposed to HBV, perform hepatitis surface antigen testing. If this is positive, then the individual has been vaccinated and is a known responder; no further treatment is required.

For the person exposed to a HCV-positive source, baseline testing for anti-HCV and alanine aminotransferase

(ALT) activity is performed, with repeat testing at 4–6 months. If earlier detection is desired, testing for HCV RNA can be performed at 4–6 months. For the person exposed to HIV, HIV-antibody testing should be performed for at least 6 months postexposure (at 6 weeks, 12 weeks, and 6 months). Extended HIV follow-up (for 12 months) is recommended for health care professionals who become infected with HCV after exposure to a source co-infected with HIV and HCV.

MEDICAL DECISION MAKING

The decision to initiate treatment is determined by assessment of the risk of the exposure and the infectivity of the source patient (Figure 38-1). Low-risk injuries are defined by a solid needle, superficial appearance, and a low risk source, such as a patient with an HIV viral load <1,500 copies/mL. High-risk injuries include those involving a hollow bore needle with presence of visible blood on the device or exposure from a needle that was in an artery or vein of the source patient.

TREATMENT

In addition to cleaning the wound if it has not already been done, the most important treatment decision for the ED is determining whether or not to give postexposure prophylaxis for HIV. Postexposure prophylaxis should be initiated as soon as possible, with the goal being to start treatment within 1–2 hours after exposure.

Two nucleosides are recommended for low-risk exposures. The most commonly used dual nucleoside regimens include:

- Combivir (ZDV plus 3TC; 1 tablet daily) or
- Truvada (TDF plus FTC; 1 tablet daily)

For higher risk exposures, a boosted protease inhibitor is added:

- Kaletra (2 tablets twice daily; 200 mg lopinavir/50 mg ritonavir in each tablet)

These medications can be difficult to tolerate given their side effect profile (headache, asthenia, and gastrointestinal intolerance). In addition to the dose administered in the ED, the patient will require continued therapy for 1 month.

For potential HBV exposures, the health care worker's vaccination status should first be determined. If the exposed person is unvaccinated, treatment with hepatitis B immunoglobulin (HBIG) should be started as soon as possible after exposure (preferably within 24 hours). If the exposed person was vaccinated but didn't have an appropriate antibody response (HBsAb <10 mIU/mL), then proceed as if unvaccinated. If the exposed person has an appropriate antibody response after vaccination, then no treatment is needed, although a booster HBV vaccine can be considered.

CHAPTER 38

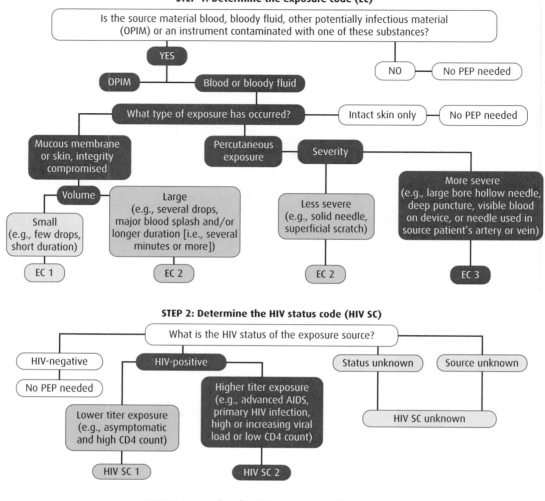

STEP 1: Determine the exposure code (EC)

Is the source material blood, bloody fluid, other potentially infectious material (OPIM) or an instrument contaminated with one of these substances?

YES → NO — No PEP needed

OPIM — Blood or bloody fluid

What type of exposure has occurred? — Intact skin only — No PEP needed

Mucous membrane or skin, integrity compromised

Percutaneous exposure — Severity

Volume

Small (e.g., few drops, short duration) — **EC 1**

Large (e.g., several drops, major blood splash and/or longer duration [i.e., several minutes or more]) — **EC 2**

Less severe (e.g., solid needle, superficial scratch) — **EC 2**

More severe (e.g., large bore hollow needle, deep puncture, visible blood on device, or needle used in source patient's artery or vein) — **EC 3**

STEP 2: Determine the HIV status code (HIV SC)

What is the HIV status of the exposure source?

HIV-negative — No PEP needed

HIV-positive

Status unknown — Source unknown

Lower titer exposure (e.g., asymptomatic and high CD4 count) — **HIV SC 1**

Higher titer exposure (e.g., advanced AIDS, primary HIV infection, high or increasing viral load or low CD4 count) — **HIV SC 2**

HIV SC unknown

STEP 3: Determine the PEP recommendation

EC	HIV SC	PEP recommendations
1	1	PEP may not be warranted. Exposure type does not pose a known risk for HIV transmission.
1	2	Consider basic regimen. Exposure type poses a negligible risk for HIV transmission.
2	1	Recommend basic regimen. Most HIV exposures are in this category; no increased risk for HIV transmission has been observed but use of PEP is appropriate.
2	2	Recommend expanded regimen. Exposure type represents an increased HIV transmission risk.
3	1 or 2	Recommend expanded regimen. Exposure type represents an increased HIV transmission risk.
Unknown		If the source or, in the case of an unknown source, the setting where the exposure occurred suggests a possible risk for HIV exposure and the EC is 2 or 3, consider PEP basic program.

▲ **Figure 38-1.** Blood and body fluid exposure diagnostic algorithm. Reprinted with permission from Public Health Service Guidelines for the Management of Health-Care Worker Exposures to HIV and Recommendations for Postexposure Prophylaxis. *MMWR Recomm Rep.* 1998 May15;47(RR-7):1-33. Available at http://wonder.cdc.gov/wonder/prevguid/m0052722/m0052722.asp.

For potential HCV exposures, baseline testing for anti-HCV, HCV RNA, and ALT should occur with follow-up testing for HCV RNA between 4 and 6 weeks after exposure and follow-up testing for anti-HCV, HCV RNA, and ALT between 4 and 6 months after exposure. Currently there is no proven effective postexposure prophylaxis treatment available. Immunoglobulins and antiviral agents are not recommended.

All patients should be counseled on refraining from unprotected sexual intercourse and blood donations. Follow-up should be given with the institution's employee health departments.

DISPOSITION

Health care workers exposed to blood or body fluids can be discharged home with instructions to follow up with their hospital's employee health offices the next business day.

SUGGESTED READING

Centers for Disease Control and Prevention. Basic and expanded HIV postexposure prophylaxis regimens. http://www.cdc.gov/mmwr/preview/mmwrhtml/rr5011a4.htm. Accessed April 28, 2012.

Centers for Disease Control and Prevention. Management of occupational blood exposures. http://www.cdc.gov/mmwr/preview/mmwrhtml/rr5011a3.htm. Accessed April 28, 2012.

Centers for Disease Control and Prevention. Updated U.S. Public Health Service Guidelines for the Management of Occupational Exposures to HBV, HCV, and HIV and Recommendations for Postexposure Prophylaxis http://www.cdc.gov/mmwr/preview/mmwrhtml/rr5011a1.htm. Accessed April 28, 2012.

Centers for Disease Control and Prevention. Updated U.S. Public Health Service Guidelines for the Management of Occupational Exposures to HIV and Recommendations for Postexposure Prophylaxis. http://www.cdc.gov/mmwr/preview/mmwrhtml/rr5409a1.htm. Accessed April 28, 2012.

Nephrolithiasis

Jonathan Bankoff, MD

Key Points

- Analgesic administration should not be delayed while obtaining laboratory and radiology studies.
- Abdominal aortic aneurysm should be considered in the differential of elderly patients being evaluated for kidney stones.
- Noncontrast computed tomography of the abdomen and pelvis is the test of choice for diagnosing nephrolithiasis.
- Urologic consultation is indicated in patients with coexisting infection or worsening renal insufficiency.

INTRODUCTION

Kidney stones occur when urinary solutes precipitate out of the urine and form crystalline stones in the genitourinary (GU) tract. Nephrolithiasis is common in the United States, with an estimated prevalence of 7% in men and 3% in women. Kidney stones most often affect people in the third to fifth decades of life, but can occur at all ages. The recurrence rate is 30% within the first year and 50% at 5 years. Patients with a family history of kidney stones are more likely to develop stones, and Caucasians are affected twice as often as African Americans and Asians. Specific risk factors for kidney stones include dehydration, hypercalcemia, hyperuricemia (gout), certain urinary tract infections (*Proteus, Klebsiella, Pseudomonas*), and medications (protease inhibitors, diuretics, laxatives). The 4 main types of kidney stones are listed in Table 39-1.

The GU tract has several anatomic areas of narrowing that may limit passage of a stone. The most common areas are the renal calyx, the ureteropelvic junction (UPJ), the pelvic brim (where the ureter passes over the pelvic bone and iliac vessels), and the ureterovesical junction (UVJ). Ureteral obstruction occurs when a stone blocks the passage of urine, resulting in hydroureter (dilated ureter) and hydronephrosis (dilated renal pelvis and calices).

Timely evaluation, a broad differential, and prompt administration of appropriate analgesia is paramount to proper emergency department (ED) management. Although disposition of these patients is often uncomplicated, certain factors may warrant more extensive workup, emergent urology consultation, and hospital admission.

Table 39-1. Kidney stones by type, frequency of occurrence, and precipitants.

Stone Type	Frequency	Precipitants
Calcium + phosphate/oxalate	75%	Hyperparathyroidism, immobilization
Struvite (magnesium-ammonium-phosphate)	10%	Infection caused by urea-splitting bacteria *Proteus* (most common cause of staghorn calculi)
Uric acid	10%	Hyperuricemia
Cystine	<5%	Hypercystinuria from genetic disorder

CLINICAL PRESENTATION

History

Patients often present with rapid onset of severe sharp pain, which is usually episodic ("renal colic") and lasts minutes to hours. Pain often originates in the flank and radiates to the abdomen and groin along the course of the ureter. Nausea, vomiting, and diaphoresis are common. Urinary symptoms, such as frequency and urgency, may vary, depending on where the stone is located, and often increase in severity when the stone nears the bladder.

Physical Examination

Patients with symptomatic nephrolithiasis are often rocking or writhing on the stretcher. They are frequently unable to lie down or find a comfortable position. Elevated blood pressure and heart rate are common because of pain. Examination should focus on identifying and/or ruling out other causes of abdominal and flank pain. It should include a thorough genitourinary evaluation, including pelvic or testicular examination, when pain is located in the lower abdomen. Evidence of a pulsatile abdominal mass or peritonitis suggests an alternative diagnosis.

DIAGNOSTIC STUDIES

Laboratory

Although no single laboratory test is needed to diagnose kidney stones, there are several that are critical for management and disposition. Urinalysis is performed to assess for hematuria and the presence of concomitant infection. In 15–30% of patients, microscopic hematuria may be absent. Crystals may be present in the urine and aid in the diagnosis of stone type. Urine pH >7.6 (normal is 5.5) may indicate infection with urea-splitting organisms. Urine pregnancy test should be obtained in all females of childbearing age to rule out the possibility of ectopic pregnancy. Blood urea nitrogen and creatinine are often checked to assess renal function, especially in patients at risk for renal insufficiency (diabetics, elderly) or in patients who may receive intravenous (IV) contrast. Complete blood count may be helpful when infection is suspected, but is not routinely necessary.

Imaging

Computed tomography (CT) scan of the abdomen and pelvis is the test of choice for diagnosis of nephrolithiasis (Figure 39-1). It has a sensitivity and specificity of approximately 96% for kidney stones. CT scans can visualize all 4 types of kidney stones as well as perinephric stranding, hydroureter, and hydronephrosis. They can also identify nonurologic causes of pain (eg, abdominal aortic aneurysm [AAA]) in cases of diagnostic uncertainty. Noncontrast CT scan does not evaluate renal function or the presence of complete obstruction.

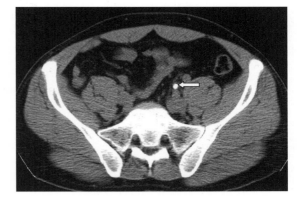

▲ **Figure 39-1.** CT scan of left ureteral stone (arrow).

Renal ultrasound may also be considered as an imaging option, particularly in patients with contraindications to CT scan (eg, pregnancy). It is highly sensitive for hydronephrosis, but only moderately sensitive for detecting stones, and provides no information regarding stone size or location.

Abdominal plain film radiography is occasionally used to diagnose kidney stones, particularly in patients with a long history of kidney stones and multiple prior imaging studies. It has similar sensitivity to renal ultrasound, with similar limitations.

MEDICAL DECISION MAKING

Although the clinical presentation of a patient with acute flank pain and suspected kidney stones may seem straightforward, particularly in a patient with a history of kidney stones, it is important to consider a broad differential diagnosis and perform a thorough history and physical exam. Immediate life-threatening conditions, such as ruptured AAA and aortic dissection, must be considered, particularly in older, hypertensive patients with no history of kidney stones. Other diagnoses to consider include biliary colic, pyelonephritis, musculoskeletal back pain, diverticulitis, and bowel obstruction. Pay specific attention to the GU exam, as both testicular/ovarian torsion and ectopic pregnancy can present with isolated flank pain and with similar clinical appearance to kidney stones (Figure 39-2).

TREATMENT

Management of suspected nephrolithiasis includes aggressive pain control, and this intervention should not be delayed pending diagnostic confirmation. Opioid analgesics are the mainstay of treatment for acute symptomatic nephrolithiasis. Nonsteroidal anti-inflammatory drugs are an excellent adjunct to opiates, but should be avoided in patients with baseline renal impairment, as this class of drugs may worsen renal insufficiency. Antiemetics are also useful in treating the nausea and vomiting often present in these patients. IV fluids are often beneficial in patients with nausea and vomiting;

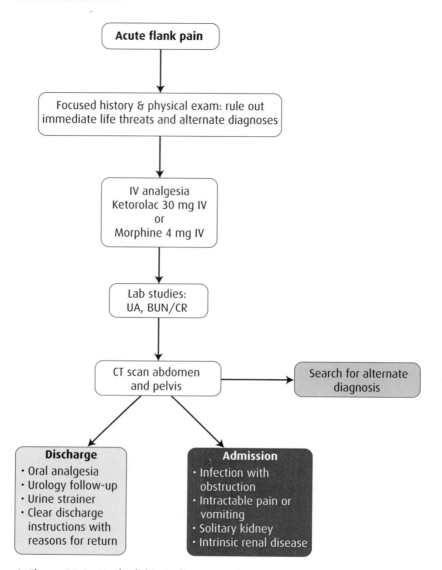

▲ Figure 39-2. Nephrolithiasis diagnostic algorithm. BUN, blood urea nitrogen; CR, creatinine; CT, computed tomography; UA, urinalysis.

however, saline boluses are no longer routinely recommended, as they do not help "flush out" the kidney stone. Additional therapeutic intervention includes antibiotics in those patients with coexisting urinary tract infections.

DISPOSITION

▶ Admission

Patients with intractable pain and/or inability to tolerate oral intake after aggressive ED management should be admitted to the hospital. Patients with kidney stones and

concomitant urinary tract infection are at high risk for developing urosepsis and require urology consultation for consideration of ureteral stenting or percutaneous nephrostomy tubes. Patients with a solitary kidney, history of renal transplant, or renal dysfunction should be discussed with urology and admitted.

▶ Discharge

Most patients with nephrolithiasis can be successfully managed in the ED and safely discharged. They should have adequate pain control and the ability to tolerate oral intake before discharge. Follow-up is recommended with a primary care provider within 1 week for small (<6 mm), uncomplicated kidney stones in patients with a known history of nephrolithiasis. Urology follow-up is recommended for patients with first time stones and large (>6 mm) proximal stones, as these stones have a low likelihood (<10%) of spontaneous passage. Patients should be given prescriptions for opioid analgesics and a urine strainer with instructions to strain all urine until stone passage and to bring passed stones to their follow-up appointment. Alpha blockers (tamulosin, terazosin, or doxazosin) are prescribed for up to four weeks to relax ureteral smooth muscles and increase the rate of stone passage and decrease pain. Lastly, patients should be given clear and specific discharge instructions to return to the ED if they have fever, persistent vomiting, intractable pain, or inability to urinate.

SUGGESTED READING

Manthey DE, Nicks BA. Urologic stone disease. In: Tintinalli JE, Stapczynski JS, Ma OJ, Cline DM, Cydulka, RK, Meckler GD. *Tintinalli's Emergency Medicine: A Comprehensive Study Guide.* 7th ed. New York, NY: McGraw-Hill, 2011, 651–657.

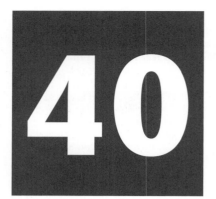

Urinary Tract Infections

40

Rebecca R. Roberts, MD

Key Points

- Differentiate a contaminated urinalysis from urinary tract infection (UTI). Obtain a catheterized urine specimen when the diagnosis is in question.
- Send a urine culture only when appropriate (pregnancy, recurrent UTI, pyelonephritis, urosepsis,

immunosuppression, fever without a source, indwelling bladder catheter).
- Treat asymptomatic bacteriuria in pregnant patients.
- Be aware of local bacterial resistance patterns when treating UTI.

INTRODUCTION

A urinary tract infection (UTI) refers to an infection anywhere in the urinary system in the presence of bacteriuria and symptoms. Cystitis is a lower tract infection of the bladder. Pyelonephritis is an upper tract infection of the kidney. An uncomplicated UTI occurs in patients without comorbidities and with an anatomically and functionally normal urinary tract. Complicated UTI occurs in patients with a functional or anatomic abnormality of their urinary tract or with the presence of serious comorbidities that place the patient at risk for serious adverse outcomes. These comorbidities include pregnancy, diabetes, immunocompromise, cancer, advanced age, and recent hospitalization or instrumentation. Anatomic factors that cause obstruction of urine flow resulting in complicated UTI include prostate enlargement, renal stones, obstructing tumors, and ureteral reflux, compression, or stricture.

UTI is one of the most common bacterial infections. In 2007, nearly 1.7 million UTIs were diagnosed in U.S. emergency departments (EDs), and 12% required hospital admission. Neonates, girls, and young women are at increased risk for infection. UTI is uncommon in young men; however, men older than 55 years have an increased risk due to incomplete bladder emptying from prostatic hypertrophy. UTI is the leading cause of sepsis

in the elderly and the most common hospital-acquired infection.

The bacterial organisms that usually cause UTI are the enteric flora that colonize the perineum. Gram-negative aerobic organisms and *Escherichia coli* are the most common, causing more than 80% of infections. *Staphylococcus saprophyticus* has the ability to adhere to urinary tract tissue, even with normal urinary flow, and causes 10–15% of UTIs. Other less common causative bacteria include the gram-negative species *Klebsiella*, *Proteus*, *Serratia*, and *Pseudomonas*.

CLINICAL PRESENTATION

▶ History

The patient history should be used to determine the presence of UTI, differentiation of upper versus lower tract infection, and the presence of any complicating factors. Uncomplicated cystitis symptoms include urinary frequency, urgency, dysuria, and mild suprapubic pain. Upper tract infection often begins with similar symptoms followed by pain extending to the back or abdomen and may have additional symptoms of fever and vomiting. Other important historical information includes pregnancy, recent hospitalization, immunosuppression, prostatic hypertrophy, urinary stones, and the presence of recent urinary tract instrumentation or bladder catheterization.

Physical Examination

Patients with lower urinary tract infection should be afebrile and have normal vital signs. Mild suprapubic tenderness may be present. An external genital examination should be performed to assess for extraurethral causes of dysuria. Pyelonephritis is indicated by flank tenderness over one or both kidneys. Fever and tachycardia may be present. The remainder of the examination should be directed at ruling out other diagnoses. A pelvic examination should be performed to assess for cervicitis, pelvic inflammatory disease, or pregnancy. In a male, the GU exam may reveal urethritis, epididymitis, or prostatitis. The abdominal examination should assess for possible cholecystitis, appendicitis, diverticulitis, or an abdominal mass that may be causing obstruction to urinary flow. Lung examination may reveal that fever and flank pain are due to a lower lobe pneumonia.

DIAGNOSTIC STUDIES

Laboratory

A urinalysis should be performed on all patients with symptoms consistent with UTI. The urine collection method should vary based on patient presentation. A clean-catch midstream specimen is usually adequate. Bladder catheterization should be performed for pediatric patients, the obese, women who are menstruating or have vaginal discharge, and the debilitated. Expected findings on urinalysis are listed in Table 40-1. A urine pregnancy test should be performed on all women of childbearing age. Asymptomatic bacteriuria in pregnancy should be treated, as this condition has been linked to prematurity, fetal morbidity, and stillbirth. Urine cultures should be sent if complicated UTI is suspected. Complicating factors include pregnancy, recurrent UTI, pyelonephritis, urosepsis, immunosuppression, indwelling bladder catheter, and fever without a source.

A complete blood count and renal function tests (blood urea nitrogen/creatinine) are warranted in patients with systemic symptoms such as pyelonephritis to assess for renal insufficiency, dehydration, electrolyte derangement, or sepsis, but are not indicated for simple cystitis. Other lab tests (liver function tests, lipase) may help with the differential diagnosis but are not routinely indicated. Blood cultures are obtained if the site of infection is unclear or if the patient has sepsis.

Imaging

Imaging is indicated when the clinical presentation indicates possible urinary obstruction, extensive disease with abscess, or to diagnose other conditions in the differential. Imaging may also be performed for relapses or recurrent UTIs to assess for an unsuspected nidus for infection such as renal stone. Noncontrast computed tomography (CT) of the abdomen and pelvis is the most common study obtained and readily diagnoses kidney stones and hydronephrosis. Renal ultrasound may be performed to assess for hydronephrosis in patients in whom CT is contraindicated (pregnancy), but is less sensitive for the presence of stones.

MEDICAL DECISION MAKING

The differential diagnosis for patients with lower tract UTI includes urethritis, vaginitis, and cervicitis. For patients with systemic symptoms and possible upper tract UTI, the differential includes nephrolithiasis, pneumonia, diverticulitis, appendicitis, cholecystitis, and pelvic inflammatory disease (Figure 40-1).

TREATMENT

Treatment of UTI is based on the type of infection, simple versus complicated, severity of illness, and local resistance patterns. Ideally, treatment for all complicated UTIs should be based on urine culture results; however, these results are not usually available at the time of empiric antibiotic administration in the ED. Also local and hospital bacterial resistance patterns should be considered when prescribing empiric treatment. Table 40-2 is a general guide to empiric treatment in the ED.

Table 40-1. Urinalysis interpretation.

Urinalysis Results	Bacteria	WBCs	RBCs	Nitrite	Leukocyte Esterase	Epithelial Cells
Normal	None	<5 per HPF	None	Negative	Negative	<5 per HPF
UTI	Any	>5–10 per HPF	Variable	Positive (specific but insensitive)	Positive (sensitive but nonspecific)	<5 per HPF
Contaminated Sample						>5 per HPF

HPF, high-power field; RBCs, red blood cells; WBCs, white blood cells.

CHAPTER 40

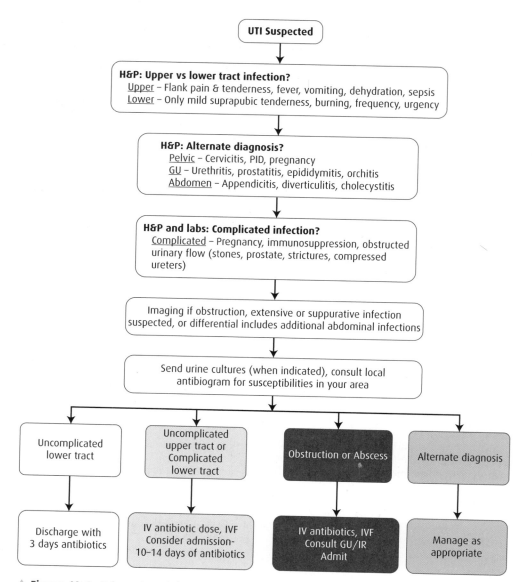

▲ **Figure 40-1.** Urinary tract infections diagnostic algorithm. GU, genitourinary; H&P, history and physical exam; PID, pelvic inflammatory disease.

DISPOSITION

▶ Admission

Admission is advised for patients with UTI complicated by urinary obstruction, immunosuppression, urosepsis, or associated unremitting vomiting, severe dehydration, renal insufficiency, or electrolyte derangements. Pregnant patients with any upper tract disease should be admitted for observation with an obstetrics consultation.

▶ Discharge

Patients with uncomplicated lower tract infection or uncomplicated upper tract infection may be discharged home with follow-up instructions to return to the ED for any complicating factors.

Table 40-2. Treatment of UTI.

Type of Infection	Pathogens	Antibiotic Regimen	Dose and Duration of Treatment
Acute cystitis	E. coli, S. saprophyticus, P. mirabilis	Trimethoprim/sulfamethoxazole OR ciprofloxacin	1 DS tab BID for 3 days 500 mg BID for 3 days
Asymptomatic bacteriuria and cystitis of pregnancy	E. coli, S. saprophyticus, P. mirabilis	Nitrofurantoin OR amoxicillin- clavulanate	100 mg BID for 5 days 500mg BID for 7 days
Pyelonephritis (outpatient)	E. coli, S. saprophyticus, P. mirabilis	Ciprofloxacin First dose IV in ED	500 mg BID for 10–14 days
Pyelonephritis (Inpatient)	E. coli, S. saprophyticus, P. mirabilis	Ciprofloxacin OR ceftriaxone	500 mg IV BID 1g IV QD Continue IV until improved
Urosepsis	E. coli, Proteus, Klebsiella, Pseudomonas	Ampicillin and gentamicin OR ceftriaxone	1 g and 5 mg/kg/day IV 1 g IV QD

SUGGESTED READINGS

Gupta K, Hooton TM, Naber KG, et al. International Clinical Practice Guidelines for the Treatment of Acute Uncomplicated Cystitis and Pyelonephritis in Women: A 2010 update by the Infectious Disease Society of America and the European Society for Microbiology and Infectious Disease. *Clin Infect Dis.* 2011;52:e103-3120.

Howes DS, Bogner MP. Urinary tract infections and hematuria. In: Tintinalli JE, Stapczynski JS, Ma OJ, Cline DM, Cydulka RK, Meckler GD. *Tintinalli's Emergency Medicine: A Comprehensive Study Guide.* 7th ed. New York, NY: McGraw-Hill, 2011.

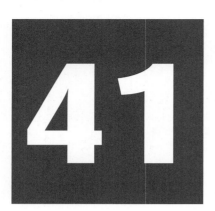

Testicular Torsion

Lynne M. Yancey, MD

Key Points

- Consider the diagnosis of testicular torsion in any male with abdominal pain.
- Perform a genitourinary (GU) examination on males complaining of abdominal pain, even if they have no GU complaints. This is especially important in adolescent males.
- When considering testicular torsion as a diagnosis, never allow an imaging study or laboratory test to delay an emergent urologic consultation.
- When attempting manual detorsion, remember the direction to turn the testicle is like opening a book.

INTRODUCTION

Testicular torsion is a primary concern in a male with acute scrotal pain and should be considered in all males with abdominal pain. Torsion is due to twisting of the testicle around the spermatic cord. It initially compromises venous outflow, and later arterial blood flow to the testicle, resulting in ischemia and infarction. The longer the torsion persists, the less chance of testicular survival. Hence, time is of the essence in the diagnosis and management of suspected torsion.

Peak incidence of testicular torsion occurs in the first year of life, before the testes descend into the scrotum, with a second peak at puberty, when the volume of the testes rapidly increases. It occurs in about 1 in 4,000 males a year. Testicular torsion is 10 times more likely to occur in a male with an undescended testis.

The initial effect of torsion is obstruction of venous return. If torsion persists, venous obstruction leads to worsening edema and ultimately to arterial obstruction and ischemia. The amount of venous obstruction is related to the degree of rotation of the testis on the spermatic cord and vascular supply. Incomplete rotation causes a lesser degree of edema and vascular congestion, whereas complete rotation leads to immediate complete obstruction and ischemia. The amount of testicular damage is related to the degree and duration of venous and arterial obstruction. If pain has been present for <6 hours, the testicular salvage rate is 80–100%.

CLINICAL PRESENTATION

History

Abnormal development of the fixation of the tunica vaginalis to the posterior scrotal wall can cause the testicle to hang freely in the scrotum like the clapper of a bell, aligned in a horizontal rather than vertical axis (Figure 41-1). This predisposes the testicle to torse, frequently in the context of strenuous physical activity or scrotal trauma. Torsion can also occur during sleep, when the cremaster muscle contracts. Other risk factors for testicular torsion include incomplete descent of the testes and testicular atrophy.

Patients will present with acute onset of unilateral scrotal pain. The pain is usually severe and noted in the lower abdomen, the inguinal canal, or the testis. Nausea and vomiting are often associated. Because it is an ischemic vascular event, the pain is not positional initially. Later, with significant testicular and scrotal edema, the pain may become more positional.

Physical Examination

Examination of the opposite testis may be helpful because anatomic abnormalities are often bilateral. Examine the patient in both the supine and standing positions. When the patient is standing, look for the affected testicle to be aligned in a horizontal (bell-clapper deformity) rather

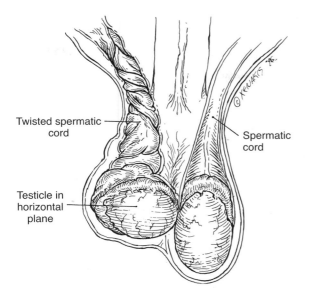

▲ Figure 41-1. Bell-clapper deformity. Reprinted with permission from Bondesson JD. Chapter 8. Urologic Conditions. In: Knoop KJ, Stack LB, Storrow AB, Thurman RJ, eds. *The Atlas of Emergency Medicine*. 3rd ed. New York: McGraw-Hill, 2010.

than vertical axis (normal). The involved testicle will often lie higher in the scrotum than the opposite side.

The involved testicle will be firm, swollen, tender, and the scrotum will usually be edematous. The size of the scrotal mass is an unreliable indicator of the underlying etiology, and the examination may occasionally be unremarkable.

Prehn sign (relief of pain with elevation and support of the scrotum) is more indicative of epididymo-orchitis than testicular torsion; however, this distinction is unreliable.

The cremasteric reflex is tested by lightly scratching the inner aspect of the thigh. A positive reflex is elicited when the ipsilateral testicle retracts upward. This reflex may be normally absent in infants and toddlers, however, absence of this reflex is relatively specific for torsion.

DIAGNOSTIC STUDIES

▶ Laboratory

Urinalysis will usually be normal. Complete blood count most often reveals an absence of a leukocytosis.

▶ Imaging

Color Doppler ultrasound is the preferred diagnostic study and has a sensitivity of 85–100% and a specificity of 100%. Ultrasound is also helpful for diagnosing other conditions that are part of the differential diagnosis of torsion, such as epididymitis, torsion of a testicular appendage, testicular rupture, hydrocele, hematocele, or hernia.

Nuclear radioisotope scanning has similar sensitivity to ultrasound; however, the specificity of nuclear scans is much lower. In addition, nuclear scans are more time-consuming than ultrasound.

MEDICAL DECISION MAKING

Testicular torsion is a time-sensitive condition that can result in loss of the testicle with associated loss of fertility. Therefore, assume acute testicular pain is torsion until proven otherwise.

Perform a focused history and physical examination as soon as possible. If your clinical suspicion for torsion is high, obtain an immediate urology consult and attempt manual detorsion.

Factors associated with testicular torsion include abrupt onset of pain, pain for less than 24 hours at the time of presentation, nausea and vomiting, high position of the testis, and abnormal cremasteric reflex. Torsion of a testicular appendage typically presents as pain that is more localized to one point on the testicle, more gradual in onset, and without nausea and vomiting. These small developmental remnants may be located at various positions on the testicle and on exam may be palpable as a hard tender nodule, most often at the upper pole of the testicle.

Epididymitis may be associated with dysuria, urgency, and pyuria. Ultrasound will show preserved or increased blood flow. A positive Prehn sign is helpful but is not always present. Epididymitis can extend to become epididymo-orchitis, which is more likely to be associated with signs of systemic illness such as fever, nausea, and vomiting. Isolated orchitis is rare and usually viral in origin. These infectious processes are all more likely to be gradual in onset.

An incarcerated inguinal hernia is another diagnostic consideration. However, the patient is likely to have a history of hernia or scrotal swelling before the episode of incarceration. Similarly, a tumor is usually gradual in onset and is often painless.

Direct testicular trauma can precipitate torsion or cause testicular contusion or rupture. Ultrasound will demonstrate rupture and possibly a hematocele. Consider torsion in any patient with testicular trauma who still has pain 1–2 hours after what seems like a relatively minor injury.

There is no single feature of the history, physical examination, or diagnostic studies that is completely reliable in diagnosing or excluding testicular torsion. Because this is a fertility-threatening diagnosis, high clinical suspicion mandates immediate urologic consultation (Figure 41-2). If ultrasound is rapidly available, it may be helpful in confirming a diagnosis, but should not delay urologic consult.

TREATMENT

Most testicular torsions occur in the lateral to medial direction. Manual detorsion should be performed by rotating the affected testis in the lateral direction 1.5 rotations

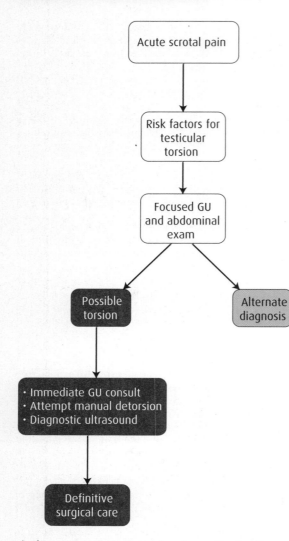

Figure 41-2. Testicular torsion diagnostic algorithm.

(540 degrees). To remember the direction to detorse, think of opening a book (Figure 41-3). The end point of the maneuver is relief of pain. If pain becomes more severe, attempt detorsion in the opposite direction. If manual detorsion is successful (ie, relief of pain), emergent consultation with a urologist is still required.

Manual detorsion is a painful procedure. You should warn your patient and consider administering intravenous (IV) narcotics before the procedure. A single dose of IV narcotics is not likely to ameliorate the pain of testicular torsion or remove the clinical end point (ie, relief of pain) of the detorsion maneuver.

When manual detorsion is unsuccessful, emergent surgical exploration and detorsion is indicated. Patients usually require surgical fixation of both the affected and the unaffected testes to avoid future torsion.

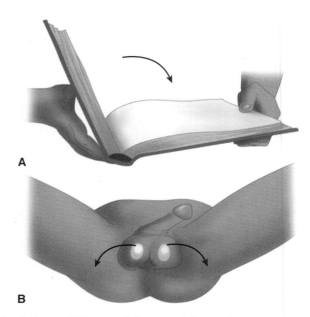

Figure 41-3. Manual detorsion of the testicle. Reprinted with permission from Gausche-Hill M, Williams JW. Chapter 82. Male Genitourinary Problems. In: Strange GR, Ahrens WR, Schafermeyer RW, Wiebe RA, eds. *Pediatric Emergency Medicine*. 3rd ed. New York: McGraw-Hill, 2009.

DISPOSITION

▶ Admission

Admission for operative urologic intervention is indicated in testicular torsion or suspected torsion with an equivocal ultrasound.

▶ Discharge

If no torsion is noted on ultrasound and an alternative diagnosis is established, the patient may be discharged with treatment as indicated (antibiotics for epididymitis, pain medications for torsion of a testicular appendage) and return precautions.

SUGGESTED READING

Cokkinos, DD, Antypa E, Tserotas P, et al. Emergency ultrasound of the scrotum: A review of the commonest pathologic conditions. *Curr Prob Diagnost Radiol.* 2011;40:1–14.

Davis JE, Silverman M. Scrotal emergencies. *Emerg Med Clin North Am.* 2011;29:469–484.

Schneider RE. Male genital problems. In: Tintinalli JE, Stapczynski JS, Ma OJ, Cline DM, Cydulka RK, Meckler GD. *Tintinalli's Emergency Medicine: A Comprehensive Study Guide.* 7th ed. New York, NY: McGraw-Hill, 2011, pp. 613–620.

Schmitz D, Safranek S. How useful is a physical exam in diagnosing testicular torsion? *J Fam Pract.* 2009;58:433–434.

Penile Disorders

S. Spencer Topp, MD

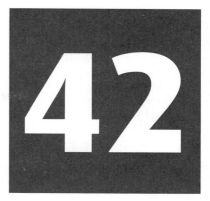

Key Points

- Priapism and paraphimosis are urologic emergencies.
- Prolonged priapism (>6 hours) may result in impotence.
- Paraphimosis may lead to glans ischemia and necrosis.

- Corpus cavernosum aspiration and dorsal slit are used by the emergency physician to prevent the complications of priapism and paraphimosis, respectively, until urology consultation is available.

INTRODUCTION

Penile disorders are a relatively uncommon presentation to the emergency department (ED); however, a few of these conditions are truly emergent. The penis is composed of 3 external anatomic parts—the shaft, glans, and foreskin. Penile disorders can be classified according to how these anatomic areas are affected. This chapter focuses on priapism, phimosis and paraphimosis, and balanoposthitis.

▶ Priapism

Priapism is a persistent, often times painful, erection in which both sides of the corpus cavernosa are engorged with blood. Priapism is subdivided into 2 classifications based on the source of blood—high flow versus low flow. Most commonly, oxygen-deprived, venous blood becomes entrapped in the cavernosa; this is termed "low-flow" priapism, or ischemic priapism. "High-flow" priapism, less often seen, results from a communication or fistula between the cavernosal arterial supply and the cavernosa itself. Because of the oxygen-rich arterial supply, this type of priapism is also called nonischemic priapism. High-flow priapism presents less of a time-sensitive risk and is often nonpainful.

▶ Phimosis and Paraphimosis

Phimosis is the inability to retract the foreskin proximally over the glans. Causes include infection, poor hygiene, and trauma, which lead to scarring and fibrosis of the foreskin and resultant loss of normal movement. This can infrequently lead to urinary retention owing to blockage of the urethral meatus. Phimosis may be normal in pre-pubertal males (physiologic phimosis). By age 4, 90% of foreskins are fully retractable. A foreskin that is not fully retractable by the end of puberty is considered pathologic phimosis.

Paraphimosis is the inability to return a retracted foreskin to its original, anatomic position. Paraphimosis results when the foreskin is not returned to its normal position overlying the glans penis. This commonly occurs as an iatrogenic complication, such as after an exam of the glans or Foley catheter placement in a debilitated patient. The retracted foreskin acts in a tourniquet manner, restricting venous outflow from the glans penis. This eventually leads to local swelling, inflammation, ischemia, and necrosis of the involved tissue, causing a urologic emergency.

▶ Balanoposthitis

Balanoposthitis is a combination of inflammation of the glans penis (balanitis) and inflammation of the foreskin (posthitis). This condition occurs most commonly in uncircumcised males as a result of poor hygiene, local/recurrent irritation, or infection (usually *Candida*, *Gardnerella*, or *Streptococcus pyogenes* species). Balanoposthitis may be the sole presenting symptom of diabetes mellitus.

CHAPTER 42

CLINICAL PRESENTATION

▶ History

Important historical features of priapism include past medical history, duration of symptoms, causative events, and medications. Medical causes of priapism include sickle cell disease or thalassemia (particularly in children) and leukemia or multiple myeloma in the elderly. The duration of priapism is also of significance. Prolonged veno-occlusive priapism (usually >6 hours) leads to fibrosis of the corporal tissue resulting in impotence. Patients should additionally be questioned about possible trauma to the penis, as high-flow priapism usually results from a traumatic fistula between arterial and venous supply. A thorough medication history should also be obtained. Medications implicated in priapism include antipsychotics (trazodone, thioridazine) and agents for erectile dysfunction (papaverine, prostaglandin E1, sildenafil). Cocaine use is also a common cause of priapism.

For phimosis and paraphimosis, patients should be questioned about duration of symptoms, general hygiene, and foreskin care. Duration of symptoms is particularly important for paraphimosis, as arterial compromise can lead to glans ischemia and necrosis.

Because of the strong association between diabetes and balanoposthitis, a thorough past medical and family history should be sought. Additionally, symptoms such as fevers, myalgias, and lymphadenopathy may suggest possible systemic involvement.

▶ Physical Examination

For any of the penile disorders, a general exam of all male genitourinary organs (penis, scrotum, testicles, perineum, anus/rectum, and prostate) should be performed. Inspection alone will often lead one to the diagnosis of priapism, paraphimosis, or balanoposthitis (Figure 42-1). If the penile foreskin is present, check for proper retraction/replacement. Inspect the underlying glans, looking for erythema, warmth, or discharge. Do not mistake paraphimosis with balanoposthitis, as both may present as a painful, edematous foreskin and glans. The key difference is that the foreskin is retracted and nonreducible in paraphimosis.

DIAGNOSTIC STUDIES

Because most penile disorders can be diagnosed by history and physical exam alone, few diagnostic measures are necessary. To help distinguish between high- and low-flow priapism, an arterial blood gas (ABG) of corporal aspirate may be obtained. Because low-flow priapism is an ischemic process, the ABG will show deoxygenated blood. If the ABG resembles a normal, oxygenated sample, the patient likely has high-flow priapism. Bedside ultrasound also has a role in priapism. If arterial flow can be seen using the color Doppler mode, then high-flow priapism is likely present. A complete blood count and reticulocyte

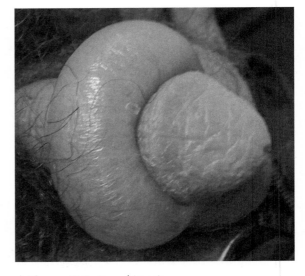

▲ **Figure 42-1.** Paraphimosis.

count can be helpful in sickle cell disease or to rule out leukemia.

Paraphimosis and phimosis are generally bedside diagnoses and require no further diagnostic testing.

Because of the strong association of diabetes mellitus and balanoposthitis, a bedside glucose test is warranted. For recurrent or difficult to treat infection, a culture may help to better guide treatment.

MEDICAL DECISION MAKING

Of the penile disorders discussed, low-flow priapism and paraphimosis are the two that require time-sensitive diagnosis and treatment or permanent penile damage may ensue. Urgent urologic consultation should be sought; however, the emergency physician should also be prepared to intervene when a urologist is not immediately available. Uncomplicated phimosis and balanoposthitis are generally treated in the ED with prompt urologic follow-up (Figure 42-2).

TREATMENT

Treatment of priapism begins with pain control. If low-flow priapism is suspected, treatment with subcutaneous terbutaline in the deltoid region can be effective. If priapism persists, corporal injection with an alpha-adrenergic agonist, such as phenylephrine, is performed.

If unsuccessful, corporal aspiration and irrigation can be attempted. First, a penile nerve block is performed for anesthesia. A 21-gauge or larger needle is inserted into the cavernosum (lateral sides of the penis), proximal to the

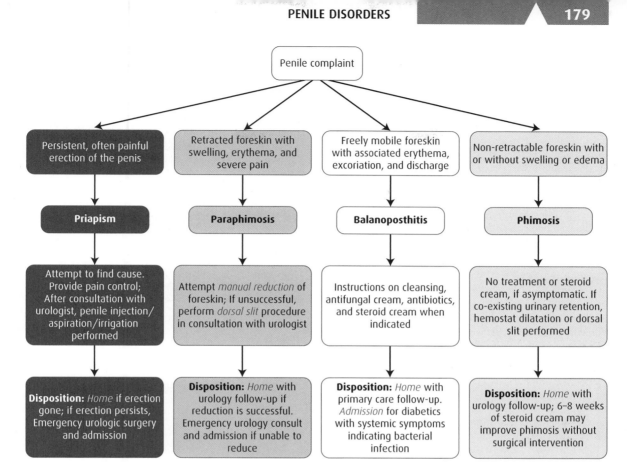

Figure 42-2. Penile disorders diagnostic algorithm.

glans. Blood is then allowed to drain, or if needed, aspirated, typically until detumescence begins. If necessary, aspiration is then followed by irrigation with 10–20 mL of sterile normal saline, with or without an alpha-adrenergic agent such as phenylephrine.

For priapism related to sickle cell disease, simple or exchange transfusion may be necessary.

Treatment of paraphimosis involves reducing the retracted foreskin. Ice packs or cold water immersion of the penis may be helpful with edema and inflammation. Compression wrapping with elastic bandage around the glans for 5–10 minutes will also help with the swelling. The glans may then be manually "pushed" back into the foreskin (Figure 42-3). Local injection with lidocaine may help the patient tolerate the compression dressing better, but will also contribute more fluid to the already swollen penis.

If manual reduction fails, the dorsal slit procedure can be attempted. A penile block or ring block is first performed for anesthesia. Next, hemostats are placed at the 11 and 1 o'clock positions on the edematous foreskin and clamped down for hemostasis. Scissors or scalpel are then used to cut the paraphimotic ring at the 12 o'clock position,

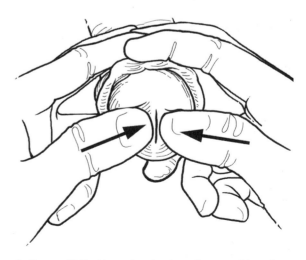

Figure 42-3. Manual reduction of a paraphimosis. Reproduced with permission from Reichman EF & Simon RR: *Emergency Medicine Procedures*, 1st edition. McGraw-Hill, New York, 2004.

between the 2 clamped hemostats. Manual reduction of the foreskin over the glans is then achieved. The reduced foreskin is then repaired with sutures, or a circumcision can then be performed by a urologist.

Phimosis requires far less emergent treatment because no vascular risk exists. If manual retraction is unable to be performed, topical steroid treatment applied under the foreskin to the tip of the penis for 4–6 weeks can be effective. If urinary retention develops, a dorsal slit procedure or full circumcision should be performed.

The treatment of balanoposthitis consists of regular cleaning of the glans with soap and water, with the foreskin retracted. Topical antifungal cream (nystatin, clotrimazole) should also be used. If bacterial infection is suspected, an oral antibiotic (ie, first-generation cephalosporin) should be added to the above treatments.

DISPOSITION

Patients with persistent, ischemic priapism require emergent urologic consultation. If corporal injection, aspiration, and irrigation (performed by either the urologist or ED physician) fail to achieve detumescence, surgery to perform a cavernosal shunt will most often be necessary. If the preceding treatment options are successful, the patient should be watched in the ED for 4–6 hours to ensure symptoms do not return. If an inciting cause was identified, the patient should also be thoroughly educated about future avoidance.

The disposition of paraphimosis is much like priapism. Urgent urologic consultation is required for nonreducible paraphimosis. Admission and surgery may be necessary if manual reduction or dorsal slit are unsuccessful. Patients with phimosis, as long as they can urinate, can generally be treated as an outpatient with good patient instructions, education, and urologic follow-up.

Most patients with balanoposthitis can also be safely discharged home. Patients with signs of systemic illness or severe comorbid disease may require admission and intravenous antibiotics. Patient education is also very important as the best preventative medicine is good personal hygiene.

▼ SUGGESTED READINGS

Dubin J, Davis JE. Penile emergencies. *Emerg Med Clin North Am.* 2011;29:485–499.

Nicks BA, Manthey DE. Male genital problems. In: *Tintinalli's Emergency Medicine: A Comprehensive Study Guide.* 7th ed. New York, NY: McGraw-Hill, 2011, pp. 645–651.

Vaginal Bleeding

Steven H. Bowman, MD

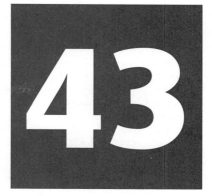

Key Points

- Obtain a pregnancy test in any woman of childbearing age who presents with vaginal bleeding or abdominal pain.
- Risk factors are absent in more than 40% of women who have an ectopic pregnancy.

- Ruptured ectopic pregnancy is a surgical emergency requiring prompt intervention and gynecologic consultation.
- Patients with postmenopausal bleeding should be referred to a gynecologist for endometrial biopsy to exclude malignancy.

INTRODUCTION

Menarche, the onset of menstruation, occurs in girls at approximately age 12. Normal menstruation continues until menopause, which occurs on average at age 51. The adult menstrual cycle is 28 days (±7 days), with menstruation lasting 4–6 days. Normal menstrual blood flow is approximately 30–60 mL; >80 mL of bleeding is considered abnormal. Dysfunctional uterine bleeding (DUB) is due to prolonged or excessive estrogen stimulation or ineffective progesterone production. **Menorrhagia** is an increased volume or duration of bleeding that occurs at the typical time of menstruation. **Metrorrhagia** is bleeding that occurs at irregular intervals outside of the normal menstrual cycle. **Menometrorrhagia** is irregular bleeding that is also of increased duration or flow.

Pregnancy must be excluded in women of childbearing age who present with vaginal bleeding.

Vaginal bleeding complicates 20% of early pregnancies. When bleeding occurs, 50% of patients will have a spontaneous abortion. In the United States, about 2% of all pregnancies are ectopic pregnancies. Mortality in these women is due to shock from intra-abdominal hemorrhage. In postmenopausal women with vaginal bleeding, 10% will be diagnosed with cancer, the majority being endometrial cancer.

Ectopic pregnancy is one of the most important causes of vaginal bleeding. Ectopic pregnancy occurs when a trophoblast implants at a site outside of the endometrium. In most cases, the ectopic site is within the lateral two thirds of the fallopian tube. Other sites include the medial third of the fallopian tube, cornu (junction of the tube and uterus), ovary, fimbria, cervix, and abdomen (Figure 43-1). Risk factors for ectopic pregnancy include a history of salpingitis, use of an intrauterine device, a prior ectopic pregnancy, increased maternal age, use of fertility drugs, and history of tubal ligation. Up to 42% of women with an ectopic pregnancy have no risk factors.

CLINICAL PRESENTATION

▶ History

A detailed history is essential. Determine the onset of bleeding, the date and duration of the last normal menstrual period, the number of previous pregnancies, and the presence of any prior history of abnormal vaginal bleeding. Pain may or may not be present. If pain is present, determine pain characteristics such as location, quality, and duration. Approximately 10% of patients with ectopic pregnancy will present with bleeding only. Attempt to have the patient quantify the amount of bleeding. Although variable, a tampon or pad absorbs approximately 30 mL of blood. The presence of clotted blood suggests brisk vaginal bleeding.

Inquire about previous gynecologic problems and assess the risk factors for ectopic pregnancy.

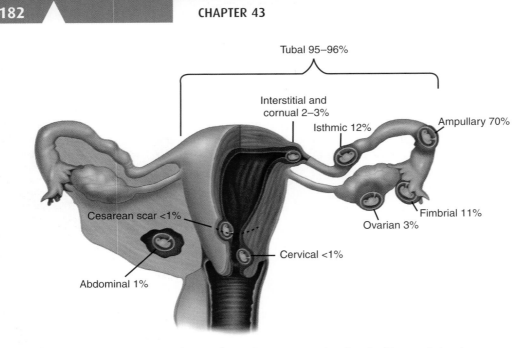

Tubal 95–96%

Interstitial and
cornual 2–3%

Isthmic 12%

Ampullary 70%

Cesarean scar <1%

Fimbrial 11%

Ovarian 3%

Cervical <1%

Abdominal 1%

▲ **Figure 43-1.** Frequency of sites of ectopic pregnancy. Reprinted with permission from Cunningham FG, Leveno KJ, Bloom SL, Hauth JC, Rouse DJ, Spong CY. Chapter 10. Ectopic Pregnancy. In: Cunningham FG, Leveno KJ, Bloom SL, Hauth JC, Rouse DJ, Spong CY, eds. *Williams Obstetrics.* 23rd ed. New York: McGraw-Hill, 2010.

Symptoms of weakness, lightheadedness, shortness of breath, or syncope suggest anemia from significant blood loss. Determine the presence of other medical conditions (eg, coagulopathies) or medications (eg, anticoagulants) that may exacerbate vaginal bleeding.

▶ Physical Examination

Note the patient's blood pressure and pulse, specifically to identify hypotension or a resting tachycardia. Look for other signs of anemia such as general, mucosal, or nail bed pallor. Before performing a pelvic examination, perform a focused general examination, including the heart, lungs, abdomen, and flank. Assess the abdomen for the presence of tenderness, masses, guarding, and rebound. Peritoneal signs may suggest infection or intraperitoneal blood.

For the pelvic examination, obtain the patient's consent and ensure her privacy during the exam. Explain what you are going to do. Ideally, both male and female examiners should request that a chaperone be present. Perform the exam with the patient in the lithotomy position. First, inspect the external genitalia. Then, using a warmed, lubricated, and appropriately sized vaginal speculum, determine the presence of blood, blood clots, tissue (products of conception), or discharge in the vaginal vault. Visually inspect the cervix.

On bimanual examination, determine whether the cervical os is open or closed. An open os is present when the tip of the examiner's index finger can easily pass through the cervix. Women with a closed internal os should be

Table 43-1. Classification of spontaneous abortion.

Type	Internal Cervical Os	Products of Conception
Threatened	Closed	Not passed
Inevitable	Open	Not passed
Incomplete	Usually open	Partially passed
Complete	Closed	Completely passed

considered to have a closed os, even if the external portion of the os is open. The internal os and the presence of products of conception will allow classification of different types of spontaneous abortions (Table 43-1).

Next, estimate the size of the uterus (12 weeks at the symphysis, 20 weeks at the umbilicus) by palpating the uterine fundus on the abdomen with one hand and palpating the cervix with the index and middle fingers on the other hand. Assess the cervix, uterus, and adnexa for tenderness or masses. Tenderness on pelvic examination is present in more than 80% of patients with a ruptured ectopic pregnancy.

DIAGNOSTIC STUDIES

▶ Laboratory

Urine pregnancy test is 99.4% sensitive for diagnosing pregnancy at the time that a woman "misses" her period.

It detects the presence of the beta subunit of human chorionic gonadotropin hormone (β-hCG) produced by the trophoblast in the patient's urine. A serum β-hCG level is also obtained. In a normal pregnancy, β-hCG levels double approximately every 2 days, peaking at 100,000 mIU/mL. Higher levels suggest trophoblastic disease. An ectopic pregnancy can be present at any β-hCG level; therefore, the initial β-hCG level cannot be used to exclude ectopic pregnancy. Patients with repeat β-hCG levels that decrease by >50% are at low risk for ectopic pregnancy, whereas those with levels that do not increase >66% are at high risk.

A serum hemoglobin is indicated in most patients with vaginal bleeding, but especially those with a resting tachycardia, lightheadedness, or prolonged duration of bleeding (≥3 weeks). Rh status should be obtained in pregnant patients with vaginal bleeding.

▶ Imaging

In pregnant patients with vaginal bleeding, the presence of an ectopic pregnancy must be excluded with a pelvic ultrasound performed by an emergency medicine physician or radiology personnel. Ectopic pregnancy is excluded when an intrauterine pregnancy (IUP) is visualized on pelvic ultrasound. A heterotopic pregnancy (a simultaneous IUP and an ectopic pregnancy), traditionally considered rare, is more common in women receiving treatment for infertility. Patients with pelvic ultrasounds that demonstrate a noncystic adnexal mass, moderate-large fluid in the cul-de-sac, an extrauterine gestational sac, or an empty uterus (with β-hCG >1,000 mIU/mL) should be considered high risk for ectopic pregnancy. In 15–20% of patients, the initial pelvic ultrasound will be indeterminate (no evidence of an IUP or an ectopic pregnancy). Of these indeterminate ultrasounds, 20% eventually will be diagnosed with an ectopic pregnancy.

MEDICAL DECISION MAKING

In a patient with vaginal bleeding, the most essential information to determine is the hemodynamic status and a urine pregnancy test. In the pregnant patient, the most important role of the emergency department is to exclude an ectopic pregnancy (Figure 43-2).

In patients with vaginal bleeding during the first trimester of pregnancy, the diagnostic possibilities include continuation of what will be a normal pregnancy or an abnormal pregnancy (ie, spontaneous abortion; ectopic pregnancy; trophoblastic disease). In nonpregnant patients, diagnostic possibilities include dysfunctional uterine bleeding, uterine fibroids, malignancy (cervical, uterine or vaginal), infection (PID, vaginal infections), trauma (assault, sexual intercourse), foreign body (IUD, tampon, sexual devices), and coagulopathies (genetic disorders, medical conditions, medications).

TREATMENT

When shock is present in a young woman with a positive pregnancy test, ruptured ectopic pregnancy is presumed. Initiate resuscitative measures immediately, including oxygen administration, intravenous (IV) fluids, and/or blood transfusion. Perform a bedside ultrasound and obtain gynecology consultation for surgical intervention. A similar work-up is pursued in women with a positive pregnancy test and an acute abdomen (presumed ruptured ectopic pregnancy), even when the initial vital signs are normal.

In pregnant patients with vaginal bleeding, always obtain the Rh status. If the woman is Rh-negative (15% of the white population), administer RhoGAM 50 mcg intramuscularly (IM). Complete and threatened abortions require no further treatment. In incomplete abortion, bleeding will continue until all products of conception have passed. Dilatation and curettage may be indicated if the abortion does not complete on its own. Patients with a ruptured ectopic pregnancy require surgery. Some patients with unruptured ectopic pregnancy are candidates for nonsurgical treatment by the gynecologist with use of methotrexate and leucovorin (IV, orally [PO], or IM as a single dose).

In patients with vaginal bleeding unrelated to pregnancy, consider blood transfusion in patients with symptomatic anemia, especially when the hemoglobin is <7 gm/dL. When bleeding is severe in patients with chronic anovulatory bleeding, relief may be obtained with hormonal therapy (eg, medroxyprogesterone 10 mg PO for 10 days or Ortho-Novum 1/35 1 tablet QID for 5 days).

DISPOSITION
▶ Admission

Patients with hemodynamic instability, peritoneal findings, severe anemia (hemoglobin <7 gm/dL), or a confirmed ectopic pregnancy on ultrasound should be admitted. Pregnant patients with a closed cervical os, no fetal tissue passed, no IUP visualized on ultrasound, and β-hCG >1,000 mIU/mL are at high risk of ectopic pregnancy; disposition should be made in consultation with a gynecologist. Admission may be warranted.

▶ Discharge

Discharge patients with mild to moderate vaginal bleeding, who are hemodynamically stable, and in whom ectopic pregnancy has been excluded. Discharge with gynecology follow-up, and a repeat β-hCG level in 48 hours is also appropriate for reliable patients with no IUP seen on ultrasound when the β-hCG is <1,000 mIU/mL. This assumes the patient is hemodynamically stable, has no significant abdominal tenderness, and has no other ultrasound findings that suggest an ectopic pregnancy (moderate to large amount of free fluid or a noncystic adnexal mass). In patients with postmenopausal bleeding, refer to a gynecologist for endometrial biopsy.

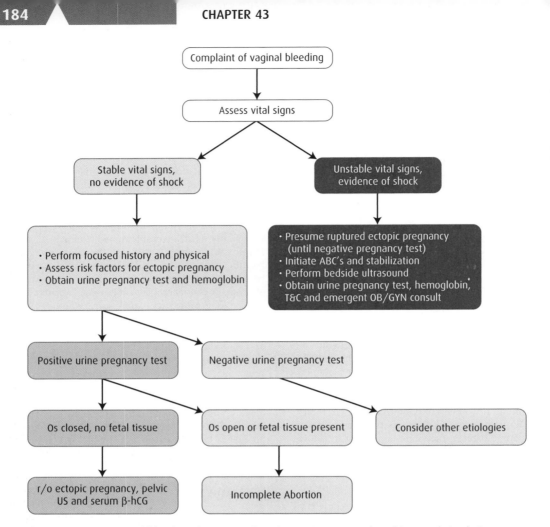

▲ **Figure 43-2.** Vaginal bleeding diagnostic algorithm. ABCs, airway, breathing, and circulation; β-hCG, beta human chorionic gonadotropin; T&C, Type and Cross; US, ultrasound.

▼ SUGGESTED READING

Clinical Policy: Critical Issues in the Initial Evaluation and Management of Patients Presenting to the Emergency Department in Early Pregnancy. Irving, TX: American College of Emergency Physicians, April 10, 2012.

Krause RS, Janicke DM, Cydulka RK. Ectopic pregnancies and emergencies in the first 20 weeks of pregnancy. In: Tintinalli JE, Stapczynski JS, Ma OJ, Cline DM, Cydulka RK, Meckler GD. *Tintinalli's Emergency Medicine: A Comprehensive Study Guide.* 7th ed. New York, NY: McGraw-Hill, 2011, pp. 676–684.

Morrison LJ, Spence JM. Vaginal bleeding in the nonpregnant patient. In: Tintinalli JE, Stapczynski JS, Ma OJ, Cline DM, Cydulka RK, Meckler GD. *Tintinalli's Emergency Medicine: A Comprehensive Study Guide.* 7th ed. New York, NY: McGraw-Hill, 2011, pp. 665–676.

Promes SB, Nobay F. Pitfalls in first-trimester bleeding. *Emerg Med Clin North Am.* 2010;28:219–234.

Vaginal Discharge

Joanna Wieczorek Davidson, MD

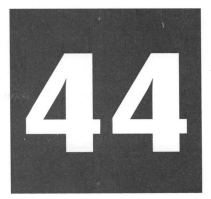

Key Points

- Vaginal discharge is a common presenting complaint in reproductive-age women.
- Possible diagnoses include vaginitis, cervicitis, or pelvic inflammatory disease (PID).
- Clinical evaluation for the diagnosis of PID is not sensitive. Maintain a high suspicion and low threshold to treat.

INTRODUCTION

Many women come to the emergency department (ED) with the chief complaint of vaginal discharge. It may be accompanied by other symptoms such as fever, abdominal or pelvic pain, malodor, itching, and dysuria. Vaginal discharge is usually due to vaginitis, cervicitis, or pelvic inflammatory disease (PID).

Vaginitis is a spectrum of diseases causing vulvovaginal symptoms including burning, irritation, and itching, with or without vaginal discharge. Normal vaginal flora maintains the vaginal pH at 3.8–4.5. Changes in the pH or disruption of the vaginal flora may result in the overgrowth of pathogenic organisms, ultimately resulting in a change in the appearance, consistency, or odor of vaginal secretions. Noninfectious causes like atrophy and contact vaginitis are fairly common—particularly in sexually inactive and postmenopausal women. The most common infectious causes of vaginitis in descending order of frequency include bacterial vaginosis (BV), vaginal candidiasis, and trichomonas vaginitis. BV is caused by a pathologic overgrowth of normal vaginal flora—*Gardnerella vaginalis*.

Infections of the upper reproductive tract (cervix, uterus, fallopian tubes, adnexa) will also cause discharge. Cervicitis is the term used when infection is present within the cervix only. Pelvic inflammatory disease (PID) is a spectrum of upper genital tract infections that includes endometritis, salpingitis, tubo-ovarian abscess, and pelvic peritonitis. Sexually transmitted organisms, especially *Neisseria gonorrhoeae* and *Chlamydia trachomatis*, are implicated in the majority of cases of both cervicitis and PID; however, other organisms (*Gardnerella vaginalis*, *Haemophilus influenza*, anaerobic and gram-negative bacteria, and *Streptococcus agalactia*) are also causative. PID affects 11% of women of reproductive age and requires hospital admission in 20%. Inflammation and infection can lead to scarring and adhesions within the fallopian tubes, leading to major long-term sequelae including infertility, ectopic pregnancy, and chronic pelvic pain. The risk of ectopic pregnancy is 12–15% higher in women who have had PID. Tubal factor infertility is increased 12–50% in women with a past diagnosis of PID. Prevention of complications is dependent on early recognition and effective treatment.

CLINICAL PRESENTATION

▶ History

Any complaint of vaginal discharge or pelvic pain requires a detailed gynecologic history. Inquire about history of sexually transmitted infections (STIs), intrauterine device use, pregnancies, last menstrual period, and any previous gynecologic procedure. History should include details of vaginal discharge, odor, irritation, itching, burning, bleeding, dysuria, and dyspareunia. In addition, determine the presence of abdominal pain, nausea, vomiting, fevers, rash, or joint aches.

Patients with vaginitis lack significant abdominal pain or fevers and do not appear systemically ill. BV typically presents with thin, whitish gray discharge that has a fishy smell. In candidiasis, pruritus is the most common and specific symptom; discharge tends to be white and occasionally thick and "cottage-cheese" like. It is important to ask about risk factors for candidal colonization: uncontrolled diabetes mellitus, recent antibiotic use, immunosuppression, and pregnancy. Patients with trichomonas vaginitis (a sexually transmitted protozoan parasite) are asymptomatic in 50% of cases, but the classic discharge is described as yellow, frothy and malodorous.

Vaginal atrophy is present in 60% of women 4 years after menopause. Symptoms of atrophic vaginitis include vaginal dryness, soreness, itching and occasional thin, scant, yellowish discharge.

Acute PID can be difficult to diagnose because of the wide variation in symptoms and signs. The most common presenting symptom is lower abdominal pain that tends to be bilateral, dull or crampy. Approximately 75% of patients with PID have abnormal vaginal discharge. Unilateral pain should raise suspicion for a tubo-ovarian abscess or an alternate diagnosis like appendicitis. Dyspareunia may be present as well as urinary tract symptoms. Only one third of patients with PID will have fever >100.4° F.

▶ Physical Examination

Obtain the patient's vital signs, particularly noting blood pressure, pulse, and temperature. Before performing a pelvic exam, perform a focused general exam, including the abdomen and flank. During the pelvic exam, inspect the external genitalia. Make note of vulvar edema or erythema, which can be a sign of vaginitis. On the speculum exam, determine the presence of blood or discharge in the vaginal vault. Visualize the cervix, looking for inflammation, foreign body, and discharge originating from the os. Mucopurulent cervicitis is a common finding in both cervicitis and PID (Figure 44-1). On bimanual exam it is important to note cervical motion tenderness (CMT) as well as adnexal fullness or tenderness. CMT, also referred to as the *chandelier sign*, is elicited by moving the cervix up and down or laterally with the index and middle finger. This causes movement of the uterus and tubes, which will significantly reproduce pain in patients with PID. CMT is sensitive but lacks specificity, as it can be positive in patients with other sources of inflammation (appendicitis, ruptured cysts, or ectopic pregnancy). Adnexal tenderness appears to be the most sensitive finding (95%) for PID.

DIAGNOSTIC STUDIES

▶ Laboratory

Any evaluation of a woman of childbearing age in the ED should including a pregnancy test, as the possibility of ectopic pregnancy or septic abortion must be considered.

During the pelvic exam, vaginal secretions may be collected and tested. Microscopic examination of vaginal secretions and evaluation of pH are useful diagnostic tools;

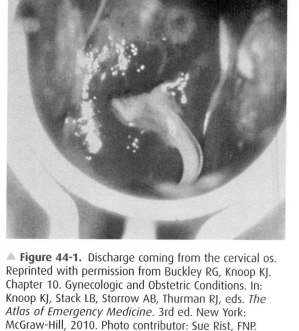

▲ **Figure 44-1.** Discharge coming from the cervical os. Reprinted with permission from Buckley RG, Knoop KJ. Chapter 10. Gynecologic and Obstetric Conditions. In: Knoop KJ, Stack LB, Storrow AB, Thurman RJ, eds. *The Atlas of Emergency Medicine.* 3rd ed. New York: McGraw-Hill, 2010. Photo contributor: Sue Rist, FNP.

however, microscopes and reagents are not available in all EDs. A slide for microscopy is prepared by mixing a sample of discharge with 1–2 drops of normal saline and then applying a coverslip. Vaginal secretions may also be prepared with 10% potassium hydroxide (KOH), often producing a fishy odor, or positive whiff test, which may provide evidence for a diagnosis (Table 44-1).

During the speculum exam, endocervical cultures should be obtained by placing a swab 1 cm into the cervix and rotating it. DNA probe swabs have a high sensitivity and specificity for both gonorrhea and chlamydia; however, the results of these tests are not immediately available in the ED.

In patients with abdominal pain or toxic appearance, blood tests may be helpful. An elevated white blood cell (WBC) count, erythrocyte sedimentation rate (ESR), or C-reactive protein (CRP) can support the diagnosis of PID. Urinalysis should be part of the laboratory evaluation;

Table 44-1. Distinguishing causes of vaginitis.

	Bacterial Vaginosis	Candidiasis	Trichomonas
Frequency	40–50%	20–25%	15–20%
Discharge color	Gray, white	White, clumped	Gray, green-yellow
Quantity	Moderate	Scant to moderate	Profuse
pH (normal ≤4.5)	≥4.5	≤4.5	≥5
Amine/fishy odor (discharge + KOH prep)	Positive	Negative	Usually positive
Microscopy (discharge + normal saline drops)	Clue cells (epithelial cells with adherent bacteria)	Mycelia or hyphae with KOH	Motile trichomonads
Treatment	Metronidazole 500 mg BID × 7 days	Fluconazole 150 mg × 1 dose	Metronidazole 2 g × 1 dose OR Metronidazole 500 mg BID × 7days

however, a positive urinalysis finding does not exclude PID, as inflammation in the pelvis can produce WBCs in the urine. Testing for other STIs such as human immunodeficiency virus, hepatitis, and syphilis may also be warranted.

▶ Imaging

Imaging may improve the accuracy of PID diagnosis. Transvaginal pelvic ultrasound demonstrates thickened, fluid-filled fallopian tubes or pelvic free fluid in severe PID. Complex adnexal masses signifying tubo-ovarian abscesses are seen on ultrasound as well. Abdominopelvic computed tomography (CT) scans can also be used for patients with toxic appearance, pain, and suspicion of tubo-ovarian abscess. CT findings in PID include cervicitis, oophoritis, salpingitis, thickening of uterosacral ligaments, simple or complex pelvic fluid, or abscess collections.

MEDICAL DECISION MAKING

In patients presenting with vaginal discharge, use the history and pelvic exam to determine the cause (Figure 44-2). Patients presenting with vulvovaginal discomfort, without evidence of cervicitis on pelvic exam or concern for STI, can be treated for vaginitis. The cause of vaginitis can be determined based on historical factors as well as composition of vaginal discharge. If there is evidence of cervical

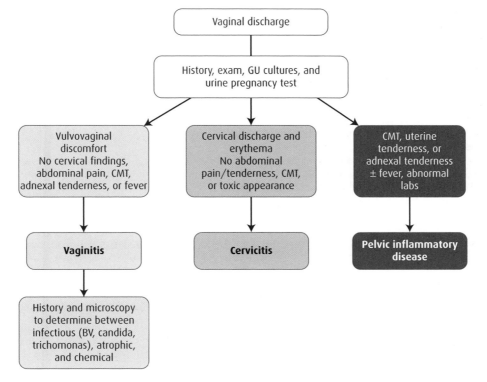

▲ **Figure 44-2.** Vaginal discharge diagnostic algorithm. BV, bacterial vaginosis; CMT, Cervical motion tenderness; GU, genitourinary.

CHAPTER 44

Table 44-2. Treatment of cervicitis: Treat for both gonorrhea and chlamydia.

	First line	Alternate
Gonorrhea	Ceftriaxone 250 mg IM OR Cefixime 400 mg PO	Cefpodoxime 400 mg PO OR Azithromycin 2 g PO
Chlamydia	Azithromycin 1 g PO	Doxycycline 100 mg PO BID × 7 days

Table 44-3. Treatment of PID.

	Option 1	Option 2
Outpatient treatment	Ceftriaxone 250 mg IM PLUS Doxycycline 100 mg PO BID × 14 days ± Metronidazole 500 mg PO BID × 14 days	Cefoxitin 2 g IM WITH Probenecid 1 g PO PLUS Doxycycline 100 mg PO BID × 14 days ± Metronidazole PO BID × 14 days
Inpatient treatment	Cefotetan 2 g IV q12hrs OR Cefoxitin 2 g IV q6hrs PLUS Doxycycline 100 mg PO or IV q12 hrs	Clindamycin 900 mg IV q8hrs PLUS Gentamicin 2 mg/kg IV followed by 1.5 mg/kg q8hrs

discharge or erythema without abdominal tenderness or toxic appearance, the patient should be treated for cervicitis. It is important to rule out PID in these patients. Given the difficulty of diagnosis and potential complications, the 2010 Centers for Disease Control and Prevention guidelines recommend that providers maintain a low threshold to treat PID. Empiric treatment for PID should be initiated in sexually active young women and other women at risk for STIs if they are experiencing pelvic or lower abdominal pain, if no other cause of pain can be identified, and if one or more of the following minimum criteria are present on pelvic exam: CMT, adnexal tenderness, or uterine tenderness. One or more of the following additional criteria can be used to enhance the specificity and support a diagnosis of PID: oral temperature >101°F, abnormal cervical or mucopurulent discharge, presence of abundant WBCs on microscopy of vaginal fluid, elevated ESR, elevated CRP, or laboratory documentation of cervical infection with *N. gonorrhoeae* or *C. trachomatis*.

TREATMENT

The treatment of vaginitis, cervicitis, and PID is outlined in Tables 44-1, 44-2, and 44-3. All regimens used to treat cervicitis and PID should be effective against *N. gonorrhoeae* and *C. trachomatis*. The need to treat anaerobes has not been completely studied. *Gardnerella* (BV) has been present in many patients with PID, so many recommend treatment regimens that include anaerobic coverage (ie, metronidazole). For women with mild to moderate severity PID, parenteral and oral regimens appear to have similar efficacy.

DISPOSITION

▶ Admission

In women with mild or moderate PID, outpatient therapy yields similar short and long-term outcomes. Hospitalization is recommended when the patient meets any of the following criteria: surgical emergencies cannot

be ruled out (eg, appendicitis, tubo-ovarian abscess), pregnancy, nonresponse to oral antimicrobial therapy, unable to tolerate oral regimen.

▶ Discharge

Patient with vaginitis and cervicitis can be safely discharged. When an STI is suspected, patients should be instructed to notify their partners. For PID, outpatient therapy is initiated in patients who do not have any of the criteria listed previously, appear nontoxic, and have reliable follow-up.

▼ SUGGESTED READING

Buckley RG, Knoop KJ. Gynecologic and obstetric conditions. In: Knoop KJ, Stack LB, Storrow AB, Thurman RJ. *The Atlas of Emergency Medicine.* 3rd ed. New York, NY: McGraw-Hill, 2010.

Centers for Disease Control and Prevention. Sexually Transmitted Diseases Treatment Guidelines, 2010. http://www.cdc.gov/std/treatment/2010/toc.htm

Kuhn, JK, Wahl RP. Vulvovaginitis. In: Tintinalli JE, Stapczynski JS, Ma OJ, Cline DM, Cydulka RK, Meckler GD. *Tintinalli's Emergency Medicine: A Comprehensive Study Guide.* 7th ed. New York, NY: McGraw-Hill, 2011, pp. 711–16.

Shepherd SM, Shoff WH, Behrman AJ. Pelvic inflammatory disease. In: Tintinalli JE, Stapczynski JS, Ma OJ, Cline DM, Cydulka RK, Meckler GD. *Tintinalli's Emergency Medicine: A Comprehensive Study Guide.* 7th ed. New York, NY: McGraw-Hill, 2011, pp. 716–720.

Sweet RL. Treatment of acute pelvic inflammatory disease. *Infect Dis Obstet Gynecol* 2011;561–909.

Preeclampsia and Eclampsia

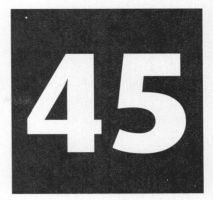

Kathleen A. Wittels, MD

Key Points

- Gestational hypertension, preeclampsia, and eclampsia represent a spectrum of potentially life-threatening diseases that must be diagnosed and treated aggressively.
- Consider preeclampsia in any pregnant patient with an elevated blood pressure.

- The degree of hypertension does not correlate with the severity of preeclampsia.
- Delivery of the fetus is the definitive treatment of preeclampsia and eclampsia.

INTRODUCTION

Hypertension in pregnancy occurs in approximately 10% of pregnancies and can be associated with significant maternal and fetal morbidity and mortality. The spectrum of disease is divided into 3 main categories: gestational hypertension, preeclampsia, and eclampsia. Preeclampsia affects 2–6% of pregnancies in the United States, with a higher incidence globally. Eclampsia occurs in <1% of patients with preeclampsia.

Gestational hypertension is defined as a blood pressure >140/90 mmHg in a pregnant patient without preexisting hypertension. The hypertension will resolve within 12 weeks postpartum. When proteinuria is also present, it is defined as preeclampsia. Preeclampsia typically occurs after 20 weeks' gestation. A subset of patients will develop severe preeclampsia, which is associated with one of more of the following: severe hypertension (>160/110 mmHg on 2 separate occasions >6 hours apart), large proteinuria, neurologic symptoms, epigastric/right upper quadrant (RUQ) pain, pulmonary edema, or thrombocytopenia. Eclampsia is preeclampsia with seizures. HELLP syndrome affects some patients with preeclampsia and eclampsia and is associated with hemolysis, elevated liver enzymes, and low platelets.

Although the exact etiology of preeclampsia is unknown, there are several factors that are thought to contribute. These include maternal immunologic intolerance, abnormal placental implantation, endothelial dysfunction, and genetic factors.

CLINICAL PRESENTATION

▶ History

Patients with gestational hypertension and preeclampsia may be asymptomatic. Some women will report facial or extremity edema, epigastric or RUQ pain, headache, or visual disturbances. Seizures in a woman with preeclampsia is pathognomonic for eclampsia and may occur in the postpartum period. Risk factors for preeclampsia that should be screened for during the history include nulliparity, advanced maternal age, a multiple gestation pregnancy, diabetes, obesity, and previous preeclampsia.

▶ Physical Examination

It is critical to pay careful attention to the vital signs, particularly the blood pressure. Edema of the face or extremities may be appreciated. Examination of the lungs may reveal rales suggestive of pulmonary edema. The abdominal exam is important to assess for tenderness as well as to estimate the gestational age of the fetus (Figure 45-1). Listen for fetal heart tones with a Doppler or

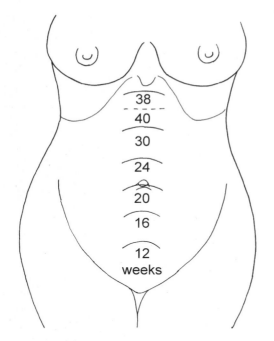

▲ **Figure 45-1.** Measurement from symphysis pubis to fundal height as a clinical estimator of gestational age.

measure the fetal heart rate with bedside ultrasound. A complete neurologic examination is performed to identify any new deficits.

DIAGNOSTIC STUDIES

▶ Laboratory

A urinalysis is indicated to identify proteinuria or infection. A 24-hour urine collection with >300 mg protein is significant and corresponds approximately to ≥1+ protein on the dipstick (although the dipstick is thought to be an unreliable measure). Additional testing includes electrolytes, renal function, and liver function tests. With HELLP syndrome, the complete blood count will reveal thrombocytopenia, and the peripheral smear may also show schistocytes. Lactate dehydrogenase will be elevated if hemolysis is present. A magnesium level should be ordered as a baseline for potential magnesium therapy. In addition, a type and cross should be sent in preparation for possible fetal delivery.

▶ Imaging

A noncontrast head computed tomography should be obtained in any patient with a new onset seizure to differentiate an intracerebral hemorrhage or mass from eclampsia as the etiology of the seizure. Ultrasonography is recommended to assess the status of the fetus. Continuous monitoring will alert providers to signs of fetal distress.

MEDICAL DECISION MAKING

In a pregnant patient with hypertension, the presence of proteinuria is enough to make a diagnosis of preeclampsia (Figure 45-2). Before confirmation of proteinuria, other diagnoses should be considered. If abdominal pain is present, the differential diagnosis includes pancreatitis, hepatitis, cholecystitis, or gastritis. Headache and neurologic deficits may be due to an intracerebral hemorrhage or stroke. Laboratory studies will help identify patients with HELLP syndrome.

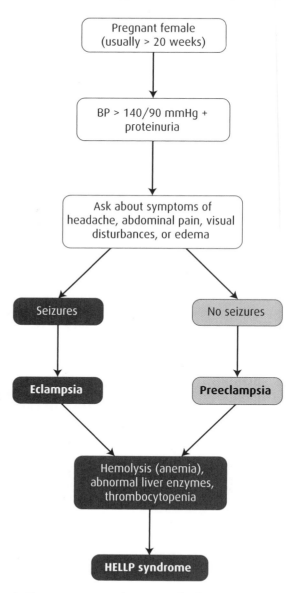

▲ **Figure 45-2.** Preeclampsia and eclampsia diagnostic algorithm. BP, blood pressure; HELLP, hemolysis, elevated liver enzymes, and low platelets.

TREATMENT

Initial treatment is focused on stabilizing the patient. Place the woman in the left lateral decubitus position to improve circulation. Apply supplemental oxygen, cardiac monitoring, and establish intravenous (IV) access. Avoid overhydration, as it may result in pulmonary edema. Antihypertensive therapy is indicated in the setting of severe hypertension (systolic blood pressure ≥160 mmHg or diastolic blood pressure ≥110 mmHg). Appropriate agents include hydralazine, labetalol, nifedipine, or nitroprusside. It is important to avoid being overly aggressive with antihypertensive agents, as a drastic drop in blood pressure can result in fetal hypoperfusion.

Magnesium remains the drug of choice for the treatment of severe preeclampsia and eclampsia. In the setting of severe preeclampsia, its primary role is prophylaxis against eclampsia, although it may also have antihypertensive effects. The initial loading dose is 4–6 g IV infused over 15 minutes, followed by 1–2 g/hr. Signs of magnesium toxicity include loss of deep tendon reflexes (8–12 mg/dL), respiratory paralysis (12–18 mg/dL), and cardiac arrest (24–30 mg/dL). Calcium gluconate should be given to counteract cardiorespiratory compromise owing to magnesium toxicity. Phenytoin is an alternate antiepileptic treatment, but is less effective than magnesium.

The definitive treatment of preeclampsia and eclampsia is delivery of the fetus. Determining the appropriate timing for this is challenging depending on the fetal age. After 37 weeks, most women with preeclampsia will be induced. In women with severe preeclampsia, delivery should be considered after 34 weeks or in the setting of worsening symptoms regardless of fetal age. If the fetus is less than 34 weeks, steroids (betamethasone) are indicated to improve fetal lung maturity.

DISPOSITION

▶ Admission

Patients with severe preeclampsia should be admitted to the hospital for management of their symptoms and determination of the ideal time for delivery. Patients with eclampsia require intensive care unit admission.

▶ Discharge

Patients with gestational hypertension or mild preeclampsia may be managed as outpatients with close obstetric follow-up. Any signs of worsening preeclampsia should result in admission. Women who are not able to easily access medical care are not good candidates for outpatient management.

▼ SUGGESTED READING

American College of Obstetricians and Gynecologists. Committee on Practice Bulletins-Obstetrics. Diagnosis and management of preeclampsia and eclampsia. *Obstet Gynecol.* 2002;99:159–167.

Echevarria MA, Kuhn GJ. Emergencies after 20 weeks of pregnancy and the postpartum period. In: Tintinalli JE, Stapczynski JS, Ma OJ, Cline DM, Cydulka RK, Meckler GD. *Tintinalli's Emergency Medicine: A Comprehensive Study Guide.* 7th ed. New York, NY: McGraw-Hill, 2011, pp. 695–702.

Sibai BM. Diagnosis and management of gestational hypertension and preeclampsia. *Obstet Gynecol.* 2003;102:181–192.

Sibai BM. Diagnosis, prevention, and management of eclampsia. *Obstet Gynecol.* 2005;105:402–410.

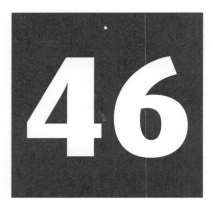

Emergency Delivery

Jessica Sime, MD

Key Points

- Assemble sufficient staff and supplies to care for both the mother and newborn.

- When vaginal bleeding is present, defer the pelvic examination until placenta previa has been excluded.

- Utilize bedside ultrasound to check fetal presentation.

- Be prepared for complications such as postpartum hemorrhage, shoulder dystocia, and breech presentation.

INTRODUCTION

Less than 1% of all deliveries are in the emergency department (ED) because most women in labor are quickly triaged to the labor and delivery unit. However, if a woman is going to precipitously deliver, or the hospital has no obstetric services, it is up to the emergency physician to be prepared to deliver the infant.

Moreover, deliveries in the ED are more likely to be considered high risk. Women who deliver in the ED more often have had little or no prenatal care, may have substance abuse problems, do not know they are pregnant, or have been victims of domestic violence. These women may have higher frequencies of complications such as premature rupture of membranes (PROM), preterm labor, malpresentation, umbilical cord prolapse, placenta previa, abruptio placentae, or postpartum hemorrhage. The emergency medicine physician must be prepared to manage these complications.

CLINICAL PRESENTATION

▶ History

Past medical, surgical, gestational age, and obstetric history should be obtained, as well as history of prenatal care. It is important to inquire about vaginal bleeding during labor. Scant, mucoid bleeding is usually termed *bloody show* and

occurs when the cervical mucus plug is expelled. Heavy vaginal bleeding is a worrisome sign and can represent placenta previa (painless vaginal bleeding from the placenta covering the cervical os) or abruptio placentae (painful bleeding owing to placental separation from the uterus). The physician should also determine whether the patient has had a spontaneous rupture of membranes (SROM). Clear, blood-tinged, or meconium-stained vaginal fluid suggests rupture of membranes.

▶ Physical Examination

As always, vital signs are the first step in examination. Fetal heart rate can be assessed with handheld Doppler or with electronic fetal monitoring, if available. The abdomen should be palpated for tenderness and fundal height. Gestational age can be estimated if the mother is unsure. At 20 weeks' gestation, the uterus is at the umbilicus, and it grows approximately 1 cm every week until 36 weeks.

Pelvic examination should begin with inspection of the perineum to determine whether the delivery is imminent (crowning). If the patient reports vaginal bleeding, examination should be deferred until an ultrasound can be performed. It is important to identify placenta previa first, as the bimanual and speculum examination can exacerbate the bleeding.

The bimanual examination determines the position of the fetus and readiness of the cervix. Sterile gloves should be used to prevent infection. A normal cervix is thick, only open at the entry to fingertip, and is firm to touch. Gradually the cervix thins; this is termed effacement. Dilation of the cervix progresses from closed to fully open (10 cm). Station indicates the location of the presenting part relative to the ischial spines. A presenting part at the ischial spines is at 0 station. If the presenting part is at the introitus, it is at +3 station. Position describes the relationship of the presenting part to the birth canal. Usually the fetal occiput is anterior.

Speculum examination can help identify spontaneous rupture of membranes. Pooling vaginal secretions should be tested with Nitrazine paper to determine pH. A dark blue color correlates to a pH of 7.0-7.4 and indicates the presence of amniotic fluid. Normal vaginal secretions have a pH of 4.5-5.5. Next, the cervical os is inspected. The examiner should identify whether it is open slightly, has bulging membranes, a visible fetal head, or other presenting part. If the examiner sees a prolapsed umbilical cord, he or she should keep a hand in the vagina and elevate the presenting part to prevent cord compression, while an assistant contacts obstetric services for an emergency cesarean section.

DIAGNOSTIC STUDIES

▶ Laboratory

If a patient is about to deliver, no laboratory studies are necessary. A complete blood count, type and screen, prothrombin time/partial thromboplastin time are useful in the event of postpartum hemorrhage. Rh type should be sent to determine the need for RhoGAM.

▶ Imaging

Bedside ultrasound is used to determine the fetal position, heart rate, and location of the placenta.

MEDICAL DECISION MAKING

Delivery of a fetus is best done by obstetricians in a labor and delivery unit. If time allows, the emergency physician should attempt to transfer the patient to an appropriate setting. In a hospital with no obstetric services, a precipitously delivering mother must be delivered by the emergency physician. If delivery is not imminent, the patient may be transferred. If a patient needs to be transferred to another hospital, she should be sent by an advanced life support–equipped ambulance, as a patient in labor is considered medically unstable (Figure 46-1).

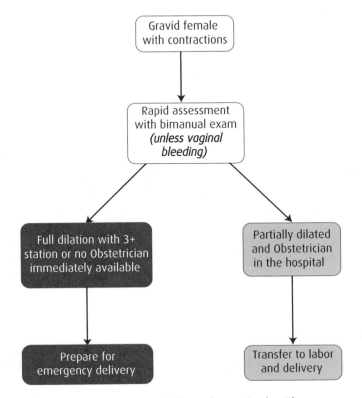

▲Figure 46-1. Emergency delivery diagnostic algorithm.

TREATMENT

If the decision is made to deliver the child in the ED, call for obstetric and pediatric support if available. Large-bore intravenous (IV) access should be obtained and fluids started. Oxygen by nasal cannula is given to the mother, especially if there are any signs of fetal distress. The infant radiant warmer should be set up and in the room. Delivery equipment should be set up including cord clamps, scissors, suction, forceps, and neonatal resuscitation equipment.

The mother is placed in the dorsal lithotomy position, and the perineum is cleaned with povidone-iodine solution. Time permitting, the physician should be dressed in gown, sterile gloves, hat, and mask. When the mother is fully dilated, and the head is at +3 station, the examiner uses a towel and supports the perineum by gently putting pressure on the fetal chin. The other hand is used to control the fetal occiput (Figure 46-2A). Slight pressure on the occiput ensures a smooth delivery of the fetal head and reduces tearing.

Once the fetal head is delivered, the physician should suction the nose and mouth and check for a nuchal cord. The mother should stop pushing at this point. If a nuchal cord is present, it is pulled over the fetal head. If unable to pull the cord over, it should be clamped in two places and cut in the middle.

Next, the anterior shoulder is delivered by guiding the head inferiorly with gentle traction. The posterior shoulder is delivered next by traction upwards. This will also deliver the rest of the infant (Figures 46-2B and 46-2C). If the shoulders are not easily delivered, the physician should consider shoulder dystocia as a complication. Once the infant is delivered, the cord is clamped in 2 locations and cut in the middle. The infant is wrapped, cleaned, and taken to the infant warmer for evaluation.

Ideally, a second physician or experienced practitioner can care for the newborn while the delivering physician

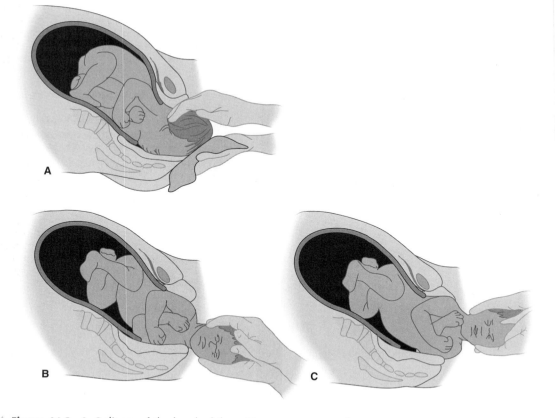

▲ **Figure 46-2. A.** Delivery of the head while putting pressure over the perineum. **B.** Delivering the anterior shoulder. **C.** Delivery of the posterior shoulder is performed with gentle upward traction, while supporting the head. Reprinted with permission from VanRooyen MJ, Scott JA. Chapter 105. Emergency Delivery. In: Tintinalli JE, Stapczynski JS, Ma OJ, Cline DM, Cydulka RK, Meckler GD, eds. *Tintinalli's Emergency Medicine: A Comprehensive Study Guide*. 7th ed. New York: McGraw-Hill, 2011.

Table 46-1. APGAR scoring.

Sign	0 Points	1 Point	2 Point
Activity	Absent	Arms and legs flexed	Active movement
Pulse	Absent	<100 bpm	> 100 bpm
Grimace	No response	Grimace	Sneeze, cough, pulls away
Appearance	Blue-gray or pale	Normal, except extremities	Normal over entire body
Respiration	Absent	Slow, irregular	Good, crying

treats the mother. The newborn should be warmed, given oxygen, and stimulated. The APGAR is performed at 1 and 5 minutes (Table 46-1). Neonatal intubation should be considered for poor tone, shallow respirations, and cyanosis. Once the infant is assessed, attention is directed back to the mother, to deliver the placenta. The placenta should deliver spontaneously, but it can be assisted with uterine massage while pulling gently on the umbilical cord. Pulling too forcefully can result in uterine inversion. Complications of delivery include postpartum hemorrhage, shoulder dystocia, and breech presentations. Although rare, these complications generally require the assistance of an obstetrician.

Postpartum hemorrhage can occur immediately after delivery or up to a few hours after delivery. The physician should check for retained products, uterine atony, uterine inversion, or vaginal lacerations that are contributing to the blood loss. In the case of uterine atony, oxytocin can be given, 20 units in 1 L of Lactated Ringer's solution. Additionally, misoprostol 1 mg can be given per rectum.

Shoulder dystocia is present when the fetus's anterior shoulder becomes caught under the mother's pubic bone. It is more common in diabetic mothers, obesity, and postmaturity of the fetus. The first clue to the physician that shoulder dystocia is occurring is a retraction of the fetal head toward the vagina immediately after it is delivered. This is called the "turtle sign." In the event of a shoulder dystocia, the mother's legs are flexed to a knee-chest position (McRobert maneuver). This rotates the pubic bone over the anterior fetal shoulder. Second, an assistant provides firm suprapubic pressure to further disengage the anterior shoulder. If this does not resolve the dystocia, an episiotomy should be performed to enlarge the opening and provide access to the posterior shoulder.

Breech presentations are ideally delivered by cesarean section. Rapid bedside ultrasound can determine whether the fetal head or another part is presenting. Breech presentations can be frank breech (legs are at the fetal face with the buttocks presenting), complete breech (the buttocks are presenting, but the fetal hips and knees are flexed), or incomplete or footling breech (one leg is the presenting part). Breech presentation is dangerous because the buttocks and legs do not fully dilate the cervix. The fetal head can become caught in the birth canal during delivery. Likewise, the cervical opening is not completely occluded by the buttocks, so cord prolapse can occur.

DISPOSITION

All mothers should be admitted to a postpartum unit, and the infant should be admitted to a neonatal nursery.

SUGGESTED READING

Lazebnik N, Lazebnik RS. The role of ultrasound in pregnancy-related emergencies. *Radiol Clin North Am.* 2004;42:315–327.

Stallard TC, Burns B. Emergency delivery and perimortem C-section. *Emerg Med Clin North Am.* 2003;21:679–693.

VanRooyen MJ, Scott JA. Emergency delivery. In: Tintinalli JE, Stapczynski JS, Ma OJ, Clince DM, Cydulka, RK, Meckler GD. *Tintinalli's Emergency Medicine: A Comprehensive Study Guide.* 7th ed. New York, NY: McGraw-Hill, 2011, pp. 703–711.

The Pediatric Patient

Joseph Walline, MD

Katrina R. Wade, MD

Key Points

- Inherent differences exist between pediatric and adult patients.
- Physicians have to treat both the parent and the child.
- The older the child, the more reliable the clinical impression.
- Disposition can be affected by unique family situations.

INTRODUCTION

Infants, children, and adolescents constitute approximately a third of all visits to emergency departments (EDs) in the United States. Of these pediatric visits, more than half are for urgent/nonemergent problems such as otitis media, respiratory and gastrointestinal infections (often viral), asthma, fractures, sprains, soft tissue trauma, and minor head trauma. The challenge of pediatric emergency medicine is to prevent mortality or increased morbidity by catching the few cases that need hospital admission or emergent intervention and ensuring proper discharge of less ill patients.

Children are considered minors up to their 18th birthday. Although no consent is needed for life-saving interventions, minors require their parent's or guardian's consent for routine medical care and discharge. An exception to this rule is the emancipated minor. "Emancipated minor" status allows a person less than 18 years of age to consent for medical care without parental knowledge, consent, or liability. The exact legal terms of what makes a minor "emancipated" varies slightly from state to state, but generally includes one or more of the following: marriage (including becoming divorced, separated, or widowed), membership in the armed forces, becoming pregnant or having children, living separately from parent(s) or guardian(s), or, finally, demonstrating the ability to manage one's own financial affairs. Of the preceding criteria, discovering a patient is pregnant is the most common

situation the authors' have encountered that leads to emancipated minor status.

Another important legal issue for clinicians working with children is our role as mandated reporters. We have a duty to protect vulnerable young patients. If there is reasonable cause to suspect that a child has been abused, neglected, or placed in imminent risk of serious harm, we are obligated to involve government agents such as child protective services, police, etc.

There are many aspects of clinical pediatric emergency medicine that differ from adult emergency medicine practice. Not only must you vary your approach to each patient based on their anatomic, physiologic, and developmental status, you also have to establish an effective relationship with the patient and his or her caregiver. In other words, physicians have to treat both the parent and the child. We review some of these differences later in this chapter.

CLINICAL PRESENTATION

▶ History

Obtain as much information as possible from the child. Questions should be direct and stated in terms the child can understand. Further details and clarifications should be sought from the parents, guardians, or caregivers. The younger the child, the greater reliance on history obtained from the parents, and the more the history may be

Table 47-1. Average quantity of feedings based on age.

Age	Volume/Feeding (every 3-4 hrs)
1-2 weeks	2-3 oz
3 weeks-2 months	4-5 oz
2-3 months	5-6 oz
3-4 months	6-7 oz
5-12 months	7-8 oz

Table 47-2. Normal vital signs in pediatric patients based on age.

Age	RR (breaths/min)	Average HR (beats/min)	Systolic BP (mmHg)
Premature	40-70	120-170	55-75
0-3 months	35-55	100-150	65-85
3-6 months	30-45	90-120	70-90
6-12 months	25-40	80-120	80-100
1-3 years	20-30	70-110	90-105
3-6 years	20-25	65-110	95-110
6-12 years	14-22	60-95	100-120
12+ years	12-18	55-85	110-135

influenced by the parent(s)' perception of symptoms. When taking the history, children can become anxious when separated from parents. Separate children from parents only when absolutely necessary (eg, in the case of an adolescent patient when a sexual and/or illicit drug history needs to be obtained) or in a younger patient when abuse or neglect is suspected. Unusual complaints such as weight loss, night sweats, headaches, or back pain in a small child should prompt concern for more indolent or life-threatening underlying pathology, particularly malignancy.

Important historical information needed in all pediatric patients includes birth history, immunizations, prior medical problems, medications, allergies, developmental milestones, usual activity, and oral intake. In particular, abnormal birth histories and immunization records can have a significant impact on the differential diagnosis for pediatric patients.

Normal oral intake for an infant depends on their age (Table 47-1). Any changes from baseline are important to discover and address. Solids are not generally initiated until the infant is approximately 6 months of age. When dehydration is a concern, you should ask about the patient's activity level, oral intake, number of wet diapers, frequency of diarrhea or vomiting, and their ability to make tears.

Finally, a mismatch between the history and physical exam or an injury not explained by the historical mechanism provided should prompt the clinician to consider abuse as a cause of the patient's complaint(s).

▶ Physical Examination

Once the history is obtained, it is time to proceed to a physical examination of the child. Because many children are nervous and afraid of strangers, especially in the unfamiliar setting of an ED, a calm, gentle approach to the child during the examination can help a great deal. Having the parent hold the child on his or her lap or hug the child against his or her chest can help to both reassure the child and immobilize him or her during the exam. If the child does start to cry, repeated examinations may be necessary to ensure a thorough and accurate assessment.

As in adult emergency medicine, we use the ABCDE (airway, breathing, circulation, disability, and exposure) approach to management with a quick general assessment. Initial assessment includes obtaining the patient's vital signs,

which will help guide your management. Normal vital signs vary significantly according to patient age (Table 47-2). For example, the normal pulse in a 6-month-old is about 110 bpm, but this rate would be considered highly abnormal in an adolescent. You should also get an accurate weight on your pediatric patient, as your treatment and medical decision making will often be based on this weight.

As mentioned previously, children have developmental and anatomical differences that must be taken into account during your examination. The pediatric airway poses some unique challenges as compared with adult patients. The larynx is more cephalad and anterior, the tongue is proportionally larger, and the epiglottis is tilted and more collapsible, all of which make visualization potentially harder. In terms of endotracheal tube selection, the narrowest portion of the pediatric airway is at the level of the cricoid cartilage, which traditionally meant that a cuffed tube was unnecessary in patients younger than 8 years. This traditional view is becoming less stringent, however, and many hospitals now use cuffed endotracheal tubes in all ages (decreasing air leak and improving ventilation efficiency).

The pediatric skeleton and surrounding ligaments and tissues are also more flexible and less protective than the adult. The pediatric head is proportionately larger than in adults, increasing the relative force of head and neck injuries. In addition, greater white matter content in the brain increases the risk of injury secondary to axonal shearing and cerebral edema. Infants also have open fontanelles in their skull until about 18 months of age. Older children have open growth plates in their long bones for many years until they close in late adolescence; these are the weakest portions of the bone and the most prone to injury. Injury to the growth plates is commonly classified by the Salter-Harris scoring system (Figure 47-1). Tenderness at the growth plate without evidence of fracture is indicative of a Salter-Harris type 1 fracture and generally should be splinted for patient comfort, improved healing, and medicolegal protection for the physician.

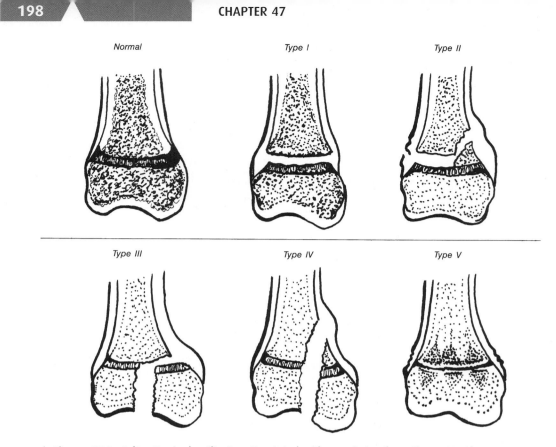

Figure 47-1. Salter-Harris classification. Reprinted with permission from Simon RR, Sherman SC, and Koenigsknecht SJ. *Emergency Orthopedics: The Extremities*. 5th ed. New York: McGraw-Hill, 2007.

Infants and children are at increased risk of hypothermia because of their high surface area to volume ratio. Pediatric patients are at risk for spinal cord injury without radiographic abnormalities (SCIWORA), because the horizontal alignment of vertebral facet joints and more elastic intervertebral ligaments predispose to subluxation without bony injury. Finally, children overall are at an increased risk for injury or disease because they are unable to communicate, are dependent on their parent(s) or guardian(s), and (especially when very young) are immunologically immature. Take seriously a parent's report of a significant change in behavior of his or her child.

DIAGNOSTIC STUDIES

▶ Laboratory

Laboratory testing in children is performed much less frequently than in adult patients. There are few instances in which laboratory testing is part of the standard of care in treating pediatric patients in the ED. These instances include febrile neonates, diabetic ketoacidosis, sickle cell crises, altered mental status, and neutropenic patients with fever. Laboratory testing, generally, should be reserved for confirming a diagnosis that is already suspected clinically, or for assisting in the final disposition of the patient.

▶ Imaging

In certain cases (eg, trauma, altered mental status, and suspected intraabdominal pathology), imaging tests such as radiographs, ultrasound, computed tomography (CT), and magnetic resonance imaging (MRI) may be necessary. Plain radiographs are usually well-tolerated by pediatric patients, as they are performed very fast and parents can be close by with lead shielding. CT scans are somewhat less tolerated, especially in younger children, as the patient is required to leave his or her parent and lie flat on a hard surface. This is even more pronounced in MRIs for these same reasons, in addition to the anxiety caused by claustrophobia and loud noises made by the MRI. Anxiety with imaging is often treated with short-acting sedatives and/or pain medications (eg, midazolam, chloral hydrate, and/or fentanyl).

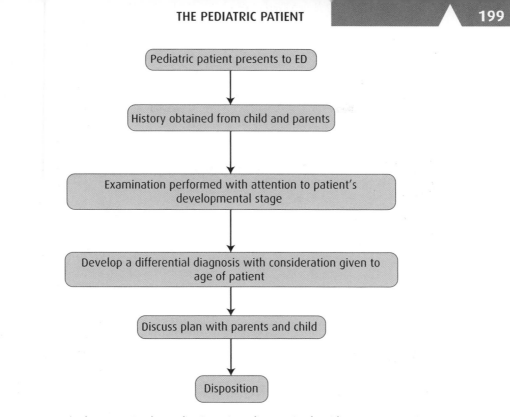

```
┌─────────────────────────────────────┐
│   Pediatric patient presents to ED   │
└─────────────────────────────────────┘
                    │
                    ▼
┌─────────────────────────────────────┐
│  History obtained from child and parents │
└─────────────────────────────────────┘
                    │
                    ▼
┌─────────────────────────────────────┐
│  Examination performed with attention to patient's │
│            developmental stage        │
└─────────────────────────────────────┘
                    │
                    ▼
┌─────────────────────────────────────┐
│  Develop a differential diagnosis with consideration given to │
│                 age of patient         │
└─────────────────────────────────────┘
                    │
                    ▼
┌─────────────────────────────────────┐
│    Discuss plan with parents and child │
└─────────────────────────────────────┘
                    │
                    ▼
┌─────────────────────────────────────┐
│              Disposition               │
└─────────────────────────────────────┘
```

▲ **Figure 47-2.** The pediatric patient diagnostic algorithm.

PROCEDURES

The general approach to procedures in children, just as in the physical exam, is less anxiety-provoking by having the parent participate as much as possible. Discussing the procedure ahead of time with the parent(s)—especially taking the time to mention key points during the procedure and important actions the parents can take to help make the procedure more comfortable for their child—can be very helpful. For example, tell parents to hold the child close, talk to the child, and help keep him or her still while using sutures to repair a laceration, and tell parents how doing so will help the child have a better experience (and cosmetic outcome).

When performing a procedure, attempts should be made to minimize pain and suffering in children through the use of anesthetic, sedative, and/or pain medications. Not only will the patient be happier, but the parents will be more satisfied with their child's care. Use of topical anesthetics during laceration repair, suprapubic bladder tap, lumbar puncture, or intravenous access is recommended. During complex laceration repair or fracture reduction, consider using procedural sedation. These protocols use stronger medications such as ketamine, midazolam, morphine, or fentanyl. Adequate pain relief can help reduce anxiety as well.

MEDICAL DECISION MAKING

In most pediatric cases, your history and physical exam are sufficient to rule out serious pathology. However, if more ominous diagnoses are suggested by the history and/or physical, testing should move into laboratory, imaging, and possibly procedures as necessary (Figure 47-2).

TREATMENT

Once treatment strategies are chosen or narrowed down to a few alternatives, it is a good time to review the options or plan with the parent(s). The parents can be very helpful in supporting the clinician in explaining the plan to the patient. If multiple alternatives are presented, the parents can help choose an option most in line with their wishes, preferences, and/or child's comfort.

Medication dosages and emergency equipment must be appropriate for the patient's weight. Getting an accurate weight as part of the initial vital signs can help speed medication calculations at this stage of the ED visit. If a directly measured weight is unavailable in an emergent situation, using a resuscitation tape (previously called Broselow tape) can be extremely helpful. The red arrow on the tape is placed at the patient's head and the tape is extended to his/her feet to measure length. There is an average weight listed on the tape for this length. It is this weight that is used for medication dosing, etc. All medication dosages must be calculated on a milligram per kilogram basis. All treatment should be performed as quickly and as gently as possible.

DISPOSITION

▶ Admission

Indications for admission in pediatric patients include suspected or confirmed acute surgical diagnoses (eg, appendicitis), any medical condition requiring further monitoring and treatment (eg, asthma, dehydration with intractable vomiting), and uncertain diagnoses requiring further work-up. Also, patients with certain social issues, including suspected abuse, neglect, and failure to thrive, should be considered for admission pending social services consultation.

▶ Discharge

Stable patients with good social supports and medical follow-up are appropriate for discharge after medical conditions have been diagnosed and treatment plans initiated and/or completed. Chronic conditions and related complex work-ups in otherwise stable patients can be completed by the patient's primary care provider. Because almost all pediatric patients have regular primary care providers, patients will benefit from contact between the emergency medicine physician and the primary care provider to have appropriate continuity of care after discharge from the ED.

The treatment of the pediatric patient presents unique challenges and requires specialized training but is easily achievable by maintaining good rapport and communication and showing patience and empathy. These skills will decrease the amount of anxiety for the patient and parent, facilitate care, and improve compliance.

▼ SUGGESTED READING

American Academy of Pediatrics Committee on Pediatric Emergency Medicine, American College of Emergency Physicians Pediatric Emergency Medicine Committee, O'Malley P, Brown K, Mace SE. Patient- and family-centered care and the role of the emergency physician providing care to a child in the emergency department. *Pediatrics*. 2006;118:2242–2244.

Corrales AY, Starr M. Assessment of the unwell child. *Aust Fam Physician*. 2010;39:270–275.

Goldman, RD, Meckler, GD. Pediatrics: Emergency care of children. In: Tintinalli JE, Stapczynski JS, Ma OJ, Cline DM, Cydulka RK, Meckler GD. *Tintinalli's Emergency Medicine: A Comprehensive Study Guide*. 7th ed. New York, NY: McGraw-Hill, 2011, pp. 731–733.

Hamm MP, Osmond M, Curran J, Scott S, Ali S, Hartling L, Gokiert R, Cappelli M, Hnatko G, Newton AS. A systematic review of crisis interventions used in the emergency department: recommendations for pediatric care and research. *Pediatr Emerg Care*. 2010;26:952–962.

Newton AS, Zou B, Hamm MP, Curran J, Gupta S, Dumonceaux C, Lewis M. Improving child protection in the emergency department: a systematic review of professional interventions for health care providers. *Acad Emerg Med*. 2010;17:117–125.

Pediatric Fever

Shannon E. Staley, MD

Alisa A. McQueen, MD

Key Points

- Regardless of age, all toxic-appearing infants and children with fever require a full septic work-up, urgent treatment with broad-spectrum antibiotics, and admission.

- Initial management of fever in infants less than 30 days old includes a complete examination of cerebrospinal fluid, blood, and urine for a serious bacterial infection, prompt empiric antibiotic administration, and hospitalization.

- Management of well-appearing febrile infants aged 1–3 months is determined by analyzing risk factors for serious bacterial infection.

- Well-appearing, low-risk, febrile infants and children who do not have a source of infection must have reliable follow-up when discharged from the emergency department.

INTRODUCTION

Fever in children is defined as a rectal temperature ≥38.0°C (100.4°F) and accounts for approximately 20% of all pediatric visits to the emergency department (ED). Fever is part of a larger, comprehensive host response to infection. Leukocytes and other phagocytic cells release pyrogens, which trigger an increase in prostaglandin synthesis, resulting in an elevation of the thermoregulatory set point. Fever occurs when the hypothalamus responds to this new set point by initiating physiologic changes involving endocrine, metabolic, autonomic, and behavioral processes. Specific physiologic changes associated with fever such as increased oxygen consumption, protein breakdown, and gluconeogenesis can quickly deplete the already limited reserves of infants and children.

Fever can be the first and only physiologic sign of illness. It can herald a serious bacterial infection (SBI) such as meningitis, bacteremia, osteomyelitis, septic arthritis, urinary tract infection (UTI), or pneumonia. These and other SBIs can rapidly lead to sepsis, an overwhelming and devastating systemic syndrome caused by infection. A child or infant with a SBI may appear "toxic" (very ill-appearing with unstable vital signs). Alternatively, well-appearing febrile children can also have an SBI

such as occult bacteremia. Occult bacteremia is the presence of pathogenic bacteria in the blood of well-appearing, febrile children without any identifiable focus of infection, also described as "fever without a source." Approximately 20% of all children presenting with fever will have no identifiable cause. Neonates (<30 days old) have immature immune systems that place them at high risk for SBI with fever.

CLINICAL PRESENTATION

▶ History

Elicit the duration, pattern, and maximum recorded temperature from caregivers. Young infants do not usually have localizing symptoms and often present with nonspecific complaints such as excessive crying, poor feeding, irritability, or lethargy. Parents of older children may report more specific complaints such as cough, rhinorrhea, sore throat, vomiting, diarrhea, dysuria, joint pain, body aches, or headache. Questions regarding oral intake and urine output will help the clinician assess the degree of associated dehydration, if present.

The presence of a seizure in a febrile infant may suggest a benign simple febrile seizure or could be an indicator of meningitis. A simple febrile seizure is defined as a single generalized tonic-clonic seizure that lasts <15 minutes in children aged 6 months to 6 years with no resulting focal neurologic deficits. These seizures occur in the setting of fever in previously healthy children with no history of epilepsy or signs of central nervous system (CNS) infection. Three percent to 5% of all children will have a simple febrile seizure. A source should be investigated for a patient presenting with a simple febrile seizure, but an extensive work-up is usually not indicated. A febrile seizure is considered complex if it has focal features, lasts longer than 15 minutes, or occurs more than once in 24 hours. A more extensive work-up including laboratory studies, imaging, and lumbar puncture should be strongly considered in those presenting with complex febrile seizures.

▶ Physical Examination

Vital signs and general appearance should always be evaluated before proceeding with the remainder of the physical exam. Heart rate can be elevated approximately 10 bpm for every 1°C of elevation in temperature. However, tachycardia out of proportion to fever can indicate sepsis. Children and infants with sepsis differ from adults as they often do not demonstrate hypotension until very late in the course due to a compensatory increase in cardiac output. Thus a normal blood pressure is not necessarily reassuring. Tachycardia and poor peripheral perfusion occur before hypotension and can be early signs of impending circulatory collapse.

Evaluating the general appearance of an infant or child with fever is also crucial. Infants or children who are lethargic or demonstrate paradoxical irritability (eg, inconsolable when held by parents) may have a CNS infection. A head-to-toe physical exam should be performed. Special attention should be paid to the anterior fontanelle in infants; a bulging tense fontanelle may indicate meningitis, whereas a sunken fontanelle may indicate severe dehydration. In older children, assessment of neck pain, stiffness, and range of motion may also be useful in helping establish a diagnosis of CNS infection. Evaluate the lung fields for crackles, asymmetry, and work of breathing. Forced expiration and percussion may assist in the detection of areas of consolidation. Carefully examine the skin to identify any rashes, petechiae, or purpura. Meningococcemia should be assumed in a febrile, ill-appearing child with a petechial or purpuric rash until proven otherwise. Additionally, jaundice in a neonate may indicate the presence of sepsis but is not a specific finding. The extremities should be examined closely for erythema, swelling, warmth, focal tenderness, and decreased range of motion, as this may indicate osteomyelitis, pyomyositis, or septic arthritis. These infections are more common in children than in adults. A reassuring clinical examination in infants <3 months does not necessarily rule out an SBI and should not be used in isolation to guide management in this age group.

DIAGNOSTIC STUDIES
▶ Laboratory

Laboratory tests to consider include a complete blood count, urinalysis, urine culture, blood culture, and cerebrospinal fluid (CSF) studies. The appropriate tests to order, if any, depend on the history and physical examination, clinical appearance, age, and risk factors for SBI.

▶ Imaging

A chest x-ray (CXR) may be helpful in identifying pulmonary infection in patients with tachypnea, cough, hypoxia, or other signs of lower respiratory tract disease. Signs of osteomyelitis may not be apparent on plain radiographs until the infection has been present for at least 7–10 days. Additional imaging, including computed tomography for intra-abdominal infection, may be helpful depending on the patient's specific signs and symptoms.

MEDICAL DECISION MAKING

The differential diagnosis for acute fever in an infant or child is broad and includes minor illnesses, such as viral infections, upper respiratory infections, and otitis media, to more significant illnesses, including pneumonia, pyelonephritis, septic arthritis, and cellulitis, to potentially life-threatening infections, including Kawasaki disease, meningitis, bacteremia, and sepsis. Because the differential diagnosis is so broad, and fever is so common, the approach to the febrile child is based on several factors, including age, clinical impression (well or ill-appearing), physical examination (source or no source), and risk stratification (high or low risk for SBI) (Figure 48-1).

Febrile infants <30 days old, even if they are well appearing, should have a full septic work-up, which includes complete blood count with manual differential, blood culture, urinalysis, urine culture, and lumbar puncture. CSF should be sent for cell count, protein and glucose levels, Gram stain, and culture. Herpes simplex virus (HSV) polymerase chain reaction should be considered in neonates and those who are high risk. Urine must be collected in a sterile manner, using bladder catheterization or suprapubic aspiration. Bagged specimens are not helpful and are frequently contaminated by skin flora. Based on symptoms, additional studies may be considered; liver function testing should be assessed if an infant presents with jaundice, and stool studies can be sent if diarrhea is present.

Well appearing infants age 1–3 months are classified as low or high risk for SBI. Their risk stratification is dependent on history, physical exam, and basic initial lab results. To qualify as low risk, an infant must be previously healthy without any comorbidity, nontoxic appearing, without a focus of infection (excluding otitis media), demonstrate normal lab values, and have reliable caregivers who can ensure close follow-up. The Rochester Criteria, the Philadelphia Protocol, and the Boston Criteria are the

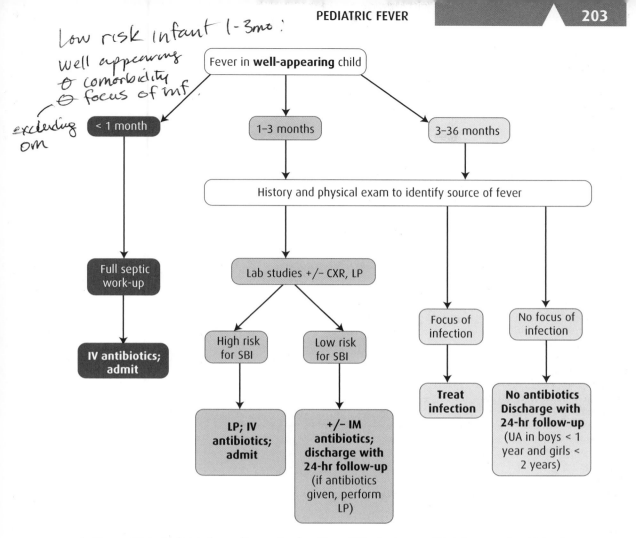

Handwritten notes (left margin):
Low risk infant 1-3mo:
well appearing
+ comorbidity
+ focus of inf.
excluding om

Figure 48-1. Pediatric fever diagnostic algorithm. CXR, chest x-ray; IM, intramuscular; LP, lumbar puncture; SBI, serious bacterial infection; UA, urinalysis.

most commonly used decision-making tools for determining management of fever in well-appearing neonates and infants (Table 48-1). Although all three have limitations, they have attempted to create sensitive, specific screening criteria to identify infants at low risk for SBI.

Lower risk stratification can be considered if the white blood cell (WBC) count is between 5 and 15,000, band to neutrophil ratio is <0.2, and urinalysis with <8 WBC per high-power field. Clinical impression alone is not sufficient to forego lumbar puncture in this age group. The decision to perform lumbar puncture depends on several factors, including laboratory results, urinalysis, vaccination status, and presence or absence of viral symptoms.

Well appearing children 3–36 months are at lower risk for disseminated infections and can generally be managed based on the nature of the infection, without an extensive

work-up for SBI. Fever in this age group is most commonly caused by viral infections. The incidence of occult bacteremia in well-appearing febrile children in this age group has steadily decreased due to routine administration of both the Hib and pneumococcal conjugate vaccine. Centers for Disease Control and Prevention data now reflect that the current rate of occult bacteremia is <1%. Furthermore, approximately 80% of pneumococcal bacteremia will resolves spontaneously without intervention. Thus several acceptable variations in management exist for this patient cohort.

The evaluation of well-appearing children age 3–36 months includes urinalysis and urine culture for girls <2 years of age and boys <1 year of age, particularly if they are uncircumcised. A CXR may be performed if there are signs of lower respiratory infection. If no source is identified after this focused evaluation, reassurance and

Table 48-1. Rochester, Philadelphia, and Boston criteria comparison.

	Rochester Criteria	Philadelphia Protocol	Boston Criteria
Age	<60 days	29–60 days	28–89 days
Qualifications	Term infant No perinatal antibiotics No underlying disease Not hospitalized longer than the mother at birth	Not specified	No immunizations within preceding 48 hours No antimicrobial within 48 hours Not dehydrated
Physical Examination	Well-appearing No ear, soft tissue, or bone infection	Well-appearing Unremarkable exam	Well-appearing No ear, soft tissue, or bone infection
Lab values to determine low-risk stratification	WBC >5,000 and <15,000/µL Absolute band count <1,500/µL UA <10 WBC/HPF	WBC <15,000/µL Band-neutrophil ratio <0.2 UA <10 WBC/HPF Urine Gram stain negative CSF <8 WBC/µL CSF Gram stain negative Chest radiograph: no infiltrate (if done)	WBC <20,000/µL CSF <10/µL UA <10 WBC/HPF Chest radiograph: no infiltrate (if done)
Treatment for **High** risk patients	Hospital admission Empiric antibiotics	Hospital admission Empiric antibiotics	Hospital admission Empiric antibiotics
Treatment for **Low** risk patients	Home No antibiotics Follow-up required	Home No antibiotics Follow-up required	Home Empiric antibiotics Follow-up required
Study outcome statistics	Sensitivity 92% Specificity 50% PPV 12.3% NPV 98.9%	Sensitivity 98% Specificity 42% PPV 14% NPV 99.7%	Sensitivity–NA Specificity 94.6% PPV–NA NPV–NA

CSF, Cerebrospinal Fluid; HPF, high-power field; NA, not available; NPV, negative predictive value; PPV, positive predictive value; UA, urinalysis; WBC, white blood cells.

supportive care with no additional laboratory studies or antibiotic therapy is appropriate.

Toxic-appearing febrile infants and children, regardless of age, require a full septic work-up, broad-spectrum antibiotics, and admission. Fever in immunocompromised children should also be aggressively managed as outlined previously followed by prompt communication with their subspecialty providers. Antibiotics should never be delayed to complete a septic evaluation.

TREATMENT

Fever may be treated with an antipyretic such as acetaminophen (10–15 mg/kg) every 4 hours or ibuprofen (5–10 mg/kg) every 6 hours as needed to ensure patient comfort. It is important to note that correlation between defervescence with an antipyretic and incidence of SBI has not been established and should not affect clinical decision making. Ample fluid intake should be encouraged. Some patients may require intravenous fluids if dehydration is present. Patients with an identifiable focus of infection should be treated with the most appropriate antibiotic regimen. For fever without a source, empiric antibiotics may be given, based largely on the patient's age and risk stratification.

Infants who are <1 month of age should be treated with antibiotic therapy directed at the most common pathogens causing SBI in this age group (*Listeria*, *Escherichia coli*, Group B Strep, and other gram-negative organisms). Ampicillin plus either gentamicin or a third-generation cephalosporin provide adequate coverage. Ceftriaxone is usually avoided in patients less than 2–4 weeks secondary to concern for biliary sludging. Acyclovir is not recommended empirically for this age group, but may be added to cover HSV if there is a history of seizures, skin lesions are present, or the patient is acutely ill.

Infants who are 1–3 months old who fully meet low-risk criteria may be given a single dose of ceftriaxone before discharge to cover occult bacteremia or UTIs. However, this dosing does not fully cover meningitis from these organisms and can complicate future decision making if the CSF has not been obtained before administration of antibiotics. Do not administer antibiotics in these patients unless a lumbar puncture has been performed. Alternatively, some providers will observe patients in this category as long as they have reliable caregivers who are able to evaluate the infant for changes in symptoms and readily access further care if the patient's condition changes. In both approaches, it is imperative that the provider has a reliable way to reach the primary caregiver and is able to communicate clearly regarding expectations. Follow-up within 24 hours should be arranged before discharge. Infants who do not meet low-risk criteria should have a full sepsis work-up, receive empiric antibiotics, and be admitted for further inpatient monitoring.

Infants and children 3–36 months with a temperature >39°C and elevated WBC >15,000 historically received ceftriaxone 50 mg/kg for possible occult bacteremia after blood cultures have been obtained. Because of decreased rates of occult bacteremia secondary to widespread pneumococcal vaccination, outpatient observation without empiric antibiotics is reasonable. Children in this age group with a urinalysis consistent with UTI who are otherwise well-appearing may be treated as outpatients with oral antibiotics (usually a third-generation cephalosporin). Children in this age group with a temperature <39°C and a reassuring physical examination can be reasonably managed as outpatients if good follow-up can be assured. Lastly, if meningitis is highly suspected or CSF Gram stain identifies an organism in any of the preceding age groups, ceftriaxone 100 mg/kg/day and vancomycin should be administered promptly in the ED.

DISPOSITION

▶ Admission

Toxic-appearing infants and children with fever require a full septic work-up, urgent treatment with broad-spectrum antibiotics, and admission. Additionally, all infants <1 month of age with documented fever or history of fever at home should be admitted for further observation and treatment after a full septic work-up. Well-appearing infants 1–3 months with a high risk of SBI or with a documented focal bacterial illness also require admission. If a patient is immunocompromised and presenting with fever, they also are also usually treated with broad-spectrum antibiotics and admitted.

▶ Discharge

Febrile patients older than 3 months who are well-appearing, vaccinated, and have access to appropriate follow-up can be discharged home. Additionally, low-risk patients who are 1–3 months old may also be discharged home as long as reliable follow-up within 24 hours can be guaranteed.

▼ SUGGESTED READING

Alpern ER, Henretig FM. Fever. In: Fleisher GR, Ludwig S. *Textbook of Pediatric Emergency Medicine.* 6th ed. Philadelphia, PA: Lippincott Williams & Wilkins, 2010, pp. 266–274.

Avner JR, Baker MD. Management of fever in infants and children. *Emerg Med Clin North Am.* 2002;20:49–67.

Wang VJ. Fever and serious bacterial illness. In: Tintinalli JE, Stapczynski JS, Ma OJ, Cline DM, Cydulka RK, Meckler GD. *Tintinalli's Emergency Medicine: A Comprehensive Study Guide.* 7th ed. New York, NY: McGraw-Hill, 2011, pp. 750–755.

Respiratory Distress

Lauren Emily Bence, MD

Alisa A. McQueen, MD

Key Points

- Respiratory disorders are potentially life-threatening and must be identified and treated rapidly.
- Certain physiologic differences make pediatric patients more at risk of respiratory failure than adults.
- Conduct patient assessment in a calm, efficient manner, attempting to localize the underlying source of distress.

- Initial treatment may be required for stabilization before a complete history and physical examination can be performed.
- Patient appearance and clinical status always supersede lab values and imaging.

INTRODUCTION

Respiratory distress is a very common presentation in the emergency department (ED). It accounts for 10% of pediatric visits to the ED, 20% of pediatric admissions, and 20% of deaths in infants. Respiratory distress can potentially lead to respiratory failure (the inability of oxygenation and ventilation to meet metabolic demands) and should be recognized and treated promptly.

Several anatomic and physiologic characteristics put pediatric patients at higher risk for respiratory compromise. Infants <4 months of age are obligate nose breathers. Nasopharyngeal obstruction significantly increases the work of breathing. The location of the narrowest part of the airway, where a foreign body is likely to lodge, differs in adults (vocal cords) and children (cricoid cartilage). The diameter of the pediatric airway is a third that of adults. Narrowing of the airway leads to a greater relative increase in resistance to airflow (1-mm occlusion decreases cross-sectional diameter by 20% in adults vs. 75% in children). Abdominal musculature is a primary contributor to respiratory effort in children. Abdominal distension and muscle fatigue can negatively impact ventilation. Pediatric lungs have a lower functional residual capacity (FRC) with less reserve potential. PaO_2 decreases more rapidly when ventilation is interrupted.

Respiratory distress may result from either upper airway obstruction, lower airway disorders, or other organ dysfunction compromising the respiratory system. Upper airway obstruction is the leading cause of life-threatening acute respiratory distress. Upper airway obstruction is defined as blockage of airflow in the larynx or trachea. It is characterized by stridor, an inspiratory sound caused by air flow through a partially obstructed upper airway. The age of the patient can aid in diagnosis.

Common causes of upper airway obstruction in children <6 months include laryngotracheomalacia (chronic, usually resolves by age 2) and vocal cord paresis or paralysis. Laryngomalacia and tracheomalacia are congenital conditions that affect the structural integrity of supporting structures in the upper airway. This leads to collapse of the affected tissues into the airway during respiration.

In children >6 months, important causes of upper airway obstruction include viral croup, foreign body aspiration, epiglottitis, bacterial tracheitis, retropharyngeal abscess, peritonsillar abscess, airway edema from trauma, thermal or chemical burn, or allergic reaction. Croup (laryngotracheobronchitis) is the most common cause of upper airway obstruction and stridor in children aged 3 months to 3 years. It occurs in 5% of children during their second year of life and is caused by a viral infection affecting the subglottic region. The patient presents with a barking cough, inspiratory stridor, and fever.

Upper airway obstruction from foreign body aspiration is most common in children aged 1 to 4 years. About 3,000 patients die each year from asphyxia related to foreign body aspiration.

Bacterial infections in the upper airway include epiglottitis and tracheitis. Epiglottitis is less common now since routine immunization against *Haemophilus influenzae* type B. Currently, tracheitis is more likely to be the cause of acute respiratory failure from airway obstruction than epiglottitis.

Lower airway obstruction has several causes, including asthma, bronchiolitis, pneumonia, allergic reaction, respiratory distress syndrome, aspiration, and environmental or traumatic insults. Asthma is the most common chronic disease in children, affecting 5–10% of the population. Bronchiolitis is most famously caused by respiratory syncytial virus (RSV), although other pathogens include parainfluenza, influenza, and adenovirus. It is a respiratory infection that causes inflammation of the bronchioles. Edema and mucous production lead to obstruction of the airways with V/Q mismatch and hypoxia. It is most common in infants 2 to 6 months and is associated with increased likelihood of asthma developing in the future. Pneumonia incidence varies inversely with age, whereas the etiology changes based on the season and age of the patient.

Important secondary causes of respiratory distress include congenital heart disease, cardiac tamponade, myocarditis/pericarditis, tension pneumothorax, central nervous system infection, toxic ingestion, peripheral nervous system disease (eg, Guillain-Barré syndrome, myasthenia gravis, botulism), metabolic disorders (eg, diabetic ketoacidosis), hyperammonemia, and anemia.

CLINICAL PRESENTATION

History

Initial treatment may be required for stabilization before a complete history and physical examination can be performed.

Ask for a description of respiratory problems, including onset, duration, and progression of symptoms. Keep in mind that respiratory distress can present as difficulty with feedings in infants and decreased activity or feeding in toddlers. Inquire about precipitating or exacerbating factors. Ask if there was any recent history of choking, as this may be the only clue for a foreign body aspiration. Inquire if they have ever had a similar presentation in the past. Review all prior medications (chronic and acute) and note time of administration. For example, how many times albuterol was given per day in the past several days and the last time given before coming to the ED. Ask if immunizations are up to date, as failure to do so could put the child at risk for rare diseases (ie, epiglottitis, pertussis). Review in detail all past medical history. Infants born prematurely may have bronchopulmonary dysplasia (BPD), making reactive airway disease, respiratory infections, hypoxia, and

hypercarbia more likely. When treating children with asthma, ask about frequency of exacerbations, if they ever required intubation or positive pressure ventilation, previous admissions (ED, general floor, intensive care unit) and the last time they were on steroids. A history of chronic cough or multiple previous episodes of pneumonias may be suggestive of a congenital condition, undiagnosed reactive airway disease, or foreign body aspiration.

Physical Examination

The assessment should be conducted in a calm, efficient manner, with assistance from parents. Agitating a child can worsen symptoms and even precipitate acute decompensation, especially in suspected upper airway obstruction. Allow the child to assume a position of comfort. Take extra caution if the patient is presenting in the sniffing position (head and chin are positioned slightly forward), as this may indicate severe upper airway obstruction. Likewise, if the patient is presenting in the tripod position (leaning forward and supporting the upper body with their hands), this indicates severe lower airway obstruction, and this position will optimize their accessory muscle use. Respiratory rate varies in relation to age: newborn (30–60); 1–6 months (30–40); 6–12 months (25–30); 1–6 years (20–30); > 6 years (15–20). Heart rate also varies with age: newborn (140–160), 6 months (120–160), 1 year (100–140), 2 years (90–140), 4 years (80–110), 6–14 years (75–100), >14 years (60–90). Keep in mind that tachycardia is typical with albuterol treatment.

Skin exam can show diaphoresis, cyanosis (peripheral or central), rash (eg, hives), bruising, or trauma and can be a clue to the cause of respiratory distress. Make sure to fully unclothe the patient, taking care not to worsen distress.

Stridor indicates upper airway obstruction, and the phase of the respiratory cycle in which it occurs is a clue to the location of obstruction. Inspiratory stridor is seen with subglottic/glottis obstruction above the larynx (eg, epiglottitis). Nasal flaring, dysphonia, and hoarseness also suggest upper airway obstruction. Expiratory stridor is consistent with obstruction below the larynx, in the bronchi or lower trachea. Croup is the most common cause, but also consider foreign body, epiglottitis, anaphylaxis, angioedema, peritonsillar abscess, retropharyngeal abscess, tracheomalacia, laryngomalacia, or obstructing mass.

Inspect the chest for depth, rhythm, and symmetry of respirations. Retractions indicate accessory muscle use. As the involved muscle groups move more superiorly (subcostal, intercostal, suprasternal, supraclavicular), airway obstruction is more severe. Also examine the chest and neck for any crepitus.

Lung exam is particularly important. Pneumothorax is suggested by unilateral decreased or absent breath sounds, but this finding is not always present. Wheezing and a prolonged expiratory phase indicate lower airway obstruction. It is important to note that in patients with very severe lower airway obstruction, wheezing may be absent as a result of poor aeration. Crackles, rhonchi, and decreased or asymmetric breath sounds are found with alveolar disease. Grunting prevents alveolar collapse and preserves functional residual capacity (FRC). Its presence implies severe respiratory compromise.

The remainder of the physical exam should focus on localizing the underlying source of distress, especially if there is no evidence of airway disease. Poor respiratory effort or apnea with depressed airway reflexes suggests central nervous system disease. Congestive heart failure can present with diminished heart sounds, a murmur or gallop, venous distension, or hepatosplenomegaly. Pallor or cyanosis suggests anemia. Consider sepsis or metabolic acidosis with isolated tachypnea. Look for any signs of ingestion or inhalation injury, such as burns or soot in the oropharynx or nares.

DIAGNOSTIC STUDIES

▶ Laboratory

The majority of causes of respiratory distress can be determined with a careful history and physical exam, and clinical appearance always supersedes lab studies. Arterial blood gas (ABG) analysis may be useful for moderate/severe respiratory distress, diabetic ketoacidosis, or other metabolic disorders. It is important to note that a "normal" ABG in severe respiratory distress is actually quite worrisome, because this may indicate that the patient is starting to tire out and retain more CO_2, thus normalizing the CO_2 and pH but heading toward impending respiratory failure. Respiratory failure can be defined as PaO_2 <60 mmHg despite supplemental O_2 of 60% or $PaCO_2$ >60 mmHg. The complete blood count identifies anemia and provides supportive evidence of an infectious process when leukocytosis or a left shift is present. Electrolytes may be useful if the suspected cause of distress is metabolic in origin. RSV and influenza testing are rarely helpful in the ED setting.

▶ Imaging

Chest x-ray may reveal an infiltrate, pleural effusion, hyperinflation, atelectasis, pneumothorax, pneumomediastinum, foreign body, or cardiomegaly. The location (esophagus vs. trachea) of an aspirated coin in a child can be determined by the orientation of the coin on the radiograph. When the coin is in the esophagus, it lies in the frontal (coronal) plane and is round on posteroanterior view (Figure 49-1). The opposite is true when the coin is in the trachea. It appears round on the lateral radiograph. This is because the incomplete cartilaginous rings of the trachea open posteriorly.

The majority of aspirated foreign bodies are radiolucent (eg, peanut), but radiographs may still provide clues to its presence. Complete bronchial obstruction produces resorption atelectasis distally. Pulmonary infiltrates may be seen because of an inflammatory reaction to the foreign body. Partial obstruction in a bronchus is identified on an expiratory film when there is air trapping and limited

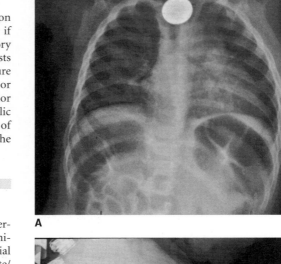

A

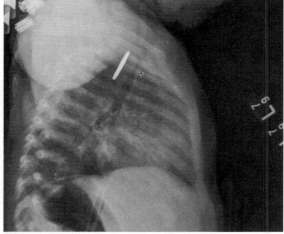

B

▲ **Figure 49-1. A, B.** Coin in the esophagus of a 10-month-old infant who presented with wheezing. Note the airway compression on the lateral view (arrow).

expiration on the affected side. In young children it is very difficult to get the patient to cooperate for expiratory films, so if there is a suspicion of air trapping, bilateral lateral decubitus films can be very useful instead (Figure 49-2).

Soft tissue neck radiograph may reveal a thumbprint sign of epiglottitis (Figure 49-3), the steeple sign of croup, or a widened retropharyngeal space seen in retropharyngeal abscess (Figure 49-4). Neck computed tomography may be required for definitive diagnosis of retropharyngeal abscess or other deep space infections of the neck causing airway obstruction.

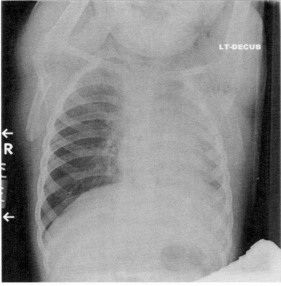

A

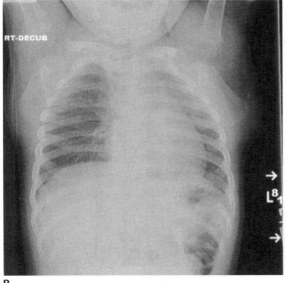

B

▲ **Figure 49-2.** Bilateral decubitus chest x-rays in a patient showing right-sided air trapping. Note that on the left lateral decubitus view **(A)** the left lung is compressed as expected. However, when the child is placed right-side down **(B)**, the right lung remains relatively hyperinflated. This child was taken to the operating room, where a peanut was found in the right mainstem bronchus.

Electrocardiogram may reveal decreased QRS amplitude (pericardial effusion), electrical alternans (severe pericardial effusion or cardiac tamponade), conduction delay (myocarditis), or ST segment and T wave changes (pericarditis).

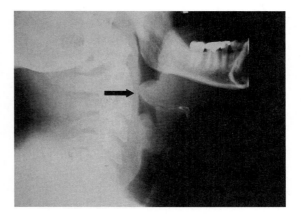

▲ **Figure 49-3.** The epiglottis is located by tracing the base of the tongue inferiorly until it reaches the vallecula. The structure immediately posterior is the epiglottis. If the epiglottis is enlarged (thumb print) and the vallecula is shallow, then epiglottitis is present (arrow).

MEDICAL DECISION MAKING

Assess and stabilize airway, breathing, and circulation as a first priority. Apply pulse oximetry, cardiac monitor, and provide supplemental oxygen and intravenous (IV) fluids immediately. Respiratory arrest means that cardiac arrest will either be present or imminent. These patients require endotracheal intubation. Jaw thrust, suction of airway secretions, and use of bag-valve mask is performed if needed before intubation.

If there are signs of impending respiratory failure (eg, depressed level of consciousness, decreased response to pain, agitation, cyanosis despite oxygen therapy, tachypnea, bradypnea, apnea, irregular respirations, absent breath sounds, stridor at rest, grunting, severe retractions,

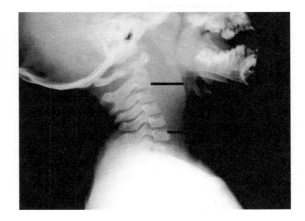

▲ **Figure 49-4.** Enlarged retropharyngeal soft tissues showing a retropharyngeal abscess (lines). The normal retropharyngeal soft tissue space is <7 mm at C2 and <22 mm at C6.

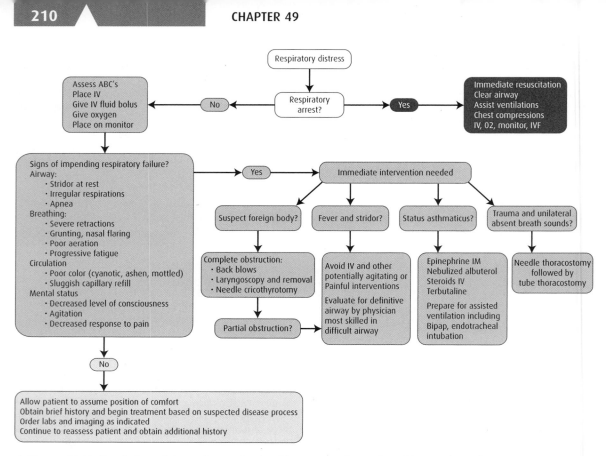

Figure 49-5. Respiratory distress diagnostic algorithm. ABCs, airway, breathing, and circulation; IM, intramuscular; IVF, Intravenous fluids.

and use of accessory muscles), direct treatment toward the suspected cause of distress.

If the patient has known trauma and unilateral decreased breath sounds, assume a tension pneumothorax and perform needle thoracostomy initially. For definitive management, then perform a tube thoracostomy (see Chapter 7). If foreign body is suspected, perform appropriate maneuvers to relieve the obstruction based on age and the size of the patient. If there is severe stridor at rest and fever, assume epiglottitis/bacterial tracheitis/retropharyngeal abscess and arrange for emergent definitive airway to be placed in the operating room with the physician most skilled in difficult airway techniques. In some cases, the ED physician must perform emergent endotracheal intubation in the ED. It is extremely important to have all difficult airway backup equipment, including a needle tracheotomy tray immediately available. If the patient is presenting with a severe asthma exacerbation or allergic reaction and does not have adequate respiratory effort, give epinephrine via intramuscular route immediately while preparing for emergent intubation, if no response to initial treatment. With severe wheezing not responsive to bronchodilator therapy alone, if the patient is at an age when they can cooperate and are still alert, an initial attempt with

positive pressure ventilation with bilevel positive airway pressure can be very helpful to decrease work of breathing and prevent need for intubation. New evidence suggests that high-flow nasal cannula with humidified oxygen can prevent need for endotracheal intubation in some cases.

If there are no signs of impending respiratory failure and no immediate life-saving intervention is needed, then let the patient assume a position of comfort to optimize respiratory effort and do not agitate. Obtain a brief history and start treatment based on the suspected disease process. Order labs and imaging that may help with the diagnosis. Sometimes, a lab result or radiograph will indicate need for emergent directed treatment (eg, foreign body). It is extremely important to frequently reassess the patient after each treatment to determine response and make decisions for further management. Clinical status can change very quickly in patients with respiratory distress (Figure 49-5).

TREATMENT

Croup. Administer humidified oxygen, and all patients should get dexamethasone 0.6 mg/kg/dose (max 16 mg) intramuscular (IM) or by mouth (PO) regardless of the severity. If there is stridor at rest, give racemic epinephrine 0.5 mL of 2.25% solution in 3 mL of normal saline (NS) via a nebulizer.

Foreign body aspiration. Definitive management is to remove in the operating room by laryngoscopy or bronchoscopy. In the setting of critical airway obstruction or impending/actual respiratory arrest, attempt to force the foreign body out with back blows or chest or abdominal thrusts depending on the age and size of the patient. These are all safer methods than the blind finger sweep, which can convert a partial obstruction to a complete obstruction. Other life-saving measures include laryngoscopy and direct retrieval with Magill forceps, passing the endotracheal tube beyond the obstruction and forcing the foreign body into either mainstem bronchus, or needle cricothyrotomy.

Epiglottitis or bacterial tracheitis. It is particularly important to allow the patient to assume a position of comfort, and if they are in the sniffing position, this is an ominous sign for severe obstruction. Ideally these patients should have a definitive airway placed in the operating room by the most skilled physician in difficult airway techniques, but if there is respiratory arrest, then immediate endotracheal intubation or needle cricothyrotomy should be performed.

Anaphylaxis and severe angioedema. Treat with epinephrine, steroids, H1 and H2 blockers.

Asthma. Treat with β-adrenergic agonists: albuterol 2.5 mg every 20 minutes as needed or 15 mg in NS nebulized over 1 hour continuously. For moderate to severe exacerbations, add anticholinergics (ipratropium bromide 500 mcg every 20 minutes for 3 doses) and steroids. If tolerating oral intake with no impending respiratory failure, administer prednisone 1–2 mg/kg/day; otherwise use IV steroids (Solu-Medrol 2 mg/kg, max 125 mg). If the patient's respiratory effort is poor and respiratory failure is imminent, administer IM epinephrine 0.01 mg/kg/dose (max 0.5 mg) 1:1,000, which can be repeated every 20 minutes for 2 more doses. Terbutaline 2–10 mcg IV loading dose then 0.1–0.6 mcg/kg/min can also be used. Magnesium sulfate (50 mg/kg over 20 minutes to max 2 g) should be considered in patients with moderate to severe exacerbations or those who do not improve after initial therapy. Heliox, a mixture of helium and oxygen, improves laminar flow through the bronchioles, resulting in decreased work of breathing. There is some evidence showing it improves pulmonary function in patients with severe obstruction. The maximum amount of oxygen in the mixture is 30%, so if the patient is hypoxic and requires more than 30% FIO_2, then Heliox is not an option.

Bronchiolitis. Attempt a trial with β-agonists and/or nebulized epinephrine. Clinical trials demonstrate that corticosteroids are of no benefit in the treatment of bronchiolitis, but they may be useful in patients with a history of reactive airway disease. High-flow humidified oxygen via nasal cannula is a more novel treatment that is showing some promising utility, especially in patients with RSV and hypoventilation. The proposed mechanisms are improvement of respiratory mechanics, washout of nasopharyngeal dead space, and decreased work of breathing. Some recent studies showed that it may decrease need for endotracheal intubation. Hypertonic saline (3–5%) with or without bronchodilators is another new therapy being studied, with minimal side effects.

Pneumonia. Administer antibiotics early and oxygen as needed.

DISPOSITION

▶ Admission

Admission is indicated in respiratory failure requiring mechanical ventilation, respiratory distress not reversible with definitive therapy or requiring intensive monitoring, pneumonia in patients <6 months, foreign body aspirations with respiratory symptoms, or new oxygen requirements.

▶ Discharge

The decision to discharge a patient is dependent on several factors: clinical response to treatment, work of breathing, hypoxia, hydration status, preexisting medical conditions, and social factors. Keep in mind that respiratory status can change quickly, and it is crucial to monitor a patient for a significant amount of time after treatment to make sure their clinical status does not deteriorate again. If the patient continues to have increased work of breathing and there is concern for impending respiratory failure, these patients should not go home. Ensure the patient is well hydrated and can tolerate oral intake before discharge. Make sure the patient has reliable caregivers who can administer treatments and medications and will bring the patient back if they worsen again. Lastly, arrange secure follow-up for the patient with his or her pediatrician or specialist.

▼ SUGGESTED READING

Cantor RM, Wittick L. Upper airway emergencies. In: Wiebe RA, Ahrens WR, Strange GR, Schafermeyer RW, eds. *Pediatric Emergency Medicine*. 3rd ed. New York, NY: McGraw-Hill, 2009. http://www.accessemergencymedicine.com/content.aspx?aID=5332700. Accessed March 29, 2012.

Rodrigo GJ, Pollack CV, Rodrigo C, Rowe BH. Heliox for nonintubated acute asthma patients. *Cochrane Database of Syst Rev*. 2006;(4):CD002884.

Schibler A, Pham TMT, Dunster KR, et al. Reduced intubation rates for infants after introduction of high-flow nasal prong oxygen delivery. *Intens Care Med*. 2011;37:847–852.

Weiner DL. Respiratory distress. In: Fleisher GR, Ludwig SL. *Textbook of Pediatric Emergency Medicine*. 6th ed. Philadelphia, PA: Lippincott Williams & Wilkins, 2010, pp. 551–563.

Zhang L, Mendoza-Sassi RA, Wainwright C, Klassen TP. Nebulized hypertonic saline solution for acute bronchiolitis in infants. *Cochrane Database Syst Rev*. 2008;(4):CD006458.

Abdominal Pain

Russ Horowitz, MD

Key Points

- Currant jelly stool is a late finding in intussusception.
- In appendicitis, young children have a very high rate of rupture on presentation.
- If bilious vomiting is present, think malrotation with volvulus.
- Nonabdominal conditions including strep pharyngitis and pneumonia often present with abdominal pain.

INTRODUCTION

Abdominal pain in children is one of the most common complaints in pediatrics. Etiologies range from benign conditions such as constipation to surgical emergencies such as malrotation with volvulus. The challenge for the clinician is to distinguish between these diseases in preverbal children and in those with limited ability to describe their symptoms. Some conditions such as pyloric stenosis are unique to young children, but others, such as appendicitis which occur in all ages, have dramatically different presentations in the very young. Although less common than in adults, children may still suffer from gallstones, peptic ulcer disease, and kidney stones. Pelvic disorders including ovarian cysts and torsion must be considered in all girls over the age of menarche.

▶ Surgical Causes of Abdominal Pain

Pyloric stenosis. Usually presents in the newborn period from 2 to 6 weeks of age. It is more common in first-born male children (4:1) and has a familial inheritance. The typical presentation is with postprandial projectile vomiting. After vomiting, children still appear hungry and will readily feed. Early on they seem well, but as symptoms progress they become dehydrated and develop the stereotypical electrolyte abnormality of hypokalemic, hypochloremic metabolic alkalosis.

Intussusception. This is a telescoping of bowel into a proximal segment. In young children 2 months to 2 years old, the condition is usually idiopathic, and the most common location is ileocolic. Over the age of 3 years, a lead point such as a polyp or Meckel diverticulum may be the culprit. The typical presentation is intermittent colicky abdominal pain of a few minutes' duration associated with vomiting. These episodes of pain are followed by periods of lethargy. Unfortunately, the classic triad of symptoms—currant jelly stools, vomiting, and colicky abdominal pain—occurs in only 20% of patients. Physical exam may reveal an empty right lower quadrant and nontender mass in the right upper quadrant. Prolonged duration leads to bowel ischemia and necrosis. Henoch-Schönlein purpura is associated with ileo-ileal intussusception. Because of this unusual location, it is neither visualizable nor reducible by standard methods and requires computed tomography (CT) scan and surgical reduction.

Meckel diverticulum. The most common congenital abnormality of the gastrointestinal tract, Meckel diverticulum is the remnant of the vitelline duct. In half of all cases there is ectopic tissue (usually gastric). Painless rectal bleeding is the most common presentation of Meckel, but other symptoms include abdominal pain, nausea, and vomiting. The rules of 2s is a good way to classify the condition (Table 50-1).

Table 50-1. Meckel diverticulum and rule of 2s.

2% of the population
2 years old most common age of presentation
2 inches long
2 feet from the ileocecal valve
2 types of ectopic tissue (gastric and pancreatic)

Malrotation and volvulus. This entity refers to abnormal intrauterine rotation and fixation of bowel within the abdomen. This abnormal development around a narrow mesenteric pedicle puts the bowel at risk of twisting around these vessels and subsequent bowel necrosis. Classic symptoms include bilious vomiting, abdominal pain, distention, and bloody diarrhea.

Appendicitis. Although uncommon in young children, more than 80% present after the appendix has ruptured. Their presentation is often atypical, with a high rate of diarrhea and absence of typical migration of pain.

Medical Causes of Abdominal Pain

Constipation. Constipation is particularly common in toddlers around potty training age. Symptoms include diffuse colicky abdominal pain, anorexia, hard stools, and straining. Constipation can be confused with intussusception because of the intermittent nature of the pain.

Gastroenteritis. This entity is prevalent in childhood, particularly in those children in daycare. The most likely agents are viral; bacterial should be considered in those with bloody diarrhea. Pain is associated with abdominal cramping. Fever, vomiting, diarrhea, and pain are all symptoms of the condition. Appendicitis particularly early in the course of illness is often mistaken for acute gastroenteritis.

CLINICAL PRESENTATION

History

A careful, detailed history is essential in the evaluation of the pediatric patient with abdominal pain. Questions should be asked of both the caregiver and child. Most preschoolers over the age of 3 or 4 years old can provide reliable information. Inquire about the location of pain (diffuse vs. localized) and whether it has remained consistent or migrated (as in the case of appendicitis from periumbilical to right lower quadrant). The duration of the pain is essential to distinguish between acute and chronic conditions. Ask about associated symptoms such as vomiting (bloody, bilious, projectile, post prandial), diarrhea (bloody, currant jelly), anorexia, dysuria, and fever (height and duration).

Physical Examination

Before focusing on the abdomen, a thorough physical examination is necessary to rule out extraabdominal conditions, which can present with abdominal pain. Assess the pharynx for exudate and skin for the stereotypical sandpaper rash, as strep pharyngitis and scarlet fever can produce diffuse abdominal pain. Carefully examine the lower extremities and buttocks for the characteristic purpuric lesions of Henoch-Schönlein purpura, which can produce abdominal pain and ileo-ileal intussusception. Auscultate the lungs, as lower lobe pneumonia will irritate the diaphragm, resulting in pain that may even overshadow the cough. A thorough genitourinary evaluation is necessary to rule out genitourinary causes, including testicular torsion and hernias.

Delicate palpation of the abdomen to assess for focal tenderness and masses will often narrow the differential diagnosis. A firm mass in the left lower quadrant or mid abdomen supports the clinical picture of constipation, as does hard stool on rectal exam. An olive-shaped mass in the epigastrium of a newborn with postprandial vomiting is pathognomonic of pyloric stenosis. Examination should include abdominal auscultation and assessment of tenderness, rebound, and guarding. Asking the child "where does it hurt the most?" and "can you show me with one finger?" enlists assistance and allows accurate identification of the most distressing location of pain. A general assessment of hydration status is essential, as decreased oral intake and vomiting often accompany pediatric abdominal pain.

DIAGNOSTIC STUDIES

Laboratory

General laboratory studies (complete blood count, electrolytes) do not often add significant information in the evaluation of children with abdominal pain. The total white blood cell count in children with appendicitis is often normal. With the correct clinical picture, an elevated absolute neutrophil count is strongly supportive of the condition. A prolonged case of pyloric stenosis will show the stereotypical hypochloremic, hypokalemic, metabolic alkalosis.

Imaging

Flat and upright abdominal radiographs are useful to look for obstruction, seen as a dilated stomach or bowel with paucity of air distally. Free air under the diaphragm is seen in the case of a ruptured viscus. In intussusception, a standard x-ray may reveal a paucity of bowel gas in the right lower quadrant (Figure 50-1).

Ultrasound is the preferred modality to diagnose appendicitis in children, intussusception, and pyloric stenosis. Classic ultrasound findings include target, bull's eye, and pseudokidney signs (Figure 50-2). Reduction of

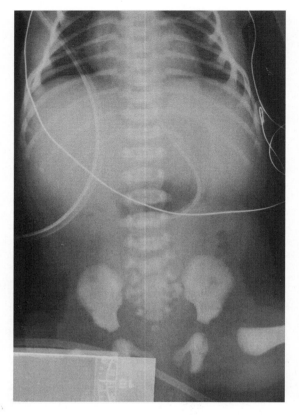

Figure 50-1. Paucity of distal bowel gas in child with malrotation.

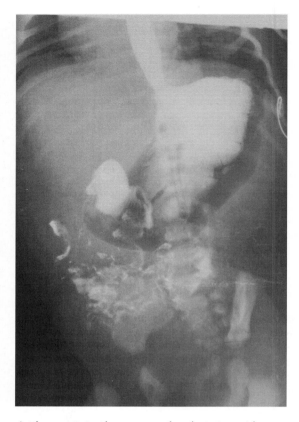

Figure 50-3. Fluoroscopy of malrotation with corkscrew sign.

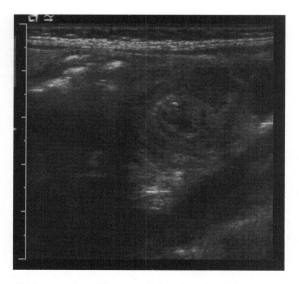

Figure 50-2. Ultrasound showing classic target sign in intussusception.

intussusception is routinely accomplished under fluoroscopy with air or barium. CT should be reserved for equivocal cases of appendicitis or when the appendix is not visualized on ultrasound. Upper GI series reveals duodenal obstruction with an abnormal course and "corkscrew" appearance in malrotation (Figure 50-3). Meckel diverticulum with ectopic gastric tissue is diagnosed with a technetium-99m pertechnetate study, commonly referred to as a Meckel scan. It can also be visualized on ultrasound or CT scan when it acts as a lead point in intussusception.

MEDICAL DECISION MAKING

Age of patient, history, and physical exam are often sufficient to narrow a differential diagnosis. Consider the following extra abdominal causes of abdominal pain in the investigation: urinary tract infection, inguinal hernia, testicular torsion, ovarian torsion and ovarian cysts, strep pharyngitis, and pneumonia. Children with bilious vomiting or peritoneal findings require immediate surgical evaluation (Figure 50-4).

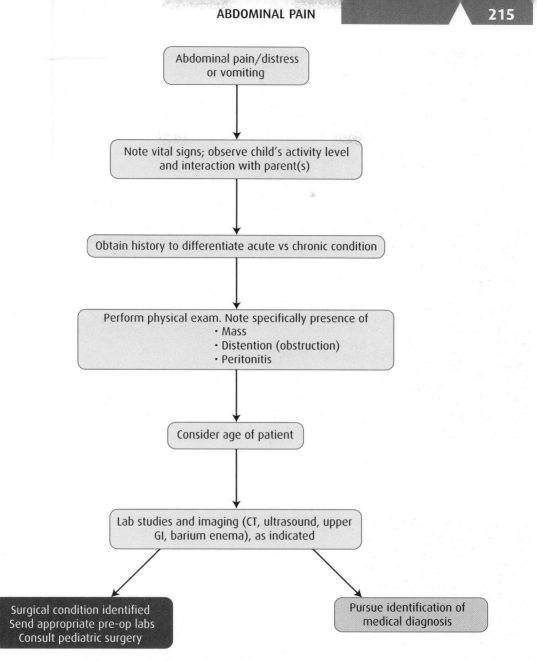

▲ **Figure 50-4.** Abdominal pain diagnostic algorithm.

TREATMENT

Pain control is essential in the care of patients. Analgesia does not interfere with the examination; on the contrary, it may even improve one's diagnostic accuracy by facilitating patient cooperation and removing less severe aspects of the pain. The treatment of the distress should proceed in parallel with the investigation of the etiology of the pain. In addition, nausea and vomiting often accompany abdominal pain and should be appropriately managed.

Intussusception. For ileo-colic intussusception, emergent radiologic reduction is necessary. In cases of unsuccessful radiologic reduction and with ileo-ileal intussusceptions, surgical reduction is indicated to prevent bowel necrosis.

Pyloric stenosis. Correction of electrolytes is a prerequisite for surgical repair. Pylorotomy is the treatment of cure.

Meckel diverticulum. Surgical resection is curative. Transfusion may be necessary in cases of significant blood loss.

Malrotation and volvulus. Emergent surgical repair is essential to minimize bowel necrosis.

Constipation. Treatments range from mild (laxatives for home use) to invasive (enema, disimpaction). Rarely, children require admission for continued enemas and nasogastric administration of laxatives.

DISPOSITION

▶ Admission

Children with surgical or suspected surgical causes of abdominal pain should be admitted to the hospital under the care of a surgeon. To prevent exposure to ionizing radiation, children with equivocal examinations or ultrasound findings may be admitted for serial abdominal examinations. Intussusception has up to a 10% recurrence risk in the first 24 hours after reduction. Most often children are admitted after reduction, but the potential exists for discharge from the ED with thorough instructions on when to return.

▶ Discharge

Children with medical causes of abdominal pain (pharyngitis, urinary tract infection, pneumonia, gastroenteritis) who tolerate oral fluids can be discharged home with close follow-up. The first presentation of etiologies of abdominal pain such as appendicitis or intussusception may be misinterpreted as viral illness. Therefore, very specific return instructions must be provided to the caregivers on discharge. These include bilious vomiting, worsening pain, localization to the right lower quadrant, and inability to tolerate oral fluids.

▼ SUGGESTED READING

Bachur RG. Abdominal emergencies. In Fleischer GR, Ludwig S. *Textbook of Pediatric Emergency Medicine.* 6th ed. Philadelphia, PA: Lippincott Williams & Wilkins, 2010, pp. 1515–1538.

Kharbanda AK, Sawaya RD. Acute abdominal pain in children. In: *Tintinalli's Emergency Medicine: A Comprehensive Study Guide.* 7th ed. New York, NY: McGraw-Hill, New York, 2011, 839–848.

Ross S, LeLeiko NS. Acute abdominal pain. *Pediatr Rev.* 2010;31:135–144.

Rothrock SG, Pagane J. Acute appendicitis in children: Emergency department diagnosis and management. *Ann Emerg Med.* 2000;36:39–51.

Dehydration

Kristine Cieslak, MD

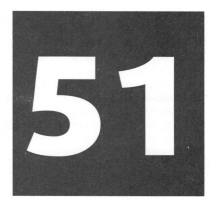

Key Points

- Dehydration is not a disease; the underlying cause must be identified and treated.
- Severity of dehydration can be classified using clinical assessment.
- Management priorities in the emergency department are stabilization of vital signs, replacement of intravascular volume deficit and ongoing losses, and correction of electrolyte abnormalities.
- Frequent reassessment of clinical status is necessary to monitor the response to treatment.

INTRODUCTION

Acute evaluation and treatment of children presenting with dehydration represents one of the most common situations in the pediatric emergency department (ED). Dehydration in sick children is often a combination of refusing to eat or drink and losing fluid from vomiting, diarrhea, or fever. In children with vomiting and diarrhea, the underlying problem is actually intravascular volume depletion, not dehydration. Volume depletion represents an equal loss of water and solutes (mainly sodium) from the blood plasma, whereas dehydration denotes a disproportional loss of plasma free water.

Children have higher morbidity and mortality rates associated with dehydration than adults due to a higher turnover of fluids and solutes (higher metabolic rates, increased body surface area/mass index, larger total body water content, immature kidneys with relative inability to produce concentrated urine, reliance on caregivers for basic needs). In clinical practice, the clinician attempts to determine the degree of volume depletion and the underlying cause of dehydration to initiate proper treatment.

Gastroenteritis is the most common cause of dehydration and is due to viruses in 80% of cases (rotavirus 30–50%). The clinical diagnosis of gastroenteritis by definition requires the presence of diarrhea. However, many infants with viral gastroenteritis present with isolated diarrhea or isolated vomiting. Rotavirus infections are responsible for approximately 3 million cases of diarrhea and 55,000 hospitalizations for diarrhea and dehydration in children <5 years of age each year in the United States. The majority of children with dehydration presenting to the ED have a benign etiology; however, there are serious causes for dehydration that should be considered.

Consider appendicitis, intussusception, volvulus, pyloric stenosis, urinary tract infection, hydrocephalus, brain tumors, and diabetes mellitus as potential underlying conditions in the pediatric patient who presents with dehydration. Other causes of dehydration include gastrointestinal (hepatitis, liver failure, drug toxicity), endocrine (congenital adrenal hyperplasia, Addisonian crisis), renal (pyelonephritis, renal tubular acidosis, thyrotoxicosis), poor oral intake (pharyngitis, stomatitis), and insensible losses (fever, burns, sweating, pulmonary processes).

CLINICAL PRESENTATION

History

A complete history is necessary to determine the severity of illness and to identify the type of dehydration present. Obtain as much information from the child, and elicit further details and clarifications from the parent or caregiver. Obtain a detailed description of intake (types of liquids and solids, volume, frequency) and output of urine (frequency, amount, color, odor, hematuria), stool (number, consistency, presence of blood or mucous), and emesis (frequency, volume, bilious or nonbilious, hematemesis). Estimate urine output by the number and saturation of wet diapers in infants and young children. Note the presence of abdominal pain (duration, location, intensity, quality, and radiation). Inquire about weight loss and activity level. Note the time interval of symptoms. The last episode of vomiting is important in determining when the initiation of an oral trial is advisable.

Ask about associated symptoms (fever, headache, neck pain, throat pain, dysuria, urinary frequency, rash). Travel and recent antibiotic use are also pertinent.

Note underlying diseases that could contribute to dehydration (kidney disease, diabetes mellitus, cystic fibrosis, hyperthyroidism). Contact with ill people and daycare attendance should be considered. Important elements of the past medical history include immunocompromise and malignancy.

▶ Physical Examination

The examination begins with assessment of the general appearance of the child. Lethargy or listlessness can warn of impending circulatory collapse. Examine the throat for erythema, ulcerations, or tonsillar exudates. Assess the abdomen for tenderness, rebound, or guarding. Neurologic exam should include mental status, cranial nerves, strength, and reflexes. Altered mental status or focal neurologic findings can indicate increased intracranial pressure. Capillary refill and skin turgor should be noted. The gold standard for the diagnosis of dehydration is measurement of acute weight loss. True pre-illness weight is rarely known in the acute care setting. An estimate of the fluid deficit is thus made based on clinical assessment (Table 51-1). Any of the two following findings

are predictive of clinically significant dehydration in children: ill appearance, absence of tears, dry mucous membranes, and delayed capillary refill (>2 seconds). Other important considerations are abnormal respiratory pattern and skin tenting.

Vital signs are an important objective measure and can be normal in a child with dehydration. The first sign of mild dehydration in children is tachycardia. Hypotension is a late sign of severe dehydration.

DIAGNOSTIC STUDIES

▶ Laboratory

Laboratory studies are not required if the etiology is apparent and mild-to-moderate dehydration is present. A bedside glucose is indicated for all infants and children with altered mental status. Blood sugar may be low (poor intake) or high (diabetic ketoacidosis [DKA]). With moderate-to-severe dehydration, electrolyte abnormalities may point to a specific diagnosis: high K (congenital adrenal hyperplasia, renal failure), low K (pyloric stenosis), low bicarbonate (acidosis, HCO_3 loss in diarrhea), high blood urea nitrogen/creatinine (renal hypoperfusion). Urinalysis may show glucose, ketones, or signs of infection. Urine-specific gravity may be elevated in patients with dehydration, but it is not a reliable measure. Serum sodium should be determined because hypo/hypernatremia requires specific treatment regimens.

▶ Imaging

No imaging is required for most patients presenting to the ED with dehydration. Consider flat/upright abdominal x-rays if there is suspicion for obstruction. Ultrasound or computed tomography (CT) scan of the pelvis is indicated if appendicitis suspected. Noncontrast head CT scan is indicated when evaluating severe headache or if exam reveals signs of intracranial pressure.

Table 51-1. Clinical assessment of severity of dehydration in the pediatric patient.

Signs and Symptoms	Mild (3–5% body weight)	Moderate (5–10% body weight)	Severe (>10% body weight)
Mental status	Alert/restless	Irritable and drowsy	Lethargic
Respirations	Normal	Deep ± rapid	Deep and rapid
Pulse	Normal	Rapid and weak	Weak to absent
Blood pressure	Normal	Normal with orthostasis	Low
Mucous membranes	Moist	Dry	Very dry
Tears	Present	Decreased	Absent
Skin turgor	Pinch and retract	Tenting	Tenting to doughy
Urine output	Normal	Decreased	Absent
Capillary refill	<2 sec	2–3 sec	>3 sec

MEDICAL DECISION MAKING

History and physical examination are generally sufficient to identify signs or symptoms of dehydration. Shock needs immediate recognition and treatment with fluid resuscitation. Determine severity of dehydration using clinical assessment (Figure 51-1).

The underlying cause of dehydration should be identified, and electrolyte abnormalities require correction. Further testing is guided by clinical suspicion of more serious problems.

TREATMENT

Identify patients with signs of shock and resuscitate with fluid immediately (20 mL/kg normal saline [NS] or Lactated Ringer's over a 20- to 30-minute period). Reassess and repeat fluid bolus until perfusion is adequate and vital

signs normalize (fluid bolus × 3 if necessary). Urine output is the most important indicator of restored intravascular volume (minimum = l mL/kg/hr). If 60–80 mL/kg of isotonic fluid is given with no improvement, consider other causes of shock (sepsis, hemorrhage, cardiac disease). Treat hypoglycemia promptly (2.5 mL/kg of 10% dextrose or 1 mL/kg of 25% dextrose). Once vital sign abnormalities are corrected, the rate of fluid administration for treatment is determined by the estimated fluid losses plus ongoing maintenance fluid requirements (Table 51-2).

The literature supports the use of a single dose of oral ondansetron in combination with oral rehydration for patients with dehydration due to nausea and vomiting. Ondansetron can be given as an oral dissolving tablet or intravenously (IV; 2 mg, 4 mg). Antidiarrheal agents are not recommended. Rapid oral rehydration has been shown to be as effective as IV fluid therapy in restoring intravascular

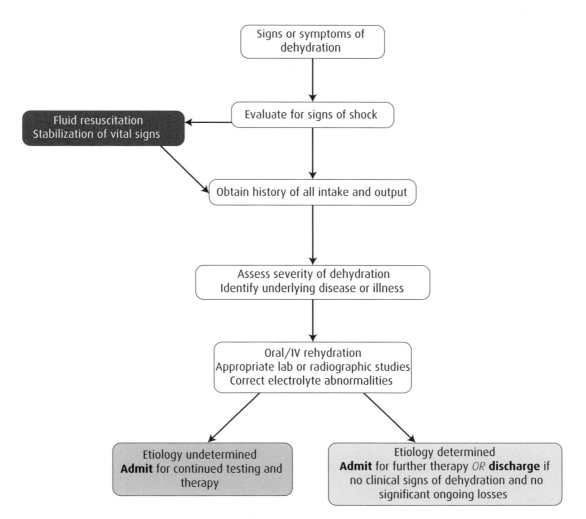

▲ **Figure 51-1.** Dehydration diagnostic algorithm.

Table 51-2. Calculations for maintenance fluid in the pediatric patient.

Patient Weight	4/2/1 Method	Holiday-Segar Method
First 10 kg	4 mL/kg/hr	100 mL/kg/day
Second 10 kg	2 mL/kg/hr	50 mL/kg/day
Each additional 10 kg	1 mL/kg/hr	20 mL/kg/day

volume and correcting acidosis in patients with moderate dehydration. For every 25 children treated with oral rehydration treatment for dehydration, 1 fails and requires IV therapy. Oral rehydration solutions for infants and toddlers should contain 45–50 mEq/L of sodium and 25–30 g/L glucose (Pedialyte, Infalyte). Give 5–10 mL of fluid every 5–10 minutes and increase as tolerated, with the goal of 30–50 mL/kg over a 4-hour period. If vomiting occurs, wait 30 minutes after last episode before reinitiating oral fluids. An estimate for fluid replacement is 10 mL/kg body weight for each watery stool and 2 mL/kg body weight for each episode of vomiting.

Dehydration can be categorized according to osmolarity and severity. Serum sodium is a good marker of osmolarity (assuming a normal glucose) and guides replenishment therapy. Isotonic dehydration is the most common (80%). Sodium and water losses are similar in intra- and extracellular compartments. Maintenance fluid requirements plus half the fluid deficit are administered over the first 8 hours, and the remaining fluid deficit over the following 16 hours. Hypotonic dehydration (Na <130 mEq/L) occurs when more sodium than water is lost. Calculate sodium deficit for replacement fluids. Sodium deficit (mEq) = (135-measured Na) × (pre-illness weight in kg) × 0.6. Sodium deficit should be replaced over a 4-hour period but should not exceed 1.5–2.0 mEq/hr; 0.9 NS is an appropriate solution. Hypertonic dehydration (Na >150 mEq/L) exists when more water is lost than sodium. The free water deficit is calculated as free water deficit (mL) = (measured serum Na-145) × 4 mL/kg × pre-illness weight (kg). Because of the risk of cerebral edema, correct the free water deficit over a 48-hour period, with a goal of reducing serum sodium by no more than 10–15 mEq/L/day; D5 ¼ to D5 ½ NS are appropriate solutions.

DISPOSITION

▶ Admission

Most patients with moderate-to-severe dehydration with significant acidosis should be admitted to the hospital (serum bicarbonate level of ≤13 is predictive of return to the ED for treatment failure as outpatient). Other indications for admission include significant ongoing fluid losses, inability to tolerate oral fluids, hypotonic or hypertonic dehydration, or undetermined etiology in need of further assessment. Patients with signs of increased intracranial pressure or DKA should be admitted to an intensive care unit.

▶ Discharge

Patients with no clinical evidence of dehydration or those with mild-to-moderate isotonic dehydration who have received adequate fluid rehydration (oral or IV) can be discharged home.

▼ SUGGESTED READING

Colletti JE, Brown KM, Sharieff GQ, Barata IA, Ishimine P. The management of children with gastroenteritis and dehydration in the emergency department. *J Emerg Med.* 2010;38:686–698.

Freedman SB, Adler M Seshadri R, Powell EC. Oral ondansetron for gastroenteritis in a pediatric emergency department. *N Engl J Med.* 2006;354:1698–1705.

Freedman SB and Thull-Freedman JD. Vomiting, diarrhea and dehydration in children. In: Tintinalli JE, Stapczynski JS, Ma OJ, Clince DM, Cydulka RK, Meckler GD. *Tintinalli's Emergency Medicine: A Comprehensive Study Guide.* 7th ed. New York, NY: McGraw-Hill, 2011, 830–839.

Otitis Media

Suzanne M. Schmidt, MD

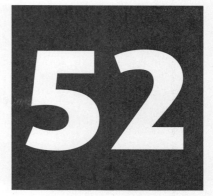

Key Points

- Distinguish between acute otitis media (AOM) and otitis media with effusion (OME), both of which present with a middle ear effusion.
- Clinical findings most suggestive of AOM are a bulging tympanic membrane (TM) with a purulent effusion, whereas the TM in OME has a clear effusion with a normal or retracted position.

- Erythema alone is a poor predictor of AOM and must be combined with other TM characteristics to make a diagnosis.
- Antibiotic treatment may be indicated for some episodes of AOM, but is not indicated for OME.
- Assess the patient for possible complications of AOM.

INTRODUCTION

Otitis media refers to the presence of inflammation or infection in the middle ear space. A middle ear effusion without infection is called otitis media with effusion (OME) or serous otitis. Infection of fluid in the middle ear is called acute otitis media (AOM). Diagnosis of AOM should be based on the acute onset of signs or symptoms of middle ear inflammation (fever, ear pain, distinct erythema of the tympanic membrane) in conjunction with a middle ear effusion seen on physical exam.

Ear disease is common in children, with 90% of children having at least 1 episode of a middle ear effusion and two thirds with at least 1 episode of AOM by school age. The peak incidence of AOM occurs between 6 and 24 months of age.

Episodes of AOM are often preceded by a viral upper respiratory tract infection (URI). The eustachian tube in children is shorter and more horizontal than in adults. Eustachian tube dysfunction associated with a URI can lead to a middle ear effusion (OME). Bacterial pathogens in the nasopharynx ascend via the eustachian tube, leading to infection of the fluid in the middle ear (AOM).

AOM is caused by bacteria in 50–80% of cases, most commonly *Streptococcus pneumoniae* or nontypable *Haemophilus*

influenzae and less commonly *Moraxella catarrhalis*. Purulent otorrhea may be caused by *Staphylococcus aureus* or *Pseudomonas aeruginosa* as well. Common complications of AOM are persistent middle ear effusion, tympanic membrane perforation, and tympanosclerosis. Other complications of AOM include cholesteatoma, hearing loss, tinnitus, balance problems, and facial nerve injury. Intracranial complications are rare and include mastoiditis, intracranial abscess, meningitis, and venous sinus thrombosis.

CLINICAL PRESENTATION

▶ History

Children with AOM usually present with acute onset of signs and symptoms of inflammation from AOM, such as fever and ear pain. This is often preceded by URI symptoms. Many symptoms associated with AOM, such as fever, irritability, restless sleep, and crying, are neither sensitive nor specific for AOM, and may be present in children with a URI with or without AOM. The presence of ear pain increases the relative risk of a patient having AOM. Purulent drainage from the ear may be present with AOM with tympanic membrane perforation or with otitis externa. Previous episodes of AOM, including timing of

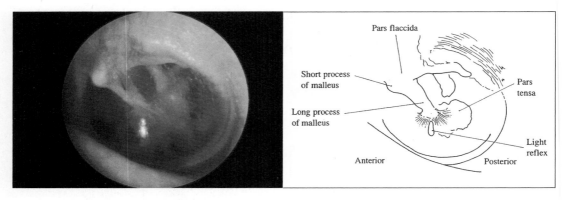

▲ **Figure 52-1.** Normal tympanic membrane. Courtesy Richard A. Chole, MD PhD

most recent infection and antibiotic use may influence choice of therapy. Persistent fever and headache may be signs of intracranial complications of AOM.

▶ Physical Examination

Fever, though nonspecific, is present in 50% of cases of AOM. Careful examination of the head and neck, including the oropharynx, teeth, jaw, and lymph nodes, should be done to search for other causes of pain that may be referred to the ear. Inspection of the pinna, tragus, and external auditory canal, as well as palpation of the tragus, should be performed. Pain with manipulation of the pinna or tragus, in conjunction with purulent otorrhea and inflammation of the external auditory canal, suggests otitis externa. The mastoid process should be examined for swelling, erythema, and tenderness, signs of mastoiditis. With mastoiditis, the pinna may also be displaced anteriorly.

Diagnosis of AOM or OME is made based on the appearance of the tympanic membrane (TM) on otoscopic examination, in conjunction with the clinical presentation. Adequate visualization of a child's TM requires good patient immobilization, typically with the child seated on the parent's lap with the head immobilized against the parent's chest, as well as use of the largest speculum that will comfortably fit in the external auditory canal. Removal of cerumen from the external auditory canal may be required for good visualization of the TM and can be accomplished with a cerumen scoop or gentle irrigation. Ear irrigation should not be performed if there is suspicion for a perforated TM. The external auditory canal in children may be narrow and tortuous, and the tympanic membrane is located anteriorly and superiorly. Gentle traction on the pinna in a posterior direction straightens the ear canal and can aid in visualization of the TM. Once adequate visualization is obtained, the following tympanic membrane characteristics should be assessed: translucency (translucent, opaque, partly opaque), color (clear/grey, white, amber, red), position (normal, retracted, bulging),

and mobility (normal, decreased or absent). A normal tympanic membrane is translucent and clear with a colorless or pearly gray color, and the bony landmarks of the middle ear are easily visible (Figure 52-1). In addition, a normal TM has a neutral position and brisk mobility with positive and negative pressure on insufflation. Opacity of the TM often obscures the bony landmarks and suggests the presence of fluid in the middle ear or another abnormality of the TM (tympanosclerosis, cholesteatoma). Other findings consistent with a middle ear effusion are an air fluid level or bubbles behind the TM, a bulging TM, decreased or absent mobility of the TM, or otorrhea. A middle ear effusion is present with both OME and AOM. Characteristics associated with OME include a normal or retracted TM, clear, or amber color, and impaired mobility on insufflation. Characteristics associated with AOM are a bulging TM, a purulent effusion, and distinct erythema of the TM with a middle ear effusion (Figure 52-2). Erythema alone is a poor predictor of AOM because the TM may

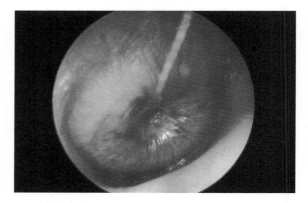

▲ **Figure 52-2.** Image showing patient with acute otitis media. Courtesy Richard A. Chole, MD PhD

appear pink or red with fever or crying. In addition, it is important to distinguish between distinct erythema of the TM itself (as in AOM) and increased vascularity with a red appearance only in the areas of the blood vessels.

DIAGNOSTIC STUDIES

▶ Laboratory

AOM is a clinical diagnosis, and laboratory studies are usually not required. Gram stain and culture of middle ear fluid obtained by tympanocentesis may be helpful in directing antibiotic therapy in complicated or resistant infections, but is not routinely performed.

▶ Imaging

A computed tomography (CT) scan of the head may be needed if there is concern for mastoiditis or other intracranial complication.

MEDICAL DECISION MAKING

History and physical examination should be sufficient to diagnose AOM and distinguish it from OME. If the tympanic membrane is normal, consider alternative causes of ear pain or fever (Figure 52-3). Inflammation of the mastoid process with anterior displacement of the pinna or other signs and symptoms of intracranial extension of infection should warrant investigation with a head CT.

TREATMENT

Antibiotics are not recommended in OME. Analgesics should be given if the child has pain associated with the middle ear effusion.

In children <2 years of age, oral antibiotic therapy is indicated in AOM because ear infections in this age group are less likely to resolve without antibiotic therapy. For children ≥2 years of age with uncomplicated AOM, a "wait-and-see" approach to treatment is an option. Because many cases of AOM will resolve without antibiotic therapy, the parent is given a prescription for antibiotics to be given to the patient if symptoms worsen or do not improve in 48–72 hours. Ear pain should always be managed with analgesics as needed, regardless of the therapeutic approach taken. Analgesics for ear pain include oral ibuprofen and acetaminophen as well as topical benzocaine/antipyrine drops. Topical analgesics should not be given if there is concern for a perforated TM.

If antibiotic therapy is chosen, high-dose amoxicillin (80–90 mg/kg/day divided BID) is recommended as first-line treatment for uncomplicated AOM. Treatment duration is 10 days in children <2 years of age and can be shortened to a 5–7 day course in children >2 years of age with uncomplicated infections. Amoxicillin-clavulanate (90/6.4 mg/kg/day divided BID) may be needed to treat β-lactamase producing *H. influenzae* and *M. catarrhalis* and should be used for AOM not responsive to amoxicillin. In addition, it may be considered as initial therapy in

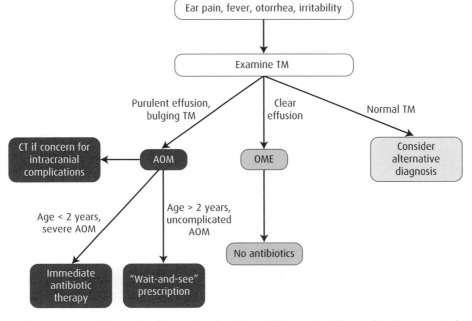

▲ **Figure 52-3.** Otitis media diagnostic algorithm. AOM, acute otitis media; CT, computed tomography; OME, otitis media with effusion; TM, tympanic membrane.

children with severe disease (fever >39°C or severe ear pain). Cephalosporins (cefdinir 14 mg/kg/day in 1–2 doses, cefuroxime 30 mg/kg/day divided bid, cefpodoxime 10 mg/kg/day once daily) may also be used for treatment failures. Ceftriaxone (50 mg/kg intramuscularly or intravenously) may be used to treat AOM in a patient with vomiting and an inability to tolerate oral medications. A single dose is adequate for initial treatment; 3 doses over 3 days are recommended for treatment failures. For patients with a penicillin allergy, a third-generation cephalosporin should be given if it is a non–type I hypersensitivity. With a type I hypersensitivity to penicillins, options include clindamycin, macrolides, erythromycin-sulfisoxazole, and trimethoprim-sulfisoxazole, but all provide suboptimal coverage.

DISPOSITION

▶ Admission

Only children with complications of AOM, such as mastoiditis or other intracranial complications, require hospitalization.

▶ Discharge

Non–toxic-appearing children without complications of AOM may be discharged home. Discharge instructions should be clear, especially if using a "wait-and-see" prescription for antibiotics, and should always include treatment of ear pain with analgesics as needed. Patients should be instructed to follow up with the primary care provider if symptoms do not improve in 48–72 hours or earlier if symptoms worsen or there are signs or symptoms of complications of AOM.

▼ SUGGESTED READING

AAP Clinical Practice Guideline. Diagnosis and management of acute otitis media. *Pediatrics*. 2004;113:1451–1465.
AAP Clinical Practice Guideline. Otitis media with effusion. *Pediatrics*. 2004;113:1412–1429.
Spiro DM, Arnold DH. Ear and mastoid disorders in infants and children. In: Tintinalli JE, Stapczynski JS, Ma OJ, Cline DM, Cydulka RK, Meckler GD. *Tintinalli's Emergency Medicine: A Comprehensive Study Guide*. 7th ed. New York, NY: McGraw-Hill, 2011.

Pharyngitis

S. Margaret Paik, MD

Key Points

- Distinguish potentially life-threatening (epiglottitis, peritonsillar, and retropharyngeal abscess) and benign (uncomplicated pharyngitis) conditions.
- Use a scoring system to guide management of pharyngitis.
- Suspected group A β-hemolytic streptococcus (GABHS) infections can be confirmed by performing a rapid antigen screening test or a throat culture.
- Antibiotic treatment is used to prevent suppurative and nonsuppurative (immune-mediated) complications GABHS.

INTRODUCTION

Sore throat is a common complaint seen in the emergency department (ED). Pharyngitis is inflammation of the throat and is usually the cause of sore throat. Inflammation of the tonsils (ie, tonsillitis) may also be present. The goal of the initial evaluation of patients with a complaint of sore throat is to exclude the most serious conditions (eg, abscess, epiglottitis).

Infectious pharyngitis involves direct invasion of the pharyngeal mucosa by bacteria or viruses leading to a local inflammatory response. Viruses are the most common cause of pharyngitis and include adenovirus, parainfluenza, influenza A and B, Coxsackie, rhinovirus, coronavirus, and Epstein-Barr virus (EBV).

Group A β-hemolytic streptococcus (GABHS) is the most common bacterial cause of pharyngitis. It accounts for 15–30% of cases of pharyngitis in children and 5–15% in adults. The peak age group is 5–15 years old. Most cases are seen in the winter and spring. GABHS pharyngitis is rare in patients younger than 2 years. Antibiotics are used to treat GABHS and to prevent suppurative and nonsuppurative complications. Suppurative complications include abscess formation. Nonsuppurative complications include scarlet fever, acute rheumatic fever (ARF), poststreptococcal glomerulonephritis, and streptococcal toxic shock syndrome. Scarlet fever, presenting with pharyngitis and a diffuse erythematous rash, is the result of the skin's reactivity to

the release of pyrogenic exotoxin by GABHS. ARF is a delayed sequela and can present with arthritis, carditis, chorea, erythema marginatum, and subcutaneous nodules. Poststreptococcal glomerulonephritis is caused by nephritogenic strains of GABHS. Children <7 years of age are at the highest risk. Streptococcal toxic shock syndrome is a severe GABHS infections presenting with shock and multisystem organ failure. The pharynx, skin, mucosa, and vagina can be portals of entry for GABHS resulting in streptococcal toxic shock syndrome.

▶ Life-Threatening Causes of Sore Throat

Epiglottitis is an infection of the epiglottis and adjacent supraglottic structures that can result in respiratory arrest and death if swelling is severe enough to airway occlusion. The widespread use of *Haemophilus influenzae* type B (HIB) conjugate vaccine in young children has dramatically changed the epidemiology of epiglottitis, and the incidence has decreased. Epiglottitis is currently more often seen in adolescents and adults. Common organisms include *Streptococcus pneumoniae*, *Staphylococcus aureus*, nontypeable *H. influenza*, and β-hemolytic streptococcus.

Retropharyngeal abscess is a deep space neck infection involving the lymph nodes that drain the nasopharynx, adenoids, posterior paranasal sinuses, and middle ear. The disease can start as an infection in these nodes (adenitis) leading to a suppurative adenitis, phlegmon formation, and finally, a retropharyngeal abscess. Incidence peaks between 2 and 4 years of age, as the retropharyngeal lymph nodes are prominent in young children but atrophy before puberty.

Peritonsillar abscess (PTA) is a collection of pus between the tonsillar capsule and the palatopharyngeal muscle. It is usually preceded by pharyngitis or tonsillitis with progression from cellulitis to phlegmon, and then abscess. It is the most common deep neck infection in children and adolescents. Infections are polymicrobial and include anaerobic and aerobic organisms (GABHS, *S. aureus*, fusiform, and bacteroides).

CLINICAL PRESENTATION

Most patients with pharyngitis will complain of sore throat and fever. Symptoms are acute in onset with GABHS pharyngitis. There is also pain on swallowing (odynophagia) or difficulty swallowing (dysphagia). Young children may not localize the pain to the throat and will complain of headache and/or abdominal pain instead of sore throat. Nausea and vomiting may also be present. Toddlers can present with fever, fussiness, or refusal to take liquids and solids.

Coryza, conjunctivitis, and hoarseness are symptoms suggestive of viral illness. Pharyngitis with fever, red eyes, and rash prompts concern for Kawasaki disease (mucocutaneous lymph node syndrome). Fatigue and anorexia are associated with infectious mononucleosis.

Drooling and the inability to handle oral secretions are seen is patients with epiglottitis, peritonsillar, or retropharyngeal abscess. Increased work of breathing (tachypnea, retractions, and stridor) is seen in patients with epiglottitis. Severe unilateral throat pain and inability to open the mouth (trismus) is seen in patients with a peritonsillar abscess. A muffled or "hot potato" voice can be heard in patients with a peritonsillar abscess, but is also present with epiglottitis and retropharyngeal abscess. Children with a retropharyngeal abscess may also have neck stiffness and pain with extension of the neck.

▶ Physical Examination

Airway patency must be assured, and impending airway compromise needs to be rapidly identified. Evaluate the hydration status, focusing on findings that have been correlated with dehydration in children. Signs and symptoms include a general "ill" appearance, the absence of tears with crying, dry mucous membranes, decreased skin turgor, tachycardia, and delayed capillary refill (>2 seconds). Auscultate the heart and document murmurs that might suggest the presence of acute rheumatic fever.

Patients with epiglottitis will be "toxic" appearing, showing signs of respiratory distress with stridor. The patient may prefer to sit in the "sniffing position" with the neck extended. Drooling, respiratory distress, and hyperextension of the neck are seen in patients with retropharyngeal abscess. Anterior bulging of the posterior pharyngeal wall may be visualized on examination. Those with a peritonsillar abscess may have trismus, "hot potato" muffled voice, and drooling with a fluctuant bulge in the

posterior aspect of soft palate with contralateral deviation of the uvula (Figure 53-1A). Classic findings in GABHS pharyngitis are fever, tender cervical adenopathy, tonsillar erythema, exudates, and hypertrophy (Figure 53-1B). Those with scarlet fever may have a fine, erythematous, "sandpaper-like" rash. Palatal petechiae (Figure 53-1C), a

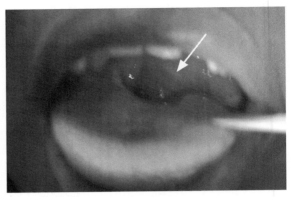

A

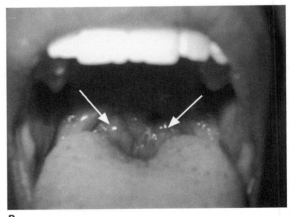

B

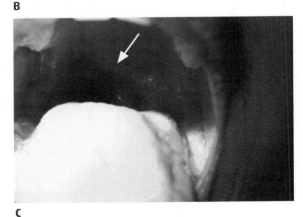

C

▲ **Figure 53-1. A.** Peritonsillar abscess. **B.** Tonsillitis. **C.** Palatal petechiae. (arrows)

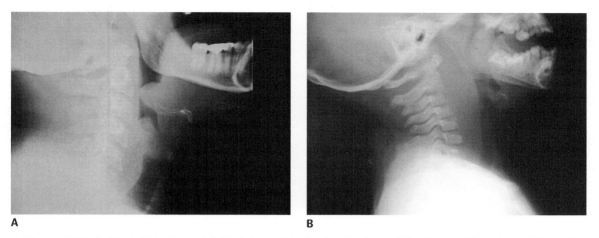

A   **B**

▲ **Figure 53-2. A.** Epiglottitis. The epiglottis is located by tracing the base of the tongue inferiorly until it reaches the vallecula. The structure immediately posterior is the epiglottis. If the epiglottis is enlarged (thumb print) and the vallecula is shallow, epiglottitis is present. **B.** Retropharyngeal abscess. The normal retropharyngeal soft tissue space is <7 mm at C2, <14 mm at C6 in children, and <22 mm at C6 in adults.

white or red "strawberry tongue" (inflamed tongue papillae), desquamating rash, and Pastia lines (accentuation of rash in flexor creases) are also suggestive of GABHS infection and scarlet fever.

Patients with infectious mononucleosis will have pharyngeal injection with exudates, posterior cervical adenopathy, and hepatosplenomegaly. A maculopapular rash is often seen in patients who are treated with amoxicillin or ampicillin.

DIAGNOSTIC STUDIES

▶ Laboratory

Rapid antigen detection of GABHS is 70–90% sensitive and 95–100% specific when performed correctly. GABHS diagnosis based solely on clinical grounds is accurate 50% of the time. A negative rapid strep test should be confirmed with a throat culture. Throat culture is the gold standard for diagnosis of GABHS pharyngitis, but results can take up to 48 hours. Approximately 20% of asymptomatic school-aged children are chronic carriers of GABHS.

In patients with infectious mononucleosis, a complete blood count will typically show lymphocytosis with a preponderance of atypical lymphocytes (>10%). Heterophile antibody (Monospot) or EBV titers are used to confirm the presence of infectious mononucleosis. Monospot is very insensitive in children younger than 4 years of age. Liver enzymes may also be elevated.

▶ Imaging

A soft tissue lateral neck radiograph may be helpful to visualize an aspirated foreign body or narrowing of the tracheal air column (masses). The "thumb print" sign is seen with epiglottitis (Figure 53-2A). Widening of the retropharyngeal space is seen with a retropharyngeal abscess (Figure 53-2B). The normal retropharyngeal soft tissue space is defined as <7 mm at C2, < 14 mm at C6 in children, and < 22 mm at C6 in adults. Computed tomography (CT) scan of the neck may be required for the definitive diagnosis of peritonsillar or retropharyngeal abscess.

MEDICAL DECISION MAKING

Patients with signs and symptoms of toxicity or severe respiratory distress need to be emergently evaluated for the possibility of epiglottitis, retropharyngeal abscess, or peritonsillar abscess. The history and physical examination will help to differentiate between these conditions.

Using either the Strep score (Table 53-1) or modified Centor criteria (Table 53-2) can help in the decision to test and treat patients with pharyngitis (Figure 53-3). Consider an alternative diagnosis of viral pharyngitis or foreign body if clinically indicated.

Table 53-1. Strep Score (each factor is worth 1 point).

- Fever >38.3°C (101°F)
- Age 5-15 years
- Season (November-May)
- Evidence of pharyngitis on exam (erythema, edema, exudates)
- Tender, enlarged >1 cm anterior cervical lymph nodes
- Absence of upper respiratory infection signs/symptoms

Scoring:

Points	PPV	Diagnosis/Treatment
0-1	2%	Supportive care
2-4	20-40%	Rapid test and treat accordingly
5-6	60-75%	Consider empiric treatment

Table 53-2. Modified Centor Criteria.

Criteria	Points
Fever >38°C (101.4°F)	1
Absence of cough	1
Tender, enlarged anterior cervical lymph nodes	1
Tonsillar exudates	1
Age	
3-14 years	1
15-44 years	0
45 years or older	-1

Points	Diagnosis/Treatment
0-1	Supportive care
2-3	Rapid test/culture and treat accordingly
4-6	Consider empiric treatment ± culture

TREATMENT

Epiglottitis. Place the patient in a position of comfort (parent's lap), avoid agitating the patient, and administer supplemental O$_2$. Obtain ear, nose, and throat (ENT) consultation with the goal to secure the airway in the operating room.

Retropharyngeal abscess. Start intravenous (IV) antibiotics (ampicillin-sulbactam 50 mg/kg or clindamycin 13 mg/kg). Obtain ENT consultation for surgical drainage if the CT reveals an abscess.

Peritonsillar abscess. Start IV antibiotics (ampicillin-sulbactam or clindamycin). Needle aspiration and/or incision and drainage in ED can be done in older children. Surgical drainage of the abscess in the operating room will be necessary for children requiring significant sedation.

Pharyngitis. Advise symptomatic treatment with warm salt water gargles (not for young children who will swallow the salt water) and acetaminophen (15 mg/kg every 4–6 hours) or ibuprofen (10 mg/kg every 6–8 hours). Antibiotics are prescribed in patients with suspected or confirmed GABHS. Oral choices of antibiotics include penicillin (25–50 mg/kg day PO TID or QID for 10 days),

amoxicillin (50 mg/kg/day PO BID-TID for 10 days), or a first-generation cephalosporin. Benzathine penicillin (<27 kg: 600,000 units; >27 kg: 1.2 million units) can be given intramuscularly to ensure compliance. Patients with penicillin or cephalosporin allergies can be given either erythromycin ethyl succinate (40 mg/kg/day PO BID or TID for 10 days), azithromycin (children: 12 mg/kg/day PO, maximum dose 500 mg/day PO for 5 days; adolescents and adults 500 mg tablet on day 1 followed by 250 mg tablet on days 2–5), or clindamycin (20 mg/kg/day PO TID for 10 days, maximum 1.8 g/day).

DISPOSITION

▶ Admission

Admit patients with epiglottitis and retropharyngeal abscess with potential airway compromise to an intensive care unit. Young patients with peritonsillar abscess who cannot be drained in the ED or are unable to tolerate liquids also require admission. When Kawasaki disease is suspected or pharyngitis causes severe dysphagia preventing adequate oral intake, admission may be necessary.

▶ Discharge

Patients with a peritonsillar abscess drained either by needle aspiration or incision and drainage who are tolerating oral fluid adequately can be discharged from the ED. The first dose of antibiotics should be given IV. Uncomplicated pharyngitis in patients tolerating oral fluids can also be discharged from the ED.

SUGGESTED READING

Caglar D, Kwun R. The mouth and throat. In Tintinalli JE, Stapczynski JS, Cline DM, Ma OJ, Cydulka RK, Meckler GD. *Tintinalli's Emergency Medicine: A Comprehensive Study Guide.* 7th ed. New York, NY: McGraw-Hill, 2011, pp. 774–782.

Fleischer GR. Sore throat. In: Fleisher GR, Ludwig S. *Textbook of Pediatric Emergency Medicine.* 6th ed. Philadelphia, PA: Lippincott Williams & Wilkins, 2010, pp. 579–583.

Gunn JD III. Stridor and drooling. In Tintinalli JE, Stapczynski JS, Cline DM, Ma OJ, Cydulka RK, Meckler GD. *Tintinalli's Emergency Medicine: A Comprehensive Study Guide.* 7th ed. New York, NY: McGraw-Hill, 2011, pp. 788–796.

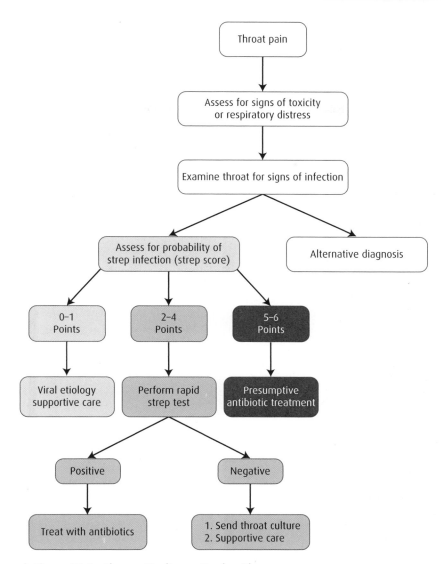

▲ **Figure 53-3.** Pharyngitis diagnostic algorithm.

The Poisoned Patient

Sean M. Bryant, MD

Key Points

- A thorough history of present illness including information gathered from available friends, family, and emergency medical service personnel can be invaluable in the management of poisoned patients.

- Perform a comprehensive physical exam including a full set of vital signs to help classify the patient's clinical presentation into a particular toxidrome.

- Always focus on supportive measures first in the clinical management of poisoned patients.

- Consult your regional poison center (1-800-222-1222) to ensure the appropriate management of poisoned patients.

INTRODUCTION

More than 2 million toxic exposures and poisonings are reported to U.S. regional poison centers annually. Consequently, all emergency physicians should possess a basic fundamental comprehension of emergency toxicology and a sound clinical approach for managing the poisoned patient. Depending on the absolute dose and/or duration of exposure, all substances have the potential for harm. Factors including the absorption, distribution, and elimination rate of the inciting agent help determine its overall toxicity. In poisoned patients, the pharmacokinetic features of the toxin (eg, circulating half-life) can be markedly prolonged secondary to extended absorption times and the saturation of metabolizing enzymes. These toxicokinetic principles often result in an unpredictable onset of symptoms and overall duration of toxicity.

The initial goal in managing a poisoned patient is to provide excellent supportive care. Contact your regional poison center (1-800-222-1222) early in the management of your patient as they can provide invaluable support. To aid in making the diagnosis, attempt to classify the patient's clinical presentation into a specific toxidrome (a syndrome complex that characterizes certain classes of poisonings) (Table 54-1). Only by following the preceding guidelines will certain patients be suitable for decontamination measures and possibly focused antidotal care.

CLINICAL PRESENTATION

▶ History

When possible, obtain a thorough history, including the location of the exposure and the patient's occupation. Pill bottles found at the scene or chemical containers noted by emergency medical service, family, or friends may provide the necessary clues to identify the causative toxin. Attempt to establish the exact time of exposure, although this is often limited to when the patient was last seen in a "normal" condition. Try to discern the amount that was ingested and whether it was in a regular or extended release formulation. Finally, try to establish the chronicity of the exposure, the immediate symptoms after the exposure, a history of previous suicide attempts, a thorough past medical history, and a history of any illicit drug abuse. If known, contacting the patient's regular pharmacy may provide further insight into the case.

Table 54-1. Common toxidromes.

Toxidrome	Representative agent(s)	Most Common Findings	Additional Signs/ Symptoms	Potential Interventions
Opioid	Heroin, morphine	CNS depression, miosis, respiratory depression	Hypothermia, bradycardia, respiratory arrest, acute lung injury	Ventilation or naloxone
Sympathomimetic	Cocaine, amphetamine	Psychomotor agitation, mydriasis, diaphoresis, tachycardia, hypertension, hyperthermia	Seizures, rhabdomyolysis, myocardial infarction, cardiac arrest	Cooling, sedation with benzodiazepine, hydration
Cholinergic	Organophosphate insecticides, carbamate insecticides	Salivation, lacrimation, diaphoresis, nausea, vomiting, urination, defecation, muscle fascicula- tions, weakness, bronchorrhea	Bradycardia, seizures, respiratory failure	Airway protection and ventilation, atropine, pralidoxime
Anticholinergic	Scopolamine, atropine	AMS, mydriasis, dry/flushed skin, urinary retention, decreased bowel sounds, hyperthermia, dry mucous membranes	Seizures, dysrhythmias, rhabdomyolysis	Physostigmine (if applicable), sedation with benzodiazepine, cooling, supportive management
Salicylates	Aspirin, oil of wintergreen	AMS, respiratory alkalosis, metabolic acidosis, tinnitus, hyperpnea, tachycardia, diaphoresis, nausea, vomiting	Low-grade fever, ketonuria, acute lung injury	MDAC, alkalinization of the urine with K+ repletion, hemodialysis, hydration
Hypoglycemia	Sulfonylureas, insulin	AMS, diaphoresis, tachycardia, hypertension	Paralysis, slurring of speech, seizures	Glucose, octreotide
Serotonin syndrome	Meperidine or dextro- methorphan and MAOI; SSRI and TCA; SSRI/TCA/MAOI and amphetamines; SSRI alone	AMS, increased muscle tone, hyperreflexia, hyperthermia	Intermittent whole-body tremor	Cooling, sedation with benzodiazepine, supportive management

AMS, altered mental status; CNS, central nervous syndrome; MAOI, monoamine oxidase inhibitor; MDAC, multi-dose activated charcoal; SSRI, serotonin reuptake inhibitor; TCA, tricyclic antidepressant.

▶ Physical Examination

Examination findings are very important to help recognize potential toxidromes and identify to what class of agent the patient might have been exposed. Obtain a full set of vital signs to evaluate for evidence of hyperpyrexia, hemodynamic instability, and tachypnea/hyperpnea (which could indicate compensation for significant acidemia). Characterize the patient's mental status and note any neurologic deficits. Findings such as delirium, central nervous system (CNS) hyperactivity, or frank obtundation/ coma may help to determine the responsible toxin. Perform a careful ocular exam focusing on pupillary size and responsiveness, the presence of nystagmus, and evidence of abnormal lacrimation (Table 54-2). Finally, noting the absence or presence of bowel sounds and whether the skin is dry or wet may help differentiate anticholinergic from sympathomimetic poisoning, respectively.

DIAGNOSTIC STUDIES

▶ Laboratory

Obtain a basic metabolic panel looking for electrolyte abnormalities or evidence of renal insufficiency. Check a serum creatine phosphokinase in all patients with ongoing seizures, prolonged down times, or renal abnormalities, as rhabdomyolysis is a serious concern. Calculation of an anion gap coupled to venous or arterial blood gas analysis may help differentiate acid–base disorders. Co-oximetry with blood gas analysis is also useful to determine

Table 54-2. Agents that affect pupil size.

Miosis (COPS)	Mydriasis (AAAS)
Cholinergics, clonidine	**A**ntihistamines
Opioids, organophosphates	**A**ntidepressants
Phenothiazine, pilocarpine	**A**tropine (anticholinergics)
Sedative-hypnotics	**S**ympathomimetics

methemoglobin and carboxyhemoglobin concentrations. A markedly elevated serum lactate level (>8–10 mmol/L) often indicates serious toxicity from an inhibitor of cellular metabolism (eg, cyanide).

Quantitative blood screens for determining the serum concentrations of multiple potential toxins including acetaminophen, salicylates, lithium, carbamazepine, valproic acid, lead, iron, and digoxin are usually very helpful to guide the management of poisoned patients. That said, qualitative urine toxicology screening rarely changes the work-up, management, or disposition of emergency department patients. The frequent false-positive results (eg, positive for PCP due to dextromethorphan use) and tests that remain persistently positive for several days after the actual exposure (eg, positive opiates × 7 days after heroin use; positive cocaine × 3 days after cocaine use; positive cannabinoids × 30 days after marijuana use) render urine toxicology screens challenging to interpret.

▶ Electrocardiogram

Obtain an electrocardiogram looking for any evidence of dysrhythmias, conduction blocks, or abnormal intervals. These findings may assist in both the diagnosis and treatment of patients poisoned by cardiotoxic agents.

▶ Imaging

Obtain computed tomography imaging of the brain when either mental status changes or neurologic deficits are present that are not consistent with the type of poisoning being entertained (eg, focal or lateralizing signs). Order a chest x-ray for all patients complaining of either shortness of breath, hypoxia, toxic fume inhalation, or potential aspiration (eg, hydrocarbon ingestion). Check abdominal x-rays, looking for radio-opaque ingestions (eg, leaded paint chips or toys, batteries, selected drug packets) as indicated to help complete the work-up.

MEDICAL DECISION MAKING

The first priority must always be supportive care in the management of the poisoned patient. Use all available historical items to help identify the possible toxin. A thorough physical exam including careful attention to the patient's mental status, vital signs, pupillary size and responsiveness, the presence of seizures, or abnormal changes in skin color, temperature, and moisture may help classify the patient's presentation into a specific toxidrome. Use the ancillary studies described previously to help clarify the diagnosis and guide further management (Figure 54-1).

TREATMENT

The treatment of poisoned patients can be broken down into a very systematic approach outlined by the mnemonic ABCDEFGH. First and foremost, initiate aggressive supportive care. The **airway** and **breathing** must be secured and addressed without delay. Intubation may be prevented

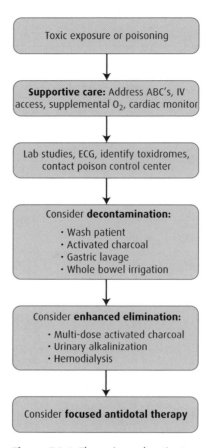

Figure 54-1 The poisoned patient diagnostic algorithm. ABCs, airway, breathing, and circulation; ECG, electrocardiogram; IV, intravenous.

with the successful use of a focused therapy such as naloxone in opioid toxicity or supplemental dextrose in hypoglycemic patients. Likewise, correct any **circulatory** compromise in the form of hypotension or bradycardia with standard fluid and/or vasopressor administration. Pay careful attention to the core temperature. Aggressively and expeditiously correct hyperpyrexia with active cooling measures and not systemic antipyretics. These measures, rather than the early search for specific antidotes, are the cornerstone of the initial management of the poisoned patient. The basic goal of **decontamination** is to remove the poison from the patient and the patient from the poison. Attempt decontamination as early as possible to achieve maximal benefit. Washing a patient's skin with soap and water to prevent further absorption and/or prevent harm to the emergency staff (eg, a patient covered with an organophosphate) is the simplest form of decontamination. Activated charcoal (1 g/kg or a 10:1 ratio of charcoal to toxin) can be given orally to bind ingested poisons and limit further gastrointestinal (GI) absorption. Although most drugs are amenable to this, lithium, iron and other metals, hydrocarbons, caustics, and toxic alcohols are not. Consider gastric lavage in patients who present very early (within 1 hour) after a potentially lethal ingestion. Additionally, any potentially fatal ingestions that don't have available antidotes may warrant lavage regardless of the timing of ingestion (eg, massive colchicine overdose). Contraindications to gastric lavage include the ingestion of hydrocarbons or other caustic agents, and potential complications include increased intracranial pressure, aspiration, and esophageal rupture. Whole-bowel irrigation with polyethylene glycol (GoLYTELY), given at a rate between 0.5 L/hr (pediatrics) and 2 L/hr, may help to "flush" toxins that won't bind to charcoal (eg, leaded paint chips) out of the GI tract and therefore limit total absorption. Contraindications to whole-bowel irrigation include hemodynamic instability (hypotension = lack of GI perfusion) and decreased bowel sounds (impaired GI motility). Of note, pulmonary aspiration is the most common adverse side effect for all forms of GI decontamination, and patients must have an intact airway for these procedures to be pursued.

There are several different modalities available to enhance the **elimination** of poisons. Hemodialysis is ideal for smaller-sized poisons with small volumes of distribution (<1 L/kg) and low degrees of protein-binding. Ideal agents for hemodialysis include aspirin, toxic alcohols, and lithium. Hemodialysis should also be performed in all patients with profound acidemia regardless of the etiology. Alkalinization of the urine is commonly initiated for ingestions of weak acids such as aspirin and phenobarbital. The proposed mechanism depends on increasing the urinary pH by giving doses of intravenous (IV) sodium bicarbonate. Circulating toxins will be preferentially converted to their conjugate bases in the alkaline environment and consequently trapped in the renal tubules, where they will be excreted in the urine. Alkalinization can also benefit patients in select cases (eg, salicylate overdose) by keeping the poison preferentially out of the CNS, as the ionized form cannot enter through the blood–brain barrier. Finally, multiple doses of oral activated charcoal (MDAC) can be administered to patients poisoned with select agents including theophylline, phenobarbital, carbamazepine, dapsone, or quinine. The proposed mechanism relies on the use of the GI tract wall as a dialysis membrane. The intraluminal charcoal functions to pull circulating toxins back into the GI tract where they are bound to the charcoal and excreted. MDAC can also be employed to further decontaminate the gut of agents that have erratic and prolonged absorption (eg, salicylates, valproic acid). If MDAC is entertained, ensure that the charcoal is not premixed with sorbitol, as cathartics (unlike polyethylene glycol) can cause marked fluid and electrolyte shifts, resulting in significant morbidity and/or mortality.

Antidotal therapy is important and necessary when managing the poisoned patient, but should never take priority over the supportive measures already mentioned. Examples of selected **focused therapy** along with general indications are listed in Table 54-3. The final portion of the

Table 54-3. Specific antidotes for toxicologic agents.

Poison	Antidote
Acetaminophen	N-acetylcysteine
Crotalidae bite	Antivenom Fab
Hydrofluoric acid, calcium channel antagonists	Calcium gluconate or calcium chloride
Cyanide	Sodium nitrite, thiosulfate
Iron	Deferoxamine
Digoxin	Digoxin Fab
Ethylene glycol, methanol	Fomepizole or ethanol
Methanol, methotrexate	Folic acid/leucovorin
Calcium channel blocker, β blocker	Glucagon
Oxidizing chemicals (nitrites, benzocaine, sulfonamides)	Methylene blue
Refractory hypoglycemia after oral hypoglycemic	Octreotide
Opioid, clonidine	Naloxone
Anticholinergic (not TCA)	Physostigmine
Cholinergic	Pralidoxime (2-PAM)
Heparin	Protamine
Isoniazid	Pyridoxine
Anticoagulants	Vitamin K

TCA, tricyclic antidepressant.

management algorithm includes **G** and **H**. This is a reminder for clinicians to never hesitate in calling their regional poison center (1-800-222-1222) for assistance during any point in the care of the poisoned patient. **Getting help** early may facilitate a more focused work-up, prevent unnecessary laboratory and/or diagnostic studies, provide insight into potentially life-saving antidotal therapy, and assist with appropriate disposition making.

DISPOSITION

▶ Admission

All patients with hemodynamic abnormalities, persistent mental status changes, and metabolic or acid–base irregularities should be admitted to an intensive care setting. Additionally, those who ingested medications that either require antidotal therapy or have prolonged or delayed toxic effects (eg, sulfonylureas, extended-release calcium channel blockers, or beta-blockers) also require admission to a critical care setting. All suicidal patients will require psychiatric consultation for clearance.

▶ Discharge

Patients with accidental ingestions of innocuous substances, those with no evidence of acute toxicity, and those who have no potential for delayed detrimental effects can be discharged.

▼ SUGGESTED READING

Barry JD. Diagnosis and management of the poisoned child. *Pediatr Ann.* 2005;34:937–946.

Erickson TB, Thompson TM, Lu JJ. The approach to the patient with the unknown overdose. *Emerg Med Clin North Am.* 2007;25:249–281.

Hack JB, Hoffman RS. General management of poisoned patients. In: Tintinalli JE, Cline DM, Cydukla RK, et al., eds. *Tintinalli's Emergency Medicine: A Comprehensive Study Guide.* 7th ed. New York, NY: McGraw Hill, 2011:1187–1193.

Toxic Alcohols

Mark B. Mycyk, MD

Key Points

- Consider toxic alcohol poisoning in cases of an unexplained anion gap acidosis or an elevated osmol gap.
- Focus your initial treatment on the early inhibition of alcohol dehydrogenase (ADH) in cases of ethylene glycol or methanol poisoning to prevent the accumulation of toxic metabolites.

- Consult your local poison center (800-222-1222) or local toxicologist in all suspected cases for help initiating antidotal therapy and obtaining confirmatory toxic alcohol levels.
- Consult a nephrologist early to prepare for hemodialysis in cases involving large ingestions or severe metabolic acidosis.

INTRODUCTION

With the exception of ethanol, no other alcohols are safe for human consumption and are therefore considered toxic alcohols. Ethylene glycol, methanol, and isopropanol are the most common toxic alcohols associated with human poisoning. Toxic alcohols are often ingested in 1 of 2 ways, either unintentionally if placed in an inappropriately labeled container, or intentionally by patients either attempting suicide or trying to become intoxicated when regular ethanol is not readily available. Of note, each of the 3 is capable of causing inebriation, with isopropanol being twice as intoxicating as ethanol.

According to the National Poison Data System, more than 35,000 toxic alcohol exposures are reported to the American Association of Poison Control Centers yearly. Isopropanol is the most frequently ingested but causes the fewest number of deaths, whereas methanol is the least commonly ingested toxic alcohol but associated with the highest number of fatalities.

Although the parent compound is responsible for inebriation, toxicity results from the metabolism of these compounds via alcohol dehydrogenase (ADH) into toxic organic acid byproducts with consequent end organ injury. Ethylene glycol is metabolized to glycolic acid, glyoxylic acid, and oxalic acid, all of which can produce systemic acidosis and acute kidney injury. Methanol is converted to formic acid which can produce systemic acidosis and retinal toxicity. Isopropanol is not converted to an organic acid but is rather metabolized into acetone, which can produce hemorrhagic gastritis and systemic hypotension in the absence of a concurrent acidosis. If either are unrecognized or untreated, all toxic alcohol ingestions can result in patient fatality.

CLINICAL PRESENTATION

▶ History

Obtaining a history of toxic alcohol ingestion is often challenging. Patients may be obtunded on arrival to the emergency department (ED), not forthcoming with the ingestion history, or too young to be appropriately descriptive (children). Reading the ingredient lists on the labels of any empty bottles found at the scene or brought to the ED can be extremely helpful. If a bottle or label is not available, ask the patient what kind of product was ingested. For example, antifreeze usually contains ethylene glycol, windshield-washing fluid usually contains methanol, and rubbing alcohol usually contains isopropanol.

That said, remember that some products may contain different types of toxic alcohols (eg, some gas-line antifreeze products contain methanol). Beyond attempting to identify exactly what was ingested, it is critically important to determine the time of ingestion, as this will affect the interpretation of laboratory results and impact patient management priorities.

Physical Examination

Most patients poisoned with a toxic alcohol will demonstrate some level of central nervous system (CNS) depression analogous to inebriation. Patients arriving soon after an ingestion may appear well with unremarkable physical exams, whereas those who arrive many hours after ingestion may be obtunded with unstable vital signs. Of note, the peak serum level of a toxic alcohol correlates poorly with the physical exam findings. As with all overdoses, perform a careful neurologic examination (mental status, cranial nerves, cerebellar findings, and motor strength). Ocular examination may reveal blurred vision, decreased visual acuity, retinal edema, optic atrophy, or hyperemia of the optic disc in methanol poisoning. Abdominal tenderness or blood on rectal examination may indicate isopropanol ingestion as it is classically associated with hemorrhagic gastritis.

DIAGNOSTIC STUDIES

Laboratory

A basic metabolic panel is indicated to determine renal function, acid–base status, and calculate an anion gap (the normal range is 8–12 mEq/L). Obtain an arterial blood gas to ascertain the degree of acidosis. A serum ethanol level is required in all cases of suspected toxic alcohol poisoning, as this result impacts the osmol gap equation and helps determine the timing of ADH inhibition.

An osmol gap can be a useful screening test for toxic alcohol poisoning if calculated early after the ingestion. Send a serum sample to the laboratory to measure osmolality. The osmol gap is equal to this value minus the calculated osmolality ($2*Na$ + glucose/18 + blood urea nitrogen/2.8 + ethanol/4.6). Traditionally a normal osmol gap is <10 mEq/L, but in actuality will normally range between −7 to +14. It is the toxic alcohol parent compound that contributes to the osmol gap, and elevated gaps occur early after ingestion before the metabolism of the toxic alcohols into their poisonous byproducts. Later, as the toxic organic acid metabolites build up and the parent compound levels decrease, an anion gap metabolic acidosis becomes the predominant finding, with the osmol gap becoming less significant (Figure 55-1). Ethylene glycol and methanol can result in a simultaneous anion gap metabolic acidosis and elevated osmol gap. Because isopropanol is not metabolized into an organic acid, ingestion typically results in an elevated osmol gap in the absence of an elevated anion gap. Because isopropanol is rapidly converted to acetone, a serum acetone level can help identify isopropanol poisoning in this setting.

Calcium oxalate crystals on urine microscopy or urine fluorescence under ultraviolet light (due to the addition of fluorescein to most commercial antifreeze) may be clues for ethylene glycol poisoning, but the absence of either should *not* be used to rule out exposure.

Most importantly, serum toxic alcohol levels (quantitative ethylene glycol, methanol, and isopropanol) should be ordered STAT in cases of suspected toxic alcohol poisoning to confirm ingestion and guide management. It is important to recognize that toxic alcohol tests are rarely performed in hospital laboratories and must be sent to an off-site reference lab in most cases, so results may not be available for several hours.

Imaging Studies

Although imaging studies do not help diagnose toxic alcohol poisoning, methanol exposure has been reported to cause basal ganglia hemorrhage or infarct. Computed tomography imaging of the head should also be considered when the mental status does not correlate with the presumed exposure or associated trauma is a concern.

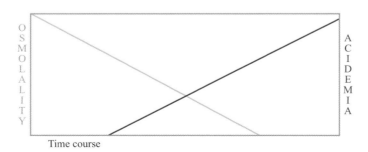

▲ **Figure 55-1.** Relationship of degree of osmolality and acidosis during the course of ethylene glycol or methanol poisoning. Used with permission from Mark B. Mycyk, MD.

MEDICAL DECISION MAKING

History alone may be sufficient to prompt a work-up for toxic alcohol poisoning. In the absence of a reported ingestion, an unexplained anion gap acidosis or elevated osmol gap should prompt further evaluation for a toxic alcohol. Order STAT serum tests for all toxic alcohols (ethylene glycol, methanol, and isopropanol). Initiate care based on the presumptive clinical diagnosis and do not delay ED treatment awaiting laboratory confirmation, as even in ideal scenarios these levels will often take several hours to measure. The initiation of antidotal therapy to inhibit ADH should be the management priority early after an ingestion before the onset of acidosis, whereas hemodialysis should be the priority in cases with a delayed presentation when severe acidosis is already present (Figure 55-2).

TREATMENT

Attention to the airway in cases of CNS depression should take precedence. IV fluids should be administered to treat hypotension and maintain renal perfusion in all cases of toxic alcohol poisoning. In cases of isopropanol ingestion, no additional treatment is necessary. In cases of ethylene glycol or methanol poisoning, initiate ADH inhibition until the ethylene glycol or methanol level is <20 mg/dL and no acidosis is present. ADH may be inhibited with either IV fomepizole (load = 15 mg/kg) or an IV ethanol infusion (to achieve a serum ethanol level between 100–150 mg/dL).

Obtain early nephrology consultation to facilitate emergent hemodialysis if the ethylene glycol or methanol level is >50 mg/dL to filter out the parent compound and any accumulated toxic metabolites. Emergent dialysis is also indicated in cases of renal failure or severe acidosis irrespective of the ethylene glycol or methanol level to remove any remaining toxic metabolites and improve the systemic acid–base status. In cases of ethylene glycol poisoning, both thiamine 10 mg IV and pyridoxine 50 mg IV every 6 hours may help convert glyoxylic acid to nontoxic metabolites. In cases of methanol poisoning, folic acid 50 mg IV every 4 hours may help convert formic acid to CO_2 and H_2O.

DISPOSITION

▶ Admission

Admit all patients who are either suicidal, require hemodialysis, or require ADH inhibition. All patients with abnor-

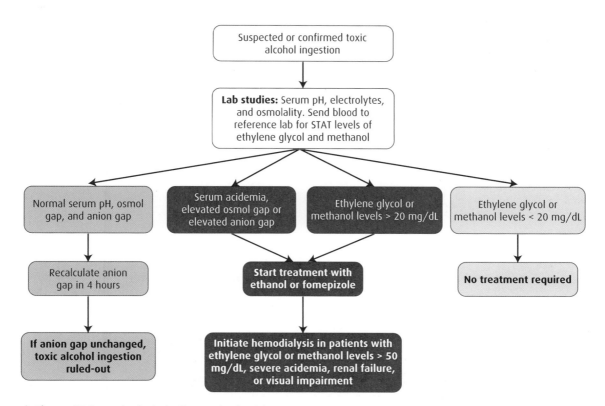

▲ **Figure 55-2.** Toxic alcohols diagnostic algorithm.

mal vital signs, systemic acidosis, or evidence of end-organ damage require admission to an intensive care unit setting, as do patients requiring an ethanol infusion for ADH inhibition to follow serial ethanol levels and monitor CNS depression. Patients receiving fomepizole can typically be admitted to a regular hospital bed.

▶ Discharge

Unintentional ingestions with no evidence of acidosis or indications for antidotal treatment or hemodialysis may be safely discharged after appropriate poison prevention counseling.

▼ SUGGESTED READING

Brent J. Fomepizole for ethylene glycol and methanol poisoning. *N Engl J Med*. 2009;360:2216–23.

Mycyk MB. Toxic alcohols. In: Barton C, Collings J, DeBlieux P, et al., eds. *Adams' Emergency Medicine*. 2nd ed. Philadelphia, PA: Elsevier, 2012, pp. 1292–1298.

Mycyk MB, Aks SE. A visual schematic for clarifying the temporal relationship between the anion gap and the osmol gap in cases of toxic alcohol poisoning. *Am J Emerg Med*. 2003;21:333–335.

Smith JC, Quan D. Alcohols. In: Tintinalli JE, Stapczynski JS, Cline DM, Ma OJ, Cydulka RK, Meckler GD, eds. *Tintinalli's Emergency Medicine: A Comprehensive Study Guide*. 7th ed. New York, NY: McGraw-Hill, 2011:1222–1230.

Acetaminophen Toxicity

Jenny J. Lu, MD

Key Points

- Acetaminophen is the most popular over-the-counter analgesic in the United States and is widely prescribed in combination form with alternative pain relievers, resulting in frequent unintentional overdose.

- Treatment with N-acetylcysteine detoxifies NAPQI, the hepatotoxic byproduct of acetaminophen metabolism.

- The Rumack-Matthew nomogram should only be used in acute overdoses with reliable times of ingestion. Pay careful attention to all *units of measurement*.

- Consider early transfer to a liver transplant center for patients with worsening hepatic function or general signs of deterioration *before* they meet criteria for liver transplantation.

INTRODUCTION

Acetaminophen (APAP) is the most commonly used over-the-counter (OTC) analgesic in the United States. It is found in more than 100 combination pharmaceuticals (eg, cold and cough agents, sleep agents) and is present in multiple prescription opioid analgesics (eg, Vicodin, Darvocet). Toxic exposures to analgesics as a class have increased rapidly over the last decade. According to the National Poison Data System (NPDS) database of exposures reported to poison centers nationwide, there were 139,780 exposures to all APAP-containing products in the year 2010, with 1,142 cases exhibiting "major" effects and 125 fatalities. APAP toxicity is the most common cause of medication-induced liver failure in the United States and accounts for a significant portion of liver transplants.

The maximum recommended safe dose is 4 g per day for adults and 60–90 mg/kg/day for children. Toxicity may result after an ingestion of 7 g in adults or 140 mg/kg in a child and is due to the conversion of APAP into toxic byproducts. APAP is normally metabolized via multiple pathways in healthy individuals. Sulfonation and glucuronidation are the two primary mechanisms and produce nontoxic metabolites that are cleared in the urine. Approximately 10–15%, though, is metabolized via the cytochrome P450 system into the toxic metabolite N-acetyl-p-benzoquinoneimine (NAPQI).

After a therapeutic ingestion, endogenous stores of hepatic glutathione will rapidly detoxify any accumulating NAPQI. However, in cases of APAP overdose, the sulfonation and glucuronidation pathways are overwhelmed, and a greater percentage of APAP is metabolized via cytochrome P450 into NAPQI. Glutathione stores can become rapidly depleted, resulting in elevated levels of intrahepatic NAPQI with secondary toxicity. Furthermore, in overdose scenarios, a small percentage of APAP can be metabolized into NAPQI within the kidneys, resulting in consequent renal toxicity. Patients with lower glutathione stores (chronically ill, malnourished, and alcoholics) and those with upregulated cytochrome P450 activity (patients on certain medications including anticonvulsants and antituberculosis agents, chronic alcoholics) are more likely to suffer significant toxicity.

Clinically, APAP poisoning progresses through 4 distinct stages. Although all patients may not progress beyond the first stage after a toxic exposure, those that do tend to follow the following timeline. Stage 1 is generally encountered within the first 24 hours postexposure. Symptoms of gastrointestinal (GI) irritation predominate, including abdominal pain and vomiting, although patients may remain asymptomatic. Stage 2 occurs between 24–48 hours post exposure and is known as the latent stage. GI symptoms resolve, but ongoing hepatotoxicity can lead to significantly elevating serum transaminases. The third stage occurs within 3–4 days after exposure. Abdominal symptoms return, including pain and vomiting along with jaundice and potential encephalopathy. Laboratory studies may reveal acidemia, hypoglycemia, renal failure, and coagulopathy. Stage 4 lasts between 4 days and 2 weeks of the exposure and involves a progression to outright liver failure and death or complete patient recovery. The hepatic function of those patients who survive APAP poisoning will also recover completely.

CLINICAL PRESENTATION

▶ History

Always attempt to identify the exact formulation, amount, and timing of the ingestion. Ask about any coingestants (eg, ethanol) that might impact the metabolism of APAP and clarify the number and frequency of ingestions to rule out chronic toxicity. Ask about risk factors for increased toxicity, including chronically ill and alcoholic patients and those taking medications that activate the cytochrome P450 system (eg, anticonvulsants, antituberculosis).

The majority of symptoms are abdominal and neurologic in nature. Ask about the presence of any abdominal pain, nausea, and vomiting. Inquire about any symptoms of altered mental status and decreased levels of consciousness, as these portent a more serious clinical course.

▶ Physical Examination

Pay careful attention to the patient's vital signs. Hemodynamic instability suggests a significant poisoning. Significant tachypnea may indicate an attempt to compensate for an ongoing metabolic acidosis. Coingestions or combination products (eg, APAP + opioid or APAP + diphenhydramine) may cause marked abnormalities due to concurrent opioid or anticholinergic toxidromes.

Note the patient's general appearance, mental status, and level of consciousness. Carefully examine the abdomen. Diffuse abdominal tenderness is common after significant overdose, and tender hepatomegaly may be evident beginning in the latent stage. Finally, examine the skin and sclera, looking for signs of jaundice.

DIAGNOSTIC STUDIES

▶ Laboratory

Obtain an immediate serum APAP level in all patients and follow with serial testing to establish an upward or downtrending value. In patients with clearly timed acute ingestions, order a second level at the 4-hour mark postexposure. These values can be plotted on the Rumack-Matthew nomogram to help determine treatment (Figure 56-1). Check a full panel of liver studies (aspartate aminotransferase, alanine aminotransferase, albumin, bilirubin) in all patients and follow serially, looking for evidence of worsening hepatotoxicity. Order a coagulation profile (prothrombin time [PT], international normalized ratio and partial thromboplastin time) to determine the degree of liver synthetic dysfunction.

Check a baseline complete blood count and follow serial hemoglobin levels in patients who develop coagulopathies. Order a metabolic panel to assess for electrolyte abnormalities and to calculate the anion gap, as a significantly elevated anion gap metabolic acidosis may be present. Confirm the degree of acidosis with blood gas sampling. Finally, check the renal function in all patients, as acute kidney injury is common secondary to intra-renal NAPQI production.

▶ Imaging

Consider a head computed tomography (CT) in patients whose mental status does not correlate with an isolated ingestion. Cerebral edema secondary to hyperammonemia may occur in hepatic failure. Abdominal CT imaging is usually of limited utility in APAP poisoning but should be considered in patients with signs of peritonitis.

MEDICAL DECISION MAKING

Many exposures and overdoses have the potential for significant hepatotoxicity. In most cases, a thorough history will be sufficient to identify APAP as the culprit. In patients presenting with elevated transaminases or signs of hepatic failure and no obvious source, there is usually little downside in empirically starting therapy with N-acetylcysteine (NAC) until more information is obtained.

Draw baseline APAP and liver function tests and follow serially to determine whether the levels are rising or falling. In patients with acute ingestions of reliable timing, plot their 4-hour APAP level on the Rumack-Matthew nomogram to determine treatment. Of note, the nomogram cannot be used if either the time of ingestion is unknown or the ingestion is chronic (occurring over hours/days). The nomogram may also be unreliable in cases of coingestions with products that alter APAP absorption and pharmacokinetics.

Use the King's College liver transplant criteria early to estimate the severity of exposure and identify which patients may require transfer for specialty care. Patients with either a pH <7.3 after fluid resuscitation or a combination of PT >100, creatinine >3.3 mg/dL, and grade 3 or 4 encephalopathy are considered to meet these criteria. Consult your regional poison control center for all patients with significant hepatotoxicity to help determine the ideal treatment (Figure 56-2).

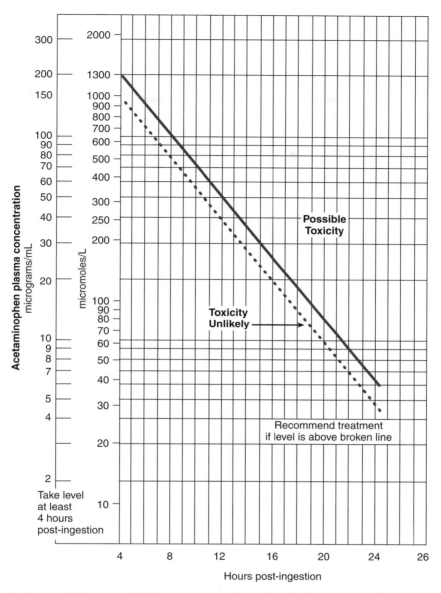

▲ Figure 56-1. Rumack-Matthew nomogram. Reprinted with permission from
Tintinalli JE, Stapczynski JS, Ma OJ, Cline DM, Cydulka RK, Meckler GD. Chapter 184.
Acetaminophen. In: Tintinalli JE, Stapczynski JS, Ma OJ, Cline DM, Cydulka RK,
Meckler GD, eds. *Tintinalli's Emergency Medicine: A Comprehensive Study Guide.*
7th ed. New York: McGraw-Hill, 2011.

TREATMENT

As with all cases of acute poisoning, address the patient's
airway, breathing, and circulation. Gastric decontamination
is occasionally indicated and generally performed with
activated charcoal (AC). AC readily absorbs APAP and
should be given in cases with recent ingestions (within

8–12 hours of exposure) or those with evidence of ongoing
absorption, provided there are no contraindications. Give
a starting dose of 1 g/kg and consider repeated dosing in
patients with significantly large ingestions. Beware AC
products containing sorbitol with repeated dosing to
avoid significant fluid and electrolyte abnormalities.
Gastric lavage and whole-bowel irrigation are rarely

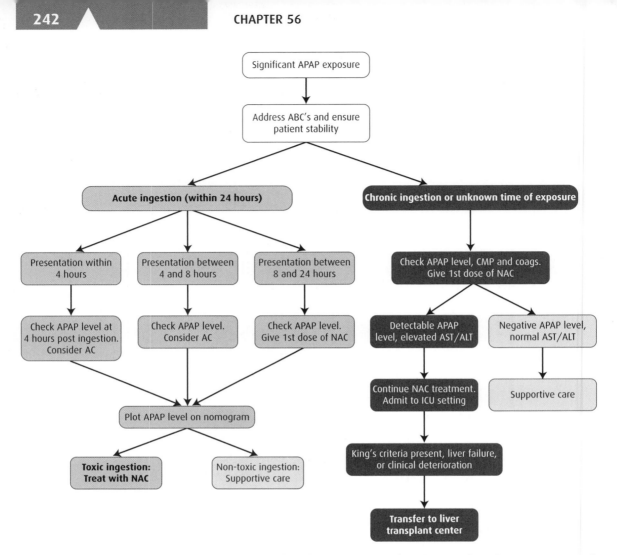

▲ **Figure 56-2.** Acetaminophen toxicity diagnostic algorithm. ABCs, airway, breathing, and circulation; AC, activated charcoal; ALT, alanine aminotransferase; APAP, acetaminophen; AST, aspartate aminotransferase; CMP, comprehensive metabolic panel; ICU, intensive care unit; NAC, N-acetylcysteine.

utilized due to the effective binding qualities of AC and the ready availability of an effective antidote.

NAC detoxifies NAPQI via multiple pathways, including functioning as a glutathione precursor. It is given orally in a loading dose of 140 mg/kg and subsequent doses of 70 mg/kg every 4 hours. NAC is adsorbed by charcoal, but there is no evidence that there is less effectiveness when NAC and charcoal are given together orally. Of note, oral NAC can be given by the intravenous (IV) route if passed through a 0.22-micron filter, and multiple protocols exist taking advantage of this. There is also a Food and Drug Administration–approved IV NAC formulation, Acetadote, that doesn't require the use of a filter and has a lower likelihood of anaphylactoid reaction compared with giving

the oral compound intravenously. IV NAC can be used in all patients (including pregnancy) and is particularly useful in patients who cannot tolerate anything by mouth due to vomiting or altered mental status. Regardless of route, current guidelines recommend to continue NAC treatment until the liver function has normalized and APAP levels are undetectable.

NAC therapy is generally indicated in 3 different patient cohorts. Start NAC in patients with (1) acute ingestions and 4-hour levels that lie above the nomogram cutoff, (2) in patients who report significant ingestions if obtaining a level will be significantly delayed, and (3) in those with evidence of hepatotoxicity presumed secondary to APAP regardless of APAP level.

Seek early consultation with a liver transplant center if the patient shows any signs of deterioration (eg, altered mental status, acidosis, worsening liver function). Ideally, the patient should be transferred before meeting liver transplantation criteria.

DISPOSITION

Admission

Admit all patients who require treatment with NAC or demonstrate any signs of hepatotoxicity. Patients with hemodynamic instability, altered mental status, systemic acid–base derangements, and evidence of end-organ damage require admission to a critical care setting. Patients with intentional overdoses require psychiatric assessment.

Discharge

Patients with unintentional ingestions who exhibit no signs of hepatotoxicity and have downtrending serum APAP levels in the nontoxic range can be safely discharged home.

SUGGESTED READING

Dart RC, Rumack BH. Patient-tailored acetylcysteine administration. *Ann Emerg Med.* 2007;50:280–281.

Kanter MZ. Comparison of oral and IV acetylcysteine in the treatment of acetaminophen poisoning. *Am J Health Syst Pharm.* 2006;63:1821–1827.

Rumack BH. Acetaminophen hepatotoxicity: the first 35 years. *J Toxicol Clin Toxicol.* 2002;40:3–20

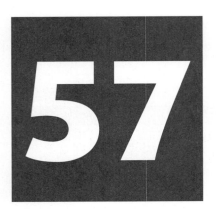

Salicylate Toxicity

Steven E. Aks, DO

Key Points

- Salicylate toxicity causes a mixed respiratory alkalosis, metabolic alkalosis, and elevated anion gap metabolic acidosis.
- Chronically intoxicated patients will be more seriously ill at lower salicylate concentrations than their acutely poisoned counterparts.
- Pursue hemodialysis in patients with refractory acidosis, pulmonary edema, renal insufficiency, and altered

mental status or seizure, regardless of the actual serum salicylate level.
- Match the ventilation rate in intubated patients with severe salicylate poisoning to their pre-intubation minute ventilation, as most require remarkably high rates for adequate respiratory compensation.

INTRODUCTION

Analgesics are among the most commonly ingested substances in patient overdose. According to the National Poison Data System, there were more than 300,000 cases of analgesic overdose reported in the year 2009, with salicylates accounting for the 13th most common cause of isolated drug ingestion and 62 total fatalities. Aspirin is most often ingested in some form of aspirin-containing combination product such as over-the-counter cold remedies. It can also be found as a component in various prescribed combination products such as Fiorinal, Soma Compound, and Percodan. Methyl salicylate, the major component of oil of wintergreen, is commonly found as a rubefacient in various medical products such as Ben Gay and in multiple household items, including air fresheners and mouthwash. One teaspoon of 98% methyl salicylate can contain as much as 7 g of salicylate (>20 tablets of 325 mg aspirin).

Aspirin absorption can be very erratic with peak concentrations occurring >20 hours after ingestion. That said, levels obtained six hours after ingestion generally reveal evidence of toxicity. Salicylate metabolism follows Michaelis-Menten kinetics. At concentrations over 30 mg/dL, salicylates are metabolized by zero-order kinetics due to enzyme saturation. This means that a constant

amount will be eliminated per unit of time. Below this concentration, salicylate metabolism follows first-order kinetics, with elimination rates proportional to serum salicylate concentrations.

In overdose scenarios, salicylates induce a mixed acid–base disorder. They cause an initial respiratory alkalosis by directly stimulating the medullary respiratory center. In addition, excessive circulating salicylate induces lipolysis, inhibits the Krebs cycle, and uncouples oxidative phosphorylation. This process impairs normal cellular respiration, resulting in the accumulation of organic acids and a secondary elevation in the anion gap. Furthermore, volume depletion secondary to excessive vomiting can lead to a concurrent metabolic alkalosis. Therefore, the classic (although far from uniformly present) acid–base disorder with salicylate poisoning is a mixed respiratory alkalosis, metabolic alkalosis, and elevated anion gap metabolic acidosis.

CLINICAL PRESENTATION

▶ History

It is very important to determine the amount ingested and the timing of exposure. In addition, try to distinguish between acute, chronic, and acute on chronic ingestions.

Patients with chronic intoxication often present with more subtle signs of toxicity. For example, elderly patients may present with isolated signs of altered mental status or tinnitus. Conversely, acutely poisoned patients typically present with more dramatic findings, including nausea, vomiting, tachypnea, diaphoresis, and altered mental status. Attempt to identify the exact type of product ingested. Immediate-release aspirin will produce much more rapid symptom onsets and elevated salicylate concentrations compared to the enteric-coated variety. Patients who ingest combination products may exhibit toxic effects from the secondary agent (eg, a concurrent opiate toxidrome from ingestion of a combined salicylate-opioid analgesic).

▶ Physical Examination

Pay very careful attention to patient vital signs. Patients are frequently tachycardic due to significant volume loss. Tachypnea is common secondary to stimulation of the medullary respiratory center and as a compensation for the metabolic acidosis. Fever can occur as a result of uncoupling of the oxidative phosphorylation chain. Finally, hypoxia may be present secondary to salicylate-induced acute lung injury (ALI).

The remainder of the exam should focus on the skin, abdomen, and neurologic systems. Diaphoresis is an important sign in moderate to severe salicylate toxicity. Abdominal tenderness can be present because of the erosive effects of salicylate on the gastric mucosa. Patients may display alterations in their mental status. This can be a presenting sign in the chronically intoxicated patient or may accompany significant acute poisonings. Seizures may also be present in advanced cases.

DIAGNOSTIC STUDIES

▶ Laboratory

Obtain a complete blood count, chemistry panel, urinalysis, and bedside urinary pregnancy test. Calculate the anion gap and follow it serially. Order a serum blood gas to look for evidence of a mixed acid–base disorder. Check salicylate concentrations every 2 hours until a peak concentration and subsequent decline has been observed, as pharmacobezoar formation is not uncommon with secondary erratic absorption. It is also wise to obtain a serum acetaminophen concentration because of the prevalence of readily available combination analgesics and their high rates of use in patient overdoses.

▶ Imaging

Imaging studies are generally unrewarding to detect ingested salicylates. A routine chest radiograph should be obtained to assess for ALI.

PROCEDURES

Meticulous attention should be paid to the airway. The decision to intubate a patient in the face of salicylate over-dose is truly a life or death decision. Many patients with severe salicylate poisoning have very high minute ventilations exhibited by both an increased depth of respiration and a high respiratory rate. It is sometimes difficult, if not impossible, to mechanically reproduce a salicylate-poisoned patient's minute ventilation. If you are forced to intubate a salicylate-poisoned patient, the ventilator rate needs to be set very high to replicate the pre-intubation minute ventilation. Frequent post-intubation blood gases should be obtained to be sure that the pH does not drop.

MEDICAL DECISION MAKING

Always obtain a thorough history from the patient, family, and paramedics on what substances may be ingested. Determine whether the patient's presentation is consistent with an acute or chronic exposure. Be alert for the co-ingestion of alternative analgesics including acetaminophen. Patients with the classic picture of salicylate poisoning may mimic the systemic inflammatory response syndrome, and one must consider alternative causes including sepsis. Obtain salicylate concentrations every 2 hours until a peak value has been obtained. In patients with salicylate levels <30 mg/dL, follow until <20 mg/dL and treat supportively. Initiate urinary alkalinization for patients with levels >30 mg/dL to facilitate urinary clearance and limit central nervous system penetration.

One must observe vigilantly for any signs of clinical deterioration and initiate early hemodialysis, as this may be a life-saving intervention. Such findings include patients with altered mental status, seizures, severe acid–base derangements, pulmonary edema, and renal insufficiency. Furthermore, patients with salicylate levels >90 mg/dL after an acute ingestion and those with levels >60 mg/dL with chronic exposures warrant hemodialysis. These thresholds should be lowered for patients with significant comorbidities (Figures 57–1).

TREATMENT

As with all poisonings, the initial focus should be on aggressive supportive care. Pay meticulous attention to the patient's airway, breathing, and circulation. Intubate patients only if absolutely necessary because of the difficulty in attaining the required minute ventilation with mechanical respiration. Because most patients are significantly dehydrated, initiate aggressive volume resuscitation with 1–2 L of normal saline to ensure an adequate urine output (1–2 mL/kg/hr).

There are several available modalities for patient decontamination. Administer activated charcoal at a dose of 1 g/kg to awake and alert patients with intact airway reflexes and no concern for vomiting. This can be repeated as needed to adsorb salicylates that form a concretion. Urinary alkalinization is performed by injecting 3 ampules of sodium bicarbonate into a 1-L bag of 5% dextrose solution to create an isotonic solution. Infuse this solution

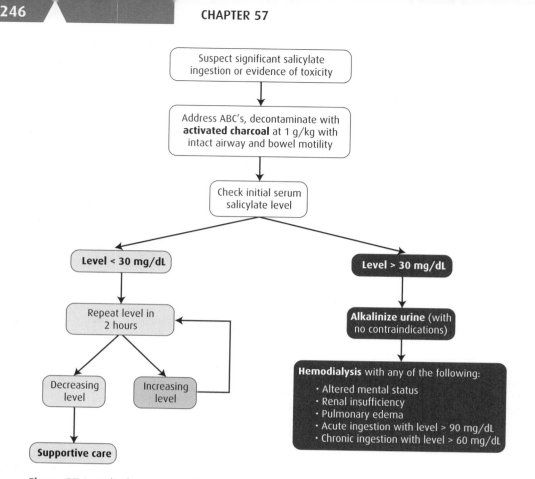

Figure 57-1. Salicylate toxicity diagnostic algorithm.

at 200 mL/hr. Pay careful attention to potassium levels and replete as necessary, as hypokalemic patients will excrete hydrogen ions into the distal renal tubules to retain potassium, thereby impairing successful alkalinization of the urine. The goal of alkalinization is to raise the urine pH >7.5-8. Avoid alkalinization in patients with congestive heart failure and renal failure, as they will be unable to tolerate the necessary volume load.

DISPOSITION

▶ Admission

All symptomatic patients will require hospitalization. Patients who require urinary alkalinization or hemodialysis should be admitted to a critical care setting. All patients with a suicidal ingestion will require psychiatric evaluation.

▶ Discharge

Patients with a detectable serum salicylate level require serial testing to rule out continued absorption. An asymptomatic patient with an undetectable salicylate concentration at the 6-hour mark can be safely cleared from a toxicologic perspective.

SUGGESTED READING

Bronstein AC, Spyker DA, Cantilena LR, et al. 2010 Annual report of the American Association of Poison Control Centers' National Poison Data system (NPDS): 28th annual report. *Clin Toxicol.* 2011;49:910–941.

Chyka PA, Erdman AR, Christianson G, et al. Salicylate poisoning: An evidence-base consensus guideline for out-of-hospital management. *Clin Toxicol.* 2007;45:95–131.

O'Malley G. Emergency department management of the salicylate-poisoned patient. *Emerg Med Clin North Am.* 2007;25:333–346.

Yip L. Aspirin and salicylates. In: Tintinalli JE, Stapczynski JS, Ma OJ, Cline DM, Cydulka RK, Meckler GD. *Tintinalli's Emergency Medicine: A Comprehensive Study Guide.* 7th ed. New York, NY: McGraw-Hill, 2011, pp. 1243–1245.

Carbon Monoxide Poisoning

Vinodinee L. Dissanayake, MD

Key Points

- Consider carbon monoxide (CO) poisoning in all patients with headaches, flu-like symptoms, altered mental status, or an unexplained anion gap metabolic acidosis.

- Immediately administer supplemental O_2 to all patients with potential CO poisoning before any confirmatory studies.

- Pulse oximetry values will be falsely elevated in patients with CO poisoning as a result of the inability of standard oximetry to distinguish between oxyhemoglobin and carboxyhemoglobin.

- Symptomatology is often more important than the absolute carboxyhemoglobin level when determining treatment and disposition.

INTRODUCTION

Carbon monoxide (CO) is an invisible killer; it is an odorless, colorless, and nonirritating gas. It is generally encountered as a byproduct of the incomplete combustion of carbon-based fuels (eg, coal, gasoline, natural gas). Faulty furnaces and vehicle exhaust fumes are common sources for clinical CO poisoning. Methylene chloride, a substance found in paint stripper and bubbling holiday lights, is metabolized in vivo into CO and may account for cases of delayed poisoning. According to 2010 US Poison Control Center data, more than 13,000 cases of possible CO poisoning were reported. Approximately 5,000 of these cases were treated in medical facilities, and CO is the leading cause of toxin-related fatalities in children less than 5 years of age. In survivors of CO poisoning, it is not uncommon to develop delayed neurologic sequelae, including recurrent headaches, cognitive deficits, and motor disorders.

CO exposure produces toxicity by 3 major pathways. The first of these is an inhibition of systemic O_2 delivery. CO binds to hemoglobin (Hb) with an affinity roughly 240 times greater than O_2. Systemic O_2 delivery plummets as the majority of circulating Hb binding sites are now occupied by CO. In addition, Hb that has bound CO has an increased affinity for concurrently bound O_2, resulting in the impaired release of O_2 as it reaches the target tissues. This results in a leftward shift and altered shape of the oxyhemoglobin dissociation curve (Figure 58-1).

The ability of CO to inhibit normal cellular respiration accounts for its second mechanism of toxicity. CO binds to cytochrome aa3 and inhibits normal transit through the electron transport chain. The resulting shutdown in the oxidative phosphorylation pathway leads to a rapid decimation of stored ATP and secondary cellular death.

The binding of CO to myoglobin accounts for the third mechanism of toxicity. Myoglobin binds to CO with an affinity 40 times that of O_2, impairing the adequate delivery of oxygen to muscle tissues. When myocardial cells are affected, a global reduction in cardiac contractility occurs. Of note, CO readily crosses the placenta and binds to fetal hemoglobin (HbF) with a 10–15% higher affinity than adult Hb, so fetal toxicity in cases of CO poisoning is often more severe than is evident on examination of the mother.

CLINICAL PRESENTATION

▶ History

The symptoms of CO poisoning are notoriously nonspecific, but typically present with some degree of neurologic and cardiovascular impairment. A vague headache is the

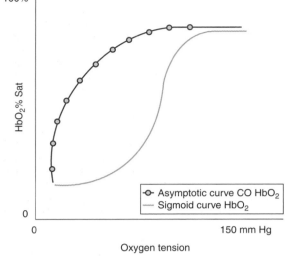

▲ **Figure 58-1.** Carboxyhemoglobin "shift to the left" reshaping of the oxyhemoglobin (HbO₂) dissociation curve. Reprinted with permission from Maloney G. Chapter 217. Carbon monoxide. In: Tintinalli JE, Stapczynski JS, Ma OJ, Cline DM, Cydulka RK, Meckler GD, eds. *Tintinalli's Emergency Medicine: A Comprehensive Study Guide.* 7th ed. New York: McGraw-Hill, 2011.

most common complaint, followed by fatigue, malaise, nausea, cognitive difficulties including memory impairment, paresthesias, weakness, altered mental status, and lethargy. Cardiovascular symptoms include ischemic chest pain, shortness of breath, and palpitations. Maintain a high index of suspicion in patients with vague symptomatology, especially in those with risk for CO exposure.

Inquire about the location of presumed exposure and whether or not anyone else in the vicinity has developed symptoms. Ask about the presence of regularly maintained CO detectors in the house. High-risk scenarios for CO exposure include fire victims, patients in older houses with faulty furnaces during the winter time and/or those using alternative forms of combustion to heat their homes, and patients in enclosed spaces with running automobiles. Finally, ask about the recent use of any paint stripper or solvents, as these compounds may contain methylene chloride.

▶ Physical Examination

As with other poisonings, rapidly assess the patient's airway, breathing, and circulation. Take careful note of a full set of vital signs, keeping in mind that standard pulse oximetry is of minimal utility in this setting. Tachypneic patients may be attempting to compensate for an underlying metabolic acidosis. Although patients with acute CO poisoning are classically described as having a "cherry red" appearance to their skin due to the bright red color of carboxyhemoglobin, this finding is absent far more often than present.

Perform a detailed neurologic exam, looking for signs of altered mental status and loss of coordination, as neurologic findings often dictate final care. Perform an ocular exam, looking for signs of retinal flame hemorrhages. The cardiovascular exam should focus on signs of hemodynamic instability and dysrhythmia, which might indicate underlying myocardial ischemia.

Carefully auscultate the lungs, noting any inspiratory crackles, which may be indicative of chemical injury to the lung parenchyma with secondary acute respiratory distress syndrome. Finally, check the skin for any signs of thermal injury in fire victims. Rarely, CO poisoning has been known to cause diffuse bullous lesion in the absence of thermal burns.

DIAGNOSTIC STUDIES

▶ Laboratory

Order an immediate COHb level on all patients to help confirm the diagnosis and estimate the severity of the exposure. COHb analysis requires co-oximetry of the blood sample and can be done on either a venous or arterial specimen. Of note, COHb levels correlate poorly with patient symptoms and should not be used in isolation to guide management. Check a metabolic panel looking for electrolyte abnormalities and to calculate the anion gap, as significant CO poisoning will result in an anion gap metabolic acidosis. Use the anion gap calculation along with a blood gas analysis to determine the severity of the acid–base derangement.

Obtain a urine pregnancy on all females of childbearing age, as a positive pregnancy test will markedly impact management. Check a serum lactate level. Significantly high levels (>10 mmol/L) indicate severe cellular toxicity or concurrent cyanide poisoning. Order serum cardiac markers in all patients complaining of chest pain or with electrocardiogram (ECG) abnormalities, as myocardial ischemia has been reported, especially in patients with underlying coronary artery disease (CAD). Finally, check a creatine phosphokinase level in patients with unknown downtimes, as rhabdomyolysis is a serious concern.

▶ Electrocardiogram

Obtain an ECG looking for signs of ischemia in patients complaining of chest pain, shortness of breath, and those with underlying CAD.

▶ Imaging

Check a chest x-ray in patients with shortness of breath or a history of smoke inhalation, as chemical injury to the lungs with secondary pulmonary edema is common. Order a computed tomography (CT) of the brain in patients with altered mental status or focal neurologic deficits to rule out alternative etiologies. Low-density lesions of the bilateral globus pallidi have been reported with CO poisoning, and patients with abnormalities on CT imaging are more likely to exhibit chronic neurologic sequelae.

MEDICAL DECISION MAKING

CO poisoning presents similar to many other conditions, including migraine headaches, influenza-like illnesses, acute gastroenteritis, vasovagal syncope, and cerebrovascular accident. Question patients about any possible exposures. Start supplemental O_2 while obtaining confirmatory studies. Send co-oximetry to measure the COHb level in patients with concerning presentations and those with an unexplained high anion gap metabolic acidosis. Consider concurrent cyanide toxicity in the unconscious and hypotensive patient who was rescued from a house or industrial fire. Rapidly exclude pregnancy with bedside urine testing, as this will significantly impact management. Use the absolute COHb in combination with the patient's symptoms to dictate further care including possible hyperbaric oxygen (HBO) therapy (Figure 58-2).

TREATMENT

Treat concomitant injuries such as smoke inhalation, trauma, myocardial injury, seizures, or neurologic deficits as you would in any other setting. Supportive care in the form of airway management, oxygen therapy, and intravenous fluids remains the most important intervention. Normobaric O_2 via a nonrebreather facemask should be administered until the COHb level is <5% and the patient is clinically stable. The circulating half-life of CO is approximately 4–6 hours in patients breathing room air, 90 minutes for those on 100% O_2, and approximately 20 minutes for those undergoing HBO therapy. The absolute indications for HBO therapy are debatable, but it is generally indicated for those patients with significant exposures (Table 58-1). The true benefit of treatment with HBO is most likely to limit the prevalence of delayed neurologic symptoms. The only absolute contraindication to HBO is an untreated pneumothorax. Because most hospitals do not have hyperbaric chambers, contacting your regional poison control center can be very helpful in the management and disposition of these patients.

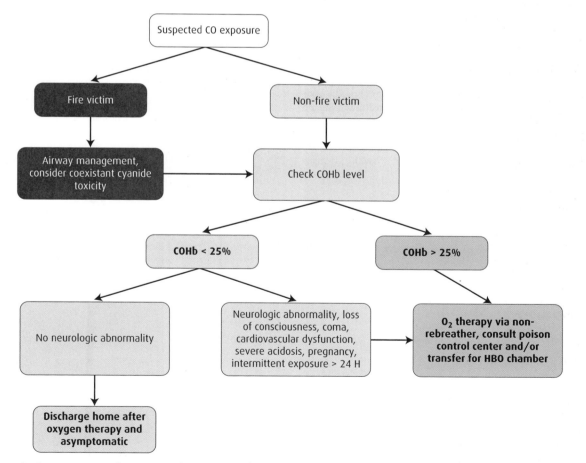

▲ **Figure 58-2.** Carbon monoxide poisoning diagnostic algorithm.

Table 58-1. Indications for hyperbaric O_2 treatment in acute CO poisoning.

Definite Indication	Relative Indication
AMS and/or abnormal neurologic examination (if patient has normal evaluation while on supplemental O_2, temporarily take patient off O_2 and repeat evaluation)	Persisting neurologic symptoms including headache and dizziness after 4 hours of 100% normobaric O_2
History of loss of consciousness or near-syncope	Persisting acidosis
History of seizure	Concurrent thermal or chemical burns
Coma	Pregnancy with history of carbon monoxide exposure regardless of COHb level
History of hypotension during or shortly after exposure	
Myocardial ischemia	
History of prolonged exposure	
Pregnancy with COHb >15%	

DISPOSITION

▶ Admission

Patients with any signs of hemodynamic instability warrant admission to a critical care setting. Furthermore, admit all patients with altered mental status or other neurologic deficits and those with indications for HBO to a critical care or monitored setting. Well-appearing patients with no signs of active toxicity whose poisoning was due to a suicide attempt require psychiatric evaluation and admission.

▶ Discharge

Patients with accidental exposures who are clinically well with COHb levels <5% after 100% O_2 treatment can be safely discharged. Educate all discharged patients about CO poisoning and encourage them to have their homes examined by the fire department or gas company. Convey the importance of a home CO detector. Provide adequate follow-up to assess for the development of delayed neurological sequelae.

▼ SUGGESTED READING

Maloney G. Carbon monoxide. In: Tintinalli JE, Kelen GD, Stapczynski JS, eds. *Tintinalli's Emergency Medicine: A Comprehensive Study Guide.* 7th ed. New York, NY: McGraw-Hill, 2011.

Nelson LS, Lewin NA, Howland MA, Hoffman RS, Goldfrank LR, Flomenbaum NE. *Goldfrank's Toxicologic Emergencies.* 9th ed. New York, NY: McGraw-Hill, 2011.

Weaver LK. Carbon monoxide poisoning. *N Engl J Med.* 2009;360:1217.

Wolf SJ, Lavonas EJ, Sloan EP, Jagoda AS, American College of Emergency Physicians. Critical issues in the management of adult patients presenting to the emergency department with acute carbon monoxide poisoning. *Ann Emerg Med.* 2008;51:138–152.

Digoxin

Michael E. Nelson, MD

Key Points

- Attempt to distinguish between acute versus chronic ingestions, as the symptoms and treatments differ.
- Electrocardiogram changes are common and include downward-sloping (scooped) ST-segment depressions, premature ventricular complexes, supraventricular dysrhythmias with slow ventricular rates, and bidirectional ventricular tachycardia.
- Although hyperkalemia can be a marker of significant digoxin poisoning, standard treatment with intravenous calcium should typically be avoided.
- Empirically administer digoxin-specific antibodies (5 vials for chronic toxicity, 10–20 vials for acute ingestions) to all patients with life-threatening dysrhythmias or hemodynamic instability.

INTRODUCTION

Digoxin, a commonly prescribed agent derived from the foxglove plant, belongs to a class of medications known as cardiac glycosides. These agents function to increase myocardial contractility and slow AV nodal conduction and are commonly used for the treatment of congestive heart failure and various cardiac dysrhythmias including atrial fibrillation. Of interest, cardiac glycosides are frequently encountered in the natural world as a predatory deterrent in both plant and animal species, including oleander, lily of the valley, red squill, and bufo toads. The relative potency of digoxin lends to a very narrow therapeutic window, and life-threatening toxicity can develop with both acute overdoses and chronic excessive exposures. Poisoned patients generally present with variable symptoms and must be viewed in light of acute versus chronic versus acute on chronic exposures. If left untreated, death will invariably result secondary to cardiac instability and hemodynamic compromise.

As a whole, cardiac glycosides were responsible for nearly 2,500 poisonings reported to the National Poison Data System in the year 2010. They were the third most common cardiovascular agent implicated in patient toxicity and were the primary agent responsible for 17 patient deaths. Of note, clinically significant toxicity is far more common in pediatric and geriatric populations. Pediatric overdoses arise from iatrogenic dosing errors or accidental ingestions of adult medications, whereas geriatric toxicity generally results from either drug–drug interactions or alterations in metabolic clearance. Intentional overdoses are most common in adult patients and can be of both the acute and chronic variety.

Orally administered digoxin begins to exhibit clinical effects within 90 minutes of ingestion and typically reaches maximal effect within 4–6 hours. Digoxin is primarily eliminated by the kidneys with a usual half-life of 36–48 hours. Although normal therapeutic concentrations generally range between 0.5 and 2 ng/mL, given the significant toxicity and narrow therapeutic window, the safest suggested concentration with maximal therapeutic benefit is between 0.5 and 1 ng/mL.

At the cellular level, digoxin inhibits the membrane-based sodium-potassium pumps, causing an increase in intracellular sodium concentrations. This rise in intracellular sodium inhibits the membrane-based sodium-calcium exchanger, causing a secondary elevation in intracellular calcium levels. The increased intracellular calcium concentration augments myocardial contractility and increases cardiac inotropy. It is this increase in cardiac inotropy that makes digoxin an attractive agent for the management of congestive heart failure. Additionally, digoxin increases the overall vagal tone of the heart and thereby decreases the electrical conduction velocity through both the SA and AV nodes. This property allows digoxin to be used as a rate-controlling agent in patients with supraventricular tachydysrhythmias (eg, atrial fibrillation). That said, this global slowing of myocardial signal conduction combined with a secondary shortening of the myocyte refractory period can potentially increase overall cardiac automaticity and excitability. Given these phenomena, toxic exposures typically present with a multitude of cardiovascular manifestations.

CLINICAL PRESENTATION

History

Ascertaining the time of exposure is extremely important with potential digoxin toxicity. As with all potential poisonings, it is extremely important to determine the total amount ingested. Elucidate the number and frequency of exposures to distinguish between acute versus chronic versus acute on chronic toxicity. Carefully clarify the circumstances of the overdose to differentiate between accidental versus more insidious etiologies. Inquire about the presence of any gastrointestinal symptoms, such as nausea, vomiting, and abdominal pain, which typically accompany most acute overdoses. Central nervous system (CNS) effects include mood changes, headache, altered mental status, lethargy, and hallucinations. Visual disturbances are common and include blurry vision, photophobia, and chromatopsia (a change of color vision), in which visualized objects are classically surrounded by yellowish-green halos.

Physical Examination

Obtain a complete set of vital signs and carefully monitor for any evidence of hemodynamic instability. Although bradydysrhythmias and systemic hypotension are most common, patients may present with any number of cardiac manifestations, including life-threatening tachycardias. Additional physical exam findings are variable and nonspecific and typically lag up to several hours after ingestion. CNS effects including confusion, generalized weakness, altered mental status, and lethargy may be present, and generalized seizures may accompany severe overdoses.

DIAGNOSTIC STUDIES

Laboratory

Obtain a STAT metabolic panel as serum electrolytes play an extremely important role in digoxin toxicity. Serum hyperkalemia (K^+ >5.5 mEq/L) indicates significant toxicity with acute overdoses and is associated with increased fatality. Serum hypokalemia (K^+ <3.5 mEq/L) is far more common with chronic toxicity and inhibits the function of

the cellular sodium-potassium pumps, thereby increasing myocardial susceptibility to digoxin-related dysrhythmias. Serum hypomagnesemia may further predispose to this increased cardiac toxicity. Finally, any decline in renal function will intensify toxicity, as digoxin is primarily eliminated via the kidneys.

Obtain a serum digoxin level, as this will guide the dosing of digoxin Fab fragments. Therapeutic digoxin levels range from 0.5 to 2.0 ng/mL. Interpret the digoxin level carefully within the clinical context. The distributive phase of digoxin lasts for ~6 hours after an ingestion, and serum levels obtained within this period may be falsely elevated.

Electrocardiogram

Obtain an emergent electrocardiogram (ECG) in all patients with potential digoxin toxicity. Prolongation of the PR interval and shortening of the QT segment are not uncommon with therapeutic digoxin concentrations. Upward "scooping" of the ST segment is also fairly common. These changes taken as a whole are referred to as the digitalis effect. In addition, excesses in intracellular calcium may produce frequent premature ventricular complexes (PVCs) and occasional U waves.

Digoxin poisoning can induce nearly every form of dysrhythmia or conduction disturbance. Classic ECG findings include supraventricular tachydysrhythmias (atrial flutter or fibrillation) combined with variable AV nodal blockade resulting in slow ventricular rates (Figure 59-1). Bidirectional ventricular tachycardia is nearly pathognomonic for serious digoxin toxicity. Additional ECG findings include sinus bradycardia, ventricular bigeminy, and ventricular fibrillation.

PROCEDURES

Cardioversion or defibrillation may be performed following Advanced Cardiovascular Life Support protocols in digoxin-poisoned patients exhibiting significant toxicity and unstable rhythms (ventricular tachycardia or

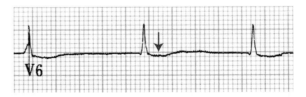

▲ **Figure 59-1.** Digitalis toxicity: Atrial fibrillation with slow ventricular rate and "scooped" ST-segment depression. Reproduced with permission from Ritchie JV, Juliano ML, Thurman RJ. Chapter 23. ECG Abnormalities. In: Knoop KJ, Stack LB, Storrow AB, Thurman RJ, eds. *The Atlas of Emergency Medicine.* 3rd ed. New York: McGraw-Hill, 2010. Photo contributor: JV Ritchie, MD.

fibrillation). Transcutaneous or transvenous pacing often fails to correct digoxin-associated bradydysrhythmias and may actually lower the threshold for life-threatening ventricular dysrhythmias.

MEDICAL DECISION MAKING

The differential diagnosis of digoxin toxicity includes any disease process or toxin capable of inducing cardiac dysrhythmias. Specific toxins include calcium channel blockers, beta-blockers, clonidine, organophosphate insecticides, class IA antidysrhythmics, and cardiotoxic plants (eg, rhododendron, monkshood). Medical conditions include underlying cardiac pathologies such as sick sinus syndrome and AV nodal blocks as well as systemic conditions such as sepsis, myxedema coma, and adrenal crisis.

The toxicologic differential of any hypotensive and/or bradycardic patient includes beta-blockers, calcium channel blockers, digoxin, and clonidine. Obtaining a thorough history frequently aids in establishing the appropriate diagnosis. The most common current presentation of digoxin toxicity is an elderly patient with an underlying cardiac history on multiple medications who experiences either significant drug–drug interactions or dehydration with secondary renal insufficiency and decreased digoxin clearance despite therapeutic usage.

The physical exam combined with appropriate ancillary testing is invaluable for identifying the correct toxidrome. Clonidine poisoning typically presents similar to an opioid toxidrome. A significantly elevated capillary blood glucose in a nondiabetic patient may indicate serious calcium channel blocker toxicity. Taken in context of the history and physical exam, classic ECG findings and abnormal serum digoxin levels may be used to direct further treatment (Figure 59-2).

TREATMENT

After addressing and stabilizing the patient's airway, breathing, and circulation status, pursue gastrointestinal (GI) decontamination with activated charcoal (AC) for cases of acute overdose. Do not give AC to patients with depressed levels of consciousness without first securing the airway to prevent aspiration. Initiate volume resuscitation in dehydrated patients but be wary of those with a history of congestive heart failure (CHF). Treat severe hyperkalemia in the standard fashion with sodium bicarbonate, albuterol nebulizers, glucose with insulin, and sodium polystyrene sulfonate (Kayexalate), but avoid empiric treatment with intravenous (IV) calcium due to the theoretical risk of "stone heart" and fatal dysrhythmias. That said, IV calcium can be given to patients with severe

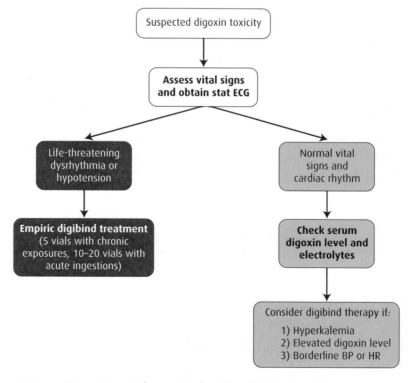

▲ **Figure 59-2.** Digoxin diagnostic algorithm. BP, blood pressure; ECG, electrocardiogram; HR, heart rate.

hyperkalemic cardiotoxicity (sinus arrest, sinusoidal rhythm) refractive to alternative treatments. In patients with chronic toxicity, carefully supplement serum hypokalemia and hypomagnesemia to prevent overcorrection. Treat significant bradycardias and/or AV nodal conduction disturbances with IV atropine (0.5–2 mg).

Digoxin-specific antibodies (Digibind, Digoxin Fab fragments) provide an eloquent and effective method for treating digoxin toxicity. Indications for use include significant dysrhythmias, hypotension, and hyperkalemia secondary to cardiac glycoside ingestion. Although no absolute contraindications exist, exercise caution in patients with a known hypersensitivity to ovine (sheep) derived products. The appropriate dose of Fab fragments can be determined by 1 of 3 ways and is based on the total body burden of digoxin. After an acute ingestion, digoxin has a roughly 80% bioavailability and each vial of Fab fragments can bind 0.5 mg of circulating digoxin. Based on this, the proper dose of Fab fragments can be calculated as follows:

1. Known quantity of ingested digoxin:

   Number of Fab vials = [(Amount of digoxin ingested (mg) × 0.8)/0.5]

   Rounded-up to the nearest whole number

2. Measured serum digoxin concentrations:

   Number of Fab vials = [Serum digoxin level (ng/mL) × patient weight (kg)]/100

   Rounded-up to the nearest whole number

3. Patients demonstrating significant toxicity (life-threatening dysrhythmias, profound hypotension, and/or severe hyperkalemia):

   Empirically treat acute ingestions with 10–20 vials of Fab fragments and chronic exposures with 5 vials. Repeated dosing may be required.

Of note, most lab assays do not distinguish between free and bound digoxin, and serum levels lose their clinical utility after the administration of Fab fragments. Furthermore, treatment with Fab fragments may lead to the secondary decompensation of underlying cardiac conditions such as CHF or atrial fibrillation, which had been previously controlled with digoxin therapy.

DISPOSITION

▶ Admission

Admit all patients after a potentially significant ingestion who either have a history of significant comorbid conditions or exhibit signs or symptoms of clinical toxicity including cardiovascular instability, dysrhythmias, GI distress, and mental status changes. Any patient with toxicity significant enough to warrant digoxin Fab fragments requires admission to an intensive care unit setting. Patients who ingest digoxin as part of a suicide attempt warrant psychiatric evaluation once they are medically stable.

▶ Discharge

Patients with accidental ingestions and no significant comorbidities who remain symptom free after an 8- to 12-hour observation period may be safely discharged home.

▼ SUGGESTED READING

Boyle JS, Kirk MA. Digitalis glycosides. In: Tintinalli JE, Stapczynski JS, Ma OJ, Cline DM, Cydulka RK, Meckler GD. *Tintinalli's Emergency Medicine: A Comprehensive Study Guide.* 7th ed. New York, NY: McGraw-Hill, 2011, pp. 1260–1264.

Hack JB. Cardioactive steroids. In: Nelson LS, Lewin NA, Howland MA, et al. *Goldrank's Toxicologic Emergencies.* 9th ed. New York, NY: McGraw-Hill, 2011, pp. 936–945.

Ma G, Brady WJ, Pollack M, Chan TC. Electrocardiographic manifestations: digitalis toxicity. *J Emerg Med.* 2001;20:145–152.

Manini AF, Nelson LS, Hoffman RS. Prognostic utility of serum potassium in chronic digoxin toxicity. *Am J Cardiovasc Drugs.* 2011;11:173–178.

Cyclic Antidepressants

Harry C. Karydes, DO

Key Points

- Cyclic antidepressants remain a leading cause of poisoning-related fatalities among psychoactive medications.
- Patients will frequently present with minimal signs and symptoms only to abruptly decompensate from life-threatening cardiovascular and central nervous system toxicity.
- Cardiovascular toxicity (specifically refractory hypotension) is the leading cause of morbidity and mortality in cyclic antidepressant overdose.
- Hypertonic sodium bicarbonate should be given in 1–2 mEq/kg boluses to reverse the wide-complex dysrhythmias commonly encountered with cyclic antidepressant poisoning.

INTRODUCTION

Cyclic antidepressants (CA) consist of a group of pharmacologically related medications that were initially developed in the late 1950s for the treatment of patients with severe depression. Although used less frequently for this purpose, their role has expanded to include the management of various alternative conditions including neuralgic pain, migraine headaches, enuresis, and attention deficit hyperactivity disorder. Traditional cyclic antidepressants have a chemical structure built on a 3-ring nucleus and include such medications such as amitriptyline, nortriptyline, doxepin, imipramine, and clomipramine. Antidepressants have historically remained a leading cause of pharmacologic self-poisoning owing to their near ubiquitous availability to a depressed patient population inherently at risk for self-harming behavior. Although the introduction of selective serotonin reuptake inhibitors (SSRIs) has decreased the overall incidence of CA poisonings, CA overdoses continue to account for a greater morbidity and mortality given their increased potential for significant toxicologic complications, especially in pediatric patients.

Cyclic antidepressants are nonselective agents that exhibit a wide array of pharmacologic effects with considerable variations in potency. The majority of clinical findings associated with CA poisoning can be attributed to ≥1 of the following pharmacologic actions:

- Competitive inhibition of acetylcholine at central and peripheral muscarinic (but not nicotinic) receptors
- Inhibition of α-adrenergic receptors
- Inhibition of norepinephrine and serotonin uptake
- Sodium channel blockade
- Antagonism of GABA-A receptors

Although it is the inhibition of norepinephrine and serotonin uptake that is believed to account for the antidepressant effects of these agents, the alternative actions just listed account for the significant toxicity associated with CA overdose, with sodium channel blockade being the most important factor contributing to patient mortality.

CLINICAL PRESENTATION

History

Patients commonly present to the emergency department with minimal clinical findings only to develop life-threatening cardiovascular and central nervous system (CNS) manifestations within the timespan of a few hours.

255

Co-ingestants are not uncommon in patients with CA overdoses, and this possibility must always be investigated.

Attempt to determine the exact amount of drug ingested, as the cyclic antidepressants have a rather narrow therapeutic window, and small excursions beyond the usual therapeutic range (2–4 mg/kg) may result in significant toxicity. Acute ingestions of more than 10–20 mg/kg will cause significant cardiovascular and CNS disturbances owing to the blockade of cardiac sodium channels and inhibition of CNS GABA-A receptors, respectively. Toxicity in children has been reported with ingestions as low as 5 mg/kg.

▶ Physical Examination

The clinical presentation of CA toxicity varies widely from mild anti-muscarinic signs and symptoms to severe

Table 60-1 Clinical manifestations of toxicity resulting from cyclic antidepressants.

Cardiovascular Toxicity
Conduction Delays
PR interval, QTc interval, and QRS complex prolongation
Terminal right access deviation (S in lead I and R in aVR)
Atrioventricular block
Dysrhythmias
Sinus tachycardia
Supraventricular tachycardia
Wide-complex tachycardia
Sinus tachycardia with rate-dependent aberrancy
Ventricular tachycardia
Torsades de pointes
Bradycardia
Ventricular fibrillation
Asystole
Hypotension
Central Nervous System Toxicity
Altered mental status
Delirium
Psychosis
Lethargy
Coma
Myoclonus
Seizures
Anticholinergic Toxicity
Altered mental status
Hyperthermia
Urinary retention
Paralytic ileus
Pulmonary Toxicity
Acute lung-injury aspiration

Reprinted with permission from Flomenbaum N, Goldfrank L, Hoffman R, et al. *Goldfrank's Toxicologic Emergencies*. 8th ed. New York: McGraw-Hill, 2006.

cardiotoxicity, coma, and death (Table 60-1). Antimuscarinic findings are commonly appreciated in poisoned patients, including dry skin and mucous membranes, diminished or absent bowel sounds, urinary retention, and sinus tachycardia. Acute cardiovascular toxicity must be recognized and treated expediently. Sinus tachycardia is a very common early finding, but typically does not result in hemodynamic compromise. That said, severe poisonings frequently progress to induce wide complex tachycardias and refractory hypotension. CNS toxicity can range from disorientation and agitation to outright lethargy. Early subtle alterations in levels of consciousness can quickly progress to obtundation and coma. Generalized tonic-clonic seizures occur in ~4% of all patients who present with CA poisoning and in 13% of those who subsequently experience cardiopulmonary arrest.

DIAGNOSTIC STUDIES

▶ Laboratory

Although quantitative assays for serum CA concentrations do exist, their limited availability and prolonged turn-around times preclude any clinical utility. Furthermore, serum levels correlate poorly with clinical significance. There are no additional laboratory studies useful for the diagnosis or management of patients with CA poisoning.

▶ Electrocardiogram

The electrocardiogram (ECG) is the most useful and readily available modality for the evaluation of patients with potential CA poisoning. It not only provides rapid, distinctive, and diagnostic findings suggestive of toxicity, but also facilitates the provision of targeted therapy. ECG abnormalities develop within the first 6 hours of ingestion and typically resolve by 36–48 hours.

The classic ECG pattern in moderate to severely poisoned patients is sinus tachycardia with right axis deviation of the terminal 40 msec of the QRS complex (terminal R-wave in lead aVR) associated with prolongation of the PR, QRS, and QT intervals (Figure 60-1). Life-threatening complications are far more likely when the QRS complex is prolonged beyond 100 msec. Thirty percent of patients will experience seizures with a QRS >100 msec, and the risk of ventricular tachycardia increases drastically when the QRS complex exceeds 160 msec.

MEDICAL DECISION MAKING

A high index of suspicion combined with a thorough history, physical examination, and ECG analysis is required to establish the diagnosis of CA toxicity. Keep in mind that patients with intentional overdoses may neither be reliable nor forthcoming regarding their ingestions. Every effort must be made to ascertain the exact time of ingestion, specific agent and amount consumed, and the presence of

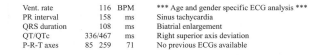

Cook County Hospital-ER

Vent. rate	116	BPM	*** Age and gender specific ECG analysis ***
PR interval	158	ms	Sinus tachycardia
QRS duration	108	ms	Biatrial enlargement
QT/QTc	336/467	ms	Right superior axis deviation
P-R-T axes	85 259	71	No previous ECGs available

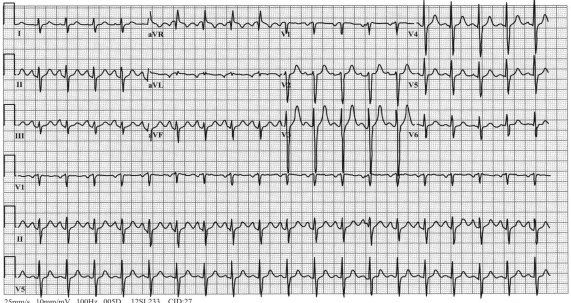

25mm/s 10mm/mV 100Hz 005D 12SL233 CID:27

▲ **Figure 60-1.** ECG findings in a patient with chronic pain who mistook his Elavil for Tylenol #3 and ingested approximately 500 mg. Note sinus tachycardia, the prolonged QRS intervals, and the terminal R-wave in aVR.

any co-ingestants. Once identified, the treatment for CA toxicity should be initiated without delay (Figure 60-2).

TREATMENT

All patients require large-bore intravenous (IV) access and continuous cardiac monitoring. Early intubation is recommended for patients with CNS depression and/or hemodynamic instability, as they have the potential for rapid deterioration. Furthermore, respiratory acidosis secondary to ventilatory insufficiency can exacerbate the cardiotoxicity of CA poisoning.

▶ Gastrointestinal Decontamination

The induction of emesis with syrup of ipecac is no longer recommended given the potential for sudden decompensation and secondary aspiration. Administer activated charcoal (1 g/kg) to all patients with intact airway reflexes as it will readily bind to and decrease the absorption of cyclic antidepressants. Orogastric lavage can be considered in symptomatic patients who present within an hour of ingestion after carefully weighing the benefits of removing a highly toxic drug against the inherent risks of the procedure.

▶ Sodium Bicarbonate Therapy

Because the cardiotoxicity of CA poisoning results from the blockade of myocardial Na^+ channels, treatment with IV sodium bicarbonate ($NaHCO_3$) remains the mainstay of therapy. Sodium bicarbonate has been shown to improve electrical conduction and increase myocardial contractility. The indications for initiation of therapy are as follows:

- QRS complex >100 msec
- Refractory hypotension
- Terminal R-wave amplitude in lead aVR >3 mm
- Ventricular dysrhythmia

Administer an initial bolus of 1–2 mEq/kg (1 ampule of $NaHCO_3$ contains 50 mEq) and repeat as necessary until the patient improves or the serum pH reaches 7.5–7.55. After the initial stabilization, continue treatment with a $NaHCO_3$ infusion at a rate of 2-3 mL/kg/hr.

▶ Hypotension

Refractory hypotension is probably the most common cause of death in cases of CA overdose. Initiate aggressive volume resuscitation with IV boluses of normal saline, but

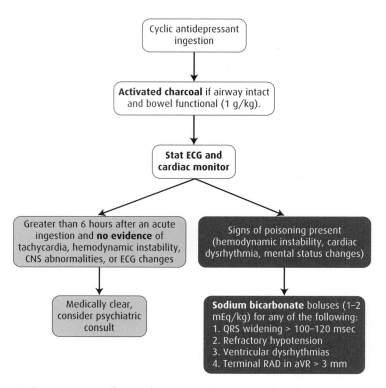

Figure 60-2. Cyclic antidepressants diagnostic algorithm. CNS, central nervous system; ECG, electrocardiogram; RAD, right axis deviation.

be wary of patients with underlying cardiopulmonary conditions so as to not precipitate life-threatening pulmonary edema. Persistent hypotension that is unresponsive to isotonic crystalloid boluses and $NaHCO_3$ therapy warrants the initiation of vasopressor support. Norepinephrine (1 mcg/min titrated to a max of 30 mcg/min) is the agent of choice as it directly antagonizes the effects of cyclic antidepressants on the α-adrenergic receptors.

Seizures

Most seizures occur within the first 3–4 hours after ingestion. Seizures are typically brief and tonic-clonic in nature. Benzodiazepines such as diazepam or lorazepam are the initial treatment of choice. Seizures that are refractive to benzodiazepines require treatment with IV phenobarbital (15 mg/kg), although careful attention must be paid to the patient's hemodynamic status. Phenytoin should be avoided because it is ineffective in patients with CA poisoning and may actually exacerbate the cardiotoxicity of these agents.

DISPOSITION

Admission

Admit all symptomatic patients to a monitored setting. Those with signs of moderate to severe poisoning

(eg, lethargy, hypotension, prolonged QRS duration) and all patients who require treatment with IV $NaHCO_3$ require admission to an intensive care unit. Obtain psychiatric consultation for all patients with intentional overdoses.

Discharge

Patients who remain symptom-free throughout an observation period of no less than 6 hours may be safely discharged home provided they are cleared from a psychiatric perspective.

SUGGESTED READING

Liebelt E. Cyclic antidepressants. In: Flomenbaum NE, Goldfrank LR, Hoffman RS et al. *Goldfrank's Toxicologic Emergencies.* 8th ed. New York, NY: McGraw-Hill, 2006, pp. 1083–1097.

Liebelt EL, Ulrich A, Francis PD, et al. Serial electrocardiogram changes in acute tricyclic antidepressant overdoses. *Crit Care Med.* 1997;25:1721.

Graudins A, Dowsett RP, Liddle C. The toxicity of antidepressant poisoning: Is it changing? A comparative study of cyclic and new serotonin-specific antidepressants. *Emerg Med (Fremantle).* 2002;14:440–446.

Mills KC. Cyclic antidepressants. In: Tintinalli JE, Stapczynski JS, Ma OJ, Cline DM, Cydulka RK, Meckler GD, eds. *Tintinalli's Emergency Medicine: A Comprehensive Study Guide.* 7th ed. New York, NY: McGraw-Hill, 2011, pp. 1193–1198.

Hypothermia

Michael T. Cudnik, MD

Key Points

- Intoxication with either alcohol or drugs is very common in patients with hypothermia.

- Most emergency thermometers cannot accurately read body temperatures below 34.4°C (94°F).

- Many hypothermic patients have serious underlying illnesses that help contribute to their presentation,

and it is imperative to aggressively identify and treat these conditions.

- Resuscitative efforts should not be terminated until defibrillation remains unsuccessful despite a rewarmed core body temperature of at least 32°C.

INTRODUCTION

Clinical hypothermia is defined as a core body temperature of less than 35°C (95°F) and can be clinically stratified by the core temperature into mild (35°–32°C/95°–89.6°F), moderate (32°–30°C/89.5°–86°F), and severe (<30°C/86°F) subtypes. Hypothermia occurs as the body loses heat from 1 of 4 major mechanisms: conduction, convection, evaporation, and radiation. Convective (windy environments) and conductive (cold and wet exposures) mechanisms are responsible for most cases of accidental hypothermia. Hypothermia can be further classified as either primary or secondary. Primary hypothermia occurs when an otherwise healthy person is unable to compensate for an excessive exposure to cold temperatures. Secondary hypothermia occurs when a comorbid medical condition (eg, hypothyroidism, sepsis, intoxication) disrupts a patient's normal thermoregulatory processes.

Although most common in colder climates, hypothermia can occur in any environment. Case reports during summer months and in hospitalized patients are not uncommon. In the United States, hypothermia is responsible for approximately 700 deaths annually, with more than half occurring in patients older than 65 years. Patients with an initial core body temperature <23°C (73.4°) typically do not survive, and the overall mortality rate of patients with hypothermia is approximately 40%.

CLINICAL PRESENTATION

▶ History

The potential for hypothermia is usually obvious in patients with significant exposures. Patients may present in wet clothing, be found outdoors in the cold weather, or be inappropriately dressed for the environment in which they live. In the United States, most hypothermic patients are either intoxicated or suffer from an underlying psychiatric illness or dementia.

The history or presentation may be less obvious for patients with mild hypothermia or unknown exposures. Said patients typically present with nonspecific neurologic findings, including dizziness, confusion, slurred speech, or ataxia. Patients with severe hyperthermia may present comatose or in cardiac arrest.

▶ Physical Examination

As with all emergency department (ED) patients, start by assessing and addressing the patient's airway, breathing, and circulation (ABCs) and vital signs. Hypothermic patients may present with unstable airways or absent pulses. Carefully measure the patient's core body temperature by inserting a specialized "low-reading" probe into the bladder, rectum, or esophagus as this will be pivotal to establish the diagnosis. Keep in mind that the majority of standard ED thermometers will not record temperatures below 34.4°C (94°F).

Physical exam findings frequently vary based on the degree of hypothermia. It is imperative to immediately and completely undress the patient to remove any wet clothing and identify any signs of coexisting frostbite, trauma, sepsis, hypothyroidism, adrenal crisis, toxidromes, or cardiac dysfunction. Refrain from any unnecessary movement of the patient to avoid precipitating life-threatening dysrhythmias, as hypothermic myocardium is exceptionally irritable. Finally, perform a comprehensive neurologic exam including an evaluation for level of consciousness, pupillary reactivity, and focal deficits. The following describes findings specific to varying degrees of hypothermia.

Mild Hypothermia

Patients tend to present with shivering, tachycardia, tachypnea, and hyperventilation. As their core temperature approaches 33°C (91.4°F), ataxia and apathy begin to develop.

Moderate Hypothermia

Patients with moderate hypothermia develop hypoventilation, hyporeflexia, and an altered sensorium or stupor. Shivering typically disappears once the core temperature drops below 32°C (89.6°F), and this should be considered an ominous finding. As the temperature approaches 30°C (86°F), the risk for dysrhythmias increases significantly.

Severe Hypothermia

Patients with severe hypothermia may present with pulmonary edema, areflexia, hypotension, and apnea and are extremely susceptible to ventricular fibrillation and cardiac arrest. Nearly all patients with a core body temperature below 27°C (80.6°F) are comatose.

DIAGNOSTIC STUDIES

▶ Laboratory

Obtain a STAT bedside glucose level on all hypothermic patients to rule out concurrent hypoglycemia. Serum hyperglycemia is actually more common secondary to a cold-induced inhibition of insulin secretion. Avoid treatment with supplemental insulin in these patients, as this may precipitate iatrogenic hypoglycemia on rewarming. Check a metabolic panel to assess electrolyte status and renal function. Hypothermia can impair the concentrating ability of the renal tubules, leading to a "cold-diuresis" with secondary dehydration and hypovolemia.

Hypothermia impairs both platelet aggregation and the coagulation cascade, and patients may become profoundly coagulopathic. In spite of this, the laboratory measurement of the prothrombin time and partial thromboplastin time will be normal as blood samples are warmed to physiologic temperatures before running these tests. In addition,

hypothermia classically induces hemoconcentration with an expected increase of the hematocrit by 2% for every 1°C drop in core temperature.

▶ Electrocardiogram

An electrocardiogram is critical for all moderately to severely hypothermic patients to assess for potentially life-threatening cardiac dysrhythmias. Sinus bradycardia and QT prolongation are the most common early findings. Although not specific for hypothermia, **Osborn J waves**, wide positive deflections at the junction of the QRS complex and ST segment, can be seen once the core temperature drops below 32°C (89.6°F) (Figure 61-1). As the hypothermia worsens, atrial fibrillation and eventually ventricular fibrillation often develop.

▶ Imaging

Imaging studies should be dictated by the clinical presentation. Obtain a head computed tomography in patients who exhibit persistent alterations in mental status despite adequate rewarming and in those with any signs of cranial trauma.

MEDICAL DECISION MAKING

The history and physical examination, coupled with a known environmental exposure, are typically adequate to establish the diagnosis of hypothermia. The absence of a known environmental exposure or any concern for secondary hypothermia should prompt an active search for potential etiologies. That said, treatment should not be delayed while awaiting the diagnostic work-up (Figure 61-2).

TREATMENT

Passive rewarming is typically adequate for patients with mild hypothermia (35°–32°C). This technique uses the body's inherent heat production mechanisms to restore a normal core temperature. To be successful, the patient needs an intact shivering response and sufficient energy stores. Remove any wet clothing and wrap the patient in warm blankets. Passive rewarming usually raises the core temperature by <1°C per hour.

Most patients with moderate hypothermia (32°–30°C) require **active external rewarming**. This includes the infusion of intravenous (IV) fluids warmed to 42°C, administering humidified supplemental O_2 warmed to 46°C, and the placement of forced-air rewarming blankets (eg, Bair Hugger). Taken as a whole, these methods can rewarm patients at a rate of approximately 3.5°C per hour. These measures are usually adequate for patients with severe hypothermia (<30°C) as well, provided they exhibit no evidence of cardiac instability. Those who do demonstrate signs of myocardial instability and/or cardiac arrest require **active core rewarming**. Available modalities include warmed isotonic saline (40°C) lavage of the stomach (only if intubated),

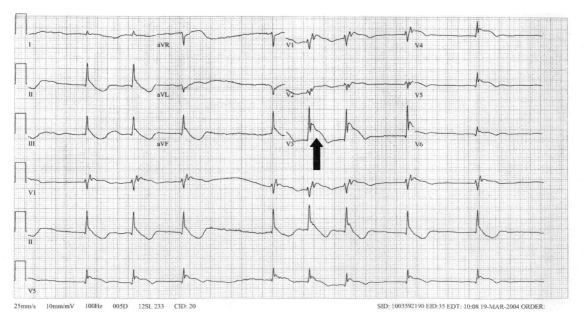

▲ **Figure 61-1.** ECG demonstrating Osborn J waves (arrow) in a hypothermic patient.

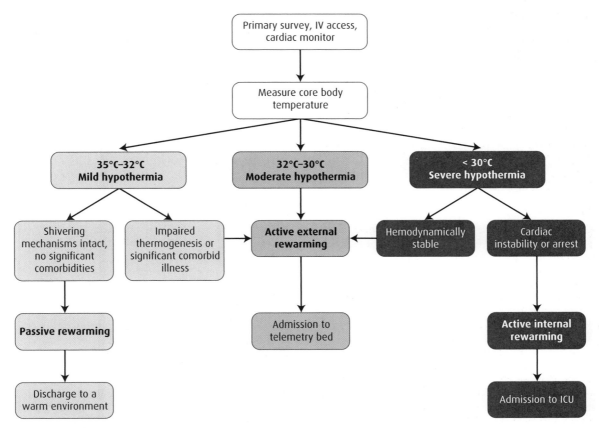

▲ **Figure 61-2.** Hypothermia diagnostic algorithm.

bladder, and colon. Peritoneal and pleural irrigation can also be performed after the insertion of percutaneous catheters. Emergent thoracotomy with internal cardiac massage and mediastinal irrigation with warmed saline is a very invasive technique, but has been used successfully in severely hypothermic patients with prolonged cardiac arrest. When available, extracorporeal rewarming with cardiopulmonary bypass remains the most rapid way (>9°C/hr) to rewarm a patient with severe symptomatic hypothermia.

Patients with ventricular fibrillation and core temperatures <30°C are often resistant to defibrillation. If the initial attempt at defibrillation is unsuccessful, begin cardiopulmonary resuscitation and actively rewarm the patient to at least 30°C before reattempting. Standard Advance Cardiac Life Support medications (eg, atropine, lidocaine, amiodarone) are typically ineffective for the management of hypothermia-induced dysrhythmias. *Remember that a patient should not be pronounced dead until first rewarmed to 32°C.*

DISPOSITION

Admission

Most patients with moderate and severe hypothermia require hospital admission for active rewarming and continued investigation into the etiology of hypothermia if not clearly environmental. Admit all patients with evidence of cardiac instability and those undergoing active core rewarming to an intensive care unit setting.

Discharge

Patients without serious comorbidities who present with mild to moderate hypothermia and successfully undergo passive rewarming can be safely discharged, provided there is a warm environment for them to go. To prevent recurrent cold exposure, obtain social work consultation to arrange placement for undomiciled patients and admit to the hospital if unsuccessful.

SUGGESTED READING

Bessen HA. Hypothermia. In: Tintinalli JE, Stapczynski JS, Ma OJ, Cline DM, Cydulka RK, Meckler GD. *Tintinalli's Emergency Medicine: A Comprehensive Study Guide.* 7th ed. New York, NY: McGraw-Hill, 2011, pp. 1231–1234.

Jurkovich GJ. Environment cold-induced injury. *Surg Clin North Am.* 2007;87:247–267.

Ulrich AS, Rathlev NK. Hypothermia and localized cold injuries. *Emerg Med Clin North Am.* 2004;22:281–298.

Vanden Hoek TL, Morrison LJ, Shuster M, Donnino M, Sinz E. Lavonas EJ, Jeejeebhoy FM, Gabrielli. Part 12: Cardiac Arrest in Special Situations: 2010 American Heart Association Guidelines for Cardiopulmonary Resuscitation and Emergency Cardiovascular Care. *Circulation.* 2010;122:S829–S861.

Wira CR, Becker JU, Martin G, Donnino MW. Anti-arrhythmic and vasopressor medications for the treatment of ventricular fibrillation in severe hypothermia: A systematic review of the literature. *Resuscitation.* 2008;78:21–29.

Cold-Induced Tissue Injuries

Christine R. Stehman, MD

Key Points

- Address hypothermia, dehydration, and any alternative life threats before focusing on cold-induced tissue injuries.
- When in doubt, treat all cold-induced tissue injuries as frostbite.
- Rewarm frostbitten extremities rapidly in a warm water bath (40–42°C) and nonfreezing injuries slowly in a dry environment.
- Do not discharge patients with cold-induced tissue injuries without first ensuring they have a warm, dry place to go.

INTRODUCTION

Previously the domain of military physicians, the prevalence of cold-induced tissue injuries in the civilian population has increased substantially over the past 20 years as a result of the growth of homelessness and an expanding interest in cold weather outdoor activities such as skiing and mountain climbing. Cold-induced tissue injuries are typically divided into 2 categories: nonfreezing cold injuries (NFCI) and frostbite. Examples of NFCIs include frostnip, chilblains/pernio, and immersion/trench foot. Of the 2 types of injury, frostbite is the more devastating and requires more aggressive treatment. That said, chilblains and immersion foot can also progress to significant disability and require prompt recognition and intervention.

Although individuals at the extremes of age are at a higher risk for cold-induced tissue injuries, frostbite is fairly uncommon in these cohorts. In fact, adults aged 30–49 are the most likely group to suffer frostbite. The hands and feet account for more than 90% of all reported frostbite injuries, whereas almost all NFCIs involve the feet. Other areas of the body at risk for cold-induced tissue injury include the face (eg, nose, ears), buttocks and perineum, and penis.

There are 3 major categories of risk factors for cold-induced tissue injury. Behavioral risk factors include homelessness, inadequate clothing or shelter, alcohol or drug use/intoxication, and psychiatric illness. Physiologic risk factors include comorbid diseases that impair distal circulation (eg, diabetes, vasculitis), the use of vasoconstrictive medications, and external conditions such as high altitude exposure. Mechanical risk factors compose the final category and are the most easily correctable. Common examples include constrictive clothing and jewelry, prolonged contact with heat conductive materials, and immobility.

Of the 3 types of NFCI, frostnip is the least severe. It typically affects the distal extremities after prolonged exposure to cold but nonfreezing temperatures. Ice crystal formation and profound vasoconstriction are common in the superficial tissues, and patients frequently complain of a dull throbbing pain during rewarming. Essentially a precursor to frostbite, overt tissue destruction is lacking.

Chilblains (pernio) involve the formation of inflammatory skin lesions after repeated intermittent exposure to a nonfreezing but cold and wet environment. Although chilblains can affect any area of the body, the face, dorsal surfaces of the hands and feet, and pretibial tissues are the most commonly involved. Permanent tissue damage secondary to vascular inflammation and tissue bed hypoxia may develop. Women, children, and patients with underlying vasculitides are most commonly affected.

Immersion foot develops after the prolonged exposure to persistently wet conditions, both warm and cold, although the latter typically results in more severe tissue injury. The long-term exposure to moisture induces tissue edema and inflammation, whereas the prolonged cold exposure leads to direct tissue injury. The consequently encountered vasospasm, intravascular thrombosis, and neuronal destruction can lead to full-thickness tissue loss. Immersion foot is most commonly seen in the homeless population.

Frostbite involves the freezing of tissues and can result in significant tissue loss and long-term disability. Ice crystal formation within the extracellular space can induce intracellular dehydration, enzymatic dysfunction, and cellular death. Microvascular occlusion secondary to profound vasospasm and intraluminal thrombosis further the severity of tissue loss. Circulating tissue inflammatory markers frequently exacerbate the intensity of tissue injury and complicate the reperfusion of warmed tissue.

CLINICAL PRESENTATION

▶ History

Taking an adequate history should never delay the removal of a patient from a cold environment. Inquire about previous medical or psychiatric illnesses, drug and alcohol use, and housing status. Any history of trauma should be documented. Try to identify the overall duration of cold exposure and elicit any previous history of frostbite or a thawing and refreezing pattern of tissue injury. The review of symptoms should attempt to discover the presence of altered sensitivity, numbness, or burning pain.

Frostnip generally presents with numbness, pain, pallor, and paresthesias of the ears, nose, fingers, and toes. Patients with chilblains typically present with complaints of erythema, edema, and an intense pruritus or burning sensation. Immersion foot is usually associated with significant pain and swelling and occasionally numbness and/or the inability to ambulate. Frostbitten patients generally complain of the inability to feel the affected areas.

▶ Physical Examination

Remove all clothing and thoroughly examine the entire body, focusing primarily on the face, hands, lower legs and feet, and buttocks and genitalia. Patients with frostnip may present with paleness of the affected areas, but a normal exam does not rule out injury. Chilblains frequently present with erythema and edema and occasionally with vesicles, bullae, and even ulcerations. The characteristic lesions are purple or bluish in hue and appear 12–24 hours after exposure. Extremities affected by immersion foot will be swollen and erythematous. Tissue sloughing is common, and there may be an associated malodor. Frostbite typically presents with mottled or violaceous tissue that may have a waxy

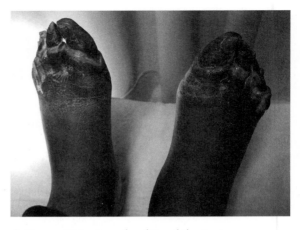

▲ **Figure 62-1.** Deep frostbite of the toes.

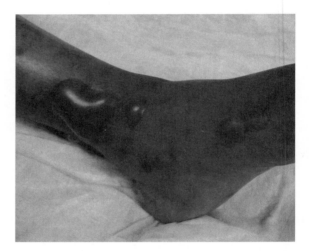

▲ **Figure 62-2.** Superficial frostbite. Note the tissue edema and clear blisters.

appearance. Although frostbite can be classified similar to burns into superficial and deep tissue injuries, this distinction often cannot be made until the tissue is properly rewarmed. Secondary blister formation is common, with the early formation of large clear blisters generally imparting a better prognosis than the delayed development of smaller hemorrhagic bullae (Figures 62-1 and 62-2). Significant tissue necrosis can complicate cases of deep tissue freezing despite minimal initial physical exam findings.

DIAGNOSTIC STUDIES

Diagnostic studies of any kind are of limited utility in the initial evaluation of patients with cold inducted tissue injuries. That said, pursue radiographic and laboratory studies as dictated for the evaluation of concurrent medical illness or traumatic injury. Radionuclide bone scanning and magnetic resonance imaging may a prognostic role in long-term management.

MEDICAL DECISION MAKING

Include cold-induced tissue injuries in the differential diagnosis of all patients exposed to freezing or near freezing temperatures, but evaluate and treat for any life-threatening conditions before dealing with these injuries. Check the core body temperature of all cold exposed patients to rule out hypothermia. Investigate for and address any concurrent trauma or dehydration. Attempt to delineate between freezing and nonfreezing injuries, as the treatments will differ. If unclear between the two, always err on the side of frostbite and treat accordingly. Consider compartment syndrome in frostbitten regions if the swelling does not resolve and pulses do not return after adequate rewarming.

Keep in mind that other injuries or illnesses can both mimic and contribute to cold-induced tissue injury. For example, the erythema of rewarmed frostnip and immersion foot can resemble cellulitis or deeper tissue infections. Peripheral vascular disease and vasculitides not only appear similar to both frostbite and chilblains but also increase their likelihood secondary to impaired microvascular circulation. Finally, the color changes and blisters of frostbite can be confused with both stasis dermatitis and autoimmune bullous forming conditions (Figure 62-3).

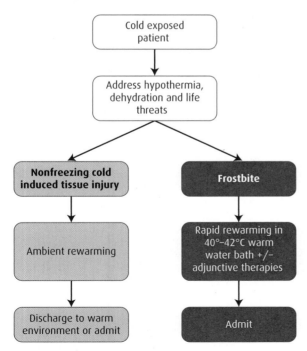

▲ **Figure 62-3.** Cold-induced tissue injuries diagnostic algorithm.

TREATMENT

All clothing should be removed and replaced with warm blankets. Wet clothing is especially problematic as it will continue to cool the patient during treatment. Dehydration is a common complicating condition and requires aggressive volume resuscitation with intravenous (IV) crystalloids to lessen blood hyperviscosity. All body parts that have suffered cold-induced tissue injury will need some type of rewarming, with the pattern of injury sustained determining the appropriate modality.

Frostnip usually resolves spontaneously with dry rewarming measures at room temperatures and requires no further intervention. Rewarm chilblains affected skin at room temperature and then wash, dry, and dress in a soft sterile bandage. Initiate pain control as needed and elevate the affected extremity to prevent excessive edema formation, as this will predispose to subsequent infection. Patients with recurrent episodes may benefit from treatment with oral nifedipine (30–60 mg/day), and topical and systemic corticosteroids have both shown promise in certain patient cohorts.

Immersion foot requires slightly more detailed care. Rewarm affected tissues at room temperature and allow them to air dry. Restrict patients to bed rest and elevate the affected extremities during the rewarming period. Certain patients may achieve adequate pain relief with oral nonsteroidal anti-inflammatory drugs, whereas others may require parental opioid analgesia. The early use of tricyclic antidepressants may help limit the future development of chronic neuropathic pain. Extreme cases of immersion foot may be indistinguishable from frostbite and should be treated as the latter until proven otherwise. Finally, all patients with NFCI require clear instructions to limit their potential for recurrent exposure and injury.

Frostbite requires more aggressive treatment to limit progressive tissue damage. Rewarm all affected areas in a warm water recirculating bath (40–42°C) with a mild antibacterial agent mixed in (eg, povidone-iodine or chlorhexidine). Do not use water warmed above 42°C to avoid superimposed thermal injury. Never initiate rewarming in the prehospital setting if there is any potential for refreezing, as this can worsen tissue injury.

A rewarming period of between 15 and 60 minutes is adequate for most patients. Use the appearance of the affected tissues to guide the duration of therapy. Appropriately rewarmed tissue should appear erythematous and pliable. Encourage active movement of the affected extremity to stimulate increased circulation. Rewarming can be exceptionally painful, and parental opioids are frequently required. Numerous adjunctive therapies have been proposed, although the evidence supporting their use is lacking (Table 62-1).

It may take many weeks for the full extent of the patient's injuries to declare. That said, certain early findings do suggest better or worse outcomes. Findings associated with a better prognosis include the rapid re-establishment of normal skin temperature and sensation and the

Table 62-1. Adjunctive therapies for frostbite.

Debride clear blisters.
Leave hemorrhagic blisters intact.
Apply aloe vera cream (Dermaide) every 6 hours to affected tissue.
Dress affected areas in soft, dry bandages.
Elevate and splint affected extremity.
Administer tetanus prophylaxis.
Administer NSAID (ibuprofen 400 mg every 8 hours).
Administer penicillin orally or intravenously every 6 hours for 48–72 hours.
Admit to hospital for daily hydrotherapy at 40°C.
Strictly prohibit smoking.

development of large clear blisters. Persistent tissue cyanosis, firm insensate skin, and the delayed formation of small hemorrhagic blisters all portent a poor prognosis.

DISPOSITION

Admission

Admit all patients with acute frostbite for a minimum of 24–48 hours, as the full extent of tissue injury may not be evident on initial presentation. Transfer to a specialized burn center may be required in severe cases where significant tissue necrosis will necessitate surgical debridement. Consider admission for all high-risk patients (young children, elderly, and homeless) with NFCI and most patients with significant immersion foot to limit further progression of disease.

Discharge

Most patients with frostnip, chilblains, and mild cases of immersion foot can be safely discharged home provided they have access to adequate cold-weather clothing and a warm, dry environment. All discharged patients require clear instructions on proper wound care and further injury prevention. Ensure adequate outpatient analgesia and arrange for close surgical follow-up as necessary.

SUGGESTED READING

Ikäheimo TM, Junila J, Hirvonen J, Hassi J. Frostbite and other localized cold injuries. In: Tintinalli JE, Stapczynski JS, Cline DM, Ma OJ, Cydulka RK, Meckler GD, eds. *Tintinalli's Emergency Medicine: A Comprehensive Study Guide.* 7th ed. New York, NY: McGraw-Hill, 2011.

Imray C, Grieve A, Shillon S, Caudwell Xtreme Everest Research Group. Cold damage to the extremities: Frostbite and non-freezing cold injuries. *Postgrad Med J.* 2009;85:481–488.

Hallam MJ, Cubison T, Dheansa B, Imray C. Managing frostbite. *BMJ.* 2010;341:1151.

Ulrich AS, Rathlev NK. Hypothermia and localized cold injuries. *Emerg Med Clin North Am.* 2004;22:281.

Heat-Related Illness

Natalie Radford, MD

Key Points

- Always consider secondary causes of hyperthermia. Heat exhaustion and heat stroke should be diagnoses of exclusion.
- Do not fluid overload elderly patients while rehydrating them in the emergency department (ED). Remember that their fluid and electrolyte deficits developed over

- days, and they do not need to be fully repleted while in the ED.
- Begin cooling the severely hyperthermic patient as soon as other life-threatening conditions and airway, breathing, and circulation have been addressed. Delays in treatment can increase morbidity and mortality.

INTRODUCTION

Heat exhaustion and heat stroke are on a continuum of disease severity. Heat exhaustion occurs when the body can no longer dissipate heat adequately, resulting in hyperthermia. Heat stroke is the result of complete thermoregulatory dysfunction. Classic heat injury occurs in the elderly or ill with prolonged exposure to high environmental temperatures. Physical exertion is not required. Elevated temperatures and high humidity overwhelm the body's normal cooling mechanisms. Exertional heat injury occurs in physically fit individuals who exert themselves during conditions with high heat and humidity. Heat gain from the environment combined with internal heat production overwhelms the body's normal cooling mechanisms, creating hyperthermia.

There are about 400 deaths from heat-related illness in the United States every year. Extremes in weather conditions can greatly affect these numbers. The Midwest heat wave in July 1995 caused 465 deaths in the city of Chicago alone. The mortality rate in patients with heat stroke can range between 10% and 70% and is affected by a patient's physical ability to adapt to changes in the ambient temperature and medical comorbidities.

The body normally maintains its core temperature between 36°C (96.8°F) and 38°C (100.4°F). In hyperthermia, as opposed to fever, there is an elevated body temperature without a resetting of the hypothalamic temperature center.

The body reacts to a heat stress to decrease body temperature via 3 main mechanisms: increased sweat production, decreased internal heat production, and removal from the hot environment. Any factors that impede these responses can lead to heat exhaustion or heat stroke.

Evaporation of sweat is the main mechanism through which the body dissipates heat. Evaporative mechanisms are impaired by both environmental and physical factors. High humidity, as seen with an elevated heat index, impedes the body's ability to evaporate sweat and cool. Elderly, infants, and those with chronic illness have decreased ability to adapt to hot conditions. Certain medications including antipsychotics, anticholinergics, beta-blockers, and diuretics also interfere with sweat evaporation and cooling. Alcoholics, those with decreased mobility, and some patients with chronic medical conditions including obesity, poor cardiac function, and scleroderma have impaired abilities to evaporate heat as well.

Radiation, conduction, and convection of heat also allow the body to lose heat, but only when the ambient temperature is lower than body temperature. Utilizing these mechanisms can aid in cooling a hyperthermic patient.

CLINICAL PRESENTATION

In patients presenting with heat exhaustion, core body temperature is usually normal, but can be elevated to 40°C

(104°F). Patients complain of nonspecific symptoms and signs including weakness, dizziness, fatigue, nausea, vomiting, headache, myalgias, tachycardia, tachypnea, hypotension, and diaphoresis. By definition, mental status remains normal. Heat stroke patients present with altered mental status (AMS) ranging from mild confusion to coma. Body temperature is elevated above 40°C (104°F), and they may or may not be sweating. Patients can exhibit a wide range of neurologic symptoms and signs, including ataxia, seizures, and hemiplegia. Multiorgan system failure consisting of hepatic, renal, and cardiac impairment may also be present in severe cases.

▶ History

Important factors to address in the history include a full description of the circumstances surrounding the heat exposure. Has the patient been in a non–air-conditioned apartment in the summer for several days, or has the patient been working outside while there is an elevated heat index? Past medical history should include questioning for medical conditions that increase the risk of heat illness and medications that impede the body's ability to cool.

▶ Physical Examination

Physical examination should involve complete exposure of the patient to remove heat-trapping clothing and to assess for any physical injuries.

DIAGNOSTIC STUDIES

▶ Laboratory

A complete metabolic panel (CMP) should be drawn to evaluate serum electrolytes. Hypo- or hypernatremia may be present as well as hyperkalemia. Prerenal azotemia may also be seen on the CMP, indicating impaired renal function. A creatine phosphokinase should be checked to rule out rhabdomyolysis. As end-organ damage occurs, patients with heat stroke may develop elevated liver enzymes (peaking at 24–72 hr), disseminated intravascular coagulopathy (DIC; thrombocytopenia, low fibrinogen levels, elevated fibrin split products, elevated D-dimer), and coagulopathy (elevated prothrombin time/partial thromboplastin time).

▶ Imaging

A noncontrast computed tomography (CT) scan of the brain should be performed on patients presenting with AMS. In heat stroke, the CT is normal. Electrocardiogram should be performed on all patients with heat exhaustion and heat stroke to evaluate for signs of ischemia or electrolyte abnormalities.

MEDICAL DECISION MAKING

When a patient presents with a potential heat-related illness, first priorities include airway, breathing, and circulation (ABCs) and vital signs with temperature (Figure 63-1). Eliminating other causes for the patient's symptoms is also

important. Differential diagnosis should include meningitis, sepsis, thyroid storm, drug intoxication (PCP, amphetamines, cocaine), cerebral hemorrhage, and status epilepticus. Neuroleptic malignant syndrome and serotonin syndrome should both be considered in any patient taking psychiatric medications. Malignant hyperthermia, although usually occurring in the context of inhalational anesthetic or succinylcholine use, should be considered if symptoms develop in a patient with a previous or family history of this condition. Vigorous exercise may precipitate this condition in susceptible individuals.

TREATMENT

Once other diagnoses are excluded, heat exhaustion is the presumed diagnosis if the patient has normal mental status. Rehydration with either oral or intravenous (IV) fluids is appropriate. Consider oral volume replacement with an electrolyte-containing solution if the symptoms are mild. If there is any concern for potential complications from comorbid conditions, IV therapy and laboratory studies should be instituted. In both cases, treat the patient with ambient cooling, removal of heavy clothing, and rest.

After eliminating other potential differential diagnoses, the diagnosis of heat stroke can be made when the patient with suspected heat illness has an elevated temperature (>40°C or 104°F) and AMS. Begin treatment immediately with IV volume and electrolyte replacement. Start with 250-500 mL of normal saline and replace other electrolytes based on laboratory values. Be careful not to fluid-overload older patients or those with cardiac problems.

Evaporative cooling should begin as soon as all life threats have been assessed and ABCs are secure. Completely expose the patient and mist with tepid water while a fan is blowing on him or her. Specially made cool mist fans are highly effective, but not available in most facilities. Alternatively, a spray bottle and a box fan are sufficient to lower the patient's temperature. The patient's core body temperature must be monitored frequently. A Foley catheter device that provides continuous temperature evaluation or rectal temperatures recorded every 10 minutes is ideal. Patients may shiver during cooling, which is counterproductive by producing heat. Treat shivering with low-dose benzodiazepines (lorazepam1 mg IV). When the patient's temperature reaches 40°C or 104°F, all active cooling measures should be discontinued. Continuing at lower temperature can cause overshoot hypothermia. Search for complications from heat stroke such as cardiac ischemia, hepatic and renal failure, DIC, and endocrine disorders. The number one factor that contributes to the morbidity and mortality of heat illness is the severity of underlying comorbid illnesses, not the absolute height of the core body temperature.

DISPOSITION

▶ Admission

If the patient has any serious comorbid conditions or illnesses, admission may be necessary. Patients with heat

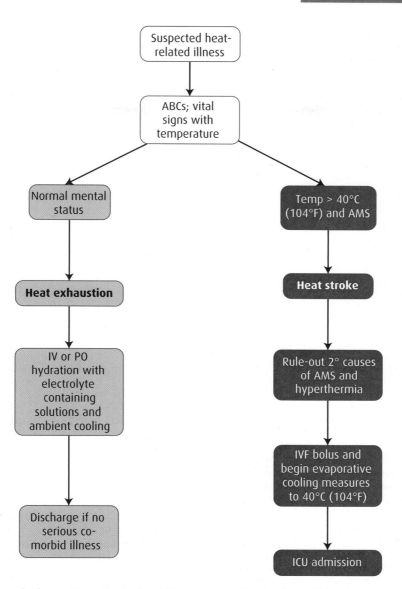

▲ **Figure 63-1.** Heat-related illness diagnostic algorithm. ABCs, airway, breathing, and circulation; AMS, altered mental status; ICU, intensive care unit; IV, intravenous; IVF, intravenous fluid; PO, by mouth.

stroke should be admitted to the intensive care unit for continued monitoring of temperature and mental status.

▶ Discharge

Discharge home is appropriate for patients with heat exhaustion if their symptoms resolve, vital signs normalize, and there are no serious derangements found in laboratory values.

▼ SUGGESTED READING

Howe AS, Boden BP. Heat-related illness in athletes. *Am J Sports Med.* 2007;35:1384.

Smith JE. Cooling methods used in the treatment of exertional heat illness. *Br J Sports Med.* 2005;39:503.

Waters TE, Al-Salamah MA. Heat emergencies. In: Tintinalli JE, Stapczynski JS, Ma OJ, Cline DM, Cydulka RK, Meckler GD. *Tintinalli's Emergency Medicine: A Comprehensive Study Guide.* 7th ed. New York, NY: McGraw-Hill, 2011, pp. 1339–1344.

Drowning Incidents

Corey R. Heitz, MD

Key Points

- Drowning is defined as the process of experiencing respiratory impairment from submersion/immersion in liquid.
- Consider that drowning may have resulted from a primary medical or traumatic insult.
- Treatment is largely supportive and stabilizing.
- Patients who present and remain asymptomatic for 6 hours may be discharged from the emergency department.

INTRODUCTION

The term "drowning incident" encompasses a variety of clinical entities. A 2005 report from the World Health Organization recommends that the term "near-drowning" be abandoned and instead to use the term "drowning incident" with a description of the outcome (death, morbidity, no morbidity). Drowning itself should be described as "the process of experiencing respiratory impairment from submersion/immersion in liquid."

Nonfatal incidents are more common than fatal incidents; in 2009, 6,519 nonfatal drowning incidents were reported, whereas 4,211 incidents resulted in death. One estimate states that there is 1 death per 13 drowning incidents, suggesting that underreporting likely occurs. Children make up the majority of fatal incidents, with peak ages of 1–4 years and seasonal variability. Freshwater drowning is more common than saltwater, with bathtubs and pool as the most common locations. Accomplished swimmers make up 35% of deaths.

CLINICAL PRESENTATION

Wide variability exists in the presentation of drowning-related injury, both in terms of time of submersion/immersion as well as how the patient is found. Children are often found face-down in small depths of water (bathtub, 5-gallon bucket, toilet). Patients may fall or jump into a body of water and their distress is immediately noted or alternatively may be found floating or at the bottom of a lake or pool after a period of time without being seen.

Symptoms also vary. Patients may be asymptomatic or may present with severe illness. Clinical effects of the submersion/immersion event itself most often manifest as respiratory abnormalities including hypoxia, tachypnea, or abnormal lung sounds. Depending on the season, patients may be hypothermic. At severe levels of illness, cardiac dysrhythmias may occur, and mental status can change. Most, if not all, drownings involve aspiration. "Dry drowning" (hypoxia from laryngospasm without aspiration) is thought to be extremely rare and physiologically difficult to explain.

▶ History

Drowned patients should be initially evaluated like major trauma patients, with attention to the airway, breathing, and circulation (ABCs) and rapid assessment of an AMPLE history. When evaluating a patient who has experienced a drowning incident, the following information must be obtained:

- Events surrounding the incident (How did they end up in the water? Did they sustain any trauma?)
- Temperature of the water and air

- Length of time in the water, length of time underwater
- Status on retrieval from the water (respiratory, mental status, cardiovascular, color)
- Was any immediate treatment needed?
- Current symptoms?

It will also be important to consider the potential of suicide; the medical status of the patient will dictate how urgently this assessment is needed.

▶ Physical Examination

The order of the physical exam will depend on patient stability. Assess the unstable patient like a trauma patient, with a primary survey and management as necessary, followed by a thorough secondary survey. In the stable patient, an examination can be conducted in a head-to-toe fashion. Areas of focus include signs of external trauma, especially the head and neck, lung sounds to evaluate for water or emesis aspiration, skin color (cyanosis), core body temperature (rectal), and a neurologic exam.

DIAGNOSTIC STUDIES

▶ Laboratory

No specific laboratory testing is universally recommended for drowned patients. If the provider feels that significant aspiration occurred, or if the patient is unstable, useful laboratory tests to determine the severity of injury include a blood count, serum electrolytes, and blood gases. To assess the pH, a venous gas is sufficient. Electrolyte changes may occur if large volumes of water are aspirated. Animal studies have shown that 11 mL/kg of aspirated hypotonic fluid are necessary before any effect is seen on hemoglobin, volume status, or electrolytes. Most drowning victims aspirate less than 4 mL/kg. In the majority of cases, hypoxia and metabolic acidosis cause the resultant morbidity and mortality.

Other laboratory studies may be indicated in certain patients. Assessment of blood alcohol level, drug ingestions, and medical causes for the patient's submersion (myocardial infarction, syncope, stroke) should be considered.

▶ Imaging

Patients in whom significant aspiration is suspected should undergo chest radiography. The most common finding is an aspiration pneumonitis (Figure 64-1). Head and cervical spine imaging should be considered if the patient dived into the water. Any other traumatic injuries noted on exam or suspected by history should be imaged and evaluated as appropriate.

MEDICAL DECISION MAKING

When a patient presents after a drowning incident, stabilization is the first priority. Once the patient is stabilized, a detailed history of events and a thorough physical

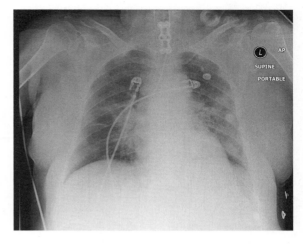

▲ **Figure 64-1.** Aspiration pneumonitis. Reprinted with permission from Heitz CR. "Drowning Incidents." CDEM Curriculum, 2009. Available at: http://www.cdemcurriculum.org/index.php/ssm/show_ssm/enviro/drowning.php.

exam should be obtained. The focus of the evaluation is 2-fold:

1. To determine types and extent of injury (aspiration, exposure, trauma)
2. To determine whether this is a primary or secondary drowning incident

Secondary drowning refers to a drowning incident that occurred as a result of a medical event, drug or alcohol ingestion, or preceding trauma. For instance, a boater who drowns in a lake may have ingested a large amount of alcohol, causing him to fall into the water. A diver may strike her head on the bottom of the pool, causing prolonged submersion. Figure 64-2 delineates a suggested algorithm for management of the drowned patient.

TREATMENT

Initial stabilization and supportive care are the mainstays of emergency department (ED) treatment for drowned patients. Airway protection, management of hypoxia and hypothermia, and urgent/emergent treatment of traumatic injuries or medical emergencies take first priority. This may include placement of an endotracheal tube, high-flow oxygen, active rewarming, and volume resuscitation. Patients who have aspirated large volumes may require positive pressure ventilation to recruit collapsed alveoli. If intubated and large-volume aspiration occurred, consider suctioning. Manage any cardiac dysrhythmias as recommended by Advanced Cardiac Life Support protocols.

Treatments once suggested but not currently recommended are prophylactic antibiotics or steroids. In addition, hyperbaric chamber use has not been shown to be beneficial unless decompression illness complicates the drowning.

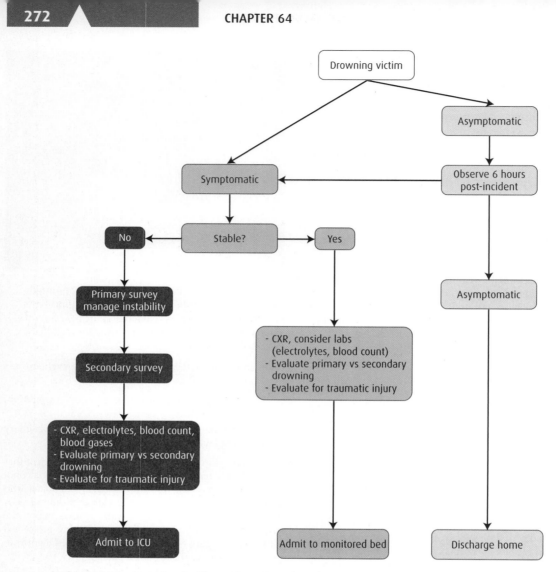

▲ **Figure 64-2.** Drowning incidents diagnostic algorithm. CXR, chest x-ray; ICU, intensive care unit.

DISPOSITION

Patient condition will largely determine disposition. Poor prognostic factors include:

- Submersion for >10 minutes
- >10 minutes before initiation of basic life support measures in an apneic/pulseless patient
- >25 minutes of pulselessness
- Initial temperature <33°C (92°F)
- Initial Glasgow score <5
- Need for cardiopulmonary resuscitation in the ED
- Submersion in water colder than 10°C (50°F)
- Initial arterial blood gas pH <7.1

▶ Admission

Admission is indicated for any symptomatic patient. Those who are intubated, have persistently altered mental status, are hypothermic, or require high-flow oxygen should be admitted to an intensive care unit. Cardiac monitoring is indicated for any patient with oxygen requirements or changes on chest radiograph.

▶ Discharge

Patients who present asymptomatic and remain asymptomatic for at least 6 hours may be safely discharged home. Discharged patients should be instructed to return for development of difficulty breathing, fever, or mental status changes.

SUGGESTED READING

Causey, AL, Nichter, MA. Drowning. In: Tintinalli JE, Stapczynski JS, Ma OJ, Cline DM, Cydulka RK, Meckler GD. *Tintinalli's Emergency Medicine: A Comprehensive Study Guide.* 7th ed. New York, NY: McGraw-Hill, 2011, pp. 1371–1374.

Causey AL, Tilelli JA, Swanson ME. Predicting discharge in uncomplicated near-drowning. *Am J Emerg Med.* 2000;18:9.

Layon AJ, Modell JH. Drowning: Update 2009. *Anesthesiology.* 2009;110:1390.

Papa L, Hoelle R, Idris A. Systematic review of definitions for drowning incidents. *Resuscitation.* 2005;65:255.

Salomez F, Vincent JL. Drowning: A review of epidemiology, pathophysiology, treatment and prevention. *Resuscitation.* 2004;63:261.

van Beeck EF, Branche CM, Szpilman D, Modell JH, Bierens JJ. A new definition of drowning: Towards documentation and prevention of a global public health problem. *Bull World Health Organ.* 2005;83:853.

Envenomation

Patrick M. Lank, MD

Key Points

- In addition to any focused or antidotal therapy available, aggressive symptom-based supportive care is important for all envenomations.
- Knowledge of local venomous species may be helpful, although be aware that patients may have contact with nonlocal or exotic venomous animals.

- North American venomous bites are rarely unprovoked.
- Contact your local poison control center (1-800-222-1222) for assistance with diagnosing and managing all envenomations.

INTRODUCTION

In 2010, there were more than 60,000 calls made to United States Poison Centers related to bites and envenomations. Although there are many venomous animal species in North America, a majority of these calls involved insects (including bees, wasps, hornets, and ants), arachnids (including spiders and scorpions), and snakes. From information provided in the 2010 Annual Report of the American Association of Poison Control Centers' National Poison Data System, there were a total of 5 fatalities related to all bites or envenomations and approximately 2,500 instances of antivenin being given.

The clinical presentations of the various forms of venom exposure vary greatly and are dependent on multiple factors including the species of the animal, the amount of venom delivered, and potential baseline medical problems in the envenomed patient. Patients presenting with an animal envenomation may therefore display a variety of symptoms ranging from local reaction to a bite or sting to generalized yet nonspecific effects (eg, vomiting, headache, hypertension) or toxin-specific findings (eg, paralysis or coagulopathy). This chapter focuses on the presentation, evaluation, and treatment of 2 of the most clinically relevant North American envenomations: snakes and spiders.

▶ Snakes

Venomous snakes found in North America are most easily divided into their 2 families: Elapidae and Viperidae (subfamily Crotalinae). The majority of venomous snakebites occurring yearly in North America are caused by snakes in the Crotalinae subfamily, which includes rattlesnakes (genus *Crotalus*), copperheads, and cottonmouths (genus *Agkistrodon*). Less than 5% of venomous snakebites are from the Elapidae family, which includes the coral snake. Fewer still may be from bites by exotic, nonnative snakes usually being kept as pets.

Venomous snakes found natively in North America are generally nonpredatory to humans. Bites, therefore, take place on provocation of the snake—either intentional or accidental. These bites are typically located on extremities, but particularly troublesome cases have been reported in which venomous bites have involved the face, neck, or tongue. The vast majority of venomous snakebites occur in young men, with an appreciable association with alcohol intoxication. Children are also at a higher risk for being bitten by a venomous snake.

There are a few characteristics that can help identify a North American snake as being part of the Crotalinae subfamily. These snakes have vertical slit-like pupils, long fangs, and a triangular head. This subfamily is also referred to as "pit vipers" because they have heat-sensing pits

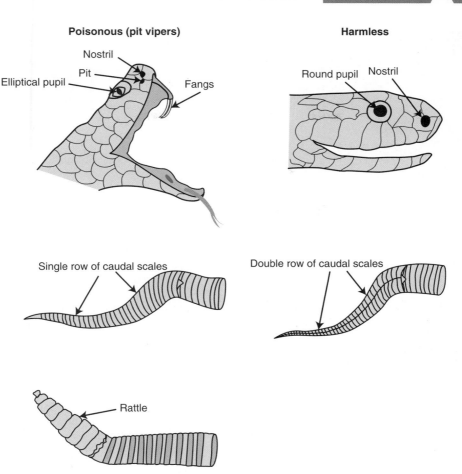

Figure 65-1. Differences between venomous pit vipers and nonvenomous North American snakes.

located on their heads just behind the nostrils and in front of the eyes (Figure 65-1). Crotaline venom contains a combination of chemicals that cause primarily local tissue damage and hematologic effects.

Elapidae native to North America are the coral snakes. These snakes, found mostly in the Southeast United States (particularly Florida and Texas), have a characteristic color pattern that distinguishes them from the similar-appearing but nonvenomous scarlet king or milk snake. People often remember this pattern difference by reciting the rhyme, "Red on yellow kills a fellow. Red on black, friend of Jack" (Figure 65-2). Elapid venom has a curare-like neurotoxic effect and is said to be one of the most potent North American venoms. However, multiple characteristics of the snake make clinically significant bites from these snakes rare. They tend to reside in remote unpopulated areas and even if confronted will attempt to flee before biting. Unlike the crotalids, the elapids' fangs are short and unlikely to penetrate thick clothing or shoes. After biting,

elapids will remain attached and "chew" on their victim to inject the venom. Although this makes it more difficult for these snakes to deliver a clinically significant amount of venom, it also makes it more difficult to clinically assess a patient with a potential bite, as there may not be bite or fang marks in a patient who has had a potentially life-threatening envenomation.

▶ Spiders

Like snakes, there are 2 major groups of spiders that cause medically significant envenomations in North America: the black widow (genus *Latrodectus*) and the brown recluse (genus *Loxosceles*). It is difficult to estimate the true incidence of spider bites, because the history of a bite is oftentimes unreliable, with many patients and physicians reasoning that a rash, abscess, or cellulitis originated from a spider bite when no spider was seen. Additionally, with the

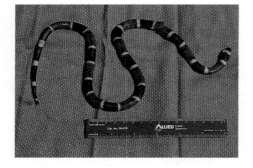

▲ **Figure 65-2.** North American coral snake. *Reproduced with permission from Knoop KJ, Stack LB, Storrow AB, et al. The Atlas of Emergency Medicine. 3rd ed. New York: McGraw-Hill Medical, 2009. Figure 16.30. Photo contributor: Steven Holt, MD.*

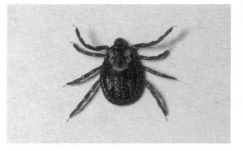

▲ **Figure 65-3.** Black widow spider, *Latrodectus mactans,* with the characteristic ventral red hourglass. Reproduced with permission from Knoop KJ, Stack LB, Storrow AB, et al. The Atlas of Emergency Medicine. 3rd ed. New York: McGraw-Hill Medical, 2009:505. Photo contributor: Lawrence B. Stack, MD.

possible exception of the female black widow spider, the general public has difficulty distinguishing medically relevant spiders from those that are generally benign. That being said, bites from brown recluse and black widow spiders can be deadly in extreme circumstances and can unquestionably cause substantial morbidity and pain.

There are 5 species of black widow spiders found in the United States. These spiders are medium-sized, typically black colored, and have species-specific ventral markings. The female *Latrodectus mactans* has the characteristic red hourglass ventral marking and has a larger body and fangs than her male counterpart, making the female more likely to cause envenomation (Figure 65-3). The clinical effects of a black widow spider envenomation in humans are thought to be caused by the neurotoxin α-latrotoxin.

There are 2 major species of recluse spiders found in the United States: the *Loxosceles reclusa* (brown recluse) and *Loxosceles deserta* (desert recluse). The brown recluse is found primarily in the southern and midwestern United States, and the desert recluse's range is in the southwestern portion of the country. North American recluse spiders are brown to gray-colored with dark dorsal markings that have a violin pattern, giving it its other names, fiddleback or violin spider (Figure 65-4). The toxin in recluse spider bites is complex, but is thought to contain proinflammatory and necrosis-inducing substances similar to phospholipase D and hyaluronidase.

CLINICAL PRESENTATION

▶ Snakes

The severity of a crotaline envenomation depends on multiple factors, including the amount of venom delivered, the potency of the venom, and the location of the venom (anatomically and by depth), as well as clinical characteristics of the envenomed patient. In 20–25% of crotaline bites, no significant amount of venom is delivered, resulting in a "dry bite." Multiple grading systems for crotaline envenomation severity have been developed, although most of these systems have limited utility in clinical practice. Instead, the clinical effects of these envenomations can be divided into 3 major categories: local/tissue, hematologic, and systemic effects. Local tissue damage from crotaline envenomation can range from minimal swelling and pain to severe edema, blistering, ecchymosis, and necrosis. Hematologic effects can be extreme after moderate to severe envenomations and include thrombocytopenia, elevated coagulation studies (prothrombin time and partial thromboplastin time), as well as degradation of fibrinogen. Even with laboratory evidence of severe coagulopathies, however, most patients do not develop clinically significant hemorrhage. Systemic effects are nonspecific; include abdominal pain, vomiting, diaphoresis, tachycardia, and hypotension; and may also be related to concomitant fear, anxiety, pain, or intoxication.

In contrast with crotaline envenomations, patients with significant elapid envenomations may initially present with minimal symptoms. The neurologic systemic symptoms that characterize North American elapid envenomations are classically delayed for hours, with reports of patients being asymptomatic up to 13 hours before developing ventilator-requiring respiratory failure. It is difficult to determine who with an elapid exposure will develop symptoms of envenomation, as it has been estimated that approximately 60% of those bitten by a coral snake did not have an envenomation. Alternatively, 15% of those with coral snake envenomations have no fang marks, and only 40% have any local swelling.

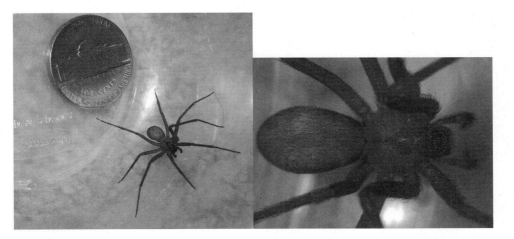

▲ **Figure 65-4.** Brown recluse spider, *Loxosceles reclusa,* with the characteristic dorsal violin-shaped marking. Photos contributed by R. Jason Thurman, MD. Reprinted from Zafren K, Thurman RJ, Jones ID. Chapter 16. Environmental conditions. In: Knoop KJ, Stack LB, Storrow AB, Thurman RJ, eds. *The Atlas of Emergency Medicine.* 3rd ed. New York: McGraw-Hill, 2010.

▶ Spiders

The clinical presentation of black widow spider bites is also referred to as latrodectism. The key feature of this syndrome is pain, which can be localized, radiating, or referred. This pain is gradual, beginning upward of an hour after the time of the bite, and is typically described as being severe muscle cramping pain in the bitten extremity, but especially with the North American black widow spider can involve the abdominal muscles, mimicking a surgical abdomen. Additional findings in latrodectism include localized areas of diaphoresis, nausea, vomiting, restlessness, fasciculations, fear of death (*pavor mortis*), and rarely priapism. The constellation of symptoms called "*facies latrodectismica*" is also specific to black widow spider envenomation and is a painful facial grimace with associated conjunctivitis, blepharitis, diaphoresis, and trismus.

"Loxoscelism" is the term used to describe envenomation from recluse spiders and can be divided into cutaneous and viscerocutaneous or systemic forms. Of significant recluse spider envenomations, the cutaneous form is the most commonly seen in North America. These patients will initially have little to no pain at the bite site, only to develop a more remarkable hemorrhagic or ulcerative painful lesion 2–8 hours after the bite. This progresses to ulceration and necrosis with surrounding erythema and induration up to 7 days after the initial bite when an eschar generally forms. This wound then slowly heals over weeks to months. Systemic loxoscelism occurs 1–3 days after the recluse spider bite and is primarily characterized by hemolytic anemia. Clinically, the patient may develop nonspecific systemic symptoms such as fever, rash, weakness, arthralgia, nausea, and vomiting. This autoimmune hemolytic anemia can be accompanied by thrombocytopenia and rhabdomyolysis and rarely progresses to renal failure and death.

HISTORY

▶ Snakes

North American snakes rarely attack unprovoked, although this provocation may be unintentional by the envenomed patient. Most bites occur during warm months, as snakes hibernate in the winter. They also more commonly occur on extremities—the areas of the body most likely to disturb a venomous snake. Young men are at particularly high risk of being bitten by a venomous snake, and it has been recognized that snakebites are frequently associated with alcohol intoxication.

▶ Spiders

North American black widow spiders tend to be nonaggressive and only attack when their web is encroached on. These areas tend to be in dark places, such as garden equipment, shoes, socks, and other clothing. Recluse spiders in North America tend to cause envenomation in domestic environments, where they hide in furniture, clothing, and sheets, particularly if they have not been used or disturbed for a while. Most recluse bites therefore happen at night or in the early morning and occur on the thigh, trunk, or proximal arm.

PHYSICAL EXAMINATION

Focused physical examination includes inspection of the possible bite area as well as screening for any associated traumatic injury. Palpation of the bite area and marking of

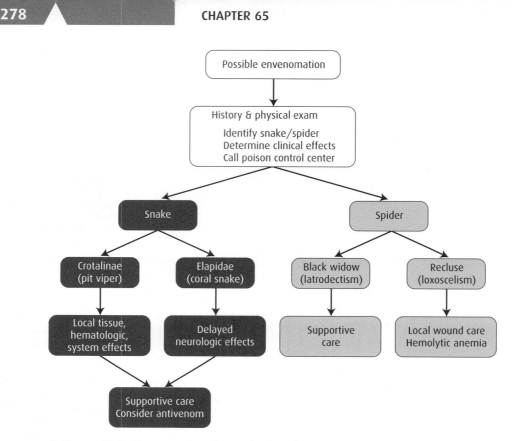

Figure 65-5. Envenomation diagnostic algorithm.

any wound margins will assist in deciding whether there is progression of local tissue injury from envenomation. However, as was discussed previously, local inspection of elapid snakebites can be deceptively reassuring. Instead, in these patients, physical examination may focus on a more detailed neurologic examination.

DIAGNOSTIC STUDIES

For crotaline envenomations, obtain a complete blood count (CBC; specifically for hemoglobin and platelet counts), coagulation studies, and fibrinogen level. If concern for retained foreign body at a bite site exists, an x-ray may be obtained.

If there is concern for systemic loxoscelism, a CBC and coagulation studies are recommended as well as chemistry panel to assess for renal dysfunction.

MEDICAL DECISION MAKING

If available, a picture of the snake/spider will aid in identification and further management. A thorough history and physical examination to determine any clinical effects, which can be local, hematologic, or systemic, is performed. Examination of the skin for bite marks to determine whether significant envenomation has occurred

is unreliable, especially in cases of a coral snake bite. Contact the poison control center for assistance in identification and management (Figure 65-5).

TREATMENT

Snakes

Many field treatments exist particularly for crotaline snakebites. However, few of them have been found to be particularly helpful, and many may be quite harmful to the patient. Such dangerous techniques include but are not limited to cutting the bite site, attempting to extract venom from the site (either orally or via commercially available devices), applying tourniquets to the bitten extremity, or applying electrical shocks to the victim. Instead, field management should consist solely of immobilization of the bitten extremity, limiting the victim's exertion, and rapidly obtaining medical evacuation and attention.

In the ED, further stabilization measures for crotaline snakebites include extremity immobilization and elevation, pain treatment, management of systemic symptoms, and assessment of tetanus vaccination status. Treatment and disposition management decisions should always involve the assistance of a poison control center (1-800-222-1222) or a local toxicologist.

Moderate to severe North American crotaline envenomations should be treated with Crotalidae polyvalent immune fab (ovine) snake antivenom (CroFab). These envenomations will be characterized by the presence of a bite site with more than minimal swelling, redness, or ecchymosis, or one with progression of any of these findings. Additionally, systemic findings and any hematologic abnormalities should prompt initiation of antivenom. Antivenom is given by intravenous infusion of 4–6 vials of antivenom in 250 mL of normal saline given over 1 hour. If initial control has been achieved with this initial dose, the patient should be admitted to an intensive care unit (ICU) for observation and consideration of maintenance dosing. If control was not achieved by the initial dose, that dose can be repeated.

Prophylactic antibiotics are not recommended for routine use in crotaline envenomations. Additionally, unless the patient develops an allergic reaction of some sort, routine use of steroids is not recommended. Because of theoretical hematologic effects of nonsteroidal anti-inflammatory drugs (NSAIDs), some experts prefer pain control with opioids.

Because of the deceptively benign appearance of potentially significant elapid snakebites, the treatment course is more reflexively conservative than that described for crotaline envenomations. It was previously recommended that any patient with bite marks or evidence of skin penetration receive elapid (equine) antivenin. However, the makers of the product have discontinued manufacture, so there is currently only very limited supply in endemic areas. In the event of a suspected elapid snakebite, the poison control center should be contacted immediately to determine need for and possible location of any available antivenin.

▶ Spiders

Although multiple therapeutic options have been investigated for black widow spider bites, aggressive supportive symptomatic care is currently recommended. Studies on the use of intravenous calcium and *Latrodectus* antivenoms have been contradictory and largely unimpressive for appreciable difference from placebo. It is therefore recommended that pain associated with black widow spider bites be managed as other painful conditions would be, with attempts at treating with NSAIDs, opioids, and/or benzodiazepines as deemed appropriate.

Multiple specific therapies have also been studied for loxoscelism. The most dangerous and ill-advised of these therapies have included shock therapy, liberal use of prophylactic surgical excision, and dapsone. These therapies, while ineffective in treating recluse envenomation, also are thought to cause worsening wound healing (for shock and surgical excision) or undesirable medication effects (such as methemoglobinemia with dapsone). Antivenoms are currently investigational and are not

available in the United States. What is instead recommended is excellent wound care, symptomatic management, and appropriate focused treatment of potential adverse effects of systemic loxoscelism.

DISPOSITION

▶ Admission

All symptomatic patients from elapid envenomation require ICU admission for anticipated respiratory failure. Asymptomatic patients receiving elapid antivenin will need to be observed for neurologic symptoms. Asymptomatic patients not receiving antivenin should also be observed for 24 hours, because risk stratification in these patients has been found to be so difficult.

▶ Discharge

For crotaline snakebites, patients with an apparent "dry bite" or those without bite marks can be observed in the ED for 8 hours and discharged without focused therapy. Patients with minor envenomations, characterized by only mild local findings on skin examination with the absence of hematologic or systemic abnormalities, should be observed for 12–24 hours with repeat blood testing and may be discharged home without antivenom administration if their symptoms remain mild. Patients requiring antivenom administration should be observed for 18–24 hours after control of symptoms was obtained. These patients will also need close outpatient follow-up for repeat laboratory work to evaluate for any worsening hematologic abnormalities and must be given very strict discharge instructions.

▼ SUGGESTED READING

Dart RC, Daly FFS. Reptile bites. In: Tintinalli JE, Stapczynski JS, Cline DM, Ma OJ, Cydulka RK, Meckler GD. *Tintinalli's Emergency Medicine: A Comprehensive Study Guide.* 7th Ed. New York, NY: McGraw-Hill, 2011, pp. 1354–1358.

Hahn IH. Arthropods. In: Nelson LS, Lewin NA, Howland MA, Hoffman RS, Goldfrank LR, Flomenbaum NE. *Goldfrank's Toxicology Emergencies.* 9th ed. New York, NY: McGraw-Hill Medical, 2011, pp. 1561–1581.

Isbister GK, Fan HW. Spider bite. *Lancet.* 2011;378: 2039.

Lavonas EJ, Ruha AM, Banner W, at al. Unified treatment algorithm for the management of crotaline snakebite in the United States: results of an evidence-informed consensus workshop. *BMC Emerg Med.* 2011;11:2.

Riley BD, Pizon AF, Ruha AM. Snakes and other reptiles. In: Nelson LS, Lewin NA, Howland MA, Hoffman RS, Goldfrank LR, Flomenbaum NE. *Goldfrank's Toxicology Emergencies.* 9th ed. New York, NY: McGraw-Hill Medical, 2011, pp. 1601–1610.

Diabetic Emergencies

Sarah E. Ronan-Bentle, MD

Key Points

- Hyperglycemia causes an osmotic diuresis that may result in dehydration.

- Patients with diabetic ketoacidosis (DKA) and hyperglycemic hyperosmolar state (HHS) are treated with intravenous fluids and insulin. Potassium supplementation should begin as soon as the potassium level is in the normal range.

- Both DKA and HHS are often precipitated by another illness, frequently infection. An attempt should be made to search for and treat any precipitating illness.

- When treating patients with HHS, it is important to follow sodium and serum osmolality measurements to document return to normal values.

INTRODUCTION

Diabetes mellitus is a common disorder and is present in 6% of the population in the United States. Diabetes mellitus is defined as fasting blood glucose >126 mg/dL on 2 separate occasions or a random glucose >200 mg/dL plus the classic symptoms of hyperglycemia (ie, polyuria, polydipsia). Derangement of glucose homeostasis is a continuum that ranges from hypoglycemia on one extreme to diabetic ketoacidosis (DKA) on the other end of the spectrum.

Hyperglycemia, even in the absence of DKA or hyperglycemic hyperosmolar state (HHS), has many deleterious effects. An osmotic diuresis occurs when an elevated glucose level overwhelms the kidneys and begins to pull electrolytes and water into the urine. In the healthy individual, serum glucose of 240 mg/dL is required before glucose is found in the urine. Additionally, hyperglycemia impairs leukocyte function and wound healing, making patients prone to infection. Chronic hyperglycemia causes renal failure, blindness, neuropathy, and atherosclerosis.

Diabetic ketosis is an intermediate metabolic state between hyperglycemia and ketoacidosis. Patients have an inadequate amount of insulin to provide the necessary energy substrates to the cell. As a result, lipolysis is stimulated to provide ketone bodies that can be used as substrates by the brain and other tissues. The ketone bodies include acetoacetate, acetone, and β-hydroxybutyrate.

DKA is defined as blood glucose >250 mg/dL, serum bicarbonate <15 mEq/L, ketonemia, and an arterial pH <7.3. DKA is present in 5–10% of hospitalized patients. It is the presenting illness of diabetes mellitus in 15–25% of patients. When making the diagnosis of DKA, the physician should attempt to determine what has precipitated the illness. The most common causes of DKA are the "3 I's": insulin lack, ischemia (cardiac), and infection. The mortality rate of patients with DKA is approximately 5% and most often is attributable to concomitant illness.

In DKA, reduced circulatory insulin levels do not allow glucose to reach the intracellular space. In response, the cell stimulates lipolysis, which provides the body with glycerol (substrate for gluconeogenesis) and free fatty acids. Free fatty acids are a precursor to the ketoacids, acetoacetate, acetone, and β-hydroxybutyrate. The ketone bodies can be used as an energy source, but when they are present in excess, metabolic acidosis results.

HHS occurs when a hyperglycemic osmotic diuresis causes extreme dehydration. Defining features include a serum glucose >600 mg/dL, plasma osmolality >320 mOsm/L, and the absence of ketoacidosis. HHS is most common in elderly individuals. It results in <1% of diabetes-related hospital admissions, but has a reported mortality rate of 20–60%. HHS occurs when a prolonged osmotic diuresis from hyperglycemia results in severe dehydration and an elevated serum osmolality. Concurrent medical illness is very common and is often a precipitating cause of HHS.

CLINICAL PRESENTATION

History

Patients with hyperglycemia report polydipsia and polyuria. They may also present with blurry vision owing to changes in the shape of the lens induced by osmotic movements of water. Recovery is spontaneous, but may take up to 1 month.

Patients with DKA present with often vague complaints such as nausea, fatigue, or generalized weakness. Vomiting and abdominal pain may be present. Altered mental status (AMS) also occurs in severe disease and is closely correlated with a high serum osmolality.

In patients with HHS, AMS is the most common presentation. Additional neurologic complaints include seizures, hemiparesis, and coma. Coma is present in only 10% of cases.

Physical Examination

Patients with hyperglycemia or diabetic ketosis may exhibit evidence of mild dehydration.

In DKA, vital signs are often abnormal, with tachycardia and tachypnea, with characteristic Kussmaul respirations. If there is severe dehydration or sepsis, hypotension or hyperthermia may be present. Hypothermia is a poor prognostic sign. Fruity odor on the breath owing to ketonemia may be present. Evidence of dehydration includes dry mucous membranes, decreased skin turgor, and tachycardia. Urine output may be maintained because of the ongoing osmotic diuresis. Physical examination may reveal a source of infection such as pneumonia, pyelonephritis, or cellulitis.

In HHS, physical examination findings are similar to those of DKA. Patients usually show evidence of severe dehydration. AMS is a hallmark. A focused neurologic examination is indicated in these patients to detect focal neurologic deficits. Searching for other precipitating causes that can be seen on physical examination such as infection is imperative.

DIAGNOSTIC STUDIES

Laboratory

The first most important test to obtain is a fingerstick blood glucose at the bedside to rapidly establish the presence of hyperglycemia. The accuracy of these machines is known to decrease at extreme elevations, and many will not read values >600 mg/dL.

Obtain serum electrolytes, renal function, serum osmolality, and urine ketones. In DKA, the bicarbonate level will be low, and there will be an elevated anion gap. The serum potassium level is frequently elevated as a result of acidemia, causing a shift of potassium into the extracellular space. As treatment is initiated, potassium is drawn back into the cells, exposing a total body potassium that is low. Sodium concentration is also frequently low, usually artificially, because water is drawn out of the intracellular space by the elevated glucose. To account for this, the sodium concentration is corrected by adding 1.6 mEq/L (correction factor) for every 100 mg/dL increase in the glucose. A correction factor of 2.4 mEq/L is more accurate for glucose levels >400 mg/dL. In HHS, the measured (uncorrected) sodium concentration, glucose level, and blood urea nitrogen (BUN) are used to calculate the serum osmolality:

$$\text{Serum osmolality (mOsm/L)} = 2(\text{Na}) + \text{glucose}/18 + \text{BUN}/2.8$$

The nitroprusside test used for the detection of ketones on urinalysis identifies acetoacetate and acetone but does not detect β-hydroxybutyrate. In DKA, there is a predominance of β-hydroxybutyrate. Despite some earlier concerns that urine ketones could be falsely normal in DKA because of the predominance of β-hydroxybutyrate, this has not turned out to be the case in clinical practice. Urine ketones can be used as an accurate screen for the presence of serum ketones. However, it should be remembered that as treatment ensues, a shift to acetoacetate and acetone makes urine ketones more positive despite adequate treatment.

The pH of a venous blood gas is an accurate estimation of the arterial pH in DKA and can be used to guide management. To determine complex acid–base disorders, an arterial blood gas can be obtained, but this test rarely impacts treatment decisions.

When there is suspicion of an underlying infection, blood cultures, urinalysis, and urine culture should also be obtained.

Electrocardiogram

An electrocardiogram is obtained to evaluate for signs of hyperkalemia or cardiac ischemia.

Imaging

A chest x-ray is indicated when clinical symptoms suggest pneumonia or another concomitant cardiopulmonary illness. Head computed tomography scan is obtained to rule out precipitating cranial pathology (ie, stroke, intracranial hemorrhage) if the patient has AMS.

MEDICAL DECISION MAKING

The differential diagnosis of DKA includes all causes of metabolic acidosis with an anion gap (methanol ingestion, uremia or renal failure, isoniazid, lactic acidosis, ethylene glycol ingestion, alcoholic ketoacidosis, salicylate toxicity). History and laboratory data should provide the clues to make the appropriate diagnosis. In determining the precipitant of DKA, the differential diagnosis includes sources of infection, cerebral vascular accident, and acute

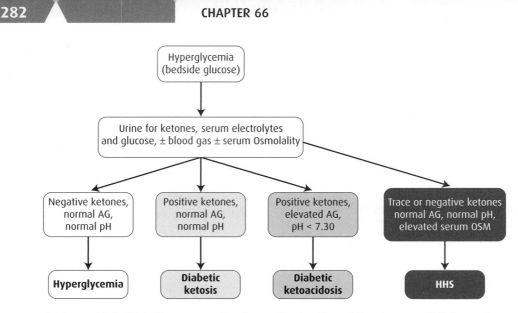

▲ **Figure 66-1.** Diabetic emergencies diagnostic algorithm. AG, anion gap; HHS, hypergly-cemic hyperosmolar state; OSM, Osmolality.

coronary syndrome. Noncompliance with insulin therapy is a diagnosis of exclusion.

Often presenting complaints of patients with DKA include abdominal pain, and thus the differential diagnosis also includes appendicitis, pancreatitis, and gastroenteritis. These are ruled in or out primarily based on history and physical exam.

In HHS, the differential diagnosis includes DKA and alcoholic ketoacidosis. Precipitating causes are varied and are included or excluded based on history and physical exam. These include multiple types of medications such as diuretics, lithium, beta-blockers, and antipsychotics; gastrointestinal hemorrhage; ischemia of bowel, myocardium, or brain; renal insufficiency; trauma; burns; and cocaine toxicity.

For differentiating hyperglycemic conditions, see Figure 66-1.

TREATMENT

Diabetic patients who are noncompliant or inadequately treated are frequently seen in the emergency department, and there is some controversy regarding the best treatment for these patients once it is determined that they do not have DKA or HHS. Treatment will depend on the degree of elevation of the glucose level and the presence of dehydration. Options include initiating or restarting an oral antihyperglycemic medication (ie, glipizide or metformin), administering IV or oral fluids and rechecking the glucose level, or administering insulin (usually regular insulin SQ) and rechecking the glucose level. Correction of dehydration prevents further osmotic diuresis.

The 3 pillars of treatment of DKA are fluids, insulin, and potassium, which are generally administered in that order. The initial IV fluid given is 1 L of 0.9 normal saline (NS)

over 30-60 minutes. Depending on the size of the patient, often a second liter of 0.9 NS is also administered. Then switch to 0.45 NS. Be careful to avoid fluid overload in patients with congestive heart failure. General total body water depletion in patients with DKA is 6–8 L.

Insulin can be initiated after the first liter of fluids. An IV bolus (0.15 U/kg) is optional. Start an IV infusion of 0.1 U/kg/hr of regular insulin. Continue IV insulin until the pH is >7.3 and the anion gap has closed. Switch to D5 0.45 NS when the glucose level is <250 mg/dL.

Treatment with supplemental potassium depends on the initial potassium level. For K >5.5 mEq/L: hold treatment. If K 3.5–5.5 mEq/L: add 10–20 mEq to each liter of IV fluids if renal function is normal. If K <3.5 mEq/L: add 40 mEq to each liter of IV fluids if renal function is normal. If K <3.5 mEq/L: do not administer insulin until the serum K is >4.0 mEq/L.

It is important to monitor serum glucose and serum electrolytes, including magnesium and phosphate regularly, as electrolyte shifts occur quickly in DKA. Obtain serum glucose once every hour after starting an insulin drip. Check electrolytes every 2–4 hours. Magnesium and phosphate replacement may be required.

In HHS, the average fluid deficit is 8–12 L. Use 0.9 NS for the initial resuscitation (1 L). Switch to 0.45 NS at a rate of 200–500 mL/hr. Goal is 3–4 L over the initial 4-hour period. The corrected serum sodium and the serum osmolarity should be gradually returned to normal over a 24- to 36-hour period. Insulin IV infusion can be started after initiating infusion of IV fluids. A total of 0.1 U/kg/hr of regular insulin is given if the K >3.3 mEq/L. Potassium replacement is similar to that in patients with DKA. Frequent monitoring of glucose and electrolytes is necessary to avoid iatrogenic electrolyte abnormalities, such as hypokalemia.

DISPOSITION

▶ Admission

Admission is indicated for patients with DKA and HHS. An intensive care unit (ICU) setting is appropriate for all patients with HHS. In DKA, AMS or pH <7.0 generally necessitate ICU admission.

▶ Discharge

Discharge is appropriate for patients with hyperglycemia once DKA and HHS have been excluded. Patients should be given instructions to obtain close follow-up.

SUGGESTED READING

Chansky ME, Lubkin CL. Diabetic ketoacidosis. In: Tintinalli JE, Stapczynski JS, Ma OJ, Cline DM, Cydulka RK, Meckler GD. *Tintinalli's Emergency Medicine: A Comprehensive Study Guide.* 7th ed. New York, NY: McGraw-Hill, 2011, pp. 1432–1438.

Graffeo CS. Hyperosmolar hyperglycemic state. In: Tintinalli JE, Stapczynski JS, Ma OJ, Cline DM, Cydulka RK, Meckler GD. *Tintinalli's Emergency Medicine: A Comprehensive Study Guide.* 7th ed. New York, NY: McGraw-Hill, 2011, pp. 1440–1444.

Kitabchi AE, Umpierrez GE, Miles JM, et al. Hyperglycemic crises in adult patients with diabetes. *Diabetes Care.* 2009;32:1335.

Nugent BW. Hyperosmolar hyperglycemic state. *Emerg Med Clin North Am.* 2005;23:629.

Potassium Disorders

Brooks L. Moore, MD

Key Points

- Obtain an electrocardiogram (ECG) early in patients with suspected hyperkalemia and never ignore a K+ >6.0 mEq/L.
- Patients with ECG changes consistent with hyperkalemia require prompt treatment to avoid a life-threatening dysrhythmia.

- The most common cause of hypokalemia in a patient in the emergency department is diuretic (loop or thiazide) use.
- Replacing K+ via the oral route is safe and is the preferred method for cases of mild to moderate hypokalemia.

INTRODUCTION

Potassium (K+) is involved in maintaining the resting cell membrane potential. Small shifts in potassium concentration result in problems with muscle and nerve conduction, leading to potentially life-threatening disorders of the cardiac and neuromuscular systems. The normal plasma concentration of potassium is 3.5–5.5 mEq/L. Hyperkalemia is defined as potassium level >5.5 mEq/L. It can be classified as mild (5.6–6.0 mEq/L), moderate (6.1–7.0 mEq/L), and severe (>7.0 mEq/L). Hyperkalemia is present in approximately 8% of hospitalized patients. If not treated promptly, two thirds of patients with severe hyperkalemia (>7.0 mEq/L) will die. Etiologies include pseudohyperkalemia (red blood cell hemolysis, white blood cell count >200,000, or platelet count >1 million), transcellular shifts (acidosis or insulin deficiency), medications (digoxin, succinylcholine, angiotensin-converting enzyme inhibitors, nonsteroidal anti-inflammatory drugs, or spironolactone), cell breakdown (crush injury, burns, tumor lysis), increased intake (consumption of fruits or salt substitutes), or impaired excretion (renal failure, Addisonian crisis, or type 4 renal tubular acidosis).

Hypokalemia is defined as potassium level <3.5 mEq/L. Mild hypokalemia is present when the serum potassium concentration is between 3.1 and 3.4 mEq/L. Moderate (2.5–3.0 mEq/L) and severe (<2.5 mEq/L) hypokalemia are less common. Approximately 15% of emergency department

patients are mildly hypokalemic. The percentage increases to 80% in patients taking diuretics, especially loop or thiazide diuretics. Etiologies for hypokalemia include decreased intake, transcellular shifts (respiratory or metabolic alkalosis), medication effects (diuretics, insulin, or β-2 adrenergic stimulation), thyrotoxicosis, hypokalemic periodic paralysis, or excessive losses from the renal (hyperaldosteronism, Cushing syndrome, type 1 renal tubular acidosis) or gastrointestinal (vomiting, diarrhea) systems.

CLINICAL PRESENTATION

▶ History

Symptoms of hyperkalemia and hypokalemia are vague and frequently include fatigue and generalized weakness. Other features include paresthesias, nausea, vomiting, constipation, abdominal pain, psychosis, or depression. A history of vomiting, diarrhea, renal failure, thyroid disease, adrenal disease, or use of offending medications should raise suspicions.

▶ Physical Examination

Patients with potassium disorders may not have any physical manifestations. In an unresponsive patient, evidence of dialysis access (arteriovenous [AV] fistulae, AV grafts, or tunneled catheters) may provide an indication of the possibility of these conditions. Patients may also display signs of illnesses that cause potassium disorders, such as paralysis, tachycardia, rashes, or striations. Patients with a hyperkalemia-induced QRS widening may appear bradycardic before degeneration into a sinusoidal rhythm (see Diagnostic Studies).

DIAGNOSTIC STUDIES

▶ Laboratory

An electrolyte panel will detect abnormalities of potassium (turnaround time is approximately 30–40 minutes). A potassium level can be obtained using many blood gas analyzers. Advantages include a more rapid turnaround time (2 minutes). However, blood gas analyzers are unable to detect a hemolyzed sample and therefore may overdiagnose hyperkalemia. A magnesium level should be obtained in patients with hypokalemia, because of the difficulty in correcting low potassium in the setting of low magnesium levels.

▶ Electrocardiogram

Symmetrical T-wave peaking, P-wave flattening, QRS widening, or a sinusoidal pattern are characteristic of hyperkalemia (Figure 67-1). Unfortunately, the electrocardiogram (ECG) lacks sensitivity to detect elevated potassium levels. Only 50–60% of patients with potassium levels >6.5 mEq/L have any of the preceding ECG findings. Hypokalemia is manifested by U-waves, T-wave flattening, and ST-segment depression. Dysrhythmias, including ven-

tricular fibrillation, may occur in patients with severe hypokalemia or in patients with moderate hypokalemia and a history of cardiac disease.

MEDICAL DECISION MAKING

Patients with a history consistent with a potassium disorder (eg, missed dialysis, profuse diarrhea) should have immediate ECG testing performed and should be placed on a cardiac monitor. An electrolyte panel or arterial blood gas with electrolytes should be drawn. If an ECG is consistent with hyperkalemia, therapy should be initiated immediately, before confirmatory tests. Before treating isolated hyperkalemia detected on an electrolyte panel, pseudohyperkalemia (hemolysis) should be ruled out by communication with the lab. Patients who are dialysis dependent or who remain hyperkalemic despite treatment should have emergent dialysis arranged. Patients with hypokalemia should have potassium and magnesium repleted (Figure 67-2).

TREATMENT

▶ Hyperkalemia

All patients with hyperkalemia should be put on a cardiac monitor, and an ECG should be performed. If QRS widening or arrhythmias are noted on a rhythm strip or ECG, calcium, given as calcium gluconate 10% (less irri-

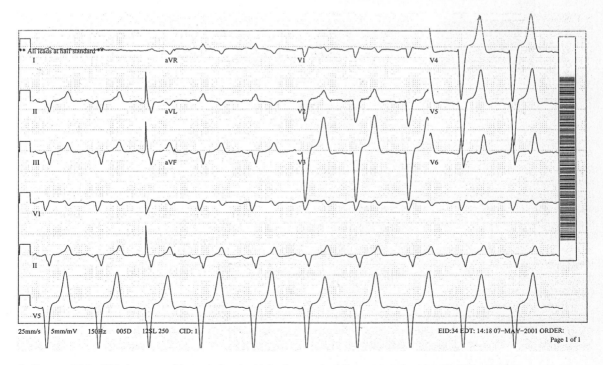

▲ **Figure 67-1.** ECG changes of hyperkalemia. Note the peaked T waves and widened QRS complex.

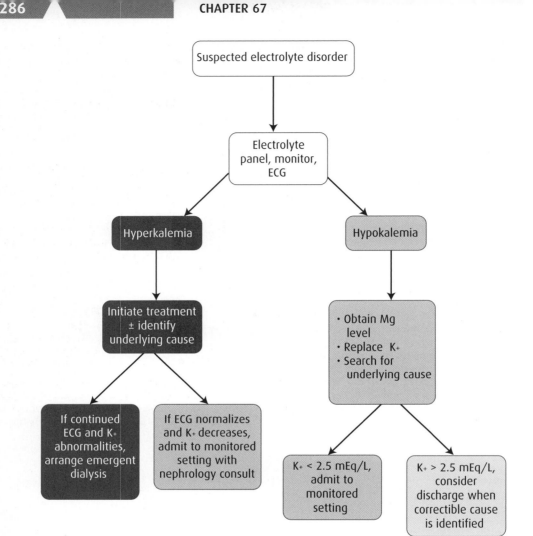

▲ **Figure 67-2.** Potassium disorders diagnostic algorithm. ECG, Electrocardiogram.

tation to peripheral veins) or calcium chloride 10% (3× more calcium) should be administered to stabilize myocardial membranes. Calcium can be repeated every 5 minutes until the ECG normalizes. The duration of action is 30–60 minutes. Calcium is not indicated in the stable patient when the ECG shows only peaked T waves. *Avoid giving calcium when treating hyperkalemia with coexisting digoxin toxicity,* because intracellular calcium is already elevated in digoxin toxicity. Further administration of calcium may cause asystole and death.

Therapy should also be instituted to induce an intracellular shift of potassium. Insulin 0.1 Unit/kg intravenously (IV) is administered to shift potassium into the cell via an intracellular messenger. Within 30 minutes, insulin will reduce the potassium level by 0.5–1.0 mEq/L. In patients with normal glucose levels, administer 25–50 g (1/2–1 amp) of dextrose IV. An alternate method in stable patients is to add 10 Units of regular insulin in 500 mL of D10W and administer this over a 1-hour period. Patients with chronic renal failure given insulin should have fingerstick glucose monitoring initiated, as hypoglycemia is not uncommon. Nebulized albuterol also shifts potassium back into cells and may work synergistically with insulin. Albuterol 10–20 mg in 4 mL of NS is given via nebulizer over 10 minutes. Sodium bicarbonate ($NaHCO_3$) also shifts potassium back into cells and leads to increased potassium excretion by the kidneys. One amp (50 mEq) infused over a 5-minute period has an onset in 5–10 minutes and lasts 2 hours.

Finally, potassium elimination therapy should be initiated. Furosemide 20–40 mg IV in patients not already taking the drug will reduce potassium levels. The onset is several hours, and the amount of decrease in the potassium level is variable. Cation exchange resins like sodium polystyrene sulfonate (Kayexalate) remove up to 1 mEq potassium per gram. A standard dose is 30 g mixed with 50 mL of 20% sorbitol to induce diarrhea. It can be administered rectally (50 g with 200 mL 20% sorbitol), if necessary. Onset is delayed and may take more than 4 hours. Dialysis should be activated early for patients in renal failure. Dialysis is also indicated in refractory cases. Treatment for the underlying disorder (eg, steroids for Addisonian crisis, Fab fragments for digoxin toxicity) should be initiated as soon as possible.

▶ Hypokalemia

Patients with hypokalemia should be put on a cardiac monitor. Oral K+ replacement (40 mEq/day) is safe and generally recommended in patients with mild to moderate hypokalemia. IV K+ should be used if cardiac dysrhythmias or severe hypokalemia are present. The rate of infusion should be no more than 20 mEq/hr, especially when the infusion is to run through a peripheral IV line. Pain and burning with peripheral IV potassium replacement can be treated by slowing down the infusion rate. Avoid IV potassium in patients in renal failure. Physicians should treat concomitant hypomagnesemia, as potassium repletion is dependent of magnesium.

DISPOSITION

▶ Admission

Because of the potential for life-threatening arrhythmias, all patients with moderate to severe hyperkalemia (K+ level >6.0 mEq/L) or severe hypokalemia (K+ level <2.5 mEq/L) should be admitted to a hospital bed with a cardiac monitor.

▶ Discharge

Patients with mild to moderate hypokalemia (K+ 2.5–3.4 mEq/L) and no clinical symptoms may be discharged with appropriate oral repletion therapy. Mildly hyperkalemic (K+ level <6.0 mEq/L) who are asymptomatic, have no ECG changes consistent with hyperkalemia, and have an identifiable and correctable cause of their hyperkalemia can be considered for discharge with early follow-up for a repeat electrolyte panel.

▾ SUGGESTED READING

Gennari FJ. Hypokalemia. *N Engl J Med.* 1998;339:451–458.

Kelen GD, Hsu E. Fluids and electrolytes. In: Tintinalli JE, Stapczynski JS, Ma OJ, Cline DM, Cydulka RK, Meckler GD. *Tintinalli's Emergency Medicine: A Comprehensive Study Guide.* 7th Ed. New York, NY: McGraw-Hill, 2011, pp. 117–129.

Mahoney BA, Smith WAD, Lo DS, Tsoi K, Tonelli M, Clase CM. Emergency interventions for hyperkalaemia. *Cochrane Database Syst Rev.* 2005;CD003235:1–28.

Thyroid Emergencies

Monika Pitzele, MD

Key Points

- In a critically ill patient with a goiter or history of hyperthyroidism, consider and treat thyroid storm early.

- Thyroid storm and myxedema coma are clinical diagnoses that do not depend on the absolute levels of thyroid-stimulating hormone and free thyroxine.

- Myxedema coma should be considered in elderly hypothyroid patients who present with hypothermia and confusion.

- For successful treatment, it is important to try to identify a trigger that pushed the patient into the extreme state of thyroid storm or myxedema coma.

INTRODUCTION

Thyroid hormone (TH) is synthesized within the follicular cells of the thyroid gland. Production begins with the uptake of iodine into the follicular lumen. Thyroglobulin, produced within the follicular cell, is bound to iodine and then coupled to produce the thyroid hormones, thyroxine (T_4) and triiodothyrinine (T_3). Release of thyroid hormone is stimulated by one of the hormones secreted by the pituitary gland, thyroid-stimulating hormone (TSH). In turn, TSH is regulated by thyroid-releasing hormone (TRH) secreted by the hypothalamus. High levels of T_4 and T_3 act to suppress production of TSH and TRH via a negative feedback loop. TH released from the thyroid gland is in its less active form, T_4, which is converted in peripheral organs (kidney and liver) into its 10 times more active derivative, T_3. The half-life of T_3 is significantly shorter, approximately a day, compared with 1 week for T_4. In the serum, the majority of TH is bound to thyroid-binding globulin (TBG), making it inactive. The only active forms are free T_3 and T_4. After TH enters cells, it binds to its nuclear receptor and regulates expression of genes involved in lipid and carbohydrates metabolism and protein synthesis. As a net result of its action, there is an increase in basal metabolic rate.

Emergencies related to the thyroid gland can be caused by both excess and deficiency of TH. Excess of TH can cause a syndrome referred to as thyrotoxicosis and can be caused either by excessive production of TH or its exogenous administration. In its extreme state, thyrotoxicosis can lead to a life-threatening condition called thyroid storm, a state manifesting with fever, tachycardia, and altered mental status.

Hyperthyroidism is the term used when excessive production of TH by the thyroid is the cause of thyrotoxicosis. One of the most common causes of hyperthyroidism is Graves disease (approximately 80% of cases), in which autoimmune antibodies that bind to TSH receptors on the surface of thyroid cells stimulate production and release of TH. Other significant causes of hyperthyroidism include toxic multinodular goiter, thyroiditis, pituitary adenoma, and reaction to drugs (eg, lithium, amiodarone and iodine). Hyperthyroidism is 10 times more common in women.

Insufficiency of TH is referred to as hypothyroidism, and 95% of the time it is caused by dysfunction of the thyroid gland. One of the more common causes of hypothyroidism is Hashimoto thyroiditis, an autoimmune condition in which the body produces antibodies to the TSH receptor, which block signaling, and does not allow production of TH. Other causes include iodine deficiency, infiltrative diseases affecting the thyroid gland, or administration of drugs (eg, amiodarone). At its extreme, hypothyroidism can manifest as myxedema coma, a severe and life-threatening state that occurs more frequently in the elderly.

CLINICAL PRESENTATION

History

Depending on the degree of abnormality, patients will present with varied severity of symptoms. Patients with earlier stages of thyrotoxicosis will report excessive sweating, weight loss, palpitations, anxiety, and heat intolerance. Patients in thyroid storm will present with symptoms of thyrotoxicosis in addition to fever, tachycardia, altered mental status, and often congestive heart failure. In elderly patients, there is a rare form of thyrotoxicosis referred to as apathetic hyperthyroidism, presenting with lethargy, altered mental status, blepharoptosis (drooping of the upper eye lid), weight loss, and atrial fibrillation leading to congestive heart failure.

On the opposite side of the spectrum, patients with hypothyroidism complain of fatigue, depression, weight gain, cold intolerance, and dry skin. In its severe state, myxedema coma, patients present with altered mental status, bradycardia, hypothermia, hypoventilation, and hypotension.

Both thyroid storm and myxedema coma usually occur in patients with previously diagnosed thyroid disorders and are usually precipitated by other factors, such as infection, trauma, diabetic ketoacidosis, stroke, surgery, or medication noncompliance.

Physical Examination

Clinical findings in both hyper- and hypothyroidism are summarized in Table 68-1. Not all the signs and symptoms will be present in every patient. Frequent findings in patients with hyperthyroidism owing to Graves disease include goiter, exopthalmos, palmar erythema, and tachycardia (Figure 68-1). In thyroid storm, in addition to those findings, patients will have altered mental status, fever, hypertension, and frequently atrial fibrillation. Hypothyroid patients will present with fatigue, periorbital edema, hair loss, and dry skin. Myxedema coma patients will have altered mental status, hypothermia, hypotension, and myxedema (non-pitting peripherial edema owing to the accumulation of mucopolysaccharides in the skin).

DIAGNOSTIC STUDIES

Laboratory

It is important to note that both thyroid storm and myxedema coma are clinical diagnoses and are not defined by absolute levels of hormones. The main test used for assessment of thyroid function is TSH level, and its use as a single test is appropriate for an initial evaluation of thyroid function. In patients with an intact hypothalamic-pituitary-thyroid axis, small changes in the level of TH will lead to significant changes in TSH levels. In a majority of cases, normal TSH effectively excludes dysfunction of

Table 68-1. Comparison of clinical presentation of patients with hyper- and hypothyroidism.

System	Hyperthyroid	Hypothyroid
Vital signs	Tachycardia Hypertension Fever	Bradycardia Hypotension Hypothermia
General	Weight loss Hyperkinesis Anxiety	Weight gain Fatigue/lethargy Depressed
HEENT	Goiter Exophthalmos Lid lag*	Periorbital edema Loss of outer third of the eyebrows Hoarse voice Hair loss
Cardiovascular	Arrhythmias (atrial fibrillation) Widened pulse pressure	Bradycardia
Lungs	Dyspnea	± pleural effusion
Abdomen	Diarrhea	Constipation
Skin	Warm Moist Palmar erythema	Cool Dry Rough skin Nonpitting edema
Neuro	Altered mental status Hyperreflexia	Altered mental status Memory impairment Delayed deep tendon reflexes**

Note: The degree of symptoms depends on severity of disease.

*Lid lag is tested by having a patient look straight and placing an object in the midline of their vision slightly above the eye level. Move the target down and ask patient to follow it with his or her eyes. Observe the upper lid in relation to the iris during the movement. Lag is present if the lid does not follow the iris immediately and white sclera is visible between the lid and the limbus.

**Change in deep tendon reflexes is described as Woltman sign. This sign consists of brief upstroke and slow relaxation.

the thyroid gland. Because of the negative feedback mechanism by TH, low TSH will indicate hyperthyroidism, and high TSH will suggest primary hypothyroidism (Table 68-2). If TSH is abnormal, free T_4 level should be ordered (FT_4). In special circumstances, for example, in severely ill patients with high suspicion of thyroid dysfunction, it is appropriate to order TSH and FT_4 ± free T_3 at the same time.

It is not useful to order total T_3 or T_4 levels from the emergency department (ED). Although only free TH is clinically active, more than 99% of both T_3 and T_4 are protein bound in the serum. Measuring the total level of the hormones does not reliably provide information about the clinical thyroid status.

Very frequently, the onset of thyroid storm or myxedema coma is triggered by non–thyroid-related illness,

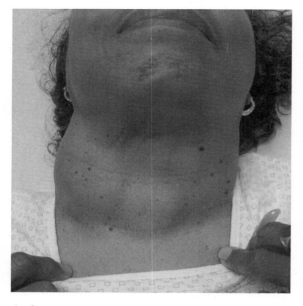

▲ **Figure 68-1.** Goiter.

such as infection, myocardial infarction, stroke, diabetic ketoacidosis, etc. Other tests should be devoted to determining the etiology of the precipitating event. Depending on the clinical presentation, those tests include complete blood count, chemistry, cardiac enzymes, electrocardiogram, urinalysis and blood, and urine cultures.

▶ **Imaging**

Imaging studies ordered from the ED will be more useful in identifying a precipitating event (for example, chest

Table 68-2. Changes in laboratory measurements of TSH and free T_4 (FT_4) in thyroid disorders.

Thyroid Disorder	TSH Level	Free T4 Level
Primary hyperthyroidism	Low	High
Primary hypothyroidism	High	Low
Secondary hyperthyroidism	High	High
Secondary hyperthyroidism	Low	Low

Primary disorders (intact hypothalamus and pituitary function, thyroid gland dysfunction) constitute a significant majority of cases. In those cases, low TSH and high FT_4 suggest thyrotoxicosis, and high TSH and low FT_4 suggest hypothyroidism. In a small percentage of cases, malfunction of pituitary gland affects the downstream function of thyroid gland (secondary hyper-or hypo-thyroid). For example, pituitary adenoma overproducing TSH will result in high TSH levels and subsequently high FT_4 levels. Panhypopituitarism resulting from tumors, hemorrhage, or infiltrative disease would cause low TSH and subsequently low FT_4.

x-ray) than in evaluation of thyroid dysfunction. Of note, use of computed tomography with iodinated contrast should be avoided whenever possible in patients with thyrotoxicosis because administration of iodinated contrast may precipitate thyroid storm. In addition, iodinated contrast diminishes the effectiveness of nuclear thyroid imaging that is used for both diagnostic and treatment purposes. This effect persists for several weeks after an iodine load.

MEDICAL DECISION MAKING

Differential diagnosis for patients presenting with severe symptoms of thyrotoxicosis includes other life-threatening conditions such as sepsis, pheochromocytoma, sympathomimetic overdose (cocaine or amphetamine), or neuroleptic malignant syndrome. Similarly, patients in myxedema coma may appear similar to patients in sepsis or adrenal crisis. If the patient has a history of thyroid problems, it should raise the index of suspicion for thyroid disorder. Of note, it is not uncommon for patients with a history of treated hyperthyroidism (eg, Graves disease treated with thyroidectomy or radioactive iodine) to present with symptoms of hypothyroidism at later stages of the disease.

A diagnostic algorithm for patients with thyroid disease is provided in Figure 68-2.

TREATMENT

Initial treatment of acutely ill patients with thyroid storm is stabilization, airway protection in cases of altered mental status, monitoring, IV fluids, and cooling blankets. Further treatment targets de novo synthesis of TH, release of TH, and adrenergic hyperactivity. There are 2 main medications that block de novo synthesis of TH: propythiouracil (PTU) and methimazole. Neither of them can be administered IV; they need to be given orally, through a nasogastric tube, or rectally. PTU also has an added advantage of blocking the peripherial conversion of T_4 to T_3. To block the release of stored TH, iodine or lithium carbonate can be used, but should be administered at least 1 hour after the initiation of blockade of de novo synthesis. Adrenergic blockers are used for symptomatic treatment, propranolol being the medication of choice. Alternative medications include esmolol, and for patients with contraindications to beta-blockers, guanethidine or reserpine. As a part of supportive treatment, IV steroids are used (hydrocortisone or dexamethasone) and acetaminophen for fever. If the patient presents in congestive heart failure, they may need diuretics and digoxin for arrhythmia control. Salicylates should not be used, because they increase the free T_4 level. As mentioned before, the precipitating cause should be treated.

Outpatient treatment of hyperthyroid patients varies with the cause and may include PTU or methimazole, pro-

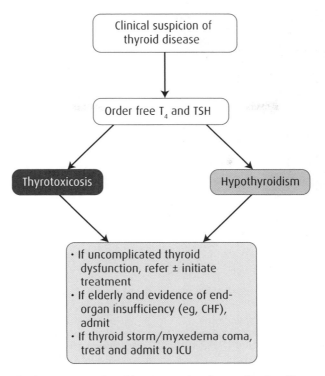

Figure 68-2. Thyroid emergencies diagnostic algorithm. CHF, congestive heart failure; ICU, intensive care unit; T₄, thyroxine; TSH, thyroid-stimulating hormone.

pranolol, radioactive iodine, subtotal thyroidectomy, and occasionally steroids.

Prompt initiation of supportive treatment for patients presenting in myxedema coma is very important and includes IV fluids, passive rewarming, and possibly pressors and mechanical ventilation. TH should be replaced by IV administration of T_4 (levothyroxine) or free T_3 (liothyronine or triiodothyronine). In severe myxedema coma, T_3 should be given, either combined with T_4 or alone (caution is necessary in patients with myocardial compromise). Administration of IV steroids is routinely recommended. A baseline cortisol level before initiating steroid therapy should be obtained.

Uncomplicated hypothyroid patients can be treated with oral replacement therapy using levothyroxine.

DISPOSITION

▶ Admission

Admit patients with concomitant illness such as CHF or dysrhythmia. An ICU setting is indicated for patients with thyroid storm or myxedema coma.

▶ Discharge

Discharge patients with uncomplicated thyrotoxicosis or hypothyroidism, with proper instructions, timely referral, and the initiation of treatment.

SUGGESTED READING

American Thyroid Association. Professional Guidelines. http://thyroidguidelines.net/

Idrose AM. Thyroid disorders: Hypothyroidism and myxedema crisis. In: Tintinalli JE et al., *Tintinalli's Emergency Medicine: A Comprehensive Study Guide.* 7th ed. New York, NY: McGraw-Hill, 2011, pp. 1444–1447.

Idrose AM. Thyroid disorders: Hyperthyroidism and thyroid storm. In: Tintinalli JE et al., *Tintinalli's Emergency Medicine: A Comprehensive Study Guide.* 7th ed. New York, NY: McGraw-Hill, 2011, pp. 1447–1453.

McKeown NJ, Tews MC, et al. Hyperthyroidism. *Emerg Med Clin North Am.* 2005;23:669.

Pimentel L, Hansen K. Thyroid disease in the emergency department: A clinical and laboratory review. *J Emerg Med.* 2005;28:201.

Tews MC, Shah SM, et al. Hypothyroidism: Mimicker of common complaints. *Emerg Med Clin North Am.* 2005;23:649.

Adrenal Emergencies

Isam F. Nasr, MD

Key Points

- Adrenal crisis is a medical emergency and must be recognized and treated promptly.
- Administration of steroids, saline, and vasopressors (as needed) should be instituted when adrenal crisis is suspected.
- Adrenal crisis should be considered in the presence of refractory hypotension.
- The preferred steroid for adrenal insufficiency is dexamethasone because it does not interfere with the cosyntropin stimulation test.

INTRODUCTION

Cortisol secretion is regulated by adrenocorticotropic hormone (ACTH), which, in turn, is regulated by corticotrophin-releasing hormone (CRH) from the hypothalamus. Aldosterone secretion is regulated by the renin-angiotensin system.

Adrenal insufficiency is the failure of the adrenal cortex to produce adequate amounts of cortisol, aldosterone, or both. Primary adrenal insufficiency (Addison disease) refers to failure of the adrenal gland as a result of tissue destruction, most frequently from an autoimmune process (70% of cases). It is uncommon, affecting 100 per 1 million persons. Risk factors for primary adrenal insufficiency include human immunodeficiency virus (HIV) infection, metastatic cancer (lung, breast, leukemia), infection (bacterial, fungal, viral, tuberculosis), sarcoidosis, or sepsis. HIV infection results in adrenal insufficiency at a much higher rate than in the general population. Up to 25% of patients with HIV have inadequate adrenal reserves. Contributing factors in HIV patients include the human immunodeficiency virus itself, opportunistic infections, and medications.

Secondary adrenal insufficiency is due to inadequate production of ACTH from the pituitary gland. Cortisol production is decreased; however, aldosterone secretion is usually intact because its production is stimulated to a much greater extent by angiotensin. Suppression of the hypothalamic-pituitary-adrenal axis by exogenous steroid administration is the most common cause of adrenal insufficiency. It is based on the dose and duration of treatment. Administrations of steroids for <2 weeks or doses <5 mg per day are unlikely to result in adrenal insufficiency. Steroid administration (withdrawal), pituitary tumors, and trauma place patients at risk for secondary adrenal insufficiency.

Acute adrenal insufficiency (Addison or adrenal crisis) is an emergent condition that occurs in a person who has underlying adrenal suppression who undergoes an acute stress or illness. Some patients have a history of chronic adrenal insufficiency; for others, adrenal crisis is the initial presentation.

Cushing syndrome refers to a situation in which there is a symptomatic excess of glucocorticoids. Prolonged exogenous administration of steroids is the most common cause of Cushing syndrome. Cushing disease is present when Cushing syndrome is due to excessive ACTH secretion from the pituitary gland. Endogenous Cushing syndrome (Cushing disease) is much less common and occurs in 13 per 1 million persons.

In addition to exogenous steroid administration, Cushing syndrome is due to an ACTH-producing tumor of the pituitary gland (70%), adrenal gland (15%), or other (15%). Other tumors producing ACTH include pancreatic cancer, small-cell lung carcinoma, and carcinoid tumors.

Prolonged steroid administration is a risk factor for exogenous Cushing syndrome. Endogenous (Cushing disease) is more common in women aged 20–40 and in the presence of malignancy (lung, pancreatic).

CLINICAL PRESENTATION

History

Patients with adrenal insufficiency report complaints of fatigue, nausea, vomiting, abdominal pain, lightheadedness, or diarrhea, whereas those with Cushing syndrome report fatigue, weakness, and menstrual irregularities.

Physical Examination

Patients with primary adrenal insufficiency will present with hyperpigmentation of the skin due to increased levels of circulating ACTH. This finding is present in 98% of these patients. Acute adrenal insufficiency is characterized by mental status changes, hypotension, and tachycardia. Hypothermia may be present, but fever can be seen in the setting of concurrent infection.

Physical findings in Cushing syndrome may include truncal obesity, moon facies, buffalo hump, hirsutism, and skin striae. Hypertension is a common finding.

DIAGNOSTIC STUDIES

Laboratory

Laboratory studies in patients with suspected adrenal insufficiency or Cushing syndrome should include complete blood count, electrolytes with glucose, cortisol, and ACTH level. In primary adrenal insufficiency, hyponatremia is present in 90% of patients, hyperkalemia in 64%, and hypercalcemia in 6–33%. In secondary adrenal insufficiency, electrolyte abnormalities are less likely because aldosterone production is not impaired. Anemia is present in 40% of patients, and an elevated white blood cell count suggests infection. Hypoglycemia is present in two thirds of patients.

A random serum cortisol level <15 mcg/dL in an acutely ill patient is diagnostic of adrenal insufficiency in most cases and can be performed in the emergency department (ED). An ACTH level can be drawn, but results are rarely available in the ED.

In Cushing syndrome, hyperglycemia is commonly present and is due to insulin resistance. Hypokalemic metabolic alkalosis is present in some patients with increased ACTH production. A random serum cortisol is not useful due to wide diurnal ranges.

The rapid ACTH stimulation test is infrequently performed in the ED, but may be used to test the responsiveness of the adrenal glands. A baseline sample of blood is drawn at time 0 for a cortisol level, then 0.25 mg of cosyntropin (synthetic ACTH) is given intravenously (IV). Plasma cortisol levels are checked at 30 minutes and 1 hour. Dexamethasone should be given empirically even without waiting for the results. In normal subjects, baseline cortisol (time 0) levels exceed 5 mcg/dL. Post–rapid ACTH stimulation test, plasma cortisol levels should rise at least7 mcg/dL and peak at >18 mcg/dL, which marks a normal response and rules out primary disorders of the adrenal glands. Subsequent measurement of the plasma ACTH level determines whether adrenal insufficiency is primary (Addison disease) or secondary. Elevated ACTH levels indicate primary adrenal insufficiency, whereas normal or low levels indicate secondary adrenal insufficiency.

Imaging

Imaging studies are not routinely indicated in adrenal insufficiency or Cushing syndrome. Chest x-ray, electrocardiogram, or head computed tomography may be useful depending on the clinical presentation (ie, altered mental status, suspected pneumonia or cardiac ischemia).

MEDICAL DECISION MAKING

The differential diagnoses for adrenal insufficiency include shock (cardiovascular, septic), dehydration, or influenza infection. Consider adrenal crisis in any patient who presents in shock, especially if they have a history of adrenal insufficiency, withdrawal of chronic steroids, characteristic electrolyte abnormalities (low Na, high K), or hypoglycemia (Figure 69-1). Acute adrenal insufficiency is usually precipitated by an underlying illness (eg, sepsis), and it is important for the clinician to identify and treat both disorders. Polycystic ovary disease, depression, diabetes mellitus, and hypothyroidism are the most common differential diagnoses for Cushing syndrome.

TREATMENT

IV 0.9 NS should be given to treat hypotension. Persistent hypotension may require vasopressors. Dextrose is administered in the setting of hypoglycemia. An ampule of D50 is given initially and is repeated as needed. Dexamethasone 4–6 mg IV is given every 6 hours or hydrocortisone 100 mg IV every 8 hours. Dexamethasone is preferred because, unlike hydrocortisone, it does not interfere with cortisol response to ACTH or the cortisol assay. If hydrocortisone is given, results of the ACTH (cosyntropin) stimulation test will be difficult to interpret. Mineralocorticoids in the form of fludrocortisone acetate (Florinef) 0.05–0.2 mg are administered. Search and treat precipitating causes (eg, sepsis).

It is not the role of the emergency physician to make the definitive diagnosis of Cushing syndrome but to suspect the condition, treat the underlying cause, and refer the patient for further testing or treatment.

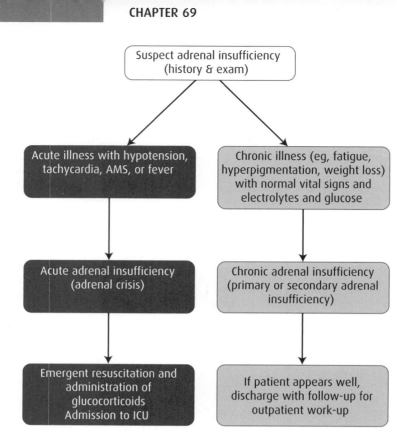

▲ **Figure 69-1.** Adrenal emergencies diagnostic algorithm. AMS, altered mental status; ICU, intensive care unit.

DISPOSITION

▶ Admission

All patients with acute adrenal insufficiency require hospital admission. Most patients will require an intensive care unit setting.

▶ Discharge

Patients with chronic symptoms of either adrenal insufficiency or Cushing syndrome may be discharged with close follow-up with a primary physician and endocrinologist.

▼ SUGGESTED READING

Idrose AM. Adrenal insufficiency and adrenal crisis. In: Tintinalli JE, Stapczynski JS, Ma OJ, Cline DM, Cydulka RK, Meckler GD. *Tintinalli's Emergency Medicine: A Comprehensive Study Guide.* 7th ed. New York, NY: McGraw-Hill, 2011, pp. 1453–1456.

Peacy SR, Guo CY, Robinson AM, et al. Glucocorticoid replacement therapy: are patients over treated and does it matter? *Clin Endocrinol (Oxf).* 1997;46:255.

Stewart PM, Krone NP. The adrenal cortex. In: Kronnenberg H, Melmed S, Polonsky K, Larson PR, eds. *Williams Textbook of Endocrinology.* 12th ed. Philadelphia, PA: Saunders Elsevier, 2011, Pages 479–544.

Oncologic Emergencies

Biswadev Mitra, MD

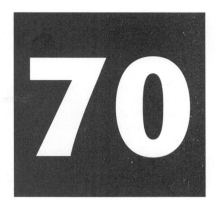

Key Points

- Spinal cord compression should be considered in any patient presenting to the emergency department with a neurologic complaint and a history of malignancy.
- Electrolyte abnormalities should be considered in all patients with malignancy and nonspecific symptoms.
- Patients undergoing chemotherapy who present with fever should be considered neutropenic until proven otherwise.

INTRODUCTION

Improvements in the management of cancer have lead to an aging population presenting to emergency departments (EDs) with complications related to malignant disease. Oncologic emergencies occur in patients with recurrence of a previously diagnosed malignancy, complications of cancer treatment, or signs and symptoms that may lead to a new diagnosis of cancer. Emergency clinicians must be aware of the common complications associated with malignancies and available treatments. These complications can be broadly divided into those created by local tumor effects, complications from hematologic derangements and biochemical abnormalities, and complications related to cancer treatment. When caring for patients with oncologic related emergencies in the ED, consideration should always be given to the nature of medical therapy warranted in view of progression of the disease. Early consultation with family members and stakeholders is advised.

Emergencies related to local tumor invasion include spinal cord compression and superior vena cava (SVC) syndrome. Both are oncologic emergencies that require prompt intervention. The most common primary tumors that metastasize to the spine are lung (29%), prostate (19%), and breast (13%). The thoracic spine is the most common site involved (77%). The lumbar spine is affected 29% of the time with the cervical (12%) and sacral (7%) regions being affected least often.

SVC syndrome is defined as obstruction of flow through the superior vena cava due to tumor-related compression. Lung cancer and non-Hodgkin lymphoma together cause about 95% of cancer-related SVC syndrome. The incidence of SVC syndrome in patients with lung cancer and non-Hodgkin lymphoma is 2–4%. Thrombosis related to central venous catheters can also cause SVC syndrome in patients with cancer as a result of their prothrombotic state.

Emergencies related to biochemical derangements in the cancer patient include hypercalcemia and tumor lysis syndrome. Hypercalcemia has been reported to occur in 20–30% of patients with cancer at some time during the course of their disease. It occurs most commonly in cancers associated with bone (multiple myeloma), bony metastasis (breast, lung, prostate, renal), or cancers that secrete parathyroid-like substance (lung) or osteoclastic factors (lymphomas). The detection of hypercalcemia in a patient with cancer signifies a very poor prognosis, with death often occurring within months.

Tumor lysis syndrome is the most common disease-related emergency encountered in patients with hematologic cancers. The syndrome occurs when tumor cells release their contents into the bloodstream, either spontaneously or in response to therapy, leading to the characteristic findings of hyperuricemia, hyperkalemia, hyperphosphatemia, and hypocalcemia. These electrolyte and metabolic disturbances can progress to clinical toxic effects, including renal insufficiency, cardiac arrhythmias, seizures, and death due to organ failure. It is most common in cancers with high cell turnover (leukemia and lymphoma).

One of the most common hematologic emergencies is neutropenic fever, which is the presence of a fever >38°C with an absolute neutrophil count of <500/μL. Febrile neutropenia is a result of bone marrow suppression, a common side effect of chemotherapy. Patients with neutropenia are susceptible to life-threatening bacterial infections. Older age has been shown to be an independent risk factor for the development of neutropenia and febrile neutropenia. A history of previous chemotherapy-induced neutropenia predicts recurrent neutropenia and neutropenic fever.

CLINICAL PRESENTATION

History

Pain is the presenting symptom of spinal cord compression in 90–95% of patients. The pain is usually constant and close to the site of the lesion. Patients complain of a band or girdle of pain/tightness radiating from back to front, exacerbated by recumbency, movement, coughing and sneezing. Symptoms may include numbness and tingling, which usually precedes weakness. Weakness often presents with "stiffness," dragging of a limb, or unsteadiness.

Facial edema is the most common symptom of SVC syndrome with patients often describing feeling bloated. Other symptoms include dyspnea, cough, chest and shoulder pain, and hoarseness. Dyspnea may be worse when leaning forward or lying down. Arm swelling and lymphedema are other common symptoms of SVC syndrome.

In both acute and chronic hypercalcemia of malignancy, the major manifestations affect gastrointestinal, renal, and neuromuscular function. Patients with acute hypercalcemia commonly present with anorexia, nausea, vomiting, polyuria, polydipsia, dehydration, weakness, and confusion. Patients with tumor lysis syndrome may have similar symptoms often related to acute renal failure.

Neutropenic patients, usually on chemotherapy, often present to the ED with fever and no clear source of infection. Tachycardia and hypotension may accompany fever and may indicate severe sepsis or septic shock. Weakness and dehydration are usually present.

Physical Examination

Patients with cancer who present to the ED require a thorough physical examination to identify potential life threats associated with malignancy. Vital signs and general assessment including mental status will often reveal whether an acute medical emergency such as neutropenic sepsis or arrhythmia exists. A thorough head-to-toe examination should follow. Head, eyes, ears, nose, and throat examination should assess for a patent airway, oropharyngeal infection, facial plethora, and cranial neuropathies. Neck

examination should assess for cervical spine tenderness and dilated neck veins. Cardiovascular and respiratory exams should assess breath sounds and cardiac rhythm. Decreased breath sounds or distant heart sounds may indicate pleural or pericardial effusions. Abdominal exam should assess for masses and possible source of occult infection. Back exam should assess for any localized tenderness or masses, and neurologic exam should identify any focal neurologic deficits. Extremities and skin should be assessed for hydration status and edema, possibly related to acute renal failure.

DIAGNOSTIC STUDIES

Electrocardiogram

An electrocardiogram should be performed in all patients with suspected electrolyte abnormalities. Patients with hypercalcemia may have a shortened QT interval due to the increased rate of cardiac repolarization. Arrhythmias such as bradycardia and first-degree atrioventricular block may occur. Tumor lysis syndrome may result in multiple electrolyte abnormalities that may manifest as arrhythmias. Hyperkalemia may demonstrate a spectrum from peaked T waves, PR and QRS prolongation, loss of P-wave and T-wave flattening, and finally a sine wave. Hypocalcemia causes a prolonged QT and may result in ventricular arrhythmias.

Laboratory

Serum basic metabolic panel (BMP) with calcium, magnesium, and phosphorous should be assessed on all patients with vague complaints, vomiting, or dehydration. BMP should also be ordered for those at risk for hypercalcemia (bony metastasis) and tumor lysis syndrome (recent cancer treatment). Patients with tumor lysis syndrome present with acute renal failure in the presence of hyperuricemia (>15 mg/dL), hyperphosphatemia (>8 mg/dL), hyperkalemia, and hypocalcemia. A complete blood count should be obtained on all patients to assess for neutropenia (absolute neutrophil count <500/μL), anemia, and thrombocytopenia. The absolute neutrophil count is determined by multiplying the total white blood cell count times the percentage of neutrophils plus bands. Multiple sets of blood cultures and a urine culture should be collected in all febrile neutropenic patients in the ED.

Imaging

Patients with signs or symptoms suggestive of spinal cord metastasis should have their spine imaged. Plain radiographs may identify bony metastasis or pathologic fractures but are not sufficiently sensitive to rule out the presence of spinal disease. Computed tomography (CT) scan of the spine is more sensitive than plain films; however, magnetic resonance imaging of the spine is the test of choice to assess for spinal metastasis and cord involvement. Similarly, chest radiograph may be used as an initial test for patients with suspected SVC syndrome, but CT chest with contrast is the test of choice for identification.

MEDICAL DECISION MAKING

Identification of common emergencies associated with malignant disease is key to the expeditious ED care of the cancer patient. Patients with acute shortness of breath should be assessed for malignant pleural or pericardial effusions or pulmonary embolus. Generalized weakness may be from dehydration, electrolyte abnormalities associated with tumor lysis syndrome or renal failure, or an occult infection owing to immunosuppression from chemotherapy. Brain or spinal cord metastasis should be considered for any focal neurologic sign or symptom, and appropriate imaging should be performed in the ED (Figure 70-1).

TREATMENT

For patients with acute spinal cord compression from spinal metastasis, IV corticosteroids relieve pain, reduce edema, and may improve neurologic function. They may also tem-

porarily prevent the onset of cord ischemia. Radiation therapy provides more definitive treatment in most patients. Indications for radiation therapy include known radiosensitive tumor with no spinal instability and palliative therapy in patients who present with paraplegia.

SVC syndrome is treated in the ED with IV steroids (dexamethasone 10 mg IV) and furosemide IV in an attempt to reduce venous pressures. Patients with cardiac or respiratory compromise or central nervous system dysfunction may require emergent endotracheal intubation or radiation therapy. Vascular surgery should be consulted for possible SVC stenting.

Hypercalcemia is treated in the ED with IV fluid administration. Levels >13 mg/dL usually require treatment. An initial bolus of 1–2 L of normal saline (NS) is initiated. Loop diuretics (furosemide) can also be given in a dose of 40-80 mg IV. Bisphosphonates may also be used, but their maximum effect does not occur for 2–4 days. Hemodialysis may be indicated in severe cases.

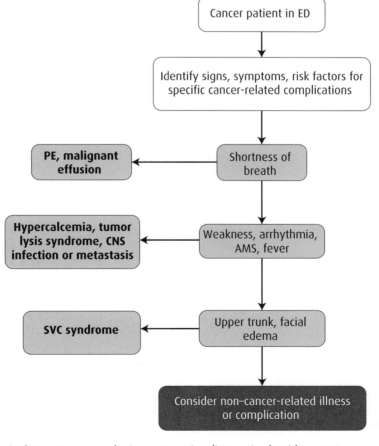

▲ **Figure 70-1.** Oncologic emergencies diagnostic algorithm. AMS, altered mental status; CNS, central nervous system; ED, emergency department; PE, pulmonary embolism; SVC, superior vena cava.

Tumor lysis syndrome is treated with IV hydration (NS), loop diuretics, and allopurinol. Hyperkalemia remains the most dangerous component of tumor lysis syndrome, causing life-threatening dysrhythmias. Hemodialysis may be needed in patients with renal failure, severe electrolyte abnormalities, or fluid overload.

If not treated in the first 48 hours, the mortality for neutropenic sepsis approaches 50%. The prompt administration of empiric antibiotic therapy has resulted in a decrease in mortality to 10%. Neutropenic fever should be treated expeditiously with ceftazidime 2 g IV. Vancomycin should be added for patients with sepsis, known methicillin-resistant *Staphylococcus aureus*, or indwelling venous catheters.

DISPOSITION

▶ Admission

Patients with acute spinal cord compression will often require intensive care unit (ICU) admission for frequent neurologic evaluation. Neutropenic patients may also require an ICU if they have signs of sepsis or septic shock.

If admitted to the floor, they should have reverse isolation precautions to protect them from hospital acquired infections. Patients with renal failure or severe electrolyte abnormalities will require an ICU or telemetry monitored bed.

▶ Discharge

Cancer patients with a febrile illness who are not neutropenic may be considered for discharge depending on the source of the fever. Patients with mild dehydration and correctable electrolyte abnormalities may also be considered for discharge.

▼ SUGGESTED READING

Blackburn P. Emergency complications of malignancy. In: Tintinalli JE, Stapczynski JS, Ma OJ, Cline DM, Cydulka RK, Meckler GD. *Tintinalli's Emergency Medicine: A Comprehensive Study Guide.* 7th ed.New York, NY: McGraw-Hill, 2011, pp. 1508–1516.

McCurdy MT, Shanholtz CB. Oncologic emergencies. *Crit Care Med.* 2012;40:2212–2222.

Sickle Cell Emergencies

Brian R. Sellers, MD

Amy V. Kontrick, MD

Key Points

- Control pain aggressively.
- Search for and treat the precipitants of pain crisis.

- Complications of sickle cell disease, both typical and atypical, must be aggressively sought after and treated.
- Have a low threshold for admission when patients may have an occult infection.

INTRODUCTION

Sickle cell disease (SCD) is an inherited chronic disease found primarily in those of African, Middle Eastern, Indian, or Mediterranean ancestry. SCD is characterized by a defect in the hemoglobin molecule, which normally consists of two pairs of α and β globin. A single amino acid substitution (valine for glutamine) on the β-globin gene results in sickle hemoglobin (Hb S). The mutation that causes the amino acid substitution is inherited as an autosomal recessive trait. Patients with sickle cell trait have one abnormal β-globin gene (heterozygous HbAS), whereas those with SCD have 2 abnormal β-globin genes (homozygous HbSS). During states of biologic stress (eg, low O_2 state, infection, dehydration, pregnancy, cold exposure, trauma) the Hb S polymerizes, resulting in deformation (sickling) of the red blood cell (RBC). This sickled RBC has reduced ability to pass through small blood vessels, resulting in vasoocclusion, hemolysis, and end-organ damage. Premature destruction of the sickled RBC results in a shorter than normal life span of the cell.

Two million people in the United States have sickle cell trait, and 70,000 have sickle cell disease. Although survival has improved dramatically recently, life expectancy of patients with SCD is shorter than average, now just greater than 50 years.

Most patients with SCD present to the emergency department (ED) with either a painful vasoocclusive crisis or sequela from vaso-occlusion, some of which may be life-threatening. It is the role of the emergency physician to not only control pain but also diagnose and treat potential life threats. Acute sickle cell emergencies can be divided into several classifications: acute pain crisis, acute chest syndrome, infection, neurologic, splenic sequestration, aplastic crisis, hemolytic anemia, and priapism.

▶ Acute Pain Crisis

Vaso-occlusive pain crises account for approximately 90% of ED visits. Severe back and extremity pain results from micro-infarction of the bones and joints. Abdominal pain crises result from ischemia to the mesentery, spleen, and liver.

▶ Acute Chest Syndrome

Acute chest syndrome is the most common cause of death in patients with SCD. Although it is more common in children, it is more severe in adults. Acute chest syndrome is characterized by fever, chest pain, respiratory symptoms, hypoxia, and an infiltrate seen on chest x-ray (CXR). It is a result of pulmonary ischemia and infarction. Acute chest is frequently a complication of pneumonia. *Chlamydia* and *Mycoplasma* are the 2 most common organisms, but viruses, *Streptococcus pneumoniae*, *Staphylococcus aureus*, and *Haemophilus influenzae* are all potential causes.

Infection

Patients with SCD are at increased risk of infection as a result of the loss of splenic function secondary to recurrent splenic infarcts. Children as young as 6 months of age may be functionally asplenic, and most patients with SCD are by the age of 5 or 6 years. This makes them more vulnerable to infections with encapsulated organisms such as *S. pneumoniae* and *H. influenzae.S. aureus, Escherichia coli,* and *Salmonella typhimurium* are also common pathogens. Bone, pulmonary, and central nervous system (CNS) infections are common and must be considered in any febrile patient with SCD.

Neurologic

Patients with SCD are at increased risk for cerebrovascular accident (CVA), ischemic and hemorrhagic, as well as subarachnoid hemorrhage. Approximately 10% of patients will have a CVA by the age of 20 years. Vasoocclusion, as well as endothelial damage, are believed to play a role in development of CVA.

Splenic Sequestration

The abnormal sickled cells become trapped in the spleen (splenic sequestration), leading to a rapid decrease in steady state hemoglobin and an enlarged spleen. A rapid decrease in hemoglobin can lead to hemodynamic instability and altered mental status. Splenic sequestration is a serious complication seen more commonly in children than adults and carries a significant morbidity and mortality potential.

Aplastic Crisis

Aplastic crisis arises when bone marrow production of RBCs stops or falls below the rate of destruction. Aplastic crisis is also associated with reticulocytopenia. Aplastic crisis in patients with SCD has been linked to infection with parvovirus as well as folic acid deficiency.

Hemolytic Anemia

Chronic hemolysis is a problem for all patients with SCD due to the deformed RBC. Hemoglobin levels range from 6–9 g/dL. Patients will also have an increased reticulocyte count due to increase RBC destruction. Under stress (eg, infection), hemolysis rates may increase and patients my have a decrease in hemoglobin from their baseline.

Priapism

Priapism, a painful failure of penile detumescence secondary to corpus cavernosum obstruction by sickled cells, has a bimodal peak (5–13 years and 21–29 years of age). Prolonged priapism can lead to impotence due to fibrosis and vascular damage.

CLINICAL PRESENTATION

History

Patients will present with pain that is usually moderate to severe and most commonly involves the extremities, back, chest, and abdomen. Important historical considerations include possible precipitants, previous complications, home analgesic regimen, and routine medical care. Common precipitants of a pain crisis include infection, cold, and dehydration. Determine whether the patient's pain is typical or atypical in relation to previous episodes in an effort to determine whether more than a simple vasoocclusive pain crisis is occurring. The presence of fever, chest pain, shortness of breath, joint swelling, or redness should prompt the clinician to look beyond a simple pain crisis.

Physical Examination

Note the presence of abnormal vital signs (VS), particularly fever, tachycardia, tachypnea, hypoxia and hypotension, which may indicate complications of SCD or another acute process. Although most patients with an acute vasoocclusive crisis will have a low-grade temperature, a fever greater than 38.3°C (100.9 F) should prompt a search for an infectious precipitant. In addition, acute chest syndrome should be suspected in patients with chest pain, shortness of breath, fever, and cough. Determination of hydration status is critical. Rehydrating the patient in crisis not only reduces sickling of the cells, but also increases the intravascular volume, thereby helping to relieve vasoocclusion. In addition to rapid and accurate VS measurements and determination of hydration status, several key organ systems must be assessed.

The general appearance of the patient should be noted for signs of respiratory distress, physical pain, and lethargy. Because of the increased rate of hemolysis, patients with SCD may have jaundice or scleral icterus. Pallor may indicate a significant drop in hemoglobin. The skin should be examined for signs of infection. Pallor, left upper quadrant pain, and splenomegaly are all concerning for splenic sequestration. Chest auscultation should be done to note any rales, rhonchi, or wheezing. The abdominal exam should note the presence of focal tenderness, especially the right or left upper quadrants. The presence of splenomegaly or hepatomegaly, or the presence of guarding or rebound tenderness, should alert the practitioner to an intra-abdominal process beyond that associated with pain crisis. Extremities and joints should be examined for focal tenderness, joint erythema, or swelling, all of which may indicate osteomyelitis or septic arthritis and not simply bone pain associated with a crisis. Patients with SCD require a thorough examination of the extremities, and it should be performed on an undressed patient to rule out these serious complications. A full neurologic exam including cranial nerves and cerebellar signs should be performed to assess for any new neurologic deficits in a patient with acute complaints.

DIAGNOSTIC STUDIES

▶ Laboratory

Initial laboratory studies in patients suspected of having vaso-occlusive crisis include complete blood count and reticulocyte count. The Hb level is usually between 6 and 9 g/dL, but should be compared with previous levels for any acute decreases that would be consistent with rapid hemolysis, splenic sequestration, or aplastic crisis. The reticulocyte count should be elevated during a typical acute vasoocclusive pain crisis to compensate for increased RBC turnover. A reticulocyte count less than 2% would be concerning for aplastic crisis. Leukocytosis (12–20 K/mm) is common and does not necessarily indicate infection. Infection should not be excluded solely on the basis of white blood cell (WBC) count. Liver function tests are indicated in patients with abdominal pain or jaundice to further evaluate evidence of hemolysis, gall bladder, or liver end-organ damage. Urinalysis is needed to assess for infection as a precipitant for the acute pain crisis. Blood and urine cultures are only needed in patients in whom infection is suspected.

▶ Imaging

Several imaging modalities can aid in the diagnosis of severe sequela of vasoocclusive crises. When fever or respiratory signs or symptoms are present, a chest x-ray should be obtained to assess for signs of infection or infarction. Should pulmonary embolus be suspected, a helical contrast computed tomography (CT) can be performed. Patients with significant abdominal pain should undergo abdominal imaging to search for evidence of gallbladder or liver infarction or infection. Patients with new neurologic symptoms or signs should have a CT scan of the brain to assess for possible CVA.

PROCEDURES

An exchange transfusion is used to reduce vasoocclusion; the abnormal Hb is removed and replaced with normal donor blood. It is used during certain crises such as stroke and priapism when the hematocrit is greater than 35%. The procedure involves removing 500 mL (adult) through one intravenous (IV) line while simultaneously infusing 500 mL of normal saline (NS) through a second. After blood is removed the patient is given one unit of donor blood.

MEDICAL DECISION MAKING

The differential diagnosis associated with sickle cell vaso-occlusive crisis is broad. It includes acute chest, pneumonia, pulmonary embolism (PE), myocardial infarction (MI), cellulitis, osteomyelitis, and septic arthritis. The clinician must differentiate a simple pain crisis from one of these potential life threats. A high level of suspicion must be maintained in each case.

Bone and joint pain during a pain crisis does not usually present with limited range of motion. When joint range of motion deficits are present, the physician should be prompted to search for osteomyelitis or septic arthritis. Although an elevated WBC may be typical of a sickle cell pain crisis, a left shift would be more concerning for infection and necessitates a closer evaluation for an infectious process. A high index of suspicion for infection is always warranted. Localized left upper quadrant pain could indicate splenic infarction, whereas right upper quadrant pain may indicate cholecystitis. Electrocardiogram (ECG) findings consistent with acute MI or ischemia (ST-segment elevation, hyperacute T waves, T-wave inversions, ST-segment depression) should prompt further cardiac evaluation. Patients whose chest pain is atypical for their pain crisis and who also exhibit vital sign abnormalities or signs of right heart strain on the ECG should be evaluated for PE. Patients with altered mental status should be evaluated for severe anemia due to splenic sequestration, meningitis, CVA/transient ischemic attack (TIA), or seizure disorder (Figure 71-1).

TREATMENT

Any identifiable precipitants of pain crisis should be treated. Even if the patient does not appear dehydrated, fluids should be replaced. If unable to tolerate oral fluids, 5% dextrose with 0.45% NS is the fluid of choice for fluid replacement. NS boluses are reserved for the hypovolemic patient. A simple blood transfusion is indicated in patients with symptomatic anemia, sequestration crisis, hemolysis, or aplastic crisis. Exchange transfusion should be considered in severe vaso-occlusive crises such as acute chest syndrome, stroke, or priapism, where the Hgb level is >10.

▶ Pain Crises

Treatment should begin with prompt analgesic administration. Supplemental oxygen is needed only for patients with low oxygen saturations or those with oxygen saturations lower than baseline. Mild pain should be treated with 1 g of acetaminophen by mouth (PO) every 4 hours (children: 15 mg/kg/dose PO), codeine 0.5–1 mg/kg/dose PO, or ibuprofen 800 mg (children: 5–10 mg/kg/dose) PO every 8 hours. IV or intramuscular ketorolac has been shown to be effective with limitations in dosing frequency. Opiates are first-line therapy for a moderate to severe pain crisis. Morphine (0.1–0.15 mg/kg/dose) and hydromorphone (0.01–0.02 mg/kg/dose) are appropriate opiates to consider. Diphenhydramine is often required to blunt histamine-induced pruritus resulting from opiate administration.

▶ Infection

Antibiotics should be used for patients with suspected infection (eg, those with suspected meningitis, urinary tract infection, acute chest syndrome, or osteomyelitis).

▶ Anemia

Transfusion should be considered for symptomatic anemia and is generally indicated in cases in which the hemoglobin

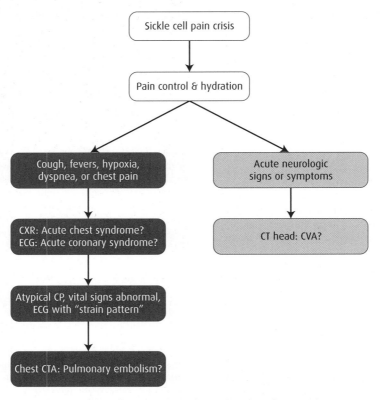

Figure 71-1. Sickle cell emergencies diagnostic algorithm. CP, chest pain; CT, computed tomography; CTA, computed tomography angiography; CVA, cerebrovascular accident; CXR, chest x-ray; ECG, electrocardiogram.

is <6 g/dL with an inappropriately low reticulocyte count. An acute crisis (acute chest, stroke, liver/gall bladder infarction, priapism) with hemoglobin <10 g/dL also merits transfusion. With regard to aplastic crisis, simple transfusion is often sufficient. Splenic sequestration is best treated with adequate hydration, analgesia, and simple transfusion. Refractory cases are treated with exchange transfusion.

Acute Chest Syndrome

Control pain, hydrate, and start oxygen therapy. Give empiric antibiotics consisting of a third-generation cephalosporin and a macrolide (eg, ceftriaxone and azithromycin). Triggers for transfusion should include a PaO_2 <70 mmHg or an oxygen saturation that falls >10% from their baseline.

Stroke

Patients with stroke related to SCD are not considered candidates for thrombolysis. Correction of hypovolemia, hypoxia, hypoglycemia, and fever are necessary. Exchange transfusion should be performed in an effort to reduce the percent of HbS to <30%. Hemorrhagic strokes warrant neurosurgical consultation.

Priapism

Hydrate, treat pain, and transfuse (refractory cases). After 4–6 hours of priapism and failure of ice packing, drainage may be necessary. Drainage should be done in conjunction with urologic consultation.

DISPOSITION

Admission

Criteria for admission include refractory pain, acute chest syndrome, CVA or TIA, unexplained fever >38.3°C or focal infection, aplastic crisis, splenic sequestration, or refractory priapism.

Discharge

If the patient's pain is well controlled and good outpatient follow-up is available, he or she may be discharged.

SUGGESTED READING

Baker M, Hafner JW. What is the best pharmacologic treatment for sickle cell disease in pain crises? *Ann Emerg Med.* 2012;59:515–516.

Claudius I. Sickle cell disease. In: Tintinalli JE, Stapczynski JS, Ma OJ, Cline DM, Cydulka RK, Meckler GD. *Tintinalli's Emergency Medicine: A Comprehensive Study Guide.* 7th ed. New York, NY: McGraw-Hill, 2011: 1480–1488.

Gladwin MT, Vichinsky E. Pulmonary complications of sickle cell disease. *N Engl J Med.* 2008;359, 2254–2265.

Kavanagh PL, Sprinz PG, Vinci SR, et al. Management of children with sickle cell disease: A comprehensive review of the literature. *Pediatrics* 2011;128:1552.

Rees DC, Williams TN, Gladwin MT. Sickle-cell disease. *Lancet* 2012;376, 2018–2031.

Roberts JR, Hedges JR. *Clinical Procedures in Emergency Medicine.* 5th ed. Philadelphia, PA: Saunders, 2009.

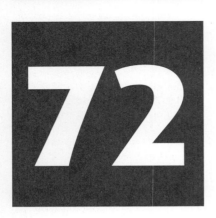

Transfusion Reactions

Christopher Reverte, MD

Jorge Fernandez, MD

Key Points

- Obtain consent when possible before administering blood transfusions and properly inform patients regarding the risk of developing complications.

- Always transfuse leukocyte-reduced blood products to recipients who are immunocompromised to prevent graft versus host disease.

- It may be difficult to clinically distinguish between benign (urticaria, simple febrile reactions) and more

- serious transfusion reactions (acute hemolysis, anaphylaxis, transfusion-associated acute lung injury, sepsis).

- Whenever a transfusion reaction is suspected, immediately stop the transfusion, confirm that the correct blood product was administered to the correct recipient, and send samples of the transfused product and the recipient's serum to the blood bank for further analysis.

INTRODUCTION

Emergency transfusion of blood products is often necessary in the emergency department (ED) for life-threatening illness or injuries. Commonly transfused blood products include packed red blood cells (PRBCs), platelets, fresh-frozen plasma (FFP), and cryoprecipitate. In the United States, approximately 30 million units of blood components are transfused annually. Approximately 1% of patients receiving transfusions will develop a transfusion-related reaction, the most common being a simple febrile reaction. Transfusion reactions must be rapidly identified to prevent morbidity and mortality.

Acute intravascular hemolysis is due to ABO blood group incompatibility between the donor and recipient. Preformed antibodies in the patient's serum react with antigens on the transfused PRBCs, resulting in complement-mediated intravascular RBC lysis. Patients present with chest pain, shortness of breath, back pain, fever, tachycardia, or shock. Complications include acute renal failure, disseminated intravascular coagulopathy (DIC), cardiovascular collapse, and death.

Delayed extravascular hemolysis is due to non-ABO blood group incompatibility between the donor and recipient.

This type of hemolysis is the result of splenic removal of RBCs, which may present days to weeks after the transfusion and in general is not life-threatening.

Simple febrile reaction is the most common type of transfusion-related reaction, occurring in about 1–7% of all transfusions. It is caused by recipient antibodies to donor leukocytes. The risk is minimized by leukoreduction. Patients present with fever *without* urticaria, bronchospasm, or shock.

Type I hypersensitivity reactions include urticaria and anaphylaxis. **Urticaria** is the result of a mild reaction due to recipient antibodies to donor blood. Patients present with hives and pruritus without fever, bronchospasm, or shock. **Anaphylaxis** is a life-threatening reaction seen most commonly in immunoglobulin A (IgA)-deficient individuals who are transfused IgA-containing blood. Patients rapidly develop fever, airway obstruction, bronchospasm, urticaria, and/or shock.

Transfusion-associated acute lung injury (TRALI) may result in a life-threatening noncardiogenic pulmonary edema. It is associated with anti-HLA antibodies (higher rates in pregnant donors). It most commonly occurs after plasma transfusion but can occur from transfusion of any type of plasma-containing blood product (including

PRBC, platelets, cryoprecipitate, etc). Signs and symptoms include fever, severe respiratory distress, noncardiogenic pulmonary edema and cardiovascular collapse.

Infectious complications to transfusion may be bacterial or viral. Bacterial infections are more common after platelet transfusion (stored at room temperature) and longer blood storage times. Organisms are most commonly skin or gastrointestinal flora. Diagnosis requires positive cultures from donor and recipient blood. Donor blood is prescreened for human immunodeficiency virus (HIV), hepatitis B virus (HBV), hepatitis C virus (HCV), cytomegalovirus (CMV), human T-lymphotropic virus (HTLV), West Nile virus (WNV), and parvovirus; nevertheless, there is a small risk of transmission of these pathogens (most commonly HCV) despite screening.

Massive transfusions put the patient at risk for developing coagulopathy, hyperkalemia, lactic acidosis, and hypothermia. Dilutional coagulopathy or thrombocytopenia can occur when >4 PRBCs are transfused within 1 hour or 10 units within 12 hours, without the addition of clotting factors or platelets. Hypocalcemia and metabolic alkalosis may occur due to the effect of citrate. Volume overload from transfusions is more common in the setting of underlying chronic cardiac or kidney disease as well as plasma transfusion. Patients present with acute pulmonary edema without fever or shock.

Graft-versus-host disease is a rare complication of transfusion seen in immunocompromised or familial recipients. It is associated with a very high mortality rate. Donor T lymphocytes attack recipient tissues. This complication is prevented by leukoreduction and irradiation. Patients may present with fever, rash, pneumonitis, abdominal pain, vomiting, diarrhea, transaminitis, and thrombocytopenia.

The incidence of transfusion-related complications is highlighted in Table 72-1.

Table 72-1. The incidence of PRBC transfusion reactions.

Acute	Incidence
Acute hemolysis	1 in 0.25–1 million
Anaphylaxis	1 in 20,000–150,000
Sepsis	1 in 5 million
TRALI	1 in 5,000–10,000
Simple febrile reaction	1 in 100
Minor allergic	1 in 1,000
Delayed	**Incidence**
Hepatitis B	1 in 137,000
Hepatitis C	1 in 1–2 million
HIV	1 in 2–3 million

CLINICAL PRESENTATION

▶ History

Fevers and chills may be seen in acute febrile reactions, acute intravascular hemolysis, anaphylaxis, sepsis due to bacterial contamination, or TRALI. Chest pain, shortness of breath, lightheadedness, or syncope may be seen in the same conditions. Isolated shortness of breath during transfusion is suggestive of volume overload, whereas generalized pruritus and rash (in the absence of other symptoms) suggests urticaria.

Risk factors for developing a transfusion-related reaction include immunocompromised recipients, those requiring massive transfusion, a history of receiving blood transfusions, preexisting congestive heart failure, or elderly patients. For example, recipients who are immunocompromised are at increased risk for graft-versus-host disease. Patients receiving massive transfusions are at significant risk for hypothermia and coagulopathy. Elderly patients or patients with congestive heart failure are at risk for pulmonary edema, particularly when blood products are transfused too rapidly. Also, patients who have been transfused blood products in the past are at increased risk of having preexisting antibodies, which may cause a variety of transfusion-related reactions. See the Introduction for classic presentations.

▶ Physical Examination

During transfusion, patients should be monitored closely for adverse reactions. New vital sign abnormalities that develop such as fever, hypotension, tachycardia, or tachypnea are all concerning for possible transfusion reaction. Even well-appearing patients who develop fever during transfusion should have the transfusion stopped and be closely monitored for more serious reactions, as they may quickly decompensate. In patients with hypotension, tachycardia, or tachypnea, it is difficult to distinguish ongoing hemorrhage (the underlying reason for many transfusions) from potentially life-threatening transfusion reactions including acute intravascular hemolysis, anaphylaxis, or sepsis. Classically, hypovolemic shock will cause cool extremities, whereas the shock states seen in acute intravascular hemolysis, anaphylaxis, or sepsis cause cardiovascular collapse and warm extremities. Patients receiving massive transfusions are at risk of hypothermia, which also may occur due to sepsis. Wheezing may be noted in anaphylaxis or pulmonary edema (due to volume overload or TRALI). Hives or rash is seen in anaphylaxis or urticaria. Dark pink or brown urine indicate hemoglobinuria after acute intravascular hemolysis.

DIAGNOSTIC STUDIES

▶ Laboratory

Laboratory studies are performed to document appropriate response to transfusion (eg, rise in hemoglobin) and to aid in identifying acute intravascular hemolysis, sepsis, or other symptoms that develop acutely during a transfusion. Transfusions should always be held pending these results, and the laboratory should be notified to test samples of both donor and recipient blood. Most hospitals have protocols to ensure that the correct blood is transfused to the correct patient and to manage a possible transfusion reaction.

Basic laboratory tests are generally not helpful in acute febrile reactions, urticaria, anaphylaxis, TRALI, or volume overload. Their utility in the ED is in identifying acute intravascular hemolysis or sepsis. In acute hemolytic reactions, complete blood count (CBC) may reveal worsening anemia and schistocytes. Other laboratory findings include a positive Coombs test, acute renal failure, DIC, and/or elevated haptoglobin, bilirubin, and lactate dehydrogenase levels. Hemoglobinuria may be seen on urinalysis.

If sepsis is suspected, Gram stain and blood cultures should be ordered. CBC may reveal leukocytosis or leukopenia; however, sepsis cannot be ruled out definitely in their absence.

During massive transfusion, dilutional thrombocytopenia or coagulopathy, metabolic acidosis, and hypocalcemia may occur.

▶ Imaging

In suspected cases of TRALI or volume overload, a chest x-ray may demonstrate acute pulmonary edema. In general, patients with volume overload will have cardiomegaly, whereas patients with TRALI will have a normal-heart size. Bedside ultrasound may help differentiate volume overload from TRALI. Volume overload is associated with poor cardiac contractility and inferior vena cava distension, whereas in TRALI, both of those features would be normal.

MEDICAL DECISION MAKING

Different transfusion reactions present similarly; however, it is important to differentiate which type of reaction is occurring to appropriately direct treatment and disposition (Figure 72-1). If there is any suspicion of a transfusion reaction, the first step is to stop the transfusion.

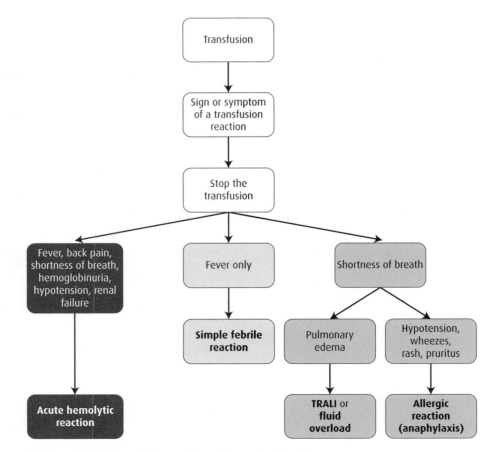

▲ **Figure 72-1.** Transfusion reactions diagnostic algorithm.

If the patient experiences a fever with no other signs or symptoms, a simple febrile reaction is likely. However, it may be difficult clinically to distinguish between other causes of fever during transfusions, including acute intravascular hemolysis, sepsis, or TRALI. The differential for hypotension during transfusion includes ongoing hemorrhage, hemolytic transfusion reaction, anaphylaxis, sepsis from bacterial contamination, and TRALI. Shortness of breath is seen in anaphylaxis, hemolytic transfusion reaction, volume overload, TRALI, and sepsis. Wheezing may be noted in anaphylaxis, volume overload, or TRALI.

Anaphylaxis is often associated with urticaria (unlike acute intravascular hemolysis or sepsis) and usually is not associated with fever. Volume overload or TRALI may present with isolated shortness of breath, pulmonary edema, and/or hypoxia without other systemic findings such as fever or hypotension. A high index of suspicion and broad differential is required in all cases, particularly when the patient experiences any new symptom in the setting of current or recent transfusion.

TREATMENT

When blood products are being transfused, they should be administered at a slow rate for the first 30 minutes to allow for early identification of a possible reaction. If a transfusion reaction is suspected, the first step is to immediately STOP the transfusion. Check the labels on the blood products and patient, and send blood samples from both the patient and the blood products to the blood bank for further analysis. Treatment modalities for each individual type of reaction follow.

Acute intravascular hemolysis. Stop the transfusion immediately. Resuscitate volume aggressively with crystalloid intravenous (IV) fluid. Administer diuretics to maintain urine output 1–2 mL/kg/hr. Vasopressors should be initiated if hypotension is refractory to IV fluids. Send blood and urine specimens to the lab per hospital protocol.

Anaphylaxis. Stop the transfusion immediately. Rapidly resuscitate with crystalloid IV fluids and administer epinephrine 0.3 mg (1:1,000) subcutaneously (SQ)/intramuscularly (IM), methylprednisolone 125 mg IV, diphenhydramine 50 mg IV, famotidine 20 mg IV, and albuterol 5 mg in 3 mL of saline nebulizer. Repeat epinephrine as needed, and consider starting an epinephrine drip if necessary.

Sepsis. Stop the transfusion immediately. Pan-culture the patient and treat with copious crystalloid IV fluids, broad-spectrum antibiotics, and vasopressors as needed for refractory hypotension. Follow the appropriate sepsis protocol at your institution.

TRALI. Stop the transfusion immediately. Administer oxygen and gently diurese. Many patients require noninvasive positive pressure ventilation, and severe cases may require intubation and mechanical ventilation.

Massive transfusion coagulopathy. Administer FFP and platelets to reverse coagulopathy and thrombocytopenia. Some hospitals have protocols in massive PRBC transfusion that include platelets and FFP in fixed ratios. Treat hypothermia by warming all blood products to room temperature, coadministration of warm crystalloid IV fluid, and external rewarming measures such as warming blankets. Treat hypocalcemia with IV calcium gluconate.

Simple febrile reaction. Stop the transfusion. Treat with antipyretics such as acetaminophen. Restart the transfusion only after ruling out acute hemolysis or sepsis from bacterial contamination.

Urticaria. Treat with an antihistamine such as diphenhydramine, and consider a short course of steroids if the rash is severe. The transfusion does *not* need to be stopped if isolated urticaria occurs, without fever or anaphylaxis.

Delayed extravascular hemolysis. Usually no specific treatment is required; often observed as outpatient.

Graft-versus-host disease. Bone marrow transplantation is the only effective treatment. Prevention is the most useful strategy by transfusing leukocyte-reduced blood in immunocompromised or related recipients.

DISPOSITION

▶ Admission

Patients with persistent vital sign abnormalities or ongoing hemorrhage require admission to a monitored setting in a telemetry or intensive care unit. Additionally, any patients with findings of intravascular hemolysis, anaphylaxis, sepsis, TRALI, massive transfusion reactions, or volume overload should be admitted to a monitored setting.

▶ Discharge

Although many patients receiving blood transfusions in the ED already require admission, hemodynamically stable patients without ongoing hemorrhage may be safely discharged home in the absence of a transfusion reaction. Patients who experience a simple febrile reaction or urticarial rash may require a period of observation, but can still be discharged safely in most circumstances.

SUGGESTED READING

Coil CJ, Santen SA. Transfusion therapy. In: Tintinalli JE, Stapczynski JS, Ma OJ, Cline DM, Cydulka RK, Meckler GD. *Tintinalli's Emergency Medicine, A Comprehensive Study Guide.* 7th ed. New York, NY: McGraw-Hill, 2011, pp. 1493–1500.

Emery M. and blood components. In: Marx JA, Hockberger RS, Walls RN. *Rosen's Emergency Medicine, Concepts and Clinical Practice.* 7th ed. Philadelphia, PA: Mosby Elsevier, 2010, pp. 42–46.

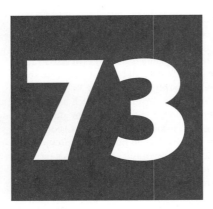

Anticoagulant Therapy and Its Complications

Joanne C. Witsil, PharmD

Key Points

- In the anticoagulated patient, have a low threshold to obtain imaging studies after trauma.
- When initiating warfarin therapy, coadministration with heparin or low-molecular-weight heparin (3–5 days) is necessary to avoid a paradoxical hypercoagulable state.

- When the international normalized ratio (INR) is supratherapeutic in a patient who is not bleeding, a cautious approach to vitamin K administration is important. Administering excess vitamin K may overcorrect the INR, leaving the patient refractory to further anticoagulation.

INTRODUCTION

Use of anticoagulation therapy and complications related to their usage are frequently encountered in the emergency department (ED). Anticoagulant therapies commonly seen include **heparin**, **low-molecular-weight heparin (LMWH)**, **warfarin**, and the direct thrombin inhibitor **dabigatran etexilate.** These agents are used frequently in patients with acute coronary syndrome (ACS), venous thromboembolism (VTE), valve replacement, and atrial fibrillation (AF). When administered in the appropriate clinical setting, anticoagulant medications prevent morbidity and mortality. For example, the risk of stroke in patients with AF and structural heart disease is 5% a year but is reduced by 70% with the use of chronic oral anticoagulation therapy.

Anticoagulants are not without complications, however. In patients taking warfarin, up to 15% will suffer a bleeding complication, 4.9% will develop a major bleeding complication, and approximately 1% will develop a fatal complication annually. The risk of a bleeding complication from heparin use is approximately 6% and is no different than the risk of bleeding from LMWH.

Heparin is a mixture of glycosaminoglycan chains of varying lengths that binds to antithrombin III, resulting in inhibition of thrombin and coagulation factors II, IX, X, XI, and XII. LMWH is prepared from unfractionated

heparin and includes only short chains. LMWH binds to antithrombin III but inhibits only factor X. LMWH is advantageous because it has a more predictable dose response and greater bioavailability. **Heparin-induced thrombocytopenia** (HIT) is due to immunoglobulin G (IgG) antibody that binds platelets and results in their activation, creating both thrombocytopenia and thrombosis. Typically, the onset of HIT is generally 5–12 days after onset of therapy. The incidence of HIT is 1–3% in patients treated with unfractionated heparin, but is much less common in patients taking LMWH.

Warfarin inhibits the cofactor of vitamin K, which normally allows for the production of anticoagulants (protein C and S) and coagulants (factors II, VII, IX, and X). Because protein C has a half-life that is much shorter than the half-life of factors II, VII, IX, and X, a hypercoagulable state is seen first, necessitating the coadministration of unfractionated or LMWH until warfarin has reached its full anticoagulant potential after 5 days. Dabigatran etexilate directly and competitively binds to free and clot-bound thrombin, which prevents further clot formation.

CLINICAL PRESENTATION

▶ History

Consider the reason the patient has presented to the ED as it relates to their anticoagulant use.

Gastrointestinal (GI) bleeding is a common complication and may not be noticed by the patient; therefore, inquire about blood in the stool or melena. Any history of trauma, especially head trauma, should be taken very seriously in the patient on anticoagulant medications. Intracranial bleeding is the most common fatal bleeding complication related to anticoagulation therapy.

If a bleeding complication is occurring, make sure to have investigated why the patient is taking anticoagulant therapy. Patients who have had a recent VTE or a prosthetic heart valve have a greater need for anticoagulation than a patient with isolated AF. This information is extremely useful when there is a severe bleeding complication that requires reversal of anticoagulation.

Consider coadministration of additional medications to patients already taking warfarin that will either increase or decrease the anticoagulant effects. Medications that increase the international normalized ratio (INR) include several antibiotics, nonsteroidal anti-inflammatory drugs, prednisone, cimetidine, amiodarone, and propanolol. A decrease in INR is induced by carbamazepine, barbiturates, haloperidol, and ranitidine. Additionally, several herbal medications may also increase or decrease the INR.

Lastly, assess for risk factors that increase the patient's chance of bleeding. For patients on warfarin, risk factors include INR >4.0, age >75 years, prior history of GI bleed, hypertension, cerebrovascular disease, renal insufficiency, alcoholism, and known malignancy. Risk factors for bleeding in patients on heparin or LMWHs include increasing dose, degree of elevation of partial thromboplastin time (PTT), recent surgery or trauma, renal failure, use of another anticoagulant (aspirin, glycoprotein inhibitor), and age >70 years.

▶ Physical Examination

Abnormal vital sign that suggest hypovolemia and shock should be addressed immediately in a patient with a bleeding complication. Look for any evidence of head trauma. Sublingual or neck hematomas are airway emergencies, especially if they are expanding. During the cardiovascular exam, listen for murmurs or an irregular heart rhythm that suggests AF. Tenderness during the abdominal exam may suggest intraperitoneal hemorrhage. A rectal examination is indicated to diagnose GI bleeding. Conduct a thorough skin assessment because patients recently started on warfarin may develop warfarin skin necrosis due to capillary thrombosis in the subcutaneous tissues. Patients with HIT may also develop similar skin lesions. Ecchymosis and hematomas should be noted.

DIAGNOSTIC STUDIES

▶ Laboratory

General laboratory studies include a complete blood count (to detect anemia and thrombocytopenia) and a prothrombin time, INR, and PTT. In addition, get a basic metabolic panel to assess renal function.

▶ Imaging

Lower the threshold to obtain an imaging study in patients on anticoagulant medications. Any patient taking oral anticoagulation therapy who suffers minor or major head trauma with or without a headache should have a head computed tomography (CT) scan to rule out intracranial hemorrhage.

MEDICAL DECISION MAKING

History, physical examination, and laboratory studies may be sufficient to arrive at a diagnosis of an anticoagulation complication. However, when indicated, intracranial, splenic, liver or retroperitoneal bleeding should be ruled out with CT. If skin lesions are noted, consider the diagnosis of warfarin skin necrosis or HIT.

TREATMENT

For patients starting on heparin therapy due to VTE disorders, the therapy begins with an 80 IU/kg bolus followed by continuous infusion of 18 IU/kg/hr. For patients receiving treatment for acute coronary syndrome or on fibrinolytic therapy or a glycoprotein inhibitor, the dose is reduced 60 IU/kg bolus, 12 IU/kg/hr infusion. PTT is measured 6 hours after initiation of the bolus, with a goal of 1.5–2.5 times normal. When clinically significant bleeding is present, stop the heparin infusion. Anticoagulation lasts up to 3 hours after the infusion is stopped. If major bleeding occurs, administer protamine (1 mg/100 IU heparin) intravenously (IV), given slowly over 5–10 minutes to a maximum dose of 50 mg.

Enoxaparin is the most commonly prescribed LMWH in the ED. The most common dosing regimen is 1 mg/kg subcutaneously every 12 hours. Dosing will need to be adjusted in morbidly obese patients or those in renal failure. Protamine (1 mg/1 mg enoxaparin) can be administered to a maximum dose of 50 mg when reversal is indicated, but reversal is not as effective as with unfractionated hepar in. If major or life-threatening bleeds occur, consider giving blood products such as PRBC and FFP.

If warfarin therapy is being initiated in the ED, the usual starting dose is 5 mg by mouth daily. Lower doses are usually required in the elderly, in patients with liver disease, or those with poor nutrition. The therapeutic range for the INR depends on the indication. Patients with mechanical valves are considered therapeutic at INR levels of 2.5–3.5, whereas other patients (eg, with AF or VTE) are therapeutic at INR levels of 2–3.

Management of bleeding complications or supratherapeutic INR with warfarin is outlined in Figure 73-1.

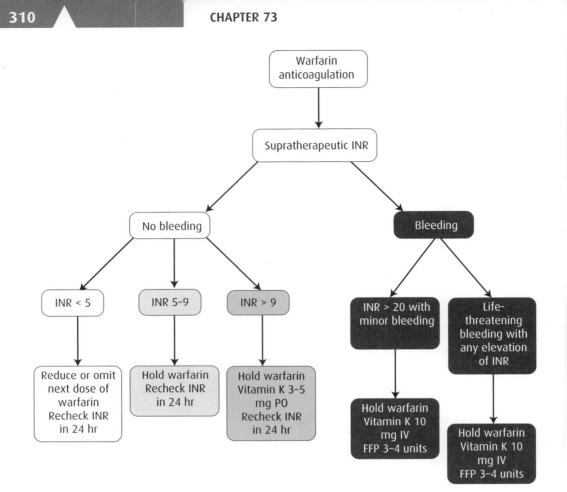

▲ **Figure 73-1.** Anticoagulant therapy and its complications diagnostic algorithm for supratherapeutic INR from warfarin. FFP, fresh-frozen plasma; INR, international normalized ratio; IV, intravenous; PO, by mouth.

For reversal, IV administration of vitamin K is most rapid, with onset within 1-2 hours, compared with 6–10 hours for oral dosing. Administer IV vitamin K over 30 minutes to minimize the small risk of anaphylaxis. Higher doses of vitamin K (10 mg) may result in warfarin resistance (up to 1 week) when it is time to restart anticoagulation therapy. FFP is used as the first-line agent for reversal of bleeding due to warfarin. The initial dose is 2–4 units. Consider giving other products such as prothrombin complex concentrate (PCC) and recombinant factor VIIa.

The oral direct thrombin inhibitor dabigatran is not routinely started in the ED. However, more patients are presenting to the ED on dabigatran with bleeding complications. Currently there is no antidote for the reversal of bleeding complications associated with its use. Therefore, clinical management consists of stopping the medication, and if a major or life-threatening bleed occurs, consider giving FFP, PRBC, or some in vitro studies suggest PCC or recombinant factor VIIa.

DISPOSITION

▶ Admission

A patient requiring anticoagulation therapy with heparin is usually admitted to the hospital for coadministration with warfarin. This is to prevent the hypercoagulable state that occurs in the early phase of warfarin treatment. Patients with a supratherapeutic INR and bleeding require admission. Patients with a supratherapeutic INR who have a poor social situation or are at risk of falling should also be admitted.

▶ Discharge

A patient with no other admission indications who requires anticoagulation may be discharged with warfarin and a 7-day course of LMWH injections. Close follow-up should be arranged within 24–48 hours, and the patient must be knowledgeable about self-injecting. Patients with supratherapeutic INR without bleeding are frequently safe to discharge if they are not at increased risk of falling.

SUGGESTED READING

Agena W, Gallus AS, Wittkowsky A, et al. Oral Anticoagulant Therapy: Antithrombotic Therapy and Prevention of Thrombosis, 9th ed: American Collage of Chest Physicians Evidence-Based Clinical Practice Guidelines. *Chest.* 2012;141(Suppl):e44s–e88s.

Garcia DA, Baglin TP, Weitz JI, et al. Parenteral Anticoagulants: Antithrombotic Therapy and Prevention of Thrombosis, 9th ed: American Collage of Chest Physicians Evidence-Based Clinical Practice Guidelines. *Chest.* 2012;141(Suppl):e24s–e43s.

Slattery DE, Pollack CV. Anticoagulants, antiplatelet agents, and fibrinolytics. In: Tintinalli JE, Stapczynski JS, Ma OJ, Cline DM, Cydulka RK, Meckler GD. *Tintinalli's Emergency Medicine: A Comprehensive Study Guide.* 7th ed. New York, NY: McGraw-Hill, 2011, pp. 1500–1507.

Slit Lamp Examination

Douglas S. Franzen, MD

Nathan J. Lewis, MD

Key Points

- Familiarity with the controls is critical to performing a slit lamp examination.
- When positioning the patient for the exam, make sure that their forehead is touching the forehead brace and encourage them to keep it there.
- When using a slit lamp to remove a corneal foreign body, first guide the removal device (eg, 25-gauge needle) to the eye under direct vision, then switch to the magnified view.
- To prevent puncturing the cornea, keep the removal device tangential to the globe at all times.

INDICATIONS

The slit lamp is used to evaluate the anterior eye including the lids, lashes, conjunctiva, cornea, visible sclera, anterior chamber, iris, and lens for signs of trauma, hemorrhage, inflammation, or foreign bodies.

CONTRAINDICATIONS

The patient must be cooperative and capable of sitting upright for the duration of the examination.

EQUIPMENT

In addition to a slit lamp, the examiner will need 2 chairs or stools, preferably of about equal height. Fluorescein allows visualization of corneal injury. Other supplies may include anesthetic drops and a needle or ophthalmic burr (for foreign body removal), cotton-tipped applicators (for lid eversion), and saline (to flush the eyes or lids).

Ideally, one should be familiar with use of the slit lamp before examining a patient. The slit lamp is a microscope in which focus is achieved by moving the lenses instead of the object being examined. The power of the microscope typically ranges from 10–25× (or higher) and is adjusted by a dial on the housing just in front of the eyepieces. The plane of focus is changed by using the joystick to move the microscope toward or away from the patient. The joystick also moves the microscope left or right. Twisting the joystick raises or lowers the microscope. If the microscope does not move when the joystick is moved, you may need to loosen the locking screw on the microscope base.

The light source is mounted on a swing arm that allows it to move independently from the microscope. Knowing how to adjust the multiple controls of the light source is critical to performing an exam. The power switch activates the lamp. Many slit lamps also have a rheostat (dimmer), usually near the power switch or on the base of the microscope. A selector switch near the base of the bulb housing allows the examiner to change from white to cobalt blue light (other options, including green, are usually available). Just below this is a dial to adjust the height of the light beam. Near the base of the microscope arm is another dial to adjust the width of the slit. The location of these controls may vary from lamp to lamp. Figure 74-1 demonstrates their position on one model.

PROCEDURE

The patient should be seated and the height of the slit lamp adjusted so the patient can place his or her chin comfortably on the chinrest and forehead against the forehead brace. The height of the chinrest should be adjusted so that the patient's lateral canthus is aligned with the eye level mark

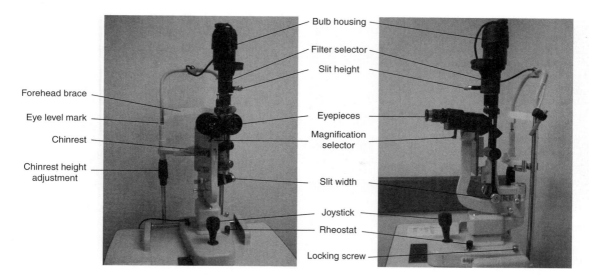

▲ **Figure 74-1.** Key components of the slit lamp.

on the chinrest support. The examiner should sit opposite the patient in a chair or stool of about the same height.

Ask the patient to close his or her eyes. Turn on the lamp with a white filter and adjust the brightness as needed. Move the microscope to grossly focus the beam on the patient's closed lid. Adjust the slit width to make the beam as narrow as possible without losing brightness. Swing the light source approximately 45 degrees to your right while leaving the microscope directly facing the patient. Ask the patient to open his or her eyes. When you look through the eyepieces, the image should be very close to focused. Two reflections will be visible: one that is curved and faint and, to the left of that, one that is straight and much brighter. The curved beam is reflecting off of the cornea. Adjust the microscope so this beam is crisply focused (usually by moving *slightly* toward the patient, about 1 mm). Protein deposits are often visible on the corneal surface when properly focused (Figure 74-2). Scan the left half of the patient's cornea by using the joystick. Move in an arc so the plane of focus follows the curve of the patient's cornea—closer to the patient as you approach the limbus and further from the patient as you move toward the pupil. Look for any corneal defects or foreign bodies. Check for ciliary flush (dilated pericorneal blood vessels, a sign of iridocyclitis) at the edges of the cornea. It may be necessary to have the patient look up, down, left, and/or right to fully view all parts of the cornea. After scanning the left half of the cornea, bring the microscope back to midline, swing the light source 45 degrees to your left, and examine the right half of the patient's cornea. The lids and conjunctiva can also be examined using this method, usually with a wider beam.

After examining the patient with white light, fluorescein should be instilled. Switch to the cobalt blue filter, widen the light beam slightly, and repeat the exam. Look for areas

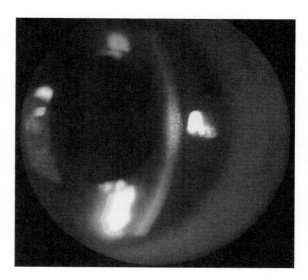

▲ **Figure 74-2.** Evaluating the corneal surface using a narrow beam at a 45-degree angle. The curved beam represents the reflection of light off the cornea. When the cornea is in focus, protein deposits are frequently visualized on its surface.

of fluorescein uptake (green fluorescence) that suggest corneal or conjunctival epithelial injury. Running or oozing of the fluorescein (Seidel sign) is caused by aqueous humor leaking from a full-thickness penetration of the cornea.

Evaluating the anterior chamber for cell and flare is the third part of the examination. The slit height should be decreased and the slit width increased to create a short, wide beam of white light. Swing the light source temporally, aiming the beam of light nasally through the anterior

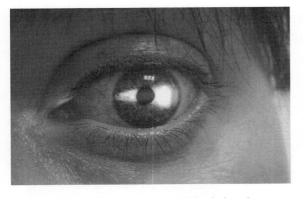

▲ **Figure 74-3.** The appearance of the light when evaluating for cell and flare.

chamber at the height of the pupil (Figure 74-3). Push the microscope forward until the patient's iris is in sharp focus, then move back *slightly* until the iris is out of focus—but not so far that the cornea comes into focus. The focal plane is now between the iris and cornea, in the anterior chamber. Using the pupil as a dark backdrop, watch for any material reflecting the light. Flare is caused by protein in the anterior chamber and creates a smoky appearance in the beam of light (a common analogy is "headlights in fog.") Cells will look like "dust particles in a sunbeam." The presence of either signifies inflammation of the anterior chamber. Use of dilating drops can cause cells to be present and applanation tonometry can cause flare, so slit lamp examination should be performed before these other tests.

If a foreign body (FB) is identified during the examination, first attempt to wash it out using saline. If this is not successful, it can be removed using a burr drill or a 25- or 27-gauge needle. Anesthetize the patient's eye using proparacaine or tetracaine. Be sure the patient's head is stabilized by full contact with the forehead brace and chin rest. Stabilize your hand on the patient's cheek or forehead so the removal device will track any movements the patient may make. Keep the removal device tangent to the surface of the patient's cornea. Guide it to the cornea under direct vision, switching to the eyepieces once the removal device is in view. If using a burr drill, press the side of the burr against the FB. When activated, the drill will "fling" the FB out of the cornea. If using a needle, place it on a small syringe (eg, insulin syringe) to provide better control. Guide the needle to the FB and use a scooping or flicking motion to pull the FB out of the cornea. *Always move tangential to the globe.*

COMPLICATIONS

When using the slit lamp and syringe/needle to remove an FB, careless attempts at removal or patient movement may result in penetration through the cornea. Additionally, in the setting of ocular trauma, avoid placing pressure on the eye when the possibility of a globe rupture exists. Excessive pressure may cause the intraocular contents to be extruded.

▼ Suggested Reading

Knoop K, Dennis W, Hedges J. Ophthalmologic procedures. In: Roberts JR, Hedges JR. *Roberts: Clinical Procedures in Emergency Medicine.* 5th ed. St. Louis, MO: Saunders, 2009, pp. 1141–1177.
Walker RA, Adhikari S. Eye emergencies. In: Tintinalli JE, Stapczynski JS, Ma OJ, Cline DM, Cydulka RK, Meckler GD. *Tintinalli's Emergency Medicine: A Comprehensive Study Guide.* 7th ed. New York, NY: McGraw-Hill, 2011, pp. 1517–1549.

Red Eye

Craig Huston, MD

Key Points

- Always begin with visual acuity, the vital sign of the eye.
- The patient should be instructed to remove contact lens and not to put them back in until the symptoms have resolved.
- The presence of pain and the relief of pain with instillation of anesthetic agents are helpful in determining the cause of red eye.

- Follow a systematic approach to the physical examination: visual acuity, lids and lashes, conjunctiva, sclera, cornea, pupil examination, and anterior chamber.
- Never prescribe topical steroids without consulting with an ophthalmologist.

INTRODUCTION

Eye complaints account for 3% of all emergency department (ED) visits. Red eye is a common complaint, and although most cases are benign, self-limited conditions, some may be vision-threatening. Conjunctivitis is the most common cause of a red eye, but other frequent problems include subconjunctival hemorrhage, corneal injuries (abrasions, keratitis, and foreign bodies), and acute uveitis.

Conjunctivitis may be viral, bacterial, or allergic. Viruses are the most frequent cause, especially adenovirus. The most common bacterial pathogens are *Staphylococcus aureus*, *Streptococcus pneumoniae*, and *Haemophilus influenzae*. *Chlamydia trachomatis* or *Neisseria gonorrhea* are unusual, but important causes of conjunctivitis. Allergic conjunctivitis is due to recurrent seasonal inflammation from allergen exposure. About 15% of the population will experience allergic conjunctivitis at one time in their life.

Subconjunctival hemorrhage is blood between the conjunctiva and sclera that results from a ruptured conjunctival blood vessel. Subconjunctival hemorrhage is caused by direct trauma or indirect injury. Although it may be alarming to the patient, it is usually a benign process that occurs with a sudden increase in pressure from sneezing, coughing, straining, or vomiting. If atraumatic, the etiology is usually hypertension or spontaneous rupture.

Corneal injury is common because the epithelium is thin and easily damaged. Corneal abrasions are particularly common, representing 10% of all ED visits for eye complaints. The cornea is resistant to infection, but when injured, a potential portal to bacteria is created. Viral infections that cause injury to the cornea include herpes simplex and varicella (ie, herpes zoster ophthalmicus). Contact lens use may predispose the patient to keratitis or a corneal ulcer due to gram-negative bacteria.

Acute anterior uveitis is defined as inflammation of the iris and ciliary body. The most common cause is trauma, with patients usually presenting 1–4 days after the precipitating event. Systemic causes include ankylosing spondylitis, Reiter syndrome, inflammatory bowel disease, and chronic granulomatous conditions like tuberculosis or sarcoidosis. Infectious ulcerations can also cause anterior uveitis.

CLINICAL PRESENTATION

History

The single most important historical feature that helps determine the cause of red eye is the presence of eye pain. Conjunctivitis is characterized by a gritty foreign body sensation and tearing or discharge, but it is usually not particularly painful. Viral (ie, adenovirus) and allergic sources tend to be pruritic with watery discharge, but suspect bacterial infection with mucopurulent discharge. An infectious source often begins unilaterally and spreads through autoinoculation. Constitutional symptoms such as fever, rhinorrhea, and myalgias suggest a systemic viral illness. Allergic conjunctivitis is associated with more intense itching and seasonal history.

Similarly, subconjunctival hemorrhage is a painless condition. Patients usually present to the ED merely because the appearance of blood on the sclera of the eye is concerning to the patient.

Eye pain is produced when the epithelium of the cornea is injured or there is inflammation to deeper structures (ie, iris). Corneal abrasions due to trauma or foreign body are characterized by pain, foreign body sensation, tearing, and photophobia. A history of working with power tools and metal should raise the suspicion of a foreign body. If the abrasion is large enough, patients may complain of decreased vision. Contact lens use or exposure to ultraviolet light should be ascertained and raises the suspicion for corneal inflammation/infection (ie, keratitis).

Acute anterior uveitis presents with a gradual onset of a painful red eye with severe photophobia and diminished vision. The patient will prefer to sit in a dark room with a hand over the eye.

▶ Physical Examination

The exam should always follow the same pattern: visual acuity, lids and lashes, conjunctiva, sclera, cornea, pupil, anterior chamber, and fluorescein staining. The characteristic findings in conjunctivitis, subconjunctival hemorrhage, corneal abrasion, and acute anterior uveitis are listed in Table 75-1. Additional characteristic features are listed here. Patients with conjunctivitis will have diffuse injection of the conjunctiva. With all causes of conjunctivitis, fluid can accumulate behind the conjunctiva known as chemosis (Figure 75-1). Allergic eyelids may be edematous and demonstrate bilateral cobblestone papillae.

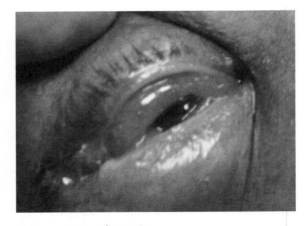

▲ **Figure 75-1.** Chemosis.

Subconjunctival hemorrhage has a characteristic appearance with bright red blood on the sclera under the thin conjunctival layer (Figure 75-2).

Corneal injury is signaled by uptake of fluorescein seen with the cobalt blue light. Corneal abrasions will affect

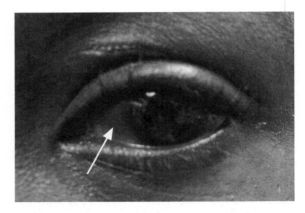

▲ **Figure 75-2.** Subconjunctival hemorrhage.

Table 75-1. Physical examination findings in patients with red eye.

Examination	Conjunctivitis	Subconjunctival Hemorrhage	Corneal Abrasion	Acute Anterior Uveitis
Visual acuity	Normal	Normal	Decreased when central	Decreased due to pain, tearing
Lids	Edema, erythema	Normal	Normal	Normal
Conjunctiva	Injection	Normal	Injection	Normal
Sclera	Normal	Erythema	Normal	Ciliary flush
Cornea (fluorescein uptake)	None, unless associated corneal ulcer	None	Yes	None
Pupil	Normal	Normal	Normal	Constricted
Anterior chamber (cell and flare)	None	None	None	Yes

visual acuity if large or there is central involvement. Lids should always be everted to look for a foreign body. If multiple lines of fluorescein uptake course together, this is highly suggestive of a foreign body under the lid that scratches the cornea with blinking. In herpes simplex virus (HSV) infection, a branching dendritic ulcer is characteristic, whereas involvement of the cornea in herpes zoster ophthalmicus causes a thin wavy lesion similar to tangled spaghetti. In patients with herpes zoster ophthalmicus, a zoster-form rash is present on the forehead in the V1 distribution of the trigeminal nerve. A bacterial cause of a corneal ulceration will also demonstrate significant uptake of fluorescein in the ulcer.

Acute anterior uveitis may affect visual acuity due to pain and tearing. The sclera may have a ciliary flush identified by redness at the limbus. No fluorescein uptake is seen, and pain is not improved with topical anesthetic application. The pupil is often constricted, and there is consensual photophobia (pain produced by shining light in the unaffected eye). On slit lamp exam, the anterior chamber will show "cell and flare." When cellular debris is significant, it can layer at the bottom of the anterior chamber between the cornea and iris. This collection is known as a hypopyon (Figure 75-3). Cell and flare and a hypopyon are also common with infectious causes of corneal ulceration.

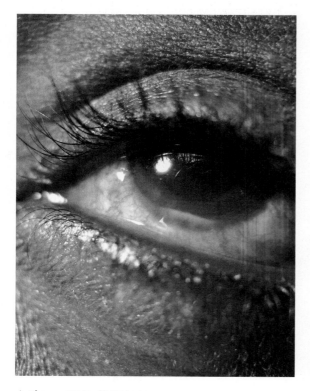

▲ **Figure 75-3.** Hypopyon.

MEDICAL DECISION MAKING

The presence of pain, response to topical anesthetic application, and the findings on the fluorescein examination are some of the most important features to determining the cause of a red eye (Figure 75-4).

TREATMENT

Uncomplicated conjunctivitis is treated with topical antibiotic drops or ointment if a bacterial source is suspected. Options include sulfacetamide, quinolones, aminoglycoside, trimethoprim, and polymyxin. The duration of treatment is 5–7 days. Remind patients of the importance of handwashing for at least 2 weeks to limit spread. Those who suffer from allergic conjunctivitis benefit from systemic antihistamines and histamine-blocking eye drops. For symptomatic relief, patients can use cool compresses and artificial tears. If *Chlamydia trachomatis* or *Neisseria gonorrhea* are suspected, patients will require systemic and topical antibiotics and must also have emergent ophthalmologic consult.

Patients with a subconjunctival hemorrhage need only reassurance that the blood will resolve within a couple weeks, similar to a bruise. If the patient has suffered recurrent subconjunctival hemorrhages, then consider coagulation studies and work-up for bleeding disorders.

Treatment of corneal injury depends on the cause. A patient with a corneal abrasion should be prescribed pain relief and infection prophylaxis. Patients benefit from a cycloplegic (cyclopentolate or homatropine) to relieve ciliary spasm and reduce pain. They will often need narcotic analgesia. To prevent secondary infections, prescribe a topical antibiotic such as 10% sulfacetamide.

Patients with herpes zoster ophthalmicus should receive oral acyclovir if treatment can be instituted within 72 hours of onset. Prompt treatment reduces the likelihood of eye involvement from 50% to 25%. Intravenous (IV) acyclovir is indicated for immunocompromised patients. Ophthalmology consultation is indicated. HSV is treated with topical antiviral drops, such as Viroptic, and consultation with an ophthalmologist. Corneal ulcers require emergent ophthalmologic consultation. Contact lens wearers should dispose of current lens and be given coverage for pseudomonas with a topical aminoglycoside or quinolone. The patient should not resume use of new lens until symptoms have resolved. Do not use an eye patch, as it is associated with an increased rate of corneal ulceration and pseudomonal infection. Tetanus prophylaxis should be updated.

Acute anterior uveitis treatment should be instituted only in consultation with an ophthalmologist, as continual monitoring and treatment is required. To eliminate ciliary spasm, use a long-acting cycloplegic such as 5% homatropine. To relieve inflammation, the

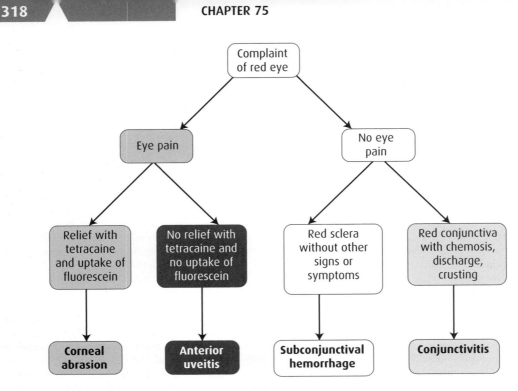

▲ **Figure 75-4.** Red eye diagnostic algorithm.

ophthalmologist may also recommend a topical steroid such as prednisolone.

DISPOSITION

▶ Admission

Patients with bacterial conjunctivitis secondary to *N. gonorrhea* should be admitted for IV antibiotic therapy. Consider admission of patients with corneal ulcers if the patient is unable to self-administer antibiotics, there is a high likelihood of noncompliance, or a large ulcer is present.

▶ Discharge

Patients with corneal abrasion, herpetic keratitis, and acute anterior uveitis should be re-evaluated by an ophthalmologist within 24–48 hours. Patients with simple conjunctivitis

and subconjunctival hemorrhage can be discharged to follow-up with their primary care physicians.

▼ **SUGGESTED READING**

Cronau H, et al. Diagnosis and management of red eye in primary care. *Am Fam Physician.* 2010;81:137–144.

Jackson WB. Acute Red Eye: Diagnosis and Treatment Guidelines. Ottawa, Ontario, Canada: University of Ottawa Eye Institute, 2004.

Kerns BL, Mason JD. Red eye: A guide through the differential diagnosis. *Emer Med.* 2004;36:31–40.

Leibowitz HM. The red eye. *N Engl J Med.* 2000;343:345–351.

Walker RA, Adhikari S. Eye emergencies. In: Tintinalli JE, Stapczynski JS, Ma OJ, Cline DM, Cydulka RK, Meckler GD. *Tintinalli's Emergency Medicine: A Comprehensive Study Guide.* 7th ed. New York, NY: McGraw-Hill, 2011, pp. 1517–1549.

Acute Visual Loss

Jordan B. Moskoff, MD

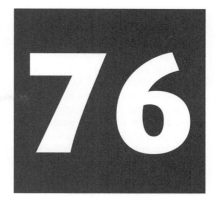

Key Points

- History and physical examination alone will lead to the diagnosis in most patients presenting with acute visual loss.
- The most important first step in addressing the patient with acute monocular visual loss is to determine whether the loss of vision is associated with pain.
- In patients with acute visual loss without pain, suspect central retinal artery occlusion (CRAO), central retinal vein occlusion (CRVO), or retinal detachment.
- Patients with acute visual loss with associated pain may have optic neuritis, temporal (giant cell) arteritis, acute angle-closure glaucoma, or a large central corneal abrasion or ulceration.
- An ophthalmologist should be consulted immediately when CRAO or acute angle-closure glaucoma are diagnosed in the emergency department.

INTRODUCTION

Central retinal artery occlusion (CRAO) and central retinal vein occlusion (CRVO) occur most frequently in elderly patients. About 90% of cases of CRVO occur in patients older than 50 years. CRAO is a result of a thrombotic plaque or more commonly an embolus of the central retinal artery, whereas CRVO is caused by thrombosis of the retinal vein.

Optic neuritis is a painful rapid reduction of central vision secondary to an inflammatory process of the optic nerve. Optic neuritis occurs more commonly in women aged 15 to 45 years. Retinal detachment results from traction of the vitreous humor on the retina. This causes a tear in the retina and a separation of the inner neuronal retina from the outer pigment epithelial layer. Retinal detachment may occur after ocular trauma, but in atraumatic cases, this condition is more prevalent in men >45 years old and in patients with significant myopia. The prevalence in the United States is 0.3%.

Temporal (giant cell) arteritis is a vasculitis that results in monocular loss of vision associated with a unilateral temporal headache. Temporal arteritis occurs most commonly in woman >50 years old. Whites are more frequently affected than are other races. Temporal arteritis is a vasculitis of medium and large arteries and can lead to optic nerve infarction and blindness.

Acute angle-closure glaucoma is a sudden painful monocular loss of vision secondary to increased pressure in the anterior chamber. Acute angle-closure glaucoma represents <10% of all cases of glaucoma in the United States. It is more common in women and is also more common in African American and Asian populations. Acute angle-closure glaucoma occurs in patients with shallow (narrow) anterior chamber angles. As the pupil dilates, the iris leaflet touches the lens. This impedes the flow of aqueous humor from the posterior to the anterior chamber with a subsequent increase in hydrostatic pressure.

CLINICAL PRESENTATION

▶ History

Painless, acute loss of vision is characteristic of CRAO, CRVO, and retinal detachment. In patients with CRAO, the monocular vision loss is usually complete and quite sudden. Risk factors include hypertension, carotid artery disease, diabetes mellitus, cardiac disease (especially atrial fibrillation and valvular disease), vasculitis, temporal arteritis, and sickle cell disease. Central retinal artery occlusion must be considered and treated early because irreversible visual loss occurs after 90 minutes.

The presentation of CRVO is more insidious than retinal artery occlusion. The patient will have a sudden painless monocular decrease in vision that is most commonly noted on awakening. Patients may also describe a sudden decrease, acutely imposed on a chronic gradual worsening over a longer period of time (eg, 1 week). Risk relates to likelihood of thrombosis. The physician should have increased suspicion in patients with diabetes mellitus, hypertension, arteriosclerosis, chronic glaucoma, and vasculitis.

Patients with retinal detachment present with painless loss of vision often described as a sensation of a curtain moving across the visual field or a shade being pulled down over the eye. Flashing lights, "spider webs," or "coal dust" in the visual field may precede visual loss. Risk is related most closely to severe myopia. Other risk factors include trauma, previous cataract surgery, family history, Marfan syndrome (or other inherited connective tissue disorders), and diabetes mellitus.

Painful loss of vision is seen in patients with optic neuritis, temporal arteritis, and acute angle closure glaucoma. Patients with optic neuritis will present with rapidly progressive reduction or blurring of their vision. Ocular pain worsens with eye movement. In patients without a previous diagnosis, 25–65% will develop multiple sclerosis.

Temporal arteritis presents as a sudden monocular loss of vision associated with a unilateral temporal headache. Eye pain usually is not present. Risk factors include polymyalgia rheumatica, female, Northern European descent, and >50 years old.

Lastly, acute angle-closure glaucoma presents as cloudy vision associated with halos around lights. In addition, the patient will complain of eye pain or headache along with nausea and vomiting and possibly abdominal pain. Often patients will have no previous history of glaucoma. Farsighted (hyperopic) persons are at risk secondary to the shape of their anterior chamber; female and elderly patients are also at increased risk.

▶ Physical Examination

For a full description of the physical examination of the eye, see Chapter 75. In acute visual loss, fluorescein staining is essential to exclude corneal abrasions or ulcerations; however, the funduscopic examination is usually most diagnostic. To perform the funduscopic exam, allow the patient to sit in a dark room for several minutes before starting. When the pupil is sufficiently dilated, ask the patient to focus on an object on the wall and ignore the examiner. Focus the ophthalmoscope on the eye and gradually approach the cornea from a lateral position. The optic disc is noted medially. If only vessels are seen, the optic disc can be located by knowing that the blood vessel's branches "point" to the direction of the disc.

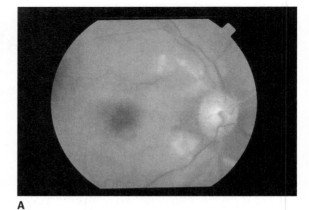

A

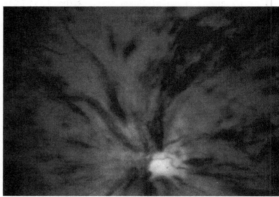

B

▲ **Figure 76-1. A.** Central retinal artery occlusion. **B.** Central retinal vein occlusion.

CRAO

Visual acuity is markedly decreased, with the patient often only able to perceive shadows or count fingers. Initial pupil examination may be normal; however, after 1–2 hours, the pupil may dilate. The pupil is poorly reactive to direct light but has a greater consensual response to light (afferent pupillary defect). On funduscopic examination, a pale retina with a cherry-red spotin the macular area (fovea) is the classic finding (Figure 76-1A).

CRVO

Visual acuity is variable but the deficit is usually less severe than retinal artery occlusion. The patient may retain the ability to see shadows or count fingers. The pupil will react sluggishly to light. On funduscopic examination, there may be retinal hemorrhage, tortuous retinal veins, and disc edema, referred to as "blood and thunder" (Figure 76-1B).

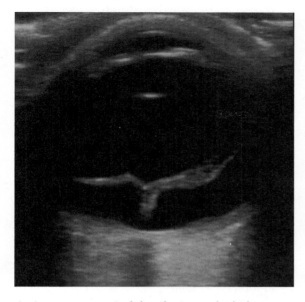

▲ **Figure 76-2.** Retinal detachment on bedside ultrasound.

Retinal detachment

The extent of the loss of vision is dependent on the degree of detachment. Visual field defects will be noted on confrontation. The pupil examination is unremarkable. Funduscopic examination reveals an undulating, dull grey, detached retina. Ocular ultrasound is a bedside procedure that is very helpful to making the diagnosis of retinal detachment (Figure 76-2).

Optic neuritis

Visual acuity varies from mildly reduced to no light perception. Often the visual deficit will be limited to the central visual field, and the patient will complain more of a defect with color vision rather than sight. This can be evaluated using the red desaturation test. Have the patient look at a dark red object with one eye and then test the other eye to see if the object looks the same color. The affected eye will often see the object as lighter or pink. An afferent pupillary defect will often be present. If the fundus is normal, the patient has retrobulbar optic neuritis. However, if the fundus is swollen or hyperemic, the patient has papillitis.

Temporal arteritis

Palpation may reveal tender, tortuous, and sometimes pulseless temporal arteries. The degree of loss of vision depends on when the diagnosis is made. If diagnosed late, visual acuity will be markedly decreased. An afferent pupillary defect may be present. On funduscopic examination, a pale, swollen optic disc will be present.

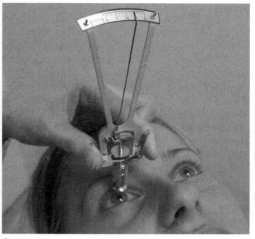

A

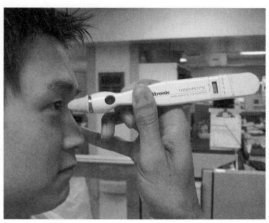

B

▲ **Figure 76-3. A.** Schiötz tonometer **B.** Tono-Pen.

Acute angle-closure glaucoma

Visual acuity is markedly decreased. The patient's sclera will be red due to ciliary injection. The cornea will be cloudy. On gentle palpation, the eye may have a rock hard consistency. The pupil is mid-dilated and nonreactive to light. Funduscopic examination is difficult to perform in the face of a cloudy cornea, but is otherwise unremarkable. To diagnose acute angle-closure glaucoma, intraocular pressure is measured with a Schiötz tonometer or Tono-Pen (Figure 76-3). Normal pressure is <20 mmHg. A pressure >40 mmHg is diagnostic.

DIAGNOSTIC FINDINGS

When temporal arteritis is suspected, an erythrocyte sedimentation rate (ESR) should be obtained. An ESR

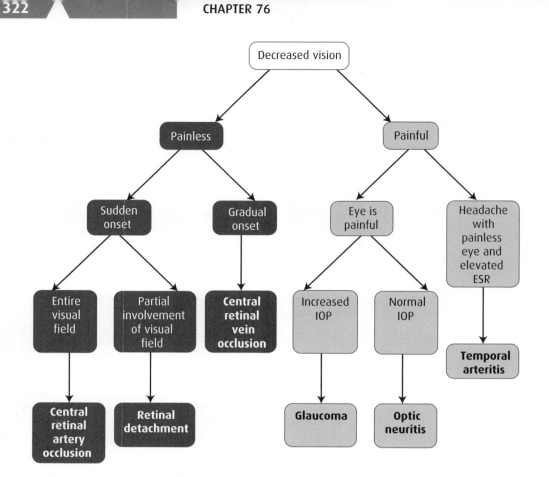

▲ **Figure 76-4.** Acute visual loss diagnostic algorithm. ESR, erythrocyte sedimentation rate; IOP, intraocular pressure.

>50 mm/hr is almost universally present in patients with temporal arteritis. Normal ESR for males is age/2; females (age + 10)/2.

MEDICAL DECISION MAKING

The first step is to determine the presence of pain associated with the acute visual loss (Figure 76-4). In the absence of pain, a history of complete sudden loss of vision versus a gradual decrease in vision in conjunction with the funduscopic examination should differentiate CRAO from CRVO. Preceding symptoms of a shade dropping or scotoma often aid in the diagnosis of retinal detachment. If retinal detachment is suspected, perform a bedside ultrasound of the eye.

If pain is associated with visual loss, then an elevated intra-ocular pressure suggests acute angle closure glaucoma. Temporal arteritis is likely when an elderly patient is complaining of headache and the ESR is elevated. Optic neuritis is best diagnosed by the funduscopic examination.

TREATMENT

Treatment of CRAO must begin as soon as the diagnosis is suspected because permanent visual loss typically occurs after 90 minutes. The goal of treatment is to restore retinal artery blood flow by dislodging the clot. This is accomplished by dilating the artery and reducing intraocular pressure through the following modalities: intermittent digital massage of the globe (5 seconds on, 5 seconds off) for 5–15 minutes; hyperventilation into a paper bag 10 minutes of every hour; acetazolamide 500 mg intravenously (IV) and a beta-blocker (timolol 0.5% drops intraocular). Immediate ophthalmology consultation is paramount for paracentesis (aspiration of aqueous fluid) of the anterior chamber.

CRVO is not as emergent as CRAO because no immediate treatment is effective. Patients should be referred to ophthalmology for confirmation of the diagnosis and monitoring of disease progression.

Patients diagnosed with retinal detachment require immediate ophthalmology consultation to evaluate for retinal reattachment surgery. The patient should be instructed to avoid activity and remain on bed rest until seen by an ophthalmologist.

Optic neuritis is treated with a short course of high-dose IV methylprednisolone followed by a rapid oral taper of prednisone. This provides a rapid recovery of symptoms in the acute phase. This treatment may also delay the short-term development of MS.

Temporal arteritis treatment begins with oral prednisone (80 mg/day) initiated in the ED when the diagnosis is suspected. Follow-up with an ophthalmologist for evaluation and a temporal artery biopsy should be arranged.

Treatment of acute angle-closure glaucoma consists of the sequential administration of several agents to decrease intraocular pressure: beta-blocker (Timoptic 0.5%) 1 drop; α agonist (Iopidine 0.1%) 1 drop; acetazolamide 500 mg by mouth or IV; steroid (pred forte 1%) 1 drop; mannitol 1–2 g/kg IV. Pilocarpine 1–2% is administered to constrict the pupil and pull the iris back, helping to prevent a recurrence. The unaffected eye should be treated prophylactically. Consult ophthalmology immediately because the definitive treatment is bilateral laser iridectomy.

DISPOSITION

▶ Admission

Optic neuritis is frequently managed as an inpatient for treatment and an expedited work-up, including magnetic resonance imaging. CRAO, retinal detachment, and acute angle-closure glaucoma require immediate ophthalmology consultation. Admission is required when definitive treatment cannot be accomplished in the ED.

▶ Discharge

Temporal arteritis can be managed on an outpatient basis after the initiation of steroids if the patient has appropriate follow-up. CRVO is managed on an outpatient basis with ophthalmology referral.

SUGGESTED READING

Graves JS, Galetta SL. Acute visual loss and other neuro-opthalmologic emergencies: Management. *Neurol Clin.* 2012;30:75–99.

Vortmann, M, Schneider JI. Acute monocular visual loss. *Emerg Med Clin North Am.* 2008;26:73–96.

Walker RA, Adhikari S. Eye emergencies. In: Tintinalli JE, Stapczynski JS, Ma OJ, Cline DM, Cydulka RK, Meckler GD. *Tintinalli's Emergency Medicine: A Comprehensive Study Guide.* 7th ed. New York, NY: McGraw-Hill, 2011, pp. 1517–1549.

Epistaxis

Emily L. Senecal, MD

Key Points

- Anterior epistaxis is more common than posterior epistaxis.
- Anterior epistaxis generally stops with pressure, but may require nasal packing.

- Posterior epistaxis requires emergent ear, nose, and throat consultation and admission.
- Any patient who requires nasal packing should be given antibiotics to prevent toxic shock syndrome or sinusitis.

INTRODUCTION

Epistaxis is common, occurring in 1 of every 7 persons in the United States. The incidence is highest in persons aged 2–10 and 50–80 years. Epistaxis, like all hemorrhage, needs prompt evaluation and treatment. The primary goal of diagnosis is to determine the location of bleeding: anterior versus posterior. Once the site of bleeding is identified, bleeding is stopped using various techniques ranging from chemical cautery (ie, silver nitrate) to nasal packing. Anterior epistaxis accounts for 90% of nosebleeds. Most commonly, the bleeding is venous from Kiesselbach plexus, which is located along the anteroinferior nasal septum. Posterior epistaxis typically originates from the posteroinferior turbinate and is more commonly arterial in origin, from the sphenopalatine artery. Posterior epistaxis represents 10% of nosebleeds.

CLINICAL PRESENTATION

▶ History

Determine the onset and duration to assess severity of blood loss. Inquire about comorbidities and medications, especially blood thinners and antiplatelet drugs. Identify mechanisms already used by the patient to attempt to stop the bleeding.

The most common etiologies of anterior epistaxis are trauma, dehumidification of the nasal mucosa (typically from dry air during winter months), and digital manipulation. Other common causes include allergies, nasal sprays,

illicit drugs, and nasal infections. Posterior epistaxis is more common in elderly debilitated patients with comorbid diseases such as a coagulopathy, atherosclerosis, neoplasm, or hypertension.

PHYSICAL EXAMINATION

Inspect the nares to identify the site of bleeding. A nasal speculum is useful to enhance visualization of the nares. If the site of bleeding cannot be identified, have the patient pinch the anterior soft portion of the nose, and examine the patient's oropharynx. If blood is trickling down the oropharynx while the patient is holding anterior pressure, a posterior bleed may be present.

DIAGNOSTIC STUDIES

▶ Laboratory

Blood work is not indicated in the majority of patients with epistaxis. Obtain a complete blood count in patients at risk for thrombocytopenia or anemia. Obtain coagulation studies in patients taking the anticoagulant warfarin and in patients with cirrhosis. Perform blood typing for patients with severe bleeding who may require transfusion.

▶ Imaging

Imaging studies are rarely indicated in the work-up and treatment of epistaxis. Angiography with interventional radiology embolization can be utilized in rare cases of refractory posterior bleeding from the sphenopalatine and greater palatine arteries.

MEDICAL DECISION MAKING

The mainstay of epistaxis evaluation and treatment is identification of the source of the bleed to facilitate prompt and effective treatment. Bleeding that ceases with pressure over the anterior soft portion of the nose is typically from an anterior source. A posterior bleed is suspected when blood continues to drain down the posterior pharynx while the anterior portion of the nose is being squeezed (Figure 77-1).

TREATMENT

If bleeding is significant, insert an intravenous line and place the patient on a cardiac monitor. Intubation is rarely necessary, but indicated if bleeding is severe and is compromising the airway. Consult ear, nose, and throat (ENT) immediately in cases with severe bleeding.

If an anterior bleed is suspected, have the patient hold continuous pressure over the soft cartilaginous portion of the nose for 15 minutes. During this time, assemble equipment including nasal speculum, headlight, suction, vasoconstrictor, lubricant, and anterior packing or balloon (Figure 77-2). If the bleeding has subsided after 15 minutes, gently apply

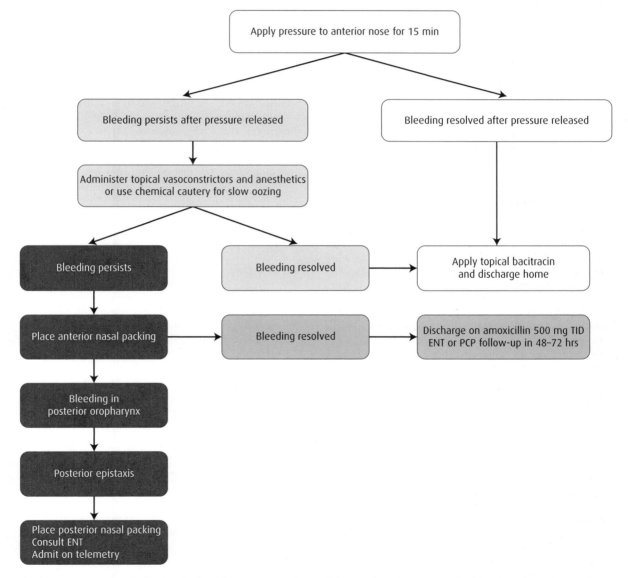

▲ **Figure 77-1.** Epistaxis diagnostic algorithm. ENT, ear, nose and throat; PCP, primary care physician; TID, three times a day.

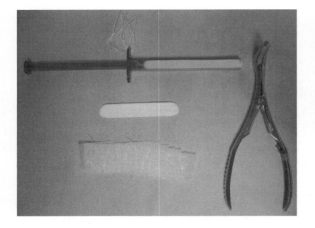

▲ **Figure 77-2.** Left, from top to bottom, anterior packs include the Rhino Rocket, Merocel, and petroleum gauze. Right, nasal speculum.

bacitracin to the anterior naris and discharge the patient. If bleeding is ongoing after 15 minutes of direct pressure, initiate topical vasoconstriction with oxymetazoline (Afrin) spray and topical anesthesia by inserting pledgets soaked in 2% lidocaine or 4% cocaine. Then hold pressure for 10–15 minutes and reassess. If slow bleeding persists, consider chemical cautery with silver nitrate sticks. Roll the stick over the area until a gray eschar is formed. Never hold the stick in one place for longer than 5 seconds, and never use silver nitrate bilaterally due to risk for nasal septal perforation.

If topical vasoconstrictors and cautery fail to stop the bleeding, pack the naris with petroleum gauze, a compressed sponge (Merocel or Rhino Rocket), or an anterior epistaxis balloon. When using a compressed sponge, apply lubricant to the sponge before inserting it into the nose, and use approximately 10 mL of saline to expand the sponge once it is in the nostril. Hemostatic material (Surgicel, Gelfoam, topical thrombin) may also be useful in controlling hemorrhage. Patients with nasal packing should be treated with prophylactic antibiotics (amoxicillin 500 mg orally 3× a day) against staphylococci to prevent toxic shock syndrome, sinusitis, and otitis media. Patients with nasal packing should follow-up with ENT or with their primary care physician in 2–3 days.

Posterior epistaxis is more challenging to treat because it is difficult to tamponade the site of bleeding, because the bleeding is often arterial, and because patients with posterior bleeds frequently have significant comorbidities. If a posterior bleed is suspected, consult ENT. In the meantime, attempt tamponade using a balloon device or a Foley catheter (Figure 77-3).

To tamponade using a balloon device, after applying topical anesthesia and vasoconstriction to the naris, apply lubricant to the catheter and insert the catheter into the nose until the tip is seen in the oropharynx. Inflate the posterior balloon with 4–8 mL of sterile saline; then pull the device

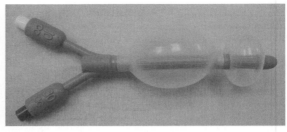

▲ **Figure 77-3.** Epistat nasal catheter for posterior epistaxis. The 30-mL balloon tamponades the anterior naris, and the 10-mL balloon is used to provide posterior tamponade of bleeding.

anteriorly to tamponade the bleeding. Inflate the anterior balloon with 10–25 mL of sterile saline. Assess the posterior oropharynx to assure cessation of bleeding. To tamponade using the Foley catheter method, obtain a 14F Foley with 30-mL balloon. Cut the tip of the catheter just *distal* to the balloon. Suction, anesthetize, and vasoconstrict the naris. Insert the catheter into the nose until the tip is seen in the oropharynx. Inflate the balloon with 10–15 mL of sterile saline. Pull back on the catheter until bleeding has stopped. Place an anterior pack. Use gauze to secure the catheter and prevent pressure necrosis on the nasal tip. If not done already, consult ENT. As with anterior bleeds, place patients with nasal packing on prophylactic antibiotics.

DISPOSITION

▶ Admission

Admission to a monitored setting is indicated for patients with posterior epistaxis, even if hemorrhage is controlled. Severe bleeding and fatal airway obstruction secondary to dislodgment of the packing can occur. Although rare, patients may develop a nasopulmonary reflex, manifested by hypoxia, hypercarbia, dysrhythmias, or coronary ischemia secondary to posterior packing placement.

▶ Discharge

Discharge is appropriate for patients with anterior epistaxis once bleeding is controlled. Remember to prescribe antibiotics to patients who have nasal packing in place. Follow-up should be arranged in 2–3 days to have the packing removed.

▼ SUGGESTED READING

Kucik CJ, Klenney T. Management of epistaxis. *Am Fam Physician.* 2005;71:305–311.
Schlosser RJ. Epistaxis. *N Engl J Med.* 2009;360:784–789.
Summers SM, Bey T. Epistaxis, nasal fractures, and rhinosinisitis. In: Tintinalli JE, Stapczynski JS, Ma OJ, Cline DM, Cydulka RK, Meckler GD. *Tintinalli's Emergency Medicine: A Comprehensive Study Guide.* 7th ed. New York, NY: McGraw-Hill, 2011, pp. 1564–1572.

Dental Emergencies

Nicholas E. Kman, MD

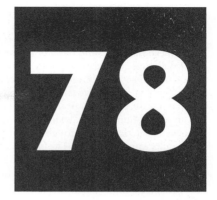

Key Points

- Dental caries are the most common dental emergency and can lead to pulpitis.
- Tooth fractures are categorized and treated according to the Ellis classification.
- Clean avulsed teeth with care to avoid dislodging the periodontal ligament.
- Permanent teeth that are avulsed should be reimplanted immediately; avulsed primary teeth are never reimplanted.
- Ludwig angina is a surgical emergency that requires prompt drainage.

INTRODUCTION

Dental complaints are common in the emergency department (ED). As much as 4% of ED workload is dental-related. Uninsured patients and even patients with basic medical coverage but no dental insurance are forced to seek care in the ED. The first step to diagnosing the dental emergency is to understand the anatomy. There are 32 teeth in most adults (2 incisors, 1 canine, 2 premolars, and 3 molars per side). The teeth are numbered from 1 to 16 on the top starting with the right-hand side. Bottom teeth are numbered 17 to 32 starting on the left and ending with the bottom right.

Dental trauma is a common complaint encountered by emergency providers. Approximately 80% of traumatized teeth are maxillary teeth. Tooth fractures are based on the Ellis classification. Ellis I fractures involve only the enamel. Ellis II fractures include the dentin, and Ellis III fractures are present when both the dentin and pulp are exposed (Figure 78-1).

Tooth avulsion is a result of disruption of the tooth's attachment apparatus. The periodontal ligament is the primary source of attachment of the tooth to the alveolar bone and is of primary concern to the emergency physician. Tooth avulsion occurs with a prevalence of up to 15% of cases. Management depends on whether the avulsed tooth is a permanent or a deciduous tooth. Preservation of the periodontal ligament and limiting the length of time out of the socket relates directly to subsequent tooth viability. A subluxed tooth refers to a tooth that is "loose" due to trauma.

Mandible fractures occur at the symphysis (16%), body (28%), angle (25%), ramus (4%), condyle (26%), and coronoid process (1%). They are most common after blunt trauma to the jaw from either an altercation or a

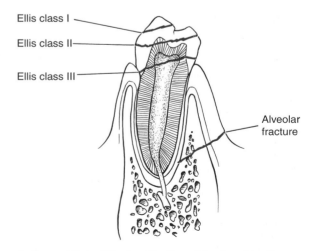

Ellis class I

Ellis class II

Ellis class III

Alveolar fracture

▲ **Figure 78-1.** Ellis classification of fractured teeth.

motor vehicle collision (MVC). Fractures are multiple in half of cases because of the ring shape of the mandible. Mandible fractures are the second most common fracture of the facial bones behind nasal bone fractures.

Dental caries are the most common dental emergency. A typical odontogenic infection originates from dental caries, which decay the protective enamel. Traumatic injury, periodontal disease, or postsurgical infections can also contribute to disruption in the enamel. Once the enamel is dissolved, bacteria travel through the microporous dentin to the pulp, causing pulpitis. The bacteria then can track to the root apex, soft tissues, and finally into the deeper fascial planes. Dental abscesses form secondary to caries (periapical) or trapped food between gums and teeth (periodontal).

Several types of dental abscesses exist. Superficial abscesses in the orofacial area include the buccal, submental, masticator, and canine spaces. If unrecognized or untreated, these infections spread to deeper spaces within the head and neck. Ludwig angina is a rapidly spreading cellulitis of the floor of the mouth involving the sublingual, submental, and submandibular spaces bilaterally. Its name originates from the sensation of choking and suffocation that a patient with this infection experiences. *Ludwig angina is an emergency because the massive swelling can result in airway obstruction.* Ludwig angina occurs secondary to an infection of the posterior mandibular molars in 75% of cases. It can also be secondary to trauma. If the infection continues to spread, the potential exists for adjacent retropharyngeal and mediastinal infection. Ludwig angina is most commonly due to anaerobic (*Bacteroides*) and aerobic (*Streptococcus, Staphylococcus*) oral flora in an immunocompromised patient who is often elderly, diabetic, or an alcoholic.

Two other dental infections that may be encountered are alveolar osteitis and acute necrotizing gingivitis (ANUG). Alveolar osteitis (dry socket) occurs after a dental extraction (usually mandibular third molars). Patients typically present on day 2 or 3. Pain is due to premature loss of healing clot with localized inflammation. ANUG (trench mouth) is the only periodontal disease in which bacteria invade nonnecrotic tissue. Etiology is usually secondary to fusobacteria and spirochete overgrowth of bacteria which is normally present. Human immunodeficiency virus infection, previous necrotizing gingivitis, poor oral hygiene, and stress are predisposing factors.

CLINICAL PRESENTATION

▶ History

Dental Trauma

Patients are typically male and were often involved in an MVC, sports activity, or assault. Ellis I fractures are painless, and the patient may only note a jagged edge to the tooth. Ellis II fractures present with the primary complaint of hot and cold sensitivity as the exposed dentin is quite sensitive. Patients with Ellis III fractures present with severe pain, although pain may be absent if there is neurovascular compromise.

When a tooth avulses, the time the tooth spends out of the socket is one of the most important pieces of information to obtain. If the tooth is out for <20 minutes, prognosis is good. If >60 minutes has elapsed, a successful re-implant is much more difficult.

Patients with a mandible fracture report jaw pain, inability to open the mouth, and possible malocclusion of the teeth. Numbness of the lower lip suggests an injury to the inferior alveolar nerve.

Odontogenic Infection

Patients with dental caries present with dull, continuous pain made worse with any stimulus. They typically have poor dental hygiene with grossly carious teeth. Pain does not occur until decay impinges on the pulp and an inflammatory process develops. If a dental abscess is present, there is excruciating pain that is made worse with tapping on the tooth. These patients may have facial swelling, especially if periapical in location.

When evaluating for an abscess, elicit a history of fever, trismus, drooling, inability to handle secretions, and recent dental infection or trauma. Predisposing factors include dental caries, alcoholism, elderly, or diabetes mellitus. Ludwig angina presents with pain, dysphagia, odynophagia, dysphonia, trismus, and drooling. The patient may also complain of severe neck and sublingual pain. By some estimates, up to 33% can result in airway obstruction.

Patients with acute necrotizing ulcerative gingivitis present with pain, metallic taste, and foul breath. They may also complain of fever and malaise.

▶ Physical Examination

Dental Trauma

Inspect the teeth for Ellis fractures. The dentin is visualized on examination as a creamy yellow color present in the center of the broken tooth. The pulp is seen as a pink tinge or drop of blood within the exposed dentin. If tooth avulsion has occurred, evaluate the socket and surrounding soft tissue for lacerations, ecchymosis, or foreign bodies. When examining an avulsed tooth, do not touch the root. Malocclusion, deformity, or bleeding in the mouth suggests a mandible fracture. An intra-oral laceration may represent an open fracture. Pain, mental nerve paresthesia, and segment mobility may also be present. Ecchymosis under the tongue is highly suggestive of a mandible fracture. The tongue blade test is used to clinically exclude a mandible fracture. The patient is asked to bite on a tongue blade. If the examiner is able to break the blade by turning it while the patient bites down, then a mandible fracture is unlikely. The sensitivity of this test is 95%.

Odontogenic Infection

Dental caries are noted on inspection. If percussion tenderness or changes in temperature cause pain, consider pulpitis.

Dental abscesses are diagnosed based on the physical examination. A submental space infection is characterized by a firm midline swelling beneath the chin. This abscess is due to infection from the mandibular incisors. A sublingual space infection is indicated by swelling and pain of the floor of the mouth and dysphagia. It is due to an anterior mandibular tooth infection.

Submandibular space infection is identified by swelling around the angle of the jaw. Mild trismus is frequently present. These abscesses are caused by an infection of the mandibular molar. Buccal space infections present with cheek swelling (Figure 78-2A). Canine space infection is characterized by anterior facial swelling and loss of the nasolabial fold. This infection can extend into the infraorbital region and be confused with ocular pathology (Figure 78-2B). Masticator space infections present with trismus. Trismus is the inability to fully open the jaw due to tonic spasm of the muscles of mastication (lockjaw). In the absence of trauma, a patient with facial swelling and trismus has a masticator space infection until proven otherwise.

Ludwig angina presents with massive swelling in the floor of the mouth that is painful to palpation. The swelling may produce an elevation of the tongue, which can occlude the oropharynx (Figure 78-3). The patient's anterior neck may be brawny in character secondary to edema.

Alveolar osteitis is identified by a fresh extraction site with absence of clot. ANUG presents with a gray pseudomembrane, ulcerations, gingival bleeding, and fetid breath. Patients often have associated regional lymphadenopathy.

DIAGNOSTIC STUDIES

No laboratory test is essential for the diagnoses of dental trauma or odontogenic infections. Panorex radiograph is useful to diagnose a mandible fracture and allows for the visualization of the entire mandible with 1 radiograph (Figure 78-4). A soft-tissue lateral neck radiograph can be used to visualize the retropharyngeal space and exclude other diagnoses. Computed tomography is used to diagnose mandible fractures and to localize odontogenic infections. In patients with potential airway compromise, evaluation and treatment should not be delayed while waiting for imaging studies.

MEDICAL DECISION MAKING

See Figure 78-5 for a diagnostic algorithm for patients with suspected odontogenic infections.

TREATMENT

▶ Dental Trauma

Ellis I fractures require no immediate treatment; patients should be referred to a dentist. For Ellis II fractures, place a calcium hydroxide paste, cement, or moist gauze over the dentin, then cover the tooth with aluminum foil to decrease contamination of the pulp. Patients will require urgent follow-up with a dentist within 24 hours. Ellis III

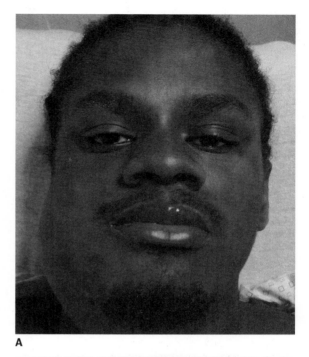

A

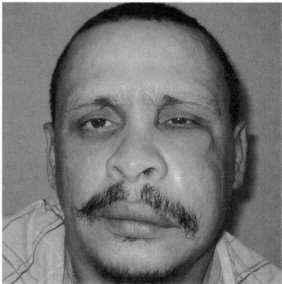

B

▲ **Figure 78-2. A.** Buccal space infection. **B.** Canine space infection.

fractures should be covered with calcium hydroxide, cement, or moist gauze and then covered with foil. These patients require immediate dental referral to avoid pulpal necrosis and loss of the tooth. Definitive treatment includes pulpotomy or pulpectomy.

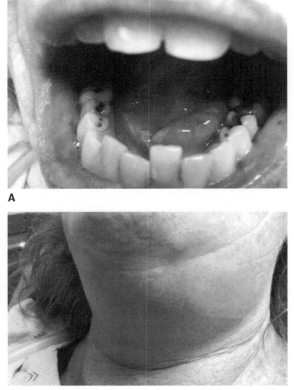

A

B

▲ **Figure 78-3.** A patient with Ludwig angina. **A.** Tongue. **B.** Neck.

Never reimplant avulsed primary teeth, as they can ankylose and block the eruption of permanent teeth. If the avulsed tooth is permanent, care should be taken to hold the tooth by the crown, carefully avoiding the periodontal ligament. If the ligament is damaged, the success of re-implantation may be compromised. In the ED, the tooth should be rinsed gently with saline; do not "brush" the

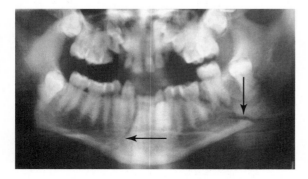

▲ **Figure 78-4.** Panorex demonstrating fractures to the right body and left angle of the mandible.

tooth clean, as this will disrupt the periodontal ligament. The socket is rinsed with normal saline to remove blood clot. Then re-implant the tooth in its socket with a firm pressure into the socket. Have the patient bite on gauze to maintain the tooth in the socket. If unable to replace the tooth, place it in Hank solution, which preserves the ligament for 4–6 hours. Milk is an acceptable alternative if Hank solution is not available. Patients require prophylactic antibiotics, soft diet, tetanus immunization, and an immediate dental referral for tooth stabilization. A tooth loosened in its socket or moved may require repositioning if the bite is impacted. Other general instructions for loose teeth include soft diet, pain control, and dental referral.

Patients with a mandibular fracture will require narcotic pain control. Antibiotics (penicillin G 2–4 million U intravenously [IV] or clindamycin 900 mg IV) are administered for open fractures. Be sure to update tetanus status. Oral surgery consultation for operative repair is indicated, with the exception of isolated nondisplaced condylar fractures, which can be managed nonoperatively.

▶ Odontogenic Infection

A nonsteroidal anti-inflammatory drug with or without narcotics is indicated for patients with dental caries. Consider dental blocks with local anesthetics as an adjunct for pain control. Most patients do not require antibiotics unless there is an obvious associated infection. Consider outpatient dental referral.

Patients with dental abscesses are treated with analgesics, antibiotics, and drainage. Most emergency physicians can drain a perigingival abscess, whereas most periapical abscesses need to be referred to an oral surgeon. Patients with localized infection should be treated with antistreptococcal oral antibiotics, such as oral penicillin (500 mg three times daily in adults or 50 mg/kg/day divided into three doses in children). In cases of penicillin allergy, erythromycin or clindamycin (Cleocin) may be substituted. Definitive therapy is root canal or extraction. Ideally, patients should be evaluated by a dentist within 1–2 days but warned to return earlier if swelling or pain worsens.

The treatment of Ludwig angina involves maintenance of the airway, IV antibiotics, and surgical drainage in the operating room (OR). The primary concern to the emergency physician is maintenance of the patient's airway. Maintain the patient in a seated position and place airway equipment at the bedside. The patient should be given IV penicillin plus metronidazole, cefoxitin, or clindamycin. Ear, nose, and throat should be consulted immediately and arrangements made for transfer to the OR for surgical decompression and possible airway intervention.

Alveolar osteitis is treated with gentle irrigation followed by packing of the socket with iodoform gauze dampened with eugenol. Consider analgesia with a nerve block before irrigation. Ensure close follow up. ANUG is treated with chlorhexidine oral rinses, analgesics, and oral antibiotics (metronidazole). Most patients require dental referral for definitive care.

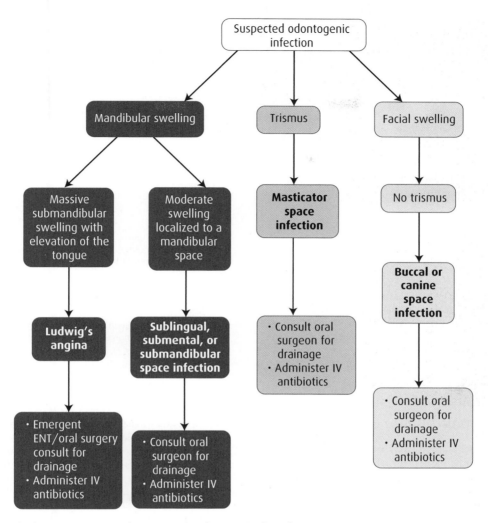

▲ **Figure 78-5.** Dental emergencies diagnostic algorithm.

DISPOSITION

▶ Admission

Patients with an open mandible fracture require admission for IV antibiotics and operative repair. Patients with mandible fractures also require admission for airway compromise (early intubation), excessive bleeding, displaced fractures, infected fractures, comorbid diseases, or if they are elderly. Patients with odontogenic deep space infections and Ludwig angina require drainage of the abscesses in a controlled setting. These patients require admission.

▶ Discharge

Most patients with dental trauma can be discharged to follow-up with a dentist. Patients with minor odontogenic abscesses can be discharged after incision and drainage by either the treating emergency physician or a consulting oral surgeon. These patients will require oral antibiotics and follow-up.

▼ SUGGESTED READING

Beaudreau RW. Oral and dental emergencies. In: Tintinalli JE, Stapczynski JS, Ma OJ, Cline DM, Cydulka RK, Meckler GD. *Tintinalli's Emergency Medicine: A Comprehensive Study Guide.* 7th ed. New York, NY: McGraw-Hill, 2011, pp. 1572–1583.

Costain N, Marrie TJ. Ludwig's angina. *Am J Med.* 2011;124: 115–117.

Douglass AB, Douglass JM. Common dental emergencies. *Am Fam Physician.* 2003;67:511–516.

Nguyen DH, Martin JT. Common dental infections in the primary care setting. *Am Fam Physician.* 2008;77:797–802.

79

Altered Mental Status

Moses S. Lee, MD

Key Points

- Do not delay bedside glucose determination, administration of glucose, and naloxone, if indicated. These interventions may prevent the need for endotracheal intubation.
- Talk to the paramedics and family; they can often identify the cause of altered mental status (AMS).
- Identify level of AMS, systemic conditions, and any focal deficits with the physical examination.
- Re-examine your patients frequently and note any changes in condition and response to therapy.

INTRODUCTION

Altered mental status (AMS) may have an organic (ie, structural, biochemical, pharmacologic) or functional (ie, psychiatric) cause. AMS accounts for 5% of emergency department (ED) visits. About 80% of patients with AMS have a systemic or metabolic cause, and about 15% have a structural lesion.

Consciousness has 2 main components: arousal and cognition. Arousal is controlled by the ascending reticular activating system (ARAS) in the brainstem. Cognition is controlled by the cerebral cortex. Lethargy, stupor, obtundation, and coma are imprecise terms used to describe alterations of arousal. A description of the patient's arousal level (eg, opens eyes to voice) is preferable. Delirium is an alteration of both arousal and cognition. Patients exhibit restlessness, agitation, and disorientation. Dementia is an alteration of cognition, not arousal.

ARAS is a complex system of nuclei in the brainstem. It may be impaired by small structural lesions in the brainstem such as ischemic or hemorrhagic stroke, shear forces from head trauma, or external compression from brain herniation. Severe toxic and/or metabolic derangements (eg, hypoxia, hypothermia, drugs) can also cause impairment. Bilateral cerebral cortex dysfunction must occur to cause decreased levels of arousal or profound AMS. This is usually caused by toxic/metabolic derangements, infection, seizures, subarachnoid hemorrhage (SAH), or increased intracranial pressure (ICP). Unilateral lesions such as stroke do not by themselves cause profound AMS.

CLINICAL PRESENTATION

▶ History

AMS represents a spectrum of disease presentations from profoundly depressed arousal requiring emergent intubation to severe agitation and confusion requiring restraint and sedation. Initial stabilizing measures are often needed before a complete history and physical examination can be performed.

If the patient is unable to give a coherent history, alternate sources of history should be sought. Prehospital providers should be questioned about the patient's condition in the field, therapies given and the response, and the condition of the home environment (eg, pill bottles, suicide note). Family members should be contacted to ascertain past history of similar episodes, medical history, trauma, substance abuse, and the last time the patient was seen in a normal state. The patient's belongings should be searched for medical identification bracelets, pill bottles, phone numbers, or other potential sources of information.

Patients presenting to the ED with AMS often include the elderly, who are more prone to infection, have comorbid illnesses, and take multiple medications; substance abusers (eg, heroin, cocaine, alcohol withdrawal, and liver failure); and psychiatric patients who may be on mood-stabilizing drugs, which, when taken in excess, have toxic effects that cause abnormal arousal or cognition.

▶ Physical Examination

Vital signs; airway, breathing, and circulation (ABCs); pulse oximetry; and bedside glucose should be assessed, looking for immediate life threats and treatable causes of AMS (ie, hypoglycemia, hypoxia or abnormal respiratory pattern, hyper- or hypotension, hyper- or hypothermia). Naloxone (Narcan), glucose, and thiamine should be administered, as dictated by history and examination.

A "head-to-toe" examination should follow, looking for systemic causes of AMS and focal neurologic deficits. The head should be examined for any signs of trauma. Pupil size, symmetry, and reactivity should be assessed. Pinpoint pupils are a sign of opiate overdose or pontine hemorrhage. An asymmetrically dilated "blown" pupil is a sign of uncal herniation. Fundi should be assessed for the presence of papilledema or subhyaloid hemorrhage associated with SAH. Neck stiffness indicates meningeal irritation caused by either SAH or infection. Cardiovascular exam should assess for dysrhythmias (atrial fibrillation), murmurs (endocarditis), or rubs (pericarditis). Lung exam should assess for symmetric breath sounds, respiratory rate, wheezes, rhonchi, and rales. Abdominal exam should assess for masses and organomegaly (alcoholic liver disease, splenic sequestration in sickle cell disease). Skin exam should assess for color, turgor (dehydration), rashes (petechiae, purpura suggesting thrombotic thrombocytopenic purpura or meningococcemia), and infection (cellulitis, fasciitis). If the neurologic examination cannot be completed because of the patient's mental status, document what you are able to do and how the patient appears. Mental status assessment should include AVPU (alert, responds to voice, responds to pain, unresponsive). If the patient responds to voice, the appropriateness and coherence of the response should be documented. The cranial nerves, motor, deep tendon reflexes (including Babinski or plantar reflex), cerebellar, and sensory examinations should be included if possible.

DIAGNOSTIC STUDIES

▶ Laboratory

Multiple laboratory tests are obtained in an attempt to gain more information, although a cause can usually be ascertained from a thorough history and physical examination. Initial laboratory tests should include complete blood count (leukocytosis, anemia, and thrombocytopenia); chemistry (electrolyte abnormalities, acidosis, and renal failure); urine (pregnancy test, toxicology screen, infection); coagulation and liver studies (liver failure, coagulopathy); blood cultures (if infection suspected); arterial blood gas (hypoxia, hypercarbia, acidosis, and lactate); alcohol level; and serum toxicology screen.

▶ Imaging

Head computed tomography (CT) scans should be performed to assess for mass lesion, hydrocephalus, and intracerebral or subarachnoid bleed. Include a chest x-ray if hypoxia, abnormal respirations, or evidence of pulmonary infection is present. Electrocardiogram should be performed on all patients, looking for ischemia, QT or QRS prolongation, or changes consistent with electrolyte abnormalities.

PROCEDURES

A lumbar puncture may be indicated when considering a central nervous system infection or bleeding after a negative head CT scan.

MEDICAL DECISION MAKING

A systematic approach to the altered mental status patient and the recognition of treatable causes (mnemonic AEIOU-TIPS) will provide optimal management (Figure 79-1 and Table 79-1). History, physical examination, and initial laboratory and imaging tests will often reveal the cause of mental status change.

TREATMENT

ED patients with AMS should be treated for any life-threatening abnormalities while ongoing patient assessment continues. Hypoglycemia, a common cause of AMS, should be treated with intravenous (IV) dextrose: adults: 1 amp D50 (50% glucose solution), pediatrics: 2–4 mL/kg D25 (25% glucose solution). Hypoxic patients should receive oxygen therapy (administer 100% O_2, mechanical ventilation as needed) while searching for a potential cause (pneumonia, congestive heart failure, pneumothorax, pulmonary embolism). Patients with

Table 79-1. AEIOU TIPS differential diagnosis of patients with AMS.

A—Alcohol
E—Epilepsy, Electrolytes, Encephalopathy (HTN and hepatic)
I—Insulin (hypo- and hyperglycemia), Intussusception (peds)
O—Opiates, Overdose
U—Uremia
T—Trauma, Temperature (hypo- and hyperthermia)
I—Infection, Intracerebral hemorrhage
P—Psychiatric, Poison
S—Shock

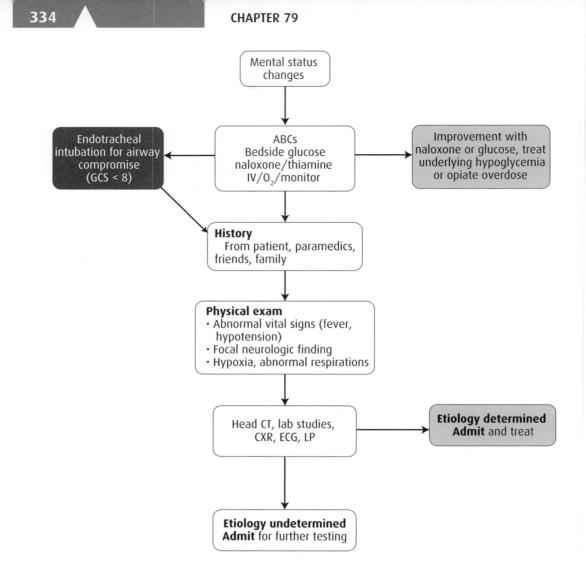

Figure 79-1. Altered mental status diagnostic algorithm. ABCs, airway, breathing, and circulation; CT, computed tomography; CXR, chest x-ray; ECG, electrocardiogram; GCS, Glasgow coma scale; LP, lumbar puncture.

suspected opiate overdose (history or pupillary examination) should be treated presumptively: adults: naloxone 2–4 mg IV given in 0.2– to 0.4-mg increments to avoid precipitating opiate withdrawal in chronic abusers. In a nonemergent setting, administer naloxone 2–4 mg in a nebulizer with 3 mL of saline. Pediatric patients should receive naloxone 0.01-0.1 mg/kg IV. Actively seizing patients should receive IV benzodiazepines: diazepam 0.1–0.2 mg/kg IV (or 0.5 mg/kg per rectum) or lorazepam 0.1 mg/kg IV. Patients with suspected meningitis or sepsis should receive IV fluid resuscitation and broad-spectrum antibiotic coverage. If hypertensive encephalopathy is a suspected cause for AMS, the mean arterial pressure should

be reduced by 25% in 30 minutes with IV antihypertensive medications.

DISPOSITION

▶ Admission

Most patients with AMS who are not immediately treatable require admission to the hospital for further work-up, therapies, and observation. The level of admission (observation unit, floor, telemetry, intensive care unit) should be guided by the patient's vital signs, reassessments in mental status, abnormalities identified, and comorbid illnesses.

Discharge

Patients with hypoglycemia caused by insulin, who are able to eat and remain normoglycemic after a period of observation, may be safely discharged. If on long-acting oral hypoglycemics, patients require admission for observation. For patients with narcotic overdose, discharge is appropriate if the patient improves with naloxone and remains stable after the duration of action of naloxone has elapsed (ie, 1–4 hours).

SUGGESTED READING

Huff JS. Altered mental status and coma. In: Tintinalli JE, Stapczynski JS, Ma OJ, Cline DM, Cydulka RK, Meckler GD. *Tintinalli's Emergency Medicine: A Comprehensive Study Guide.* 7th ed. New York, NY: McGraw-Hill, 2011, pp. 1135–1142.

Lehman RK, Mink J. Altered mental status. *Clin Pediatr Emerg Med.* 2008;9:68–75.

William K, Brady WJ, Huff JS, et al. Altered mental status: Evaluation and etiology in the ED. *Am J Emerg Med.* 2002;20:613–617.

Headache

Joseph M. Weber, MD

Key Points

- Consider emergent causes of headache first.
- Have a low threshold to perform a computed tomography (CT) scan on patients with a possible emergent cause for their headache.
- Never delay administering antibiotics while waiting for a CT scan or lumbar puncture (LP) when considering the diagnosis of bacterial meningitis.
- When subarachnoid hemorrhage is suspected, follow a normal CT scan with LP.

INTRODUCTION

Headache is the presenting complaint in 3–5% of all visits to the emergency department (ED). Headaches are classically divided into primary headache syndromes (migraine, tension, cluster) and secondary causes, which can range from benign (sinusitis) to emergent (subarachnoid hemorrhage [SAH], meningitis, tumor with increased intracranial pressure [ICP]). In clinical practice, the emergency physician attempts to classify a patient's headache as emergent or benign. The majority of headaches in patients presenting to the ED have a benign etiology; however, 5–10% of patients have a serious or potentially life-threatening cause for their headache (Table 80-1).

Brain tissue is insensate. In benign headache syndromes, pain originates from blood vessels, venous sinuses, the dura, cranial nerves, or extracranial sources (muscle tension). In emergent headaches, pain may arise from mass effect (tumor or subdural hematoma), inflammation of the meninges (meningitis and SAH), vascular inflammation (temporal arteritis), vascular dissection (carotid and vertebral artery dissection), or extracranial sources (dental caries, otitis media, sinusitis).

▶ Emergent Secondary Headaches

Subarachnoid Hemorrhage

Although SAH represents <1% of headaches in patients who present to the ED, it occurs in approximately 12% of patients with a severe sudden headache. Pain is often maximal at onset, in the occipital region, and may resolve spontaneously in the ED. The median age at presentation is 50 years. More than 50% of patients have a normal neurologic examination. Rupture of an aneurysm is the most common cause.

Meningitis

Classic triad of headache, fever, and meningismus is often *not present*. It is more difficult to diagnose at extremes of age. Immunosuppression can cause atypical subacute presentations.

Table 80-1. Headache classification by incidence.

Type of Headache	Incidence (%)
Tension	50
Unknown cause	30
Migraine	10
Serious secondary cause	3–8
Life-threatening	1

Intracranial Bleed

Subdural bleed can occur with minimal or unrecognized trauma (warfarin use, elderly). Epidural bleed usually occurs with significant trauma. Intracerebral bleed is often associated with severe hypertension.

Temporal Arteritis

Occurs in patients older than 50 years and is more frequent in women. It is caused by a systemic panarteritis. Patients present with frontotemporal throbbing headache, jaw claudication, and a nonpulsatile or tender temporal artery. It may cause visual loss from ischemic optic neuritis.

Carotid And Vertebral Artery Dissection

Together these entities cause 20% of strokes in patients younger than 45 years. Carotid dissections occur twice as often as vertebral dissections. Classically, they present as acute unilateral headache and/or neck pain, but may present atypically (lower cranial nerve deficits or C5/6 radiculopathy). The median age of onset is 40 years. Sometimes dissection occurs in association with minor trauma (yawning) or may be spontaneous.

Pseudotumor Cerebri

Benign intracranial hypertension of unclear cause. It has been linked to the use of oral contraceptives, vitamin A, tetracyclines, and thyroid disorders. Often occurs in young, obese females with chronic headaches. Papilledema is usually the only abnormal examination finding, but cranial nerve abnormalities, visual field deficits, or decreased visual acuity may also be present.

Stroke

Although 55% of patients with an intracerebral hemorrhage have a headache, less than 17% of ischemic stroke patients complain of pain. However, cerebellar infarction often presents as acute pain in the occipital area. Because of its location in the posterior fossa, there is risk of herniation as surrounding brain edema occurs.

Other

Pituitary apoplexy, acute angle-closure glaucoma, hypertensive encephalopathy, pheochromocytoma, CO poisoning, preeclampsia, venous sinus thrombosis (often in the setting of a hypercoagulable state).

▶ Primary Headaches

Migraine

Abnormal vascular activity is thought to be causal. Migraines are more common in females, with onset usually in teen years, and less commonly after age 40 years. The patient presents with unilateral pulsating headache that may have an associated aura. The pain usually follows a typical pattern for individual patients and improves during pregnancy (estrogen excess). Associated symptoms include nausea and vomiting with photophobia and phonophobia.

Tension

The most common type of primary headache. Often presents with bitemporal nonpulsating pain without associated nausea, vomiting, photophobia, or phonophobia.

Cluster

Uncommon in the general population, but more common in men beginning after age 20 years. They present with acute, severe, unilateral retro-orbital pain with associated lacrimation, eye injection, and rhinorrhea and usually occur in "clusters" over days to weeks and resolve spontaneously.

CLINICAL PRESENTATION

▶ History

A detailed history is most important to make the correct diagnosis and guide therapy. Headache pattern should be sought. Patterns that raise concern for a secondary headache include sudden onset, first ever, or a change in frequency or intensity from previous. Sudden onset of a severe headache suggests SAH, but may also be present in venous sinus thrombosis, cervical artery dissection, cerebellar infarct, and pituitary apoplexy. A headache that is worse in the mornings may indicate a tumor, whereas a headache that is worse on standing is characteristic of a post–lumbar puncture (LP) headache. Headache location is usually nonspecific. However, migraines are typically unilateral, tension headaches are bilateral, and SAH is usually occipital or nuchal. Neck pain with or without neurologic deficits may represent a carotid or vertebral artery dissection. Headache character may be pulsatile or throbbing (migraine), squeezing (tension), or sharp and acute (cluster and SAH).

Associated symptoms that may point to an emergent secondary cause include syncope, altered mental status (AMS), neck pain or stiffness, fever, hypertension, visual disturbance, weakness, seizures, or trauma. Consider carbon monoxide poisoning when multiple family members are concurrently affected during the fall or winter. Important elements of the past medical history include immunocompromise, malignancy, coagulopathy (warfarin), uncontrolled hypertension, aneurysm, connective tissue disease (cervical artery dissection), and cerebrovascular accident (CVA). Family history is also important. Migraines, SAH, and carotid/vertebral dissections are all more common if a first-degree relative has been affected.

▶ Physical Examination

Vital signs are often normal in patients with headache. However, fever may indicate meningitis or sinusitis, and severe hypertension suggests encephalopathy or intracranial bleed. General appearance should be appreciated and may aid in diagnosing a life-threatening headache or severe presentation of a primary headache syndrome. Head and neck examination should assess for sinus tenderness, dental caries, otitis media or externa, temporal artery tenderness, and meningismus. Eye exam should include visual acuity, pupil reactivity and funduscopy (papilledema from increased ICP, subhyaloid hemorrhage from SAH). On the neurologic examination, include mental status, cranial nerves, strength, sensation, reflexes, cerebellar and gait if possible. AMS or focal neurologic deficits often indicate increased ICP.

DIAGNOSTIC STUDIES

▶ Laboratory

General laboratory studies (complete blood count, chemistry panel, urinalysis) add little to the diagnosis of emergent headaches. Elevated white blood cell (WBC) count may point to an infection; elevated erythrocyte sedimentation rate (>50 mm/h) is present in cases of temporal arteritis.

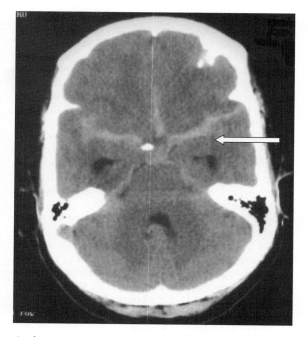

▲ **Figure 80-1.** Noncontrast head CT scan showing SAH. Note the blood (white areas) in the basal cisterns and interhemispheric fissure. This is referred to as the "star sign" (arrow).

▶ Imaging

Noncontrast head computed tomography (CT) scan is the test of choice when evaluating emergent causes of headache. It can assess for acute SAH (sensitivity 98% within 12 hours, 93% within 24 hours); acute intracerebral, subdural, and epidural hematomas; and lesions causing mass effect (Figure 80-1). Intravenous (IV) contrast is added in patients with immunocompromise, or when subacute or chronic subdural, venous sinus thrombosis, or central nervous system infections are suspected. CT scan does not diagnose idiopathic intracranial hypertension, meningitis, and some cases of venous sinus thrombosis. When considering carotid or vertebral dissection, CT angiogram of the neck, duplex ultrasonography, or magnetic resonance imaging (MRI)/magnetic resonance angiogram (MRA) of the neck should be performed.

PROCEDURES

LP should be performed when considering meningitis or SAH (if the head CT scan is nondiagnostic). It can also be performed to check the opening pressure (normal <20 cm H_2O) in patients with suspected pseudotumor cerebri. Opening pressure should also be assessed for suspected SAH; two thirds of patients will have elevated pressure. CT should be performed before LP for patients with any of the following: age >60 years, AMS, focal neurologic deficit, signs of increased ICP (papilledema), seizures, immunocompromise, or meningeal signs.

Cerebrospinal fluid (CSF) findings in acute meningitis and SAH are listed in Table 80-2. Interpreting CSF results in the face of a traumatic LP can be difficult. A decrease in red blood cells (RBCs) to near zero from tubes 1–4 suggests that the blood in tube 1 was from LP-induced trauma, not SAH. In general, there will be 1 WBC in the CSF for every 700 RBCs when from a traumatic LP. Xanthochromia (due to lysis of erythrocytes in CSF), when present, is indicative of SAH.

Table 80-2. CSF findings in meningitis and SAH.

CSF	Normal	Bacterial	Viral	SAH
Cells	<5 WBCs	200-5,000 PMN	<1,000 monocytes	100s-million RBCs
CSF/serum glucose ratio	0.6	Low	Normal	Normal
Protein	15-45 mg/dL	High	High	Normal to increased
Gram stain	Negative	Positive	Negative	Negative
Xanthochromia*	Negative	Negative	Negative	Positive

*Usually present 12 hours after SAH bleed and lasts 2-3 weeks.

MEDICAL DECISION MAKING

History and physical examination may be sufficient to arrive at a benign diagnosis (tension, migraine, cluster headache). However, when serious secondary headaches are considered, CT imaging ± lumbar puncture should be performed. Treatment of possible meningitis should not be delayed by CT or LP (Figure 80-2).

TREATMENT

For patients with a presumed benign headache, oral pain medications (nonsteroidal anti-inflammatory drug, acetaminophen, hydrocodone) may be sufficient to relieve pain. For more severe pain, especially when a migraine is suspected, IV antiemetics (prochlorperazine 5–10 mg IV) often provide relief. Sensory stimuli should be decreased (dark quiet room). IV opioids may be used for continued pain.

Patients with a presumed emergent headache usually require IV medications for pain relief concurrently with diagnostic tests (CT ± LP) and other treatments (IV antibiotics for meningitis). In general, IV antiemetics and opioids are safe for emergent headaches.

Subarachnoid Hemorrhage

Emergent neurosurgical consultation is required for aneurysm clipping or coiling. Nimodipine (60 mg by mouth [PO]) is often given to reduce subsequent vasospasm.

Meningitis

Do not delay antibiotics for CT scan or LP (ceftriaxone + vancomycin). Perform CT scan before LP if the patient meets criteria as listed previously. IV steroids should be given empirically to adult patients in whom meningitis is strongly suspected.

Intracranial Bleed

Emergent neurosurgical consultation is required for evacuation of subdural or epidural bleed. Fresh-frozen plasma should be administered if the patient is coagulopathic. Severe uncontrolled hypertension should be treated. General recommendations include reduction of the mean arterial pressure by 25% or to <150/90.

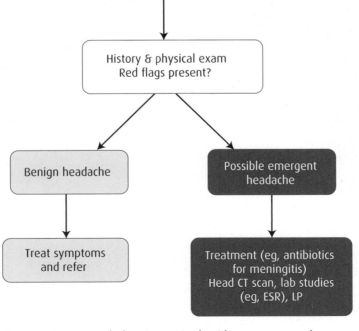

▲ **Figure 80-2.** Headache Diagnostic algorithm. CT, computed tomography; ESR, erythrocyte sedimentation rate; LP, lumbar puncture.

Temporal Arteritis

Administer oral prednisone 80 mg. The patient should be discharged home on prednisone 40 mg daily. Close follow-up for biopsy and definitive diagnosis should be arranged before the patient is discharged from the ED.

Pseudotumor Cerebri

A normal CT scan should be followed by LP to assess opening pressure. An opening pressure >25 cm H_2O suggests the diagnosis. CSF should be removed to bring ICP into the normal range (usually about 20 mL of CSF). Oral acetazolamide and steroids may be started in the ED after consulting with a neurologist.

Carotid or Vertebral Artery Dissection

For patients with only pain and no neurologic signs suggestive of CVA, head CT scan is often normal. CT angiography of neck, MRI/MRA, or duplex ultrasound may show the abnormality in the affected vessel. Treatment may include aspirin or heparin. Emergent neurologic and vascular surgery consultation is appropriate.

DISPOSITION

▶ Admission

Most patients with an emergent secondary headache should be admitted to the hospital. Patients with meningitis with AMS, SAH, intracranial hemorrhage, cervical artery dissection, or tumor with mass effect or signs of increased ICP should be admitted to an intensive care unit.

▶ Discharge

Patients with benign headache syndromes whose pain is well controlled can be discharged home. Patients with secondary headaches that are not life- or organ-threatening (temporal arteritis, pseudotumor cerebri) can be discharged home after close follow-up is arranged. These patients should be given very specific instructions to return if headache worsens or they experience any new or different symptoms, including focal weakness, numbness, speech or visual problems, or vomiting.

▼ SUGGESTED READING

Denny CJ, Schull MJ. Headache and facial pain. In: Tintinalli JE, Stapczynski JS, Ma OJ, Clince DM, Cydulka, RK, Meckler GD. *Tintinalli's Emergency Medicine: A Comprehensive Study Guide.* 7th ed. New York, NY: McGraw-Hill, 2011, pp. 1113–1118.

Edlow JA, Panagos PD, Godwin SA, et al. Clinical policy: Critical issues in the evaluation and management of adult patients presenting to the emergency department with acute headache. *Ann Emerg Med.* 2008;52:407–436.

Swadron SP. Pitfalls in the management of headache in the emergency department. *Emerg Med Clin North Am.* 2010;28:127–147.

Dizziness

William B. Lauth, MD

Key Points

- The patient's definition of "dizziness" must be clarified with a careful and explicit history taken by the health care provider.
- True vertigo must be differentiated from other types of dizziness.
- Attempt to distinguish peripheral from central vertigo.
- Consider life-threatening causes of dizziness such as cardiac syncope and cerebellar infarct or hemorrhage in all patients, especially the elderly.

INTRODUCTION

Dizziness is one of the most common emergency department (ED) presentations and one of the most difficult to characterize. Dizziness means different things to different people and crosses language and cultural boundaries. The precise definition ranges from weakness, giddiness, and anxiety to true vertigo, presyncope, disequilibrium, or nonspecific lightheadedness. A very careful history from the patient, friends, or family is the most important part of the initial evaluation of the dizzy patient.

Dizziness can be divided into 4 main types: vertigo, presyncope, disequilibrium, and lightheadedness. Vertigo is defined as the perception of movement where no movement exists. Patients often describe feeling the room spinning. It can be further divided into central and peripheral types. Peripheral vertigo is usually benign and caused by an inner ear problem, whereas central vertigo is usually serious and involves pathology within the cerebellum or brainstem. Presyncope is defined as lightheadedness derived from feeling an impending loss of consciousness. Disequilibrium refers to a feeling of unsteadiness, imbalance, or a sensation of floating while walking. Lightheadedness is the most difficult type of dizziness to characterize. Many patients in this group have vague, poorly defined symptoms, such as just not feeling right, that do not fall into one of the other categories.

The central nervous system (CNS) coordinates and interprets sensory inputs from visual, vestibular, and proprioceptive systems. These 3 systems give us the sense of position in our 3-dimensional universe. The disruption of any 1 of these 3 can produce vertigo. The most common forms of vertigo involve dysfunction of the vestibular apparatus and are thus considered peripheral vertigo. By far the most common cause of vertigo is benign paroxysmal positional vertigo (BPPV), which is caused by a mechanical disorder of the inner ear. It is due to the accumulation of floating calcium carbonate particles in either the left or right semicircular canals. These particles stimulate the labyrinth, causing asymmetric input from the normal and affected semicircular canals, which produces the sensation of vertigo. Clinically, BPPV is characterized by vertigo precipitated by certain head movements, which aggravate this unilateral dysfunction. Other causes of peripheral vertigo include Ménière disease, labyrinthitis, and vestibular neuronitis. Ménière disease is a disorder in which there is an increase in volume and pressure of the endolymph of the inner ear, eventually leading to damage of the endolymphatic system and deafness. The pathophysiology of labyrinthitis is not completely understood, although many cases are associated with systemic or viral illnesses, which is thought to cause inflammation in the vestibular apparatus. Viral infection of the vestibular nerve is believed to be the most common cause of vestibular neuronitis.

Central vertigo is much less common than peripheral vertigo and is due to CNS dysfunction. Cerebellar infarct or hemorrhage, cerebellopontine angle tumors and schwannomas, and vertebrobasilar insufficiency frequently cause central vertigo symptoms.

CLINICAL PRESENTATION

▶ History

The cause of dizziness can be elicited by history alone in more than half of all cases. Patients with vertigo complain of a sensation of movement, or "the room spinning" around them, with associated nausea and vomiting. BPPV usually has an abrupt onset, lasts <1 minute, and is provoked by head movement. ED physicians should be aware that some causes of central vertigo such as vertebrobasilar insufficiency (VBI), transient ischemic attack, and cerebellar hemorrhage may also have an acute onset. Ménière disease is associated with hearing loss and tinnitus, and the vertigo usually lasts for hours. The vertigo caused by labyrinthitis and vestibular neuronitis usually lasts for a few days. In contradistinction, the symptoms of central vertigo are usually less acute, more persistent, and may have associated neurologic symptoms (Table 81-1).

Patients with presyncope often complain of feeling as though they are going to pass out. This may be associated with a stressful event (vasovagal episode), exertion (aortic stenosis), sudden change in posture (hypovolemia), or

Table 81-1. Differentiating peripheral from central vertigo.

	Peripheral	Central
Onset	Sudden	Sudden or slow
Severity of vertigo	Intense spinning	Ill-defined, less intense
Pattern	Paroxysmal, intermittent	Constant
Aggravated by position/movement	Yes	Variable
Associated nausea/diaphoresis	Frequent	Variable
Nystagmus	Rotatory-vertical, horizontal	Vertical
Fatigue of symptoms/signs	Yes	No
Hearing loss/tinnitus	May occur	Does not occur
Abnormal tympanic membrane	May occur	Does not occur
Central nervous system symptoms/sign	Absent	Usually present

Reprinted with permission from Goldman B. Chapter 164. Vertigo and Dizziness. In: Tintinalli JE, Stapczynski JS, Cline DM, Ma OJ, Cydulka RK, Meckler GD, eds. *Tintinalli's Emergency Medicine: A Comprehensive Study Guide.* 7th ed. New York: McGraw-Hill, 2011.

palpitations (dysrhythmia). Disequilibrium is most often a complaint of elderly patients. Their sense of loss of balance is usually worse at night (limited visual acuity is further impaired) and later in the day (more fatigued). Patients with lightheadedness usually have vague complaints. Past medical history and associated chronic medical conditions should be ascertained in an attempt to find a cause for their complaints.

▶ Physical Examination

A complete physical examination should be performed, paying special attention to a few key areas. Vital signs can suggest a cause early in the evaluation. Hypotension suggests causes related to decreased cerebral perfusion, whereas hypertension may point to VBI, stroke, or hemorrhage. Bradycardia or tachycardia may cause presyncope from impaired cardiac output.

The head, eyes, ears, nose, and throat examination may reveal a possible cause for vertigo. Ears should be carefully examined for presence of a ruptured tympanic membrane, decreased hearing, infection, cerumen impaction, and foreign bodies. The cardiovascular examination should assess for signs of vascular insufficiency (carotid bruits, decreased peripheral pulses). Auscultate for any arrhythmia or the systolic murmur of aortic stenosis.

A complete neurologic examination is essential for all patients with a complaint of dizziness. Assess for the presence and type of nystagmus. While performing the cranial nerve examination, pay special attention to cranial nerves VII, VIII, and IX. Cranial neuropathies associated with cranial nerve VIII suggest brainstem involvement and a central cause of vertigo. Patients with peripheral vertigo should be able to ambulate, although they may veer to one side. Patients with cerebellar infarction or hemorrhage usually cannot ambulate. A Romberg test can be used to differentiate cerebellar from spinal cord (posterior column) dysfunction. Have the patient stand, with feet together, and then have them close their eyes. Excessive swaying or imbalance is a positive test and is seen in patients with significant proprioceptive loss from posterior column dysfunction.

DIAGNOSTIC STUDIES

▶ Laboratory

No specific laboratory test can aid in the diagnosis of vertigo (Table 81-2). However, older patients on multiple medications with nonspecific symptoms should have hemoglobin, electrolytes, and renal function evaluated. Electrocardiogram (ECG) and serial troponins should be performed in patients suspected of having a cardiac cause for their symptoms.

▶ Imaging

Head computed tomography (CT) scan is indicated in patients with a suspected central cause for their symptoms (focal neurologic findings, altered mental status, severe

Table 81-2. Ancillary testing of vertigo and dizziness.

Condition	Suggested Tests
Bacterial labyrinthitis	CBC, blood cultures, CT scan or MRI for possible abscess, lumbar puncture if meningitis suspected
Vertigo associated with closed head injury	CT scan or MRI
Near-syncope	ECG, Holter monitor, CBC, glucose, electrolytes, renal function, table tilt testing
Cardiac dysrhythmias	ECG, Holter monitor
Suspected valvular heart disease	ECG, echocardiography
Nonspecific dizziness; disequilibrium of aging	CBC, electrolytes, glucose, renal function tests
Thyrotoxicosis	Thyroid stimulating hormone, triiodothyronine, thyroxine
Cerebellar hemorrhage, infarction or tumor	CT or MRI
Vertebral artery dissection	Cerebral angiogram to include neck vessels or MRA
Vertebrobasilar insufficiency	ECG, cardiac monitoring, echocardiogram, carotid Doppler, MRI, MRA

CBC, complete blood count.

Reprinted with permission from Goldman B. Chapter 164. Vertigo and Dizziness. In: Tintinalli JE, Stapczynski JS, Cline DM, Ma OJ, Cydulka RK, Meckler GD, eds. *Tintinalli's Emergency Medicine: A Comprehensive Study Guide.* 7th ed. New York: McGraw-Hill, 2011.

headache), or significant cerebrovascular accident risk factors (Figure 81-1). Magnetic resonance imaging (MRI)/magnetic resonance angiography (MRA) may be performed if vertebral artery dissection or vertebrobasilar insufficiency is considered.

PROCEDURES

The Dix-Hallpike maneuver can be used to elicit BPPV and differentiate it from a central cause for vertigo. The procedure involves rapidly moving the patient from a seated to supine position with the head rotated 45 degrees to the right with the eyes open. If no symptoms are elicited, the procedure should be repeated with the head rotated to the left. The latency, duration, and direction of nystagmus and presence of vertigo should be noted. With BPPV, the nystagmus is horizontal or rotatory, has a latency period (up to 60 seconds), is fatigable, and suppresses with fixation (Figure 81-2).

MEDICAL DECISION MAKING

The ED evaluation of dizziness requires a broad differential diagnosis encompassing benign diagnoses such as labyrinthitis associated with an upper respiratory infection to

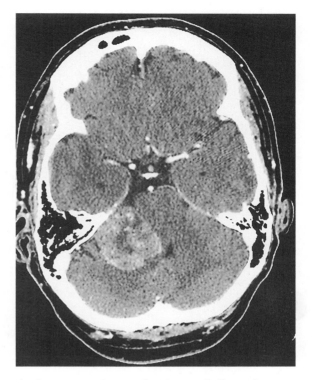

▲ **Figure 81-1.** CT scan showing cerebellopontine angle tumor (acoustic neuroma).

life-threatening emergencies such as cerebellar infarct or hemorrhage. The history and physical examination may lead to a diagnosis or point toward the need for further ED evaluation and possible admission (Figure 81-3).

TREATMENT

The treatment of patients with dizziness in the ED is dictated by the working diagnosis after evaluation. Peripheral vertigo is treated based on the suspected cause. BPPV can be treated in the ED with canalith repositioning maneuvers. The Epley maneuver is used to reposition the particulate debris from the semicircular canal to the utricle (Figure 81-4). Once the debris is repositioned, the abnormal vestibular input is eliminated. Multiple attempts at this procedure may be necessary. Vestibular suppressant medications are also used to decrease abnormal input from the affected semicircular canal (Table 81-3). For other

Table 81-3. Vestibular suppressant therapy.

Class	Medication	Dose
Antihistamine	Meclizine	25 mg PO q 8 hr
Antiemetic	Promethazine	25 mg PO q 6 hr
Benzodiazepines	Diazepam	2–5 mg PO q 8 hr

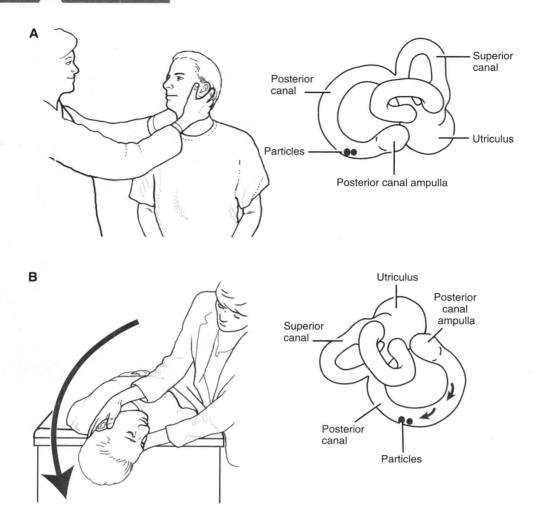

▲ **Figure 81-2.** Dix-Hallpike maneuver to elicit **benign positional vertigo** (originating in the right ear). The maneuver begins with the patient seated and the head turned to one side at 45 degrees **(A)**, which aligns the right posterior semicircular canal with the sagittal plane of the head. The patient is then helped to recline rapidly so that the head hangs over the edge of the table **(B)**, still turned 45 degrees from the midline. Within several seconds, this elicits vertigo and nystagmus that is right beating with a rotary (counterclockwise) component. If no nystagmus is elicited, the maneuver is repeated after a pause of 30 seconds, with the head turned to the left. Treatment with the canalith repositioning maneuver is shown in Figure 81-4. Reprinted with permission from Ropper AH, Samuels MA. Chapter 15. Deafness, Dizziness, and Disorders of Equilibrium. In: Ropper AH, Samuels MA, eds. *Adams and Victor's Principles of Neurology*. 9th ed. New York: McGraw-Hill, 2009.

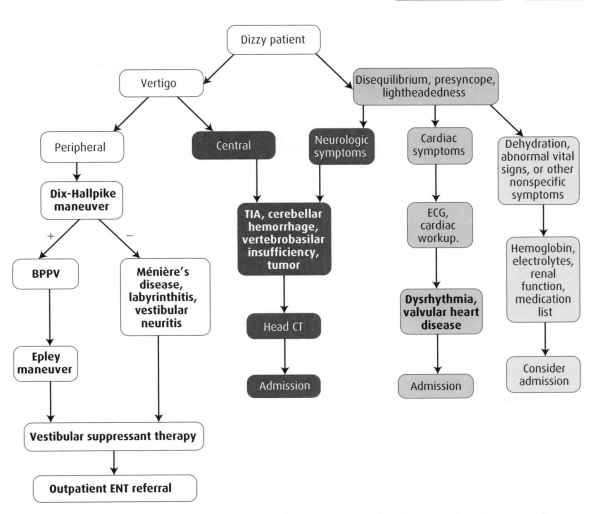

▲ **Figure 81-3.** Dizziness diagnostic algorithm. BPPV, benign paroxysmal positional vertigo; CT, computed tomography; ECG, electrocardiogram; TIA, transient ischemic attack.

causes of peripheral vertigo such as Ménière disease, labyrinthitis, and vestibular neuronitis, vestibular suppressant medications are the mainstay of treatment.

Patients with vertigo from central causes (CNS tumor, bleed, or infarct) should have appropriate neurology or neurosurgical consultation in the ED. Patients suspected of having vertebrobasilar insufficiency should be started on aspirin, and follow-up (inpatient vs outpatient) decisions should be made in consultation with their primary physician.

Patients with cardiovascular risk factors and presyncope are treated similar to patients with syncope and may require a telemetry admission to exclude an arrhythmia (see Chapter 19, Syncope). Patients found to have noncardiac causes of presyncope, such as dehydration or anemia, are treated accordingly with fluids and/or blood transfusion.

Patients with symptoms of disequilibrium or nonspecific lightheadedness with an unremarkable ED evaluation may be discharged home after consultation with their primary physician. As the majority of these patients are elderly, patients should be assessed for fall risk and home safety before discharge. Vestibular suppressants should never be used in these patients because these drugs can exacerbate their symptoms.

DISPOSITION

▶ Admission

Patients with central vertigo, focal neurologic findings, a possible cardiovascular cause (arrhythmia, ischemia), an electrolyte abnormality, or anemia should be admitted to the hospital.

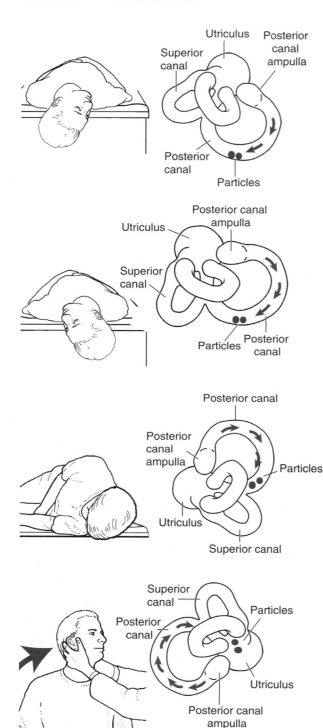

◀ **Figure 81-4.** Bedside maneuver for the treatment of a patient with benign paroxysmal positional vertigo affecting the right ear. The presumed position of the debris within the labyrinth during the maneuver is shown on each panel. The maneuver is a 4-step procedure. First, a Dix–Hallpike test is performed with the patient's head rotated 45 degrees toward the (affected) right ear and the neck slightly extended with the chin pointed slightly upward. This position results in the patient's head hanging to the right **(A)** Once the vertigo and nystagmus provoked by this maneuver cease, the patient's head is rotated about the rostral–caudal body axis until the left ear is down **(B)** Then the head and body are further rotated until the head is almost face down **(C)** The vertex of the head is kept tilted upward throughout the rotation. The patient should be kept in the final, facedown position for about 10 to 15 seconds. With the head kept turned toward the left shoulder, the patient is brought into the seated position **(D)** Reprinted with permission from Ropper AH, Samuels MA. Chapter 15. Deafness, Dizziness, and Disorders of Equilibrium. In: Ropper AH, Samuels MA, eds. *Adams and Victor's Principles of Neurology.* 9th ed. New York: McGraw-Hill, 2009.

▶ **Discharge**

Patients with peripheral vertigo may be discharged home. ENT follow-up may be necessary if the symptoms are persistent or recurrent. Patients with nonspecific symptoms without serious comorbidities and a normal ED work-up may be discharged after follow-up with their primary physician has been arranged.

▼ **SUGGESTED READING**

Goldman B. Vertigo and dizziness. In: Tintinalli JE, Stapczynski JS, Ma OJ, Clince DM, Cydulka, RK, Meckler GD. *Tintinalli's Emergency Medicine: A Comprehensive Study Guide.* 7th Ed. New York, NY: McGraw-Hill, 2011.

Cerebrovascular Accident

Tom Morrissey, MD

Key Points

- Time is brain. Time of symptom onset is key to acute stroke treatment.

- Hypoglycemia and hypoxia can mimic stroke. Assess and treat these conditions early in the evaluation of patients with stroke-like symptoms.

- Resist the urge to aggressively lower blood pressure. Hypertension is the body's attempt to maintain perfusion to ischemic tissue. Hypotension can make things worse.

- Transient ischemic attack (TIA) is a warning of a stroke to come (aborted stroke). Treat TIAs seriously and work up risk factors expediently.

INTRODUCTION

Roughly 750,000 strokes occur annually in the United States, and this will increase as the population ages. Physical, emotional, and economic damages are multifactorial. The cost of initial care is only the beginning. Many stroke survivors are not only unable to return to work, they are unable to care for themselves, placing heavy demands on family and friends.

Stroke is defined as a neurologic deficit resulting from the interruption of blood supply to neuronal tissue. The brain is highly metabolically active, consuming roughly 25% of cardiac output, but has no mechanism for storing energy reserves. This makes it extremely sensitive to even transient interruption in its supply of oxygen and glucose. Vascular compromise may be caused by several different mechanisms, but the final common pathway is impaired neuronal perfusion and tissue starvation.

Strokes are often classified in 2 different ways: etiology and location. Etiologic causes can be classified as either hemorrhagic or ischemic. Hemorrhagic strokes account for 10–20% of all strokes. They sometimes result from the rupture of an aneurysm or arteriovenous malformation (AVM), usually causing bleeding on the surface of the brain. More commonly, the bleeding comes from disruption of an intracerebral arteriole, leading to bleeding inside the parenchyma of the brain. Uncontrolled hypertension is the most common precipitant of intracerebral bleeding, but other conditions such as amyloidosis and tumors can increase the chances of intracerebral bleeding. Vasospasm can occur from the irritant effects of blood on the surface of the brain, leading to an even greater decrease in blood flow.

Ischemic strokes are caused primarily by thrombosis of a blood vessel, very similar to mechanisms involved in myocardial infarction. Conditions such as atherosclerosis, hypercoagulable states, polycythemia, and vasculitis are common precipitants. About 20% of ischemic strokes result from embolic phenomenon. The carotid bifurcation is a common source of plaque embolism. Cardiac mural thrombus and valve disease are also likely sources of embolism.

Classification by location depends on the blood vessel or vascular distribution involved (Table 82-1). The blood supply to the brain comes from paired carotid and vertebral blood vessels. The carotid distribution (ie, anterior circulation) supplies primarily cerebral and cortical structures, whereas the vertebrobasilar vascular distribution (ie, posterior circulation) feeds the cerebellum and brainstem structures. The involved vessel can often be inferred from the clinical presentation. Carotid circulation strokes commonly present with motor and sensory deficits that are fairly obvious. Visual field defects, neglect, and language difficulties (eg, aphasia) are often apparent on exam. The internal carotid bifurcates into the anterior carotid artery (ACA), which feeds areas involved in control of the leg, and the middle carotid artery (MCA), which feeds areas

Table 82-1. Vascular supply of common strokes.

Cerebral Circulation	Vascular Supply	Motor Manifestation	Sensory Manifestation	Speech
Anterior circulation	Anterior cerebral artery	Contralateral weakness of leg > arm (face and hand spared)	Minimal discrimination deficits.	Perseveration
	Middle cerebral artery	Contralateral weakness of face and arm > leg	Contralateral numbness of face and arm > leg	Aphasia, if dominant hemisphere is involved (left in 80% of patients)
Posterior circulation	Posterior cerebral artery (supplies visual cortex)	Minimal motor involvement	Visual abnormalities, light touch, and pinprick affected (patient often unaware of deficits)	
	Vertebral and basilar artery (supplies brainstem and cerebellum)	Hallmark is crossed deficits (ipsilateral cranial nerve deficits with contralateral motor weakness)		
	Vertebrobasilar artery ischemia	Cranial nerve palsies, limb weakness, diplopia	Dizziness, vertigo, ataxia	Dysarthria
	Cerebellar artery	Drop attack	Vertigo	
Lacunar infarction (4 types)	Penetrating arteries (ischemia of thalamus and internal capsule)			
Motor		Face, arm, and leg		Dysarthria
Sensory			Pure hemisensory deficit	
Clumsy hand dysarthria		Clumsiness of one hand		Dysarthria
Ataxic hemiparesis		Hemiparesis	Ataxia on same side as weakness	

more involved in control of the face and arm. Smaller branches penetrate deeper into areas such as the internal capsule. Strokes in these vessels can give pure sensory or motor deficits. Vertebrobasilar strokes cause ischemia in the brainstem or cerebellum. Large brainstem strokes are usually fatal. Smaller ones can lead to cranial nerve dysfunction and more subtle findings, such as vertigo. Cerebellar strokes can be much harder to recognize, emphasizing the importance of looking for ataxia, balance, and fine motor control on the neurologic exam. These signs are often not noticed by the patients themselves.

Until the mid 1990s, the treatment for acute ischemic stroke was almost entirely supportive care. In 1996, the Food and Drug Administration (FDA) approved the use of tissue plasminogen activator (TPA). Some facilities are employing intravascular catheter-guided clot lysis or evacuation. With the availability of these newer treatments, stroke patients now rank as true medical emergencies that warrant the focused resources of the emergency department (ED). With the time dependency of treatment options, much work has gone into increasing public awareness of stroke and enhancing prehospital recognition and transport. Many hospitals have developed dedicated stroke teams and stroke protocols to expedite care of acute stroke patients.

Transient ischemic attacks (TIAs) are defined as "a transient episode of neurologic dysfunction caused by focal brain, spinal cord or retinal ischemia, without acute infarction." Symptoms typically last less than 1–2 hours. These patients should be assessed and treated as acute strokes, with the exception of fibrinolytic treatment. TIAs are the equivalent of unstable angina in coronary disease and should be treated as "warning signs of strokes to come." Some studies estimate as many as 20% of TIA patients will suffer a stroke within 90 days, half of which may occur within 48 hours.

CLINICAL PRESENTATION

▶ History

Reperfusion strategies are both time- and situation-dependant. Gathering accurate historical information as quickly as possible is a critical facet of treatment. Issues such as aphasia and cognitive dysfunction can make it very difficult to get information directly from the patient. Make efforts to contact others (family, nursing home staff) who can provide historical details. Hemineglect and gaze deviation may cause patients not to be aware of you. Be sure you are in the patient's line of sight and touch them while you are talking to them.

One of the most important historical considerations is to determine when the symptoms began. If the patient had symptoms on awakening, or cannot clearly identify the time they started, the start time is considered the last time the patient was seen as normal. The "time last known well" is important to obtain early because it will determine whether fibrinolytics will be considered. The window to administer fibrinolytics intravenously (IV) is usually an onset of symptoms within the last 3 hours. If fibrinolytics are being considered, ask about contraindications to their administration. Is there a history of previous intracranial bleeding? Brain tumor? Head injury? Recent surgery? Is the patient on anticoagulants?

Ask the patient how he or she noticed the symptoms and what he or she was doing when it started. Is the patient dizzy, off balance, or falling? Is the patient having pain or weakness or both? Has the patient had these symptoms before? Extremity pain is an unusual feature of a stroke and suggests an alternate diagnosis. Onset of symptoms with severe headache, seizure, and syncope suggests a hemorrhage stroke. Neck pain or history of neck trauma or manipulation may indicate carotid or vertebral dissection.

When assessing the past medical history, determine whether a stroke mimic is possible. Diabetic patients may be presenting with hypoglycemia. Patients with a history of seizures may be postictal. Patients with a history of migraines may also present with stroke-like symptoms.

Lastly, elicit risk factors for stroke. Atrial fibrillation and valvular disease are common risk factors for emboli. Diabetes and hypertension are risk factors for thrombotic strokes.

▶ Physical Examination

As with history, extensive physical exam should not delay imaging and treatment. Focus on the airway, breathing, and circulation (ABCs) and pertinent neurologic findings. Of greatest importance is the patient's ability to protect his or her airway. Either decreased mental status or cranial nerve dysfunction can compromise airway protection. Check for spontaneous swallowing. Do not test gag reflex as this may induce vomiting.

Note the patient's vital signs and breathing pattern. Low blood pressure can mimic stroke symptoms. High blood pressure may be a cause or compensation. If you choose to lower blood pressure later, it will be important to know the presenting baseline pressure. Cheyne-Stokes or apneustic breathing may indicate severe brain injury. Hypoxia can cause stroke-like symptoms in the absence of a actual vascular occlusion.

Other important questions to answer on the physical examination include the following. Is the rhythm irregular (atrial fibrillation)? Are there murmurs to indicate valvular disease? Is there peripheral evidence of emboli (splinter hemorrhages in nails, on the retina)? Are carotid pulses palpable? Is there a bruit, indicating possible dissection or plaque as a source of emboli?

Is there a fever? CNS infections can be confused with stroke. Hypotension from sepsis can cause hypoperfusion and mimic stroke. Is there evidence of head trauma or other injury?

Neurologic examination need not be comprehensive initially. Tools such as the National Institute of Health stroke scale (NIHSS) are available to "quantify" the extent of the stroke and are widely available (Table 82-2).

Table 82-2. National Institute of Health stroke scale.

Category	Patient Response	Score
LOC questions	Answers both correctly	0
	Answers one correctly	1
	Answers none correctly	2
LOC commands	Obeys both correctly	0
	Obeys one correctly	1
	Obeys none correctly	2
Beat gaze	Normal	0
	Partial gaze palsy	1
	Forced deviation	2
Best visual	No visual loss	0
	Partial hemianopsia	1
	Complete hemianopsia	2
	Bilateral hemianopsia	3
Facial palsy*	Normal	0
	Minor facial weakness	1
	Partial facial weakness	2
	No facial movement	3
Best motor arm Right _____ Left _____	No drift	0
	Drift <10 seconds	1
	Falls <10 seconds	2
	No effort against gravity	3
	No movement	4
Best motor leg Right _____ Left _____	No drift	0
	Drift <5 seconds	1
	Falls <5 seconds	2
	No effort against gravity	3
	No movement	4
Limb ataxia*	Absent	0
	Ataxia in 1 limb	1
	Ataxia in 2 limbs	2
Sensory	No sensory loss	0
	Mild sensory loss	1
	Severe sensory loss	2
Neglect	Absent	0
	Mild	1
	Severe	2
Articulation	Normal	0
	Mild	1
	Severe	2
Language	Normal	0
	Mild aphasia	1
	Severe aphasia	2
	Mute or global aphasia	3

LOC, level of consciousness.

*Items deleted from the modified NIHSS.

Do not delay imaging to perform the complete examination. The details can be obtained after the computed tomography (CT). Focus on key components, including:

Level of consciousness. Is the patient alert, lethargic, obtunded, or stuporous? Rapid decline may indicate herniation.

Eye exam. Asymmetric pupils may indicate herniation or midbrain involvement. Papilledema indicates increased intracranial pressure or hypertensive encephalopathy. Retinal hemorrhages or pale spots indicate emboli. Is there a gaze deviation? Is there evidence of nystagmus?

Cranial nerve exam. The brainstem is a tightly packed area, and it is extremely rare to have a stroke that involves only one cranial nerve. Cranial nerve palsies on one side of the body and contralateral motor/sensory findings are a hallmark of brainstem strokes.

Motor exam. Assess for asymmetric weakness and classify as normal, weak, or not moving at all. Check to see if the deficit is greater in the face/arm distribution (MCA) or the leg (ACA) or both (carotid bifurcation). Checking for pronator drift is a sensitive test for subtle weakness.

Sensory exam. Compare sensation to pain and light touch bilaterally. The sensory exam is often limited by neglect, receptive aphasia, or mental status. Subtle sensory deficits may be uncovered by checking for extinction to bilateral simultaneous light touch on the arms, legs, and face.

Reflexes. Initially reflexes are decreased in the involved regions. Hyperreflexia may indicate old strokes. Assess for asymmetric release reflexes such as a Babinski sign or myoclonic jerking when feet are pushed dorsally.

Cerebellar exam. If safe, have the patient walk. Look for wide or narrow gait and perform a Romberg test. Check for smooth controlled finger-to-nose, knee-heel-shin, and rapid alternating movements to test cerebellar fine motor control.

DIAGNOSTIC STUDIES

▶ Imaging

Noncontrasted head CT is currently the test of choice for the initial evaluation of stroke patients. Most acute strokes are not visible on CT. Its role is not to "rule in stroke," but rather to rule out other entities that would be a contraindication to fibrinolytic reperfusion therapy. Bleeding is an obvious contraindication to fibrinolytics. Large strokes that show early ischemic changes (edema) on the CT scan are more likely to convert to hemorrhagic strokes and thus are a relative contraindication to fibrinolytic treatment. Plain CT is very sensitive for bleeding or mass effects from other intracranial lesions (Figure 82-1 and 82-2).

▶ Laboratory

Important lab studies include rapid blood glucose and coagulation studies (prothrombin time, partial thromboplastin time). These must be ordered as quickly as possible after

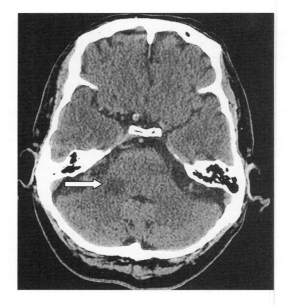

▲ **Figure 82-1.** CT scan showing an ischemic stroke. Note the hypodense area anterior and to the right of the fourth ventricle (arrow).

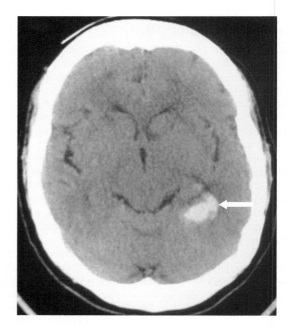

▲ **Figure 82-2.** CT scans showing hemorrhagic stroke (arrow).

patient arrival. Other common tests include complete blood count, electrolytes, and renal function. Electrocardiogram and cardiac enzymes are often ordered to assess for cardiac causes of the event.

PROCEDURES

No special procedures are required in stroke patients. It is important, however, to avoid doing procedures that could complicate the course of fibrinolytic treatment. Any central lines should be placed in areas where bleeding can be monitored and controlled with compression (jugular or femoral, not subclavian). Peripheral IVs are preferred. Do not perform a lumbar puncture unless there is a strong suspicion of subarachnoid hemorrhage or meningitis as the cause of symptoms.

MEDICAL DECISION MAKING

The first decision that should be considered with an ischemic stroke is eligibility for fibrinolytic reperfusion therapy (Figure 82-3). Critical factors include the following:

1. Is this truly an ischemic stroke (vs hemorrhagic or other stroke mimic)?
2. Is the time of the onset of symptoms clear?
3. Are there exclusion factors?
4. Is your institution capable of TPA administration, or do you need to transfer the patient to a stroke center?

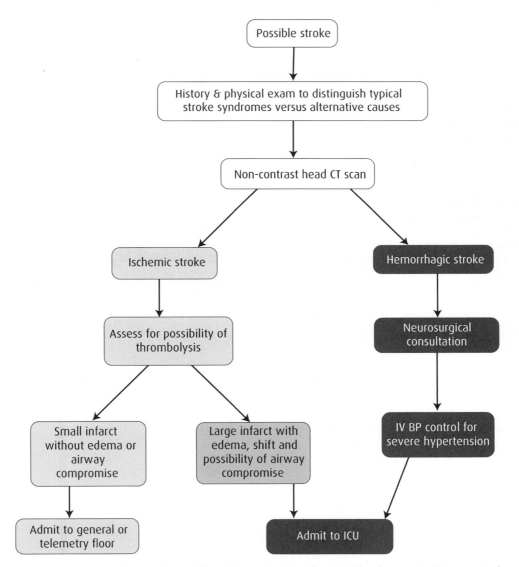

▲ **Figure 82-3.** Cerebrovascular accident diagnostic algorithm. BP, blood pressure; CT, computed tomography; ICU, intensive care unit.

TREATMENT

First, do no harm. Limit further damage by paying attention to the details of supportive care. Intubate if the patient is unable to protect his or her airway. Provide supplemental oxygen for hypoxia (generally for O_2 sats <95%; there is some evidence that *hyper*oxia can worsen neuronal damage by free radical oxidation). In addition, administer IV fluids if the patient appears hypovolemic or is hypotensive. Aim for euvolemia; volume overload can worsen cerebral edema. Severely anemic patients may need blood transfusion to assure good oxygen-carrying capability. Be very cautious lowering blood pressure, if you lower it at all. Hypotension is much worse than hypertension. Blood pressure control for ischemic strokes is not warranted unless pressures are sustained above 220/120 mmHg. Blood pressure control for hemorrhagic strokes has less evidence, but many recommend controlling any blood pressure over 150/90 mmHg.

▶ Ischemic Strokes

For patients with ischemic strokes or TIA, aspirin (325 mg orally) helps prevent platelet aggregation. Do not give until you assure that the patient does not have an intracranial hemorrhage. If you think the patient might receive fibrinolytics, hold the aspirin for the first 24 hours. Consult a neurologist and/or stroke team whenever available. If fibrinolytic therapy is administered, the FDA-approved dose is Reteplase (rTPA) 0.9 mg/kg (max dose 90 mg). Ten percent should be administered as a bolus, with the remainder of the infusion over the next hour. Intensive care monitoring is need for the first 24 hours after treatment. Any worsening of condition should prompt immediate cessation of the infusion and repeat head CT.

▶ Hemorrhagic Stroke

Mitigate elevated intracranial pressure by elevating the head of the bed to 30 degrees. Treat coagulopathy. Patients on warfarin with high international normalized ratios should be reversed with fresh-frozen plasma or prothrombin complex concentrate and vitamin K. *Do not give*

aspirin. Consult neurosurgery. Many intracerebral clots will benefit from early clot evacuation. Implement seizure precautions and consider antiepileptic administration in consultation with the admitting team.

DISPOSITION

▶ Admission

All stroke patients should be admitted to the hospital. Patients with large strokes, evidence of edema on CT scan, or decreases in mental status are at high risk for decompensation and should be admitted to an intensive care unit (ICU). All patients who receive fibrinolytic therapy should be monitored in the ICU for the first 24 hours after treatment. Patients with evidence of arrhythmias or other cardiac causes for the stroke should be admitted to a monitored setting. Patients with hemorrhagic strokes should be admitted to an ICU setting with neurosurgical consultation. In many hospitals, this will mean transfer to a facility with higher levels of care. Patients with TIA symptoms should be admitted to the hospital for an expedited evaluation.

▶ Discharge

Stable patients with obvious nonstroke etiologies may be discharged home if other medical conditions do not warrant admission. Ensure that the patient has a safe social situation and appropriate follow-up.

▼ SUGGESTED READING

Go S, Worman DJ. Stroke, transient ischemic attack and cervical artery dissection. In: Tintinalli JE, Stapczynski JS, Ma OJ, Cline DM, Cydulka RK, Meckler GD. *Tintinalli's Emergency Medicine: A Comprehensive Study Guide.* 7th ed. New York, NY: McGraw-Hill, 2011, pp. 1122–1135.

Hoffman JR, Schriger DL. A graphic reanalysis of the NINDS Trial. *Ann Emerg Med.* 2009;54:329–336.e35.

Tissue plasminogen activator for acute ischemic stroke. The National Institute of Neurological Disorders and Stroke rt-PA Stroke Study Group. *N Engl J Med.* 1995;333:1581–1588.

Seizures and Status Epilepticus

Amer Zia Aldeen, MD

Alison R. Foster, MD

Key Points

- Always check a bedside glucose level in seizure patients.
- Monitor airway, breathing, and circulation in actively seizing patients and intervene when needed.
- Intravenous lorazepam is the drug of choice for actively seizing patients.
- Search for a secondary cause of seizures in first-time seizure patients and those with a known seizure disorder who have new or different features.

INTRODUCTION

A seizure is an episode of abnormal neurologic function caused by inappropriate, excessive activation of neurons in the brain. Seizures account for up to 2% of emergency department (ED) visits and affect approximately 4 million people in the United States. The incidence of seizures is highest among those <20 and >60 years of age. Status epilepticus is continuous or intermittent seizure activity for more than 5 minutes without recovery of consciousness. It has a mortality rate of up to 20%. Half of all patients presenting to the ED in status epilepticus have no prior history of seizures. ED management of seizures should focus on cessation of seizure activity.

Seizures result from abnormal excitation or lack of inhibition of neurons in the brain. The cause may be primary (idiopathic) or secondary, with an underlying etiology that may be treatable such as hypoglycemia. In patients with a known seizure disorder, the most common cause of recurrent seizures includes medication noncompliance, sleep deprivation, alcohol or substance withdrawal, and infection. Secondary causes of seizures include head trauma, stroke, intracranial infection or mass, electrolyte abnormalities, alcohol withdrawal, drug overdose, and eclampsia.

Seizures are classified as generalized or partial. Generalized seizures are characterized by excitation of the entire cerebral cortex and always cause alteration of mental status. Generalized seizures can manifest as a staring spell (absence or petit mal), diffuse motor activity (tonic-clonic or grand mal), or drop attacks (myoclonic, tonic, clonic, or atonic). The postictal period refers to the time (lasting up to 1 hour) after a generalized seizure when the patient gradually returns to baseline mental status. The postictal period often distinguishes generalized seizures from other causes of sudden altered mental status such as syncope.

Partial seizures are caused by localized neuronal activation that may remain localized or spread to involve other areas of the brain (referred to as partial seizure with secondary generalization). Patients with simple partial seizures experience brief focal motor or sensory symptoms without altered mental status. Complex partial seizures are characterized by altered consciousness with autonomic, sensory, motor, and/or psychological manifestations (Table 83-1).

CLINICAL PRESENTATION

▶ History

While the history is performed, obtain a blood glucose level in all patients with altered mental status, including those suspected of having had a seizure. Hypoglycemic seizures are easily treated with dextrose and do not respond to standard antiepileptic drugs. To determine whether a seizure actually occurred, gather a complete and detailed history from witnesses, emergency medical service, and the patient.

CHAPTER 83

Table 83-1. Classification of seizures.

Generalized Seizures (always loss of consciousness)
Tonic-clonic seizures (grand mal)
Absence seizures (petit mal)
Myoclonic seizures
Clonic seizures
Atonic seizures
Partial (focal) Seizures
Simple partial (no alteration of consciousness)
Complex partial (impaired consciousness)
Partial seizures (simple or complex) with secondary generalization

Note the onset of symptoms, the presence of a prodrome or aura, loss of consciousness, diffuse or focal motor activity, bowel or bladder incontinence, length of the event, and postictal period. Ask about recent trauma (head injury), headaches (mass lesions), pregnancy (eclampsia), history of metabolic abnormalities such as diabetes (hypoglycemia), drug ingestions (tricyclic-antidepressants, isoniazid), alcohol use (withdrawal seizure), and sleep disturbances. If the patient has a known seizure disorder, obtain a description of the patient's typical seizure pattern and medication history.

▶ Physical Examination

As with any high-acuity patient, perform a primary survey of the patient, assessing airway, breathing, and circulation (ABCs), vital signs, bedside glucose level, basic mental status, and pupillary symmetry and reactivity. In most patients, the seizure will stop spontaneously within 2 minutes, and the initial postictal period will result in profound alteration of mental status. At this time, manage the airway by using jaw thrust/chin lift, repositioning the patient's head, or inserting a nasopharyngeal airway. Look for physical examination signs of toxidromes (eg, sympathomimetic), trauma (abrasions, contusions, fractures), increased intracranial pressure (papilledema or Cushing reflex), and any focal neurologic abnormality that would indicate a secondary cause of seizure. A complete neurologic examination should be performed as soon as possible. Transient focal muscle paralysis after a seizure is known as Todd paralysis and usually resolves within 24–48 hours. Up to 25% of patients with a generalized seizure sustain a tongue laceration, usually of the lateral tongue. Tongue biting has a 99% specificity and 24% sensitivity for diagnosis of generalized tonic-clonic seizure.

DIAGNOSTIC STUDIES

▶ Laboratory

In addition to an immediate bedside glucose for all seizure patients, check the sodium level in patients with first-time seizures. All women of child-bearing age should have a pregnancy test. In patients with significant comorbid illnesses such as renal failure, broaden laboratory testing to include renal function tests, complete blood count, alcohol, calcium, magnesium, and phosphorus levels. To differentiate between true seizures and pseudoseizures (also known as psychogenic nonepileptic seizures), check prolactin level, lactate, and electrolytes. Elevated serum prolactin level within 60 minutes of seizure onset can support the diagnosis of seizure. Additionally, an increased lactate level and anion gap with decreased bicarbonate suggests generalized seizure activity. This metabolic acidosis should resolve within 1 hour of seizure cessation. Patients with a known seizure disorder should have antiepileptic medication levels checked.

▶ Imaging

Obtain a noncontrast brain computed tomography (CT) scan in all patients with first-time seizure or those with a change in their normal seizure pattern. Other indications to perform CT include patients with a new focal neurologic deficit, severe headache, persistent altered mental status, fever, trauma, cancer, anticoagulant use, or history of immunocompromise (Figure 83-1). Magnetic resonance imaging (MRI) is more sensitive for mass lesions such as vascular malformations, certain tumors, and strokes, but is not usually necessary in the ED setting. Patients with a known seizure disorder and a typical seizure without any new secondary causes identified do not need any imaging performed in the ED.

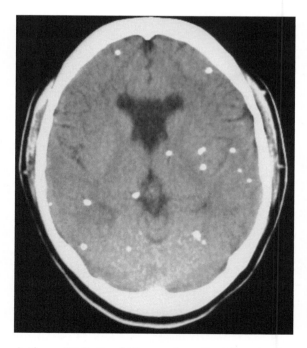

▲ **Figure 83-1.** Head CT scan of a patient from Mexico who presented to the ED with a first-time seizure. CT scan demonstrated multiple calcifications from neurocysticercosis.

Consider lumbar puncture in the setting of seizure if the patient is febrile, immunocompromised, or at high risk for subarachnoid hemorrhage despite normal CT findings. Lumbar puncture is *not* a routine part of first-time seizure evaluation. Electroencephalogram (EEG) is indicated in the ED only when nonconvulsive status epilepticus is suspected in patients with persistent altered mental status or in patients who receive paralytics or phenobarbital, both of which may mask continued seizure activity.

MEDICAL DECISION MAKING

Once normal vital signs, blood glucose, and mental status have been achieved, a patient's seizure history determines the management pathway. If the present seizure is typical of past seizure patterns, antiepileptic drug levels should be obtained and repleted. If any part of the seizure was atypical or this was a first-time seizure, the patient should be evaluated for secondary causes. If no secondary cause is identified and the seizure was an isolated event, the remainder of the evaluation can occur as an outpatient (Figure 83-2).

TREATMENT

Specific management is based on the patient's clinical scenario.

▶ First-Time Seizure, Resolved

Patients with a first-time seizure who have a normal neurologic examination, no medical comorbidities, normal diagnostic testing including a normal CT brain scan, and normal electrolytes do not require further treatment in the ED. Patients with seizures attributed to other causes (secondary seizures) will need specific treatment for the underlying etiology.

▶ Known Seizure Disorder, Resolved

If antiepileptic drug levels are very low, begin repletion in the ED. Simply resuming home dosing in these cases delays therapeutic levels for several days. Phenytoin can be loaded either intravenously (IV) or by mouth (PO) at 18 mg/kg. IV loading results in therapeutic serum levels within

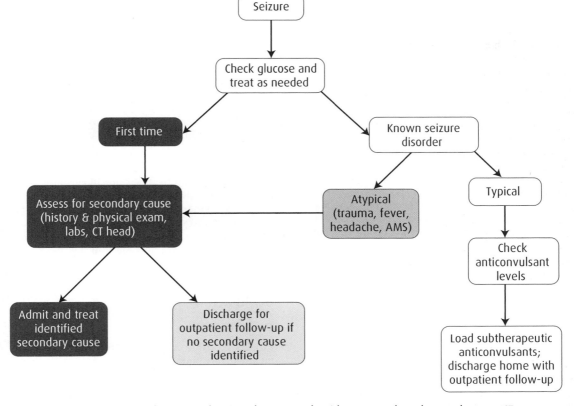

▲ **Figure 83-2.** Seizures and status epilepticus diagnostic algorithm. AMS, altered mental status; CT, computed tomography.

1 hour, and oral loading within 12 hours. In patients with subtherapeutic levels, the correct amount of phenytoin to administer is determined by the following formula:

$$Phenytoin\ load\ (mg) = (0.75\ L/kg) \times (desired\ level - current\ level) \\ \times (patient's\ weight\ in\ kg)$$

An alternative to phenytoin administration is fosphenytoin (20 mg/kg phenytoin equivalents), a prodrug of phenytoin. Fosphenytoin can be given IV or intramuscularly (IM) and has fewer side effects but is more expensive.

Actively Seizing Patient

The mainstays of treatment are to protect the patient from physical injury; reduce the risk of aspiration; monitor ABCs, vital signs, and bedside glucose; and observe the seizure for resolution. There is no indication for IV anticonvulsant medications during an uncomplicated seizure, as most are self-limited. Benzodiazepines are used for patients with frequent or continuous seizures to temporarily subdue seizure activity until a permanent solution is determined. Administer lorazepam 2 mg IV or IM (up to a total dose of 0.1 mg/kg) or diazepam (0.1 mg/kg/dose) to control seizure activity. Multiple studies have shown that lorazepam and diazepam are both equally effective at terminating seizures, although lorazepam administration decreases the occurrence of repeat seizures when compared to diazepam. If the seizure does not resolve or the patient does not return to baseline between events, treat for status epilepticus.

Status Epilepticus

Administer medications in stepwise fashion until seizure activity ceases. Benzodiazepines remain first-line agents (see preceding doses) with the addition of antiepileptic drugs as second- and third-line agents. Phenytoin (20–30 mg/kg) or fosphenytoin (20–30 mg/kg phenytoin equivalent [PE]) should be loaded IV depending on availability in ED. Fosphenytoin is preferred as it can be loaded faster. If seizure activity persists, phenobarbital is a third-line agent and is dosed at 20 mg/kg. Phenobarbital administration will result in profound respiratory depression, so a definitive airway should be secured at this time. Valproic acid (20 mg/kg) can be used instead of phenobarbital as a third-line agent. For refractory status epilepticus, use propofol, midazolam, or ketamine. Emergent EEG monitoring and neurology consultation should be obtained (Figure 83-3).

Special Cases

Seizures In HIV Patient

Seizures are a common manifestation of central nervous system (CNS) disease in an HIV-positive patient. HIV encephalopathy, CNS lymphoma, and many opportunistic infections can cause seizures. In this population, lumbar puncture should be performed with standard tests as well as specific assays for tubercular, viral, and fungal agents.

Neurocysticercosis

Neurocysticercosis is caused by the parasite Taenia solium and is the most common cause of secondary epilepsy in the developing world. CT may show 1- to 2-cm cystic lesions within the cerebral cortex. Definitive diagnosis depends on the clinical picture, serologic testing, and imaging. Noncontrast studies demonstrate calcification of inactive cysts, which is the most common finding at presentation (see Figure 83-1). In patients with active disease, contrast CT demonstrates ring enhancement signifying edema surrounding the active cysts. Seizures due to neurocysticercosis are usually controlled by antiepileptic monotherapy until definitive antiparasitic medication and/or surgical excision is successful.

Pregnancy

Test all female patients of child-bearing age for pregnancy. Pregnant patients with proteinuria, hypertension, and seizure likely have eclampsia. The treatment is IV magnesium sulfate 4- to 6-g bolus followed by a 2-g hourly infusion. Eclamptic seizures can occur postpartum and the treatment is the same.

Alcohol Withdrawal

Alcohol withdrawal seizures can occur in those with chronic alcohol dependence and are most likely to occur 12–36 hours after last alcohol intake. Benzodiazepines administered on arrival have been shown to prevent sequential seizures. It is important to remember that alcohol withdrawal seizures are a diagnosis of exclusion, and other secondary etiologies should be investigated.

Isoniazid

Patients undergoing treatment for tuberculosis are often taking isoniazid, which can cause seizures resulting from vitamin B_6 deficiency. The typical presentation will be seizures unresponsive to conventional treatment for status epilepticus. The treatment is IV vitamin B_6 (pyridoxine). Dose-dependent algorithms are available for treatment; empiric therapy if the dose of isoniazid is unknown is 5 g of B_6 IV, which can be repeated.

DISPOSITION

Admission

Patients in status epilepticus should be admitted to an intensive care unit. Patients with a first-time resolved seizure with an identified secondary cause should be admitted to the hospital for further evaluation. Patients with a known seizure disorder and atypical features should undergo further work-up and may warrant admission.

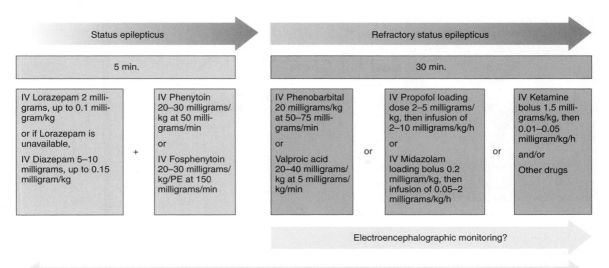

Status epilepticus → Refractory status epilepticus

5 min. | 30 min.

| IV Lorazepam 2 milligrams, up to 0.1 milligram/kg

or if Lorazepam is unavailable,

IV Diazepam 5–10 milligrams, up to 0.15 milligram/kg | + | IV Phenytoin 20–30 milligrams/kg at 50 milligrams/min

or

IV Fosphenytoin 20–30 milligrams/kg/PE at 150 milligrams/min |

| IV Phenobarbital 20 milligrams/kg at 50–75 milligrams/min

or

Valproic acid 20–40 milligrams/kg at 5 milligrams/kg/min | or | IV Propofol loading dose 2–5 milligrams/kg, then infusion of 2–10 milligrams/kg/h

or

IV Midazolam loading bolus 0.2 milligram/kg, then infusion of 0.05–2 milligrams/kg/h | or | IV Ketamine bolus 1.5 milligrams/kg, then 0.01–0.05 milligram/kg/h

and/or

Other drugs |

Electroencephalographic monitoring?

Airway, blood pressure, temperature, IV access, electrocardiography, CBC, glucose, electrolytes, AED levels, ABG, tox screen

▲ **Figure 83-3.** Guidelines for management in status epilepticus. ABG, arterial blood gases; AED, antiepileptic drug; CBC, complete blood count; PE, phenytoin equivalent. Reprinted with permission from Lung DD, Catlett CL, Tintinalli JE. Chapter 165. Seizures and Status Epilepticus in Adults. In: Tintinalli JE, Stapczynski JS, Cline DM, Ma OJ, Cydulka RK, Meckler GD, eds. *Tintinalli's Emergency Medicine: A Comprehensive Study Guide*. 7th ed. New York: McGraw-Hill, 2011.

▶ Discharge

Patients with first-time resolved seizures may be safely discharged home if no secondary cause of the seizure is identified and the patient has returned to normal mental status. Antiepileptic drugs are not indicated initially, as only one third of these patients will have a second seizure over their lifetimes. The patient should have an outpatient work-up with a neurologist including an EEG and MRI. Instruct the patient to avoid driving vehicles, swimming, or participating in any other activity that may put themselves or anyone else in danger if a second seizure occurs. Patients with a known seizure disorder may be discharged if there are no complicating factors after their antiepileptic drug levels are repleted.

SUGGESTED READING

Duvivier E, Pollack C. Seizures. In: Marx JA. *Rosen's Emergency Medicine*. 7th ed. Philadelphia, PA: Elsevier, 2009. Chapter 100, 1346–1355

Lung D, Catlett C, Tintinalli J. Seizures and status epilepticus in adults. In: Tintinalli JE, Stapczynski JS, Cline DM, Ma OJ, Cydulka RK, Meckler GD. *Tintinalli's Emergency Medicine: A Comprehensive Study Guide*. 7th ed. New York, NY: McGraw-Hill, 2011, pp. 1153–1159.

Tarabar A, Ulrich A, D'Onofrio G. Chapter 99 Seizures. In Adams J, Barton E, Collings J, DeBlieux P, Gisondi M, Nadal E. *Emergency Medicine: Clinical Essentials*. 2nd ed. Philadelphia, PA Saunders, 2013, pp. 857–69.

84

Trauma Principles

Jorge Fernandez, MD

Neil Rifenbark, MD

Key Points

- Assess all trauma patients with a rapid primary survey followed by a more comprehensive secondary evaluation.
- Address all emergent life threats in a stepwise manner during the primary survey before progressing to the next stage.

- Treat hemodynamically unstable patients as hemorrhagic shock until proven otherwise.
- Initiate aggressive volume resuscitation in all unstable patients while concurrently searching for active sources of hemorrhage.

INTRODUCTION

Trauma is currently the fourth leading cause of death in the United States across all age groups and the leading cause of death in patients under the age of 44 years. It is responsible for more deaths in patients under the age of 19 years than all other causes combined. Approximately 40% of all emergency department (ED) visits are for trauma-related complaints, and the annual costs exceed $400 billion. Adding to these costs, permanent disability is actually 3 times more likely than death in this cohort.

Trauma is broadly classified by mechanism into blunt and penetrating varieties, with the former more than twice as common as the latter. Regardless of mechanism, victims of significant trauma present with a wide range of complex problems, and their proper care necessitates a multidisciplinary approach, including emergency physicians, trauma surgeons, and the appropriate subspecialties. Most trauma care delivery systems follow the Advanced Trauma Life Support guidelines developed and maintained by the American College of Surgeons.

The mortality rates for traumatic injuries typically follow a trimodal distribution. Certain injury patterns including major vascular injuries and high cervical cord disruption with secondary apnea result in near immediate death. The second cohort of injuries, including conditions such as pneumothorax and pericardial tamponade, typically evolve over a duration of minutes to hours and are generally responsive to aggressive emergent intervention. Septicemia and multisystem organ failure account for the third peak of fatalities and typically occur weeks to months after injury.

CLINICAL PRESENTATION

▶ History

Attempt to identify the severity of mechanism, as this will predict the patterns of injury. For example, determine the approximate speed of a motor vehicle collision (MVC) and whether or not the patient was restrained. Emergency medical service personnel can be an invaluable resource, especially in amnestic and nonverbal patients. In assault patients, inquire if they can recall exactly what they were struck with and the number of times. Ask if there was any loss of consciousness, as this may portend to a significant head injury. For penetrating trauma, ask about the number of shots heard and how many times the patient felt himself or herself get shot.

Obtain a brief medical history using the **AMPLE** mnemonic. Ask about any known drug **allergies**, current **medication** use, **past medical history**, **last oral intake**, and the immediate **events** leading up to the injury. Keep in mind that regardless of past history, elderly patients have less physiologic reserve and are prone to higher rates of morbidity and mortality. In females of childbearing age, always ask about the last menstrual period and assume that they are pregnant until proven otherwise. Pregnant patients are at higher risk for domestic violence and warrant unique considerations such as placental abruption, uterine rupture, the supine hypotensive syndrome, and fetal distress or demise. Even apparently minor injuries including falls and low-speed motor vehicle accidents can induce preterm labor or placental abruption.

Always ask about any evolving symptoms and identify the exact locations of pain, as this will guide your physical exam. Patients with altered mental status should be treated as having a traumatic brain injury until proven otherwise. Shortness of breath may indicate an underlying pneumothorax (PTX), pulmonary contusion, or pericardial tamponade. Chest pain may indicate an underlying fracture of the ribs or sternum, hemothorax (HTX), or traumatic aortic injury (TAI). Assume that patients with abdominal pain, hematemesis, or rectal bleeding have an intra-abdominal visceral injury until proven otherwise. Patients complaining of hematuria should be considered at a high risk for injury to the genitourinary (GU) tract. Neurologic complaints including weakness and paresthesias may indicate an underlying spinal cord injury or vascular dissection.

▶ Physical Examination

The physical exam in major trauma patients is very systematic and can be divided into primary and secondary surveys.

Primary Survey

The primary survey is a very brief and focused exam meant to identify and address emergent life threats. It should proceed in a stepwise approach outlined by the **ABCDE** mnemonic. Always treat any encountered abnormalities before proceeding to the next step in the survey. If a patient decompensates at any point during his or her clinical course, return to the beginning of the primary survey and reassess. Assume an unstable cervical spine injury in all major trauma victims until proven otherwise and immediately immobilize on presentation.

Assess the **airway** for patency. Signs of potential airway compromise include pooling pharyngeal secretions, intraoral foreign bodies, stridulous or gurgling respirations, obvious oropharyngeal burns, significant midface, mandibular, and laryngeal fractures, and expanding neck hematomas.

Evaluate the patient's **breathing** and ventilation. Expose the chest and look for any signs of asymmetrical or paradoxical chest wall movement, obvious deformities or open wounds, tracheal deviation, and jugular venous distention. Auscultate the chest to confirm strong symmetric bilateral breath sounds. The goal is to identify the presence of emergent life threats including tension PTX, massive HTX, open PTX (sucking chest wound), and flail chest.

Rapidly assess the patient's **circulation** by evaluating for signs of altered mental status. A depressed level of consciousness should be considered hypovolemic shock until proven otherwise. Other findings concerning for hemorrhagic shock include pale, cool, and mottled extremities and thready peripheral pulses. Auscultate the heart to detect distant heart tones suggestive of an underlying pericardial effusion. Identify all sources of active bleeding and control with the application of direct pressure.

Perform a rapid neurologic exam, noting any evidence of **disability** or deficits. Document the patient's level of consciousness; note the size, symmetry, and reactivity of the pupils; and assess for any focal numbness or weakness. Perform a rectal exam to ensure adequate rectal tone and determine the patient's Glasgow Coma Scale (GCS).

Completely **expose** the patient to ensure that all potential life threats have been accounted for. Carefully log-roll the patient to examine the back and rule out any occult penetrating injuries. Once complete, immediately cover the patient with warm blankets to prevent the development of hypothermia.

Secondary Survey

The secondary survey is a complete head-to-toe examination that should be performed once the patient has been stabilized. Examine the scalp, noting any lacerations, contusions, and deformities. Check the visual acuity, visual fields, extraocular movements, and pupil size and reactivity. Assess the globe for penetrating injuries, lacerations, or proptosis. Examine the mid-face, looking for evidence of fracture, lacerations, epistaxis, or septal hematomas. Look for signs of basilar skull fracture such as hemotympanum, periorbital (raccoon eyes) or retroauricular ecchymoses (Battle sign), and cerebrospinal fluid (CSF) rhinorrhea or otorrhea. CSF rhinorrhea can be detected with the use of a bedside "halo-test." Check for dental injuries or evidence of mandibular fracture, including point tenderness, malocclusion, and sublingual hematomas.

Inspect the neck, noting any signs of obvious tracheal deviation, laryngeal fracture, subcutaneous emphysema, or expanding hematoma. Carefully palpate the cervical spine to detect any point tenderness or bony step-offs. Re-inspect the chest, noting any signs of contusions, asymmetry, paradoxical movement, or penetrating injury. Palpate the ribs and sternum, checking for point tenderness, soft tissue crepitus, and bony deformity. Repeat auscultation of the lungs and heart and document any abnormalities. Inspect the abdomen for any signs of distention, contusions, or penetrating injury. Palpate all 4 quadrants to elicit any tenderness, guarding, or rebound. Carefully assess the pelvis for signs of an unstable fracture by gently compressing the iliac crests.

Inspect the perineum for lacerations, contusions, and hematomas. Perform vaginal and rectal examinations to assess for gross blood or mucosal trauma. Note the rectal tone and check the prostate for signs of displacement. Findings consistent with urethral injury include scrotal hematomas, blood at the urethral meatus, and a high-riding prostate.

Look for any signs of blunt or penetrating trauma to the extremities. Document any open wounds, point tenderness, or obvious deformities. Range all joints, looking for abnormal movement. Palpate all muscle compartments to detect any signs of developing tension. Roll the patient and palpate the entire spine, noting any point tenderness or bony step-offs.

Assess the pulses in all 4 extremities. In penetrating trauma, the "hard" signs of arterial injury include absent distal pulses, pulsatile bleeding, expanding hematomas, and the presence of bruits or thrills. The "soft" signs of arterial injury include diminished distal pulses, visible hematomas, corresponding peripheral nerve deficits, or delayed capillary refill. Patients with soft signs for arterial injury require the measurement of the arterial pressure index (API). The API can be calculated by dividing the systolic pressure of the affected extremity by the systolic pressure of the contralateral unaffected limb. An API <0.9 is considered abnormal and suggestive of arterial injury.

Finally, perform a comprehensive motor and sensory examination, reevaluate the pupils and mental status, and recalculate the GCS.

DIAGNOSTIC STUDIES

▶ Laboratory

Check a STAT bedside capillary blood glucose level in all patients with an abnormal mental status as hypoglycemia can mimic a traumatic brain injury. Check a complete blood count to assess an initial hematocrit and follow serially to assess for occult hemorrhage and responsiveness to therapy. If available, obtain a bedside serum base deficit and lactate level and follow serially to gauge responsiveness to therapy. Send a type and screen on all trauma patients and crossmatch blood as necessary for patients likely to require transfusions or operative intervention. Obtain a urinalysis to rule out gross hematuria, a bedside urine pregnancy test in all female patients of childbearing age, and a urine toxicology screen in patients with an abnormal level of consciousness. Check coagulation studies in all patients with a clotting disorder (eg, patients on warfarin).

▶ Imaging

Portable plain radiography is readily available at most institutions for the rapid bedside evaluation of trauma patients. Plain films are useful for diagnosing bony fractures including unstable pelvic and spinal injuries; determining the trajectory of penetrating projectiles; identifying HTX, PTX, or an abnormal mediastinum; and detecting the presence of intraperitoneal free air.

Bedside ultrasonography provides a quick, highly sensitive, noninvasive, and readily repeatable modality to detect occult hemorrhage. Perform a FAST exam to look for signs of pericardial tamponade, PTX/HTX, and intraperitoneal bleeding (see Chapter 88 for further details).

Computed tomography (CT) imaging has revolutionized the care of trauma patients. That said, this modality does expose the patient to increased health care costs, potential contrast reactions, and harmful ionizing radiation, so every effort should be made to limit its use to patients whose condition truly warrants it. Furthermore, CT imaging should be pursued only in patients who are stable enough to safely leave the resuscitation area for an extended period of time. CT imaging of the head has become invaluable for the evaluation and treatment of patients with traumatic brain injury. CT imaging of the chest is now the preferred modality to evaluate patients with potential intrathoracic vascular emergencies (eg, TAI) and evolving pulmonary contusions. CT of the abdomen and pelvis can simultaneously detect solid viscus injury (eg, liver and spleen) and intraperitoneal hemorrhage and determine the severity of pelvic injuries. Finally, CT angiography has rapidly become the preferred means to exclude vascular injuries in patients whose condition warrants some form of radiographic imaging (eg, patients with "soft signs" for arterial injury).

Magnetic resonance imaging is useful for the evaluation of patients with potential spinal cord injury and to further delineate the severity of traumatic brain injury. That said, its use should be limited only to stable patients who can afford prolonged excursions outside of a resuscitation arena.

PROCEDURES

The coordinated resuscitation of a critically ill trauma patient may require a multitude of simultaneous interventions. The following procedures are described in detail in the corresponding chapters: central line placement and volume resuscitation (Chapter 3), needle thoracostomy and chest tube insertion (Chapter 7), emergent airway management (Chapter 11), pericardiocentesis and ED thoracotomy (Chapter 87), and diagnostic peritoneal lavage (Chapter 88).

Perform a retrograde **urethrogram** and **cystogram** in all patients with suspected urethral and bladder injuries. Indications include straddle injuries, pelvic fractures, scrotal hematomas, high-riding prostates, and blood at the urethral meatus. A urethrogram is performed by injecting intravenous (IV) dye into the urethral meatus while simultaneously capturing a pelvic radiograph to detect any signs of urethral disruption (ie, contrast extravasation). Avoid the insertion of a Foley catheter into any patient with a demonstrated urethral injury without GU consultation. For patients with an intact urethra, insert a catheter and distend the bladder with up to 300 mL of diluted IV contrast while simultaneously capturing a pelvic radiograph (cystogram) to detect any evidence of bladder rupture.

MEDICAL DECISION MAKING

Obtain a complete set of vital signs and note any abnormalities. Hemodynamic instability in the setting of trauma is hemorrhagic shock until proven otherwise. Initiate aggressive volume resuscitation in said patients.

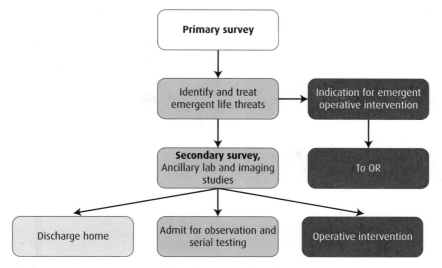

Figure 84-1. Trauma principles diagnostic algorithm. OR, operating room.

Perform an immediate primary survey and address any emergent life threats including airway obstruction, tension or open PTX, massive HTX, and pericardial tamponade. Use your laboratory and imaging studies as necessary to determine the presence and severity of injury. Following patient stabilization, perform a comprehensive secondary survey and treat all encountered injuries (Figure 84-1).

▶ Treatment

Evaluation and treatment should coincide during the primary survey. All life-threatening conditions must be stabilized before further evaluation. Secure the airway in any patient with signs of impending compromise. Patients with a GCS ≤8 require endotracheal intubation to guard against obstruction and/or aspiration. Examine the thoracic wall to identify any open PTX and cover with a 3-sided occlusive dressing to restore normal respiratory mechanics. Perform immediate needle thoracostomy in all patients with signs of tension PTX, and place a chest tube in all patients with evidence of traumatic PTX or HTX.

Patients with evidence of impaired circulation require large-bore IV access and aggressive volume resuscitation (Lactated Ringer's or normal saline). Attempt to determine the class of hypovolemic shock to guide fluid resuscitation and identify the need for packed red blood cell transfusion (Table 84-1). Concurrently attempt to identify the source of hemorrhage to determine the need for surgical intervention. Unstable patients with either clinical evidence (hypotension, distant heart sounds, jugular venous distention) or ultrasonographic confirmation of pericardial tamponade require emergent pericardiocentesis.

Provide sufficient analgesia to ensure patient comfort and facilitate further evaluation. Small boluses of IV fentanyl are ideal because of its short duration of activity and minimal hemodynamic side effects. Ketamine can be used both as an analgesic and sedative agent in lower than normal "subdissociative" doses without concern for respiratory or cardiovascular depression. Ondansetron can

Table 84-1. Classes of hypovolemic shock.

	Class I	Class II	Class III	Class IV
Blood loss (mL)	Up to 750	750–1,500	1,500–2,000	>2,000
Blood loss (% blood volume)	Up to 15%	15–30%	30–40%	>40%
Pulse rate (beats/min)	<100	>100	>120	>140
BP	Normal	Normal	Decreased	Decreased
Pulse pressure (mm Hg)	Normal or increased	Decreased	Decreased	Decreased
RR (breaths/min)	14–20	20–30	30–40	>35
Urine output (mL/hr)	>30	20–30	5–15	Negligible
CNS/mental status	Slightly anxious	Mildly anxious	Anxious, confused	Confused, lethargic
Fluid replacement (3:1 rule)*	Crystalloid	Crystalloid	Crystalloid and blood	Crystalloid and blood

*Fluid replacement should be 3× the estimated blood loss.

be given to reduce nausea and vomiting, and haloperidol may be necessary to sedate agitated patients.

DISPOSITION

▶ Admission

The majority of blunt trauma victims require admission for observation to rule out occult injuries not detected on either the primary and secondary surveys or CT imaging. Hemodynamically unstable patients with positive focused assessment with sonography for trauma (FAST) or CT imaging typically require operative intervention. Victims of penetrating trauma generally require admission and operative intervention when the implements clearly violate significant body cavities or injure vital anatomical structures.

▶ Discharge

Blunt trauma patients with minor injuries who remain hemodynamically stable on serial assessments can be safely discharged. Penetrating trauma patients may be discharged provided that the path of the implement clearly does not violate any significant body cavities nor approach any vital anatomical structures. Always ensure that the patient is able to ambulate and tolerate oral intake before discharge.

▼ SUGGESTED READINGS

Bailitz J, et al. *Emergent Management of Trauma*. 3rd ed. Chapter 3. Patient Evaluation. New York, NY: McGraw Hill, 2011.

Bonatti H, Calland J. Trauma. *Emerg Med Clin North Am*. 2008;26:625–648.

Brunett PH, Cameron PA. Trauma in adults. In: Tintinalli JE, Stapczynski JS, Ma OJ, Cline DM, Cydulka RK, Meckler GD. *Tintinalli's Emergency Medicine: A Comprehensive Study Guide*. 7th ed. New York, NY: McGraw-Hill, 2011.

Initial assessment and management. *ATLS Student Course Manual*. 9th ed. Chapter 1. Chicago, IL: American College of Surgeons, 2012, 2–28.

Head Injuries

Katie L. Tataris, MD

Key Points

- Traumatic brain injury can be classified by severity into mild (Glasgow Coma Scale [GCS] ≥14), moderate (GCS 9–13), and severe (GCS ≤ 8) categories.

- An emergent noninfused head computed tomography is the imaging modality of choice in patients with cranial trauma.

- Patients with intracranial hemorrhage can quickly deteriorate and require frequent neurological re-evaluations.

- Limit secondary brain injury by identifying and addressing concurrent hypoxemia, hypotension, and increased intracranial pressure.

INTRODUCTION

Between 1.2 and 2 million patients sustain some form of traumatic brain injury (TBI) in the United States every year. Fortunately the majority of cases (~80%) are mild, as moderate and severe TBI is associated with significant long-term disability and death. In fact, head injuries are the leading cause of traumatic death in all patients younger than 25 years. Currently more than 50,000 deaths and 370,000 hospitalizations are attributable to TBI on an annual basis. The associated costs of caring for patients with acute and chronic TBI are astronomical, exceeding $4 billion per year. TBI occurs as the normal physiologic function of the brain is disrupted by either direct (object striking the cranium) or indirect (acceleration/deceleration) forces. Patterns of injury can be classified as either primary (occur at the time of impact) or secondary (develop over time owing to neurochemical and inflammatory responses). Patients with TBI can be further stratified by their Glasgow Coma Scores (GCS) into mild (GCS ≥14), moderate (GCS 9–13), and severe (GCS ≤8) categories (Table 85-1).

Cerebral circulation is dictated by the cerebral perfusion pressure (CPP), and ensuring adequate blood flow is of the utmost importance in patients with TBI. The CPP is proportional to the difference between the mean arterial pressure (MAP and the intracranial pressure (ICP) (CPP ∝

MAP − ICP). The intracranial space is a fixed volume, and the ICP is determined by the amount of brain tissue, blood, and cerebrospinal fluid (CSF) within it. Increases in

Table 85-1. Glasgow Coma Scale (GCS).

Eye Opening	
Spontaneous	4
To verbal command	3
To pain	2
No response	1
Best Motor Response	
Obeys commands	6
Localizes to pain	5
Withdraws to pain	4
Abnormal flexion	3
Abnormal extension	2
No response	1
Best Verbal Response	
Oriented, converses	5
Confused	4
Inappropriate	3
Incomprehensible	2
No response	1

either of these variables will cause secondary elevations in the ICP. The brain can autoregulate cerebral perfusion under normal physiologic conditions, but cannot do so at the extremes of either MAP or ICP. Therefore, processes that significantly decrease the MAP (eg, traumatic shock) or increase the ICP (eg, intracranial hemorrhage) may impair cerebral perfusion and exacerbate secondary brain injury.

The following is a list of specific injury patterns seen in patients with TBI:

Concussions represent a traumatic alteration in neurologic function in the absence of abnormalities on computed tomography (CT) imaging. Symptoms including recurring headaches, sleep disturbances, and difficulties with concentration that can persist for months (postconcussive syndrome).

Skull fractures can be categorized by location (basilar vs calvarium), pattern (linear, depressed, or comminuted), and by whether they are open or closed injuries.

Cerebral contusions represent punctate intraparenchymal hemorrhages with surrounding edema and occur most commonly in the frontal, temporal, and occipital lobes. Contusions that occur both at the direct site of injury and the opposing side of the brain secondary to indirect deceleration forces are known as coup and contrecoup injuries, respectively.

Traumatic subarachnoid hemorrhage (SAH) is the most common abnormality recognized on posttraumatic CT imaging. Traumatic SAH occurs when injury to the small subarachnoid vessels leads to secondary hemorrhage within the subarachnoid space.

Subdural hematoma (SDH) is most commonly encountered in patients with significant cerebral atrophy (elderly, alcoholics). They occur when excessive shearing forces injure the small bridging veins in the subdural space. SDHs classically appear on CT imaging as crescent-shaped hematomas that freely cross suture lines. As a distinct history of trauma may not be present, always maintain a high index of suspicion in elderly patients with nonspecific mental status changes.

Epidural hematoma (EDH) is most commonly seen in patients with temporoparietal skull fractures and secondary injury to the middle meningeal artery. They occur when high-pressure arterial bleeding separates the dura from the inner table of the skull to form a hematoma. EDHs are classically lentiform or bean-shaped in appearance on CT imaging and do not cross the cranial suture lines (Figure 85-1). The classic presentation is a patient with blunt head trauma who initially appears well after the injury (the so-called lucid interval) only to rapidly decompensate several hours later.

Diffuse axonal injury (DAI) occurs when sudden deceleration mechanisms transmit shearing forces diffusely

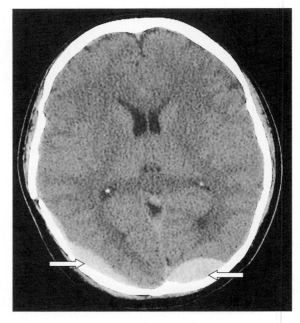

▲ **Figure 85-1.** CT scan of the head showing an epidural (patient's left) and a subdural (patient's right) hematoma.

across the axonal fibers of the brain. CT imaging is nonspecific, and patients tend to have poor outcomes.

Penetrating brain injury is usually catastrophic because of the immense amount of kinetic energy transmitted to very sensitive brain tissues. Mortality rates from gunshot wounds to the head approach 90%.

In addition to the specific injury patterns listed previously, TBI can lead to drastic increases in ICP, resulting in herniation. Transtentorial herniation of the temporal lobe uncus is the most common form and typically presents with altered mental status and a dilated or blown pupil secondary to compression of the oculomotor nerve (cranial nerve [CN] III). Transforaminal herniation of the cerebellar tonsils through the foramen magnum can occur with significant increases in the ICP, especially with posterior fossa hemorrhages, and is rapidly fatal due to compression and consequent dysfunction of the brainstem.

CLINICAL PRESENTATION

▶ History

Always attempt to identify the exact mechanism of injury, as this may predict the severity of damage to the central nervous system (CNS). For example, clarify the height of a fall, the speed of a motor vehicle collision (MVC), or the use of seatbelt restraints or airbag deployment. Emergency medical service personal can be invaluable in this setting. Inquire about any loss of consciousness, as this may portend more significant injury. The antecedent use of alcohol or illicit drugs may complicate the neurologic assessment, and their influence should be documented. Ask about the use of any prescription or over-the-counter medications, as anticoagulants can induce life-threatening bleeding despite only minor injury. Finally, look for any signs and symptoms suggestive of increased ICP (altered mental status, vomiting, headache), as this will require emergent neurosurgical intervention.

Physical Examination

As with all trauma patients, begin with a rapid primary survey, and aggressively address any emergent life threats. Carefully note vital signs, as they can predict the likelihood of secondary brain injury. Cushing reflex, defined as progressive hypertension, bradycardia, and a decreased respiratory rate, is frequently indicative of a potentially life-threatening increase in ICP.

A gross inspection of the scalp may reveal gaping lacerations or obvious cranial deformities. Carefully inspect all deep lacerations for violation of the galea, as disruption of this tough layer of connective tissue mandates careful primary closure. Palpate the skull to detect step-off deformities indicative of underlying fracture. Examine the eyes and the ears for any signs of injury. Battle sign (retroauricular ecchymosis), raccoon eyes (periorbital ecchymosis), hemotympanum, and CSF rhinorrhea or otorrhea are all signs of an underlying basilar skull fracture (Figure 85-2). Carefully palpate the cervical spine and always assume an occult C-spine injury until proven otherwise.

Perform a comprehensive neurologic exam to identify any findings suggestive of significant injury. Examine the pupils, taking care to note size, symmetry, and reactivity. A dilated unresponsive pupil in the setting of cranial trauma indicates transtentorial herniation until proven otherwise. Document an initial GCS and repeat frequently to detect any signs of decompensation. The uncoordinated flexion (decorticate) or extension (decerebrate) of one's upper extremities on painful stimulation indicates severe intracranial injury with possible brainstem compromise.

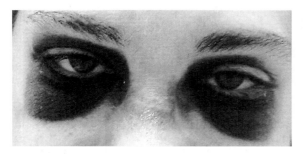

▲ **Figure 85-2.** "Raccoon eyes" suggestive of a basilar skull fracture.

DIAGNOSTIC STUDIES

▶ Laboratory

A routine trauma panel including a complete blood count, chemistry, coagulation studies, and toxicology screening should be ordered on all patients with significant multisystem trauma. That said, there are no laboratory studies specific for the diagnosis or management of TBI.

▶ Imaging

An emergent noninfused head CT is the study of choice for the evaluation of patients with potential TBI. It is quick, noninvasive, and highly sensitive for the diagnosis of both bony and intracranial injuries. Patients who present more than 48 hours after injury may require intravenous (IV) contrast to delineate the presence of isodense subdural hematomas. CT imaging does expose patients to potentially harmful ionizing radiation, and the patient's clinical presentation should always guide the decision to image.

Indications for CT imaging in adult patients are debatable, but most agree that any of the following findings warrant testing: GCS <15, age >65 years, high-energy mechanisms (fall >3 ft) focal neurologic deficits, ≥2 episodes of vomiting, evidence of depressed or basilar skull fracture, posttraumatic seizure, persistent anterograde amnesia, persistent severe headache, or the presence of coagulopathies. The indications for CT imaging in pediatric patients are similarly debatable but typically include the presence of any of the following: loss of consciousness, abnormal mental status, vomiting, palpable skull fracture or signs of basilar skull fracture, scalp hematomas, and high-energy mechanisms.

PROCEDURES

Severe TBI patients with subdural or epidural hematomas and evidence of impending or evolving herniation require intracranial decompression and clot evacuation via emergent burr-hole placement performed by a neurosurgeon or emergency physician.

MEDICAL DECISION MAKING

The primary survey and presenting GCS should guide the work-up and management of patients with TBI. The differential diagnosis should include all of the aforementioned conditions, including cerebral contusions, intracranial hemorrhage, and DAI. Rapidly decompensating patients should be considered evolving herniations until proven otherwise. Emergent CT imaging will help establish the proper diagnosis and guide further treatment (Figure 85-3).

TREATMENT

The management of TBI begins with the primary survey. Patients with severe TBI (GCS ≤8) require emergent endotracheal intubation to maintain airway protection. Perform

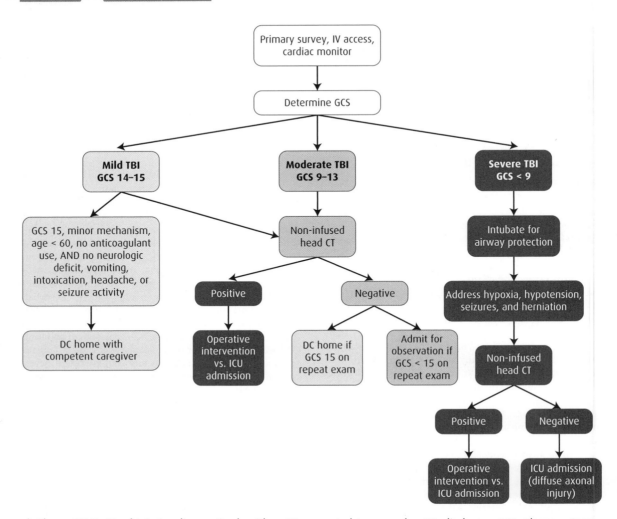

▲ **Figure 85-3.** Head injuries diagnostic algorithm. CT, computed tomography; DC, discharge; GCS, Glasgow Coma Scale; ICU, intensive care unit; TBI, traumatic brain injury.

rapid sequence intubation while following head trauma precautions (see Chapter 11). Systemic hypotension can significantly impair adequate cerebral perfusion, and patients require aggressive volume resuscitation to maintain a MAP >90 mmHg and suitable CPP. Address any uncontrolled scalp hemorrhage, as blood loss can be significant.

Patients with evidence of increased ICP and impending herniation require immediate medical intervention pending definitive neurosurgical care. Mild hyperventilation to a goal $PaCO_2$ between 30 and 35 mmHg can temporarily reduce the ICP by decreasing cerebral blood flow. Hyperosmotic agents such as IV mannitol (0.25–2 g/kg) can reduce intracerebral edema and thereby decrease the ICP. Elevating the head of the bed to 30 degrees can reduce the ICP by simple gravity. All of these interventions should be

considered temporizing measures while awaiting operative decompression or bedside extraventricular drain placement.

Posttraumatic seizures can be devastating, as they significantly exacerbate secondary brain injury. Antiepileptic drug loading (eg, phenytoin 18 mg/kg) should be pursued in all patients without known contraindications. Treat patients who are actively seizing with aggressive doses of IV benzodiazepines (eg, lorazepam 0.05 mg/kg) until their convulsions are controlled.

Patients with traumatic SAH are at an elevated risk of ischemic complications secondary to cerebral vasospasm. The careful use of peripheral arteriolar vasodilators (eg, nimodipine 60 mg orally) may limit this phenomenon in hemodynamically stable patients, although recent data suggests minimal utility at best. Finally, patients with fractures that either involve a maxillofacial sinus or are open to the environment warrant antibiotic prophylaxis to limit secondary infection and tetanus vaccination. Those with skull fractures whose margins are depressed beyond the inner table of the adjacent skull warrant neurosurgical consultation for operative elevation.

DISPOSITION

▶ Admission

Admit all patients with severe TBI (GCS ≤8) or documented injury on CT imaging to an intensive care unit setting with neurosurgical consultation, as they will require continuous ICP monitoring. Patients with a persistent GCS <15, evidence of basilar skull fracture, open or depressed fractures, and those with linear fractures that cross an arterial groove or dural sinus require admission for observation and serial neurologic exams.

▶ Discharge

Low-risk patients with a normal GCS and neurologic exam can be safely discharged from the ED. If a CT scan was not indicated at the time of the initial visit, discharge the patient with instructions to return for any changes in mental status, vomiting, or worsening headaches. Ideally, a responsible adult will be present to monitor the patient at home over the next 24 hours. If a CT scan is performed

and is negative, it is unlikely the patient will require any neurosurgical intervention in the future. These patients can also be discharged assuming normal GCS and neurologic exam. They should receive similar head injury precautions.

Patients diagnosed with a concussion should avoid any contact sports until all symptoms have completely resolved and they have been cleared by a trained physician. Postconcussive syndromes including headaches and problems concentrating or sleeping are fairly common and may persist for several weeks to months after the injury.

▼ SUGGESTED READING

Guidelines for the management of severe traumatic brain injury. *J Neurotrauma.* 2007;24(suppl 1):S1.

Jagoda AS, Bazarian JJ, Bruns JJ, et al. Clinical policy: neuroimaging and decision making in adult mild brain injury in the acute setting. *Ann Emerg Med.* 20080;52:714.

Nigrovic LE, Lee LK, Hoyle J, et al. Prevalence of clinically important traumatic brain injuries in children with minor blunt head trauma and isolated severe injury mechanisms. *Arch Pediatr Adolesc Med.* 2012;166:356–361.

Wright DW, Merk LH. Head trauma in adults and children. In: Tintinalli JE, Stapczynski JS, Ma OJ, Cline DM, Cydulka RK, Meckler GD. *Tintinalli's Emergency Medicine: A Comprehensive Study Guide.* 7th Ed. New York, NY: McGraw-Hill, 2011.

Zink BJ. Traumatic brain injury outcome: Concepts for emergency care. *Ann Emerg Med.* 2001;37:318–332.

Cervical Spine Injuries

E. Paul DeKoning, MD

Key Points

- Use the NEXUS criteria and/or Canadian C-Spine rules to determine which patients require radiographic imaging.
- Forego plain films and proceed directly to computed tomography imaging of the cervical spine for all patients with a moderate to high risk of injury.

- Consider spinal cord injury without radiologic abnormality in pediatric patients with neurologic findings despite negative initial imaging.
- The use of high-dose corticosteroids to improve long-term neurologic outcomes in patients with blunt spinal cord injury is no longer recommended.

INTRODUCTION

There are currently more than 200,000 patients living with spinal cord injury (SCI) in the United States, and between 12,000 and 20,000 new cases occur on an annual basis. The majority of patients are between 16 and 30 years of age, with motor vehicle collisions, falls, violence, and sporting injuries accounting for the bulk of cases. Fewer than 1% of patients experience complete neurologic recovery before hospital discharge, and the associated economical, physical, and emotional tolls are astronomical.

The cervical spine is composed of 7 cervical vertebrae, the first 2 of which are unique, whereas the remaining 5 (C3 through C7) are functionally similar. The anatomy of the axis (C1) is that of a bony ring without a true vertebral body. It consists of an anterior and posterior arch joined together by 2 lateral masses that articulate with the occipital condyles above and C2 below. The Atlas (C2) has a unique anterior body that extends superiorly to form the odontoid process. This structure articulates with the internal surface of the anterior ring of C1 and is held in place by the transverse ligament. The unique design of these 2 vertebrae allow for the increased flexibility and axial rotation of the upper cervical spine. The remaining cervical vertebrae are functionally similar and composed of an anterior body and a posterior arch.

The vertebrae are separated by flexible intervertebral disks and linked together by an intricate system of ligaments that allows the spine to function as a single unit. Anterior and posterior longitudinal ligaments run along the entire length of the vertebral bodies, whereas the posterior rings are linked together by the ligamentum flavum and interspinous ligaments (Figure 86-1). This network enables significant spinal column mobility while still providing adequate spinal cord protection as it courses within the spinal canal between the body and arch of each vertebra. External forces that exceed the normal physiologic range of motion can result in fractures, dislocations, and spinal cord injuries. Children and the elderly are especially prone to injury of the upper cervical spine (C1 through C3), whereas young and middle-aged adults are more likely to injure the lower cervical spine (C6 through T1). Of the cervical vertebrae, the atlas (C2) is the most frequently fractured.

Delineating between stable and unstable injury is of supreme clinical importance. The Denis 3-column theory is very helpful in this regard and divides the spine into 3 functional units. The anterior column is composed of the anterior portions of the vertebral body and annulus fibrosis together with the anterior longitudinal ligament. The middle column includes the posterior vertebral body, the posterior annulus fibrosis, and the posterior longitudinal ligament. The posterior column is composed of the

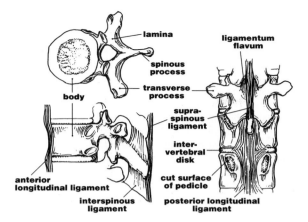

▲ **Figure 86-1.** Bony and ligamentous anatomy of the spine. Reprinted with permission from Tintinalli JE, Kelen GD, Stapczynski JS. *Tintinalli's Emergency Medicine: A Comprehensive Study Guide.* 6th ed. New York: McGraw-Hill, 2004.

posterior vertebral arch and the posterior ligamentous complex including the ligamentum flavum and the interspinous and supraspinous ligaments. Injuries to ≥2 of the columns are considered functionally unstable. In addition, acute compression fractures involving >25% of the height of the vertebral bodies of C3–C7 are considered clinically unstable.

Cervical spine fractures can be further classified by their mechanism of injury (Table 86-1). **Flexion injuries** compress the anterior column and distract the posterior column, resulting in anterior body fractures and disruption of the posterior ligamentous complex. Specific examples include anterior subluxations, bilateral facet dislocations, simple wedge fractures, spinous process avulsions (clay shoveler's fracture), and flexion teardrop fractures. A concurrent rotational mechanism results in unilateral facet dislocations. Simple wedge fractures, spinous process avulsions, and unilateral facet dislocations are generally considered stable, whereas the remainder represent unstable injuries.

Extension injuries compress the posterior column and distract the anterior column, resulting in crush injuries to the posterior elements and disruption of the anterior longitudinal ligament. Specific examples include extension teardrop fractures, hangman's fractures (traumatic spondylolisthesis of C2), laminar fractures, and hyperextension dislocations. With the exception of simple laminar fractures, these injuries are generally unstable.

Axial load injuries occur when vertical compression forces shatter the ring-like structure of a cervical vertebra, resulting in an outward burst of bony fragments. These injuries require disruption of all 3 columns and are clinically unstable. Burst fractures of C1 (Jefferson fracture) are relatively common and highly unstable.

Table 86-1. Stability of cervical spine injuries.

Flexion
Anterior subluxation (hyperflexion sprain) (stable)*
Bilateral interfacetal dislocation (unstable)
Simple wedge (compression) fracture (usually stable)
Spinous process avulsion (clay-shoveler's) fracture (stable)
Flexion teardrop fracture (unstable)
Flexion-rotation
Unilateral interfacetal dislocation (stable)
Pillar fracture
Fracture of lateral mass (can be unstable)
Vertical compression
Jefferson burst fracture of atlas (potentially unstable)
Burst (bursting, dispersion, axial-loading) fracture (unstable)
Hyperextension
Hyperextension dislocation (unstable)
Avulsion fracture of anterior arch of atlas (stable)
Extension teardrop fracture (unstable)
Fracture of posterior arch of atlas (stable)
Laminar fracture (usually stable)
Traumatic spondylolisthesis (hangman's fracture) (unstable)
Lateral flexion
Uncinate process fracture (usually stable)
Injuries caused by diverse or poorly understood mechanisms
Occipital condyle fractures (can be unstable)
Occipitoatlantal dissociation (highly unstable)
Dens fractures (type II and III are unstable)

*Usual occurrence. Overall stability is dependent on integrity of the other ligamentous structures.

Reprinted with permission from Baron BJ, McSherry KJ, Larson, Jr. JL, Scalea TM. Chapter 255. Spine and Spinal Cord Trauma. In: Tintinalli JE, Stapczynski JS, Cline DM, Ma OJ, Cydulka RK, Meckler GD, eds. *Tintinalli's Emergency Medicine: A Comprehensive Study Guide.* 7th ed. New York: McGraw-Hill, 2011.

Any significant trauma to the spinal cord generally occurs at the time of the initial injury. Although individual injuries will frequently exhibit unique neurologic findings, several classic syndromes have been described. The **central cord syndrome** occurs with hyperextension mechanisms, typically in elderly patients with severe spinal stenosis. It presents with motor weakness that is more pronounced in the upper extremities as compared with the lower. The **anterior cord syndrome** occurs with hyperflexion mechanisms and results in motor and sensory loss below the level of injury with preservation of position and vibratory sense (located in the posterior columns). The **Brown-Sequard syndrome** most commonly stems from a penetrating injury that hemisects the cord. Classic findings include the ipsilateral loss of motor function and position and vibratory sensation combined with the contralateral loss of pain and temperature sensation distal to the lesion.

Spinal cord injury without radiologic abnormality (SCIWORA) is seen in pediatric patients and should be considered in all patients with neurologic findings despite negative initial plain film or computed tomography (CT) imaging. Magnetic resonance imaging (MRI) may reveal significant pathology, including ligamentous injury, intracordal edema, and hemorrhage.

CLINICAL PRESENTATION

▶ History

Try to determine the exact mechanism of injury, as this may help predict the overall severity of pathology (Table 86-2). Inquire about the presence of neck pain and any neurologic complaints, including weakness, paresthesias, and the loss of bowel or bladder function. Review the patient's past medical history for relevant comorbid conditions, including rheumatoid arthritis, ankylosing spondylitis, or cervical degenerative joint disease.

Table 86-2. Patients at high risk for cervical spine injury.

Injury mechanism	High speed (>35 mph or 56 kph combined impact) motor vehicle crash
	Motor vehicle crash with death of an occupant
	Pedestrian struck by moving vehicle
	Fall from height >10 ft or 3 m
Primary clinical assessment	Significant or serious closed head injury*
	Neurologic symptoms or signs referable to the cervical spine
	Pelvic or multiple extremity injuries
Additional information	Intracranial hemorrhage seen on CT

*The definition of significant or serious head injury is subjective, but may include intracranial hemorrhage, parenchymal contusion, skull fracture, or persistent altered level of consciousness or unconsciousness.

Reprinted with permission from Baron BJ, McSherry KJ, Larson, Jr. JL, Scalea TM. Chapter 255. Spine and Spinal Cord Trauma. In: Tintinalli JE, Stapczynski JS, Cline DM, Ma OJ, Cydulka RK, Meckler GD, eds. *Tintinalli's Emergency Medicine: A Comprehensive Study Guide*. 7th ed. New York: McGraw-Hill, 2011.

▶ Physical Examination

As with all trauma patients, perform an initial primary survey and address all emergent life-threatening conditions. Immobilize all patients with any suspicion for cervical spine injury by applying a hard cervical collar. Visually inspect the spine for any signs of trauma, including abrasions, ecchymoses, open wounds, and deformity, and carefully palpate for any focal tenderness or bony step-offs. Keep in mind that the presence of alterations in mental status (eg, intoxication of head injury) or distracting injuries (eg, significant extremity fractures) may render the physical exam unreliable. Perform a thorough neurologic exam, including an assessment of strength, sensation (including light touch and proprioception), deep tendon reflexes, and rectal tone. The bulbocavernosus reflex can be used to differentiate between complete and incomplete SCI. With a gloved finger in the rectum, gently squeeze the glans penis or the clitoris with your opposite hand. The involuntary contraction of the anal sphincter indicates a positive reflex and rules out a complete SCI.

DIAGNOSTIC STUDIES

▶ Laboratory

There are no laboratory tests specific for the diagnosis and management of cervical spine injury.

▶ Imaging

A standard 3-view series of the cervical spine (anteroposterior [AP], lateral, and odontoid views) has been the historical standard to rule out cervical spine injury. Recent evidence has questioned the sensitivity of these films, and most patients with a moderate to high likelihood of cervical spine injury warrant noninfused CT imaging (sensitivity for bony injury >95%). Plain films are generally adequate for pediatric patients and young otherwise healthy adults with a very low pretest probability for injury. The entire cervical spine extending from the occiput to the top of T1 must be visualized to consider the imaging adequate when reviewing plain films (Table 86-3 and Figures 86-2 through 86-7). MRI is the study of choice in all patients with neurological deficits and those with presumed unstable ligamentous injuries.

Table 86-3. Key to interpretation of cervical spine radiographs.

Radiograph	Alignment	Bones	Cartilage	Soft Tissue
Lateral (Figure 86-2)	Anterior middle and posterior arcs, posterior laminar line and predental space (Figures 86-3 and 86-4)	Vertebrae and spinous process uniformity and height	Intervertebral disk space and height	Prevertebral soft tissue width (Figure 86-5)
AP	Spinous processes should be in a straight line (Figure 86-6)	Interspinous process distance should be equal (Figure 86-6)		
Open mouth (odontoid)	Lateral margins of C1 should align with lateral margins of C2 (Figure 86-7)	Space on each side of odontoid should be equal. Inspect odontoid for fractures		

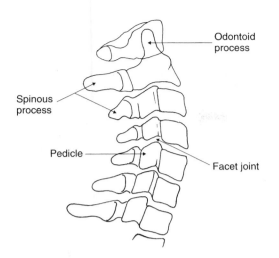

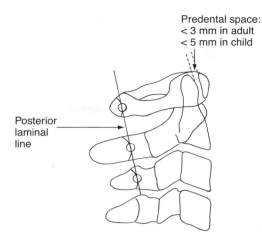

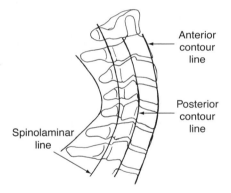

Figure 86-2. Normal lateral C-spine. Reprinted with permission from Bailitz J, Bokhari F, Scaletta TA, et al. *Emergent Management of Trauma*. 3rd ed. New York: McGraw-Hill Education, 2011.

Figure 86-4. The predental space demonstrated on a lateral C-spine radiograph. The posterior laminar line should be drawn from the base of the spinous processes of C1 to C3. The base of the spinous process of C2 should be within 2 mm of this line. This can help rule out pseudosubluxation of C2 on C3, which is commonly seen in pediatric patients. Reprinted with permission from Bailitz J, Bokhari F, Scaletta TA, et al. *Emergent Management of Trauma*. 3rd ed. New York: McGraw-Hill Education, 2011.

Figure 86-3. Normal alignment of lateral C-spine. The anterior and posterior vertebral bodies should line up to within 1 mm. The spinolaminar line can be traced through the base of the spinous process of each vertebra. Reprinted with permission from Bailitz J, Bokhari F, Scaletta TA, et al. *Emergent Management of Trauma*. 3rd ed. New York: McGraw-Hill Education, 2011.

MEDICAL DECISION MAKING

Immediately immobilize all patients at risk for cervical spine injury, perform a primary and secondary survey, and address any emergent life threats. All patients with potential cervical spine injury require some form of C-spine clearance. The NEXUS criteria and Canadian C-spine rules can be used to identify patients at a low risk of significant injury who can be clinically cleared without the need for radiographic studies (Tables 86-4 and 86-5). Patients who do not meet either criterion require radiographic clearance.

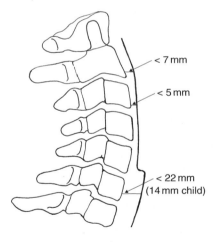

Figure 86-5. Normal prevertebral soft tissue distance on the lateral C-spine. Increased distance indicates soft tissue swelling and possible associated fracture or ligamentous injury. Reprinted with permission from Bailitz J, Bokhari F, Scaletta TA, et al. *Emergent Management of Trauma*. 3rd ed. New York: McGraw-Hill Education, 2011.

Low-risk patients with unremarkable plain films can be treated symptomatically. Pursue CT imaging in patients at a moderate to high risk for injury and those with inadequate or abnormal plain films. Proceed with MRI for any

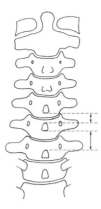

Figure 86-6. AP view of the C-spine. Note the unequal distance between the spinous processes, indicating a C-spine fracture. Reprinted with permission from Bailitz J, Bokhari F, Scaletta TA, et al. *Emergent Management of Trauma.* 3rd ed. New York: McGraw-Hill Education, 2011.

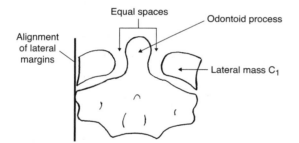

Figure 86-7. Odontoid view. Note symmetric alignment of the lateral masses of C1 and C2. Reprinted with permission from Bailitz J, Bokhari F, Scaletta TA, et al. *Emergent Management of Trauma.* 3rd ed. New York: McGraw-Hill Education, 2011.

Table 86-4. National Emergency X-Radiography Utilization Study criteria: Cervical spine imaging unnecessary in patient meeting these 5 criteria.

Absence of midline cervical tenderness
Normal level of alertness and consciousness
No evidence of intoxication
Absence of focal neurologic deficit
Absence of painful distracting injury

Reprinted with permission from Baron BJ, McSherry KJ, Larson, Jr. JL, Scalea TM. Chapter 255. Spine and Spinal Cord Trauma. In: Tintinalli JE, Stapczynski JS, Cline DM, Ma OJ, Cydulka RK, Meckler GD, eds. *Tintinalli's Emergency Medicine: A Comprehensive Study Guide.* 7th ed. New York: McGraw-Hill, 2011.

Table 86-5. Canadian C-Spine Rule for radiography: Cervical spine imaging unnecessary in patients meeting these 3 criteria.

Question or Assessment	Definitions
There are no high-risk factors that mandate radiography.	High-risk factors include: Age ≥65 years A dangerous mechanism of injury (fall from a height of >3 ft; an axial loading injury; high-speed motor vehicle crash, rollover, or ejection; motorized recreational vehicle or bicycle collision) The presence of paresthesias in the extremities
There are low-risk factors that allow a safe assessment of range of motion.	Low-risk factors include: Simple rear-end motor vehicle crashes Patient able to sit up in the ED Patient ambulatory at any time Delayed onset of neck pain Absence of midline cervical tenderness
The patient is able to actively rotate his/her neck.	Can rotate 45 degrees to the left and to the right

Reprinted with permission from Baron BJ, McSherry KJ, Larson, Jr. JL, Scalea TM. Chapter 255. Spine and Spinal Cord Trauma. In: Tintinalli JE, Stapczynski JS, Cline DM, Ma OJ, Cydulka RK, Meckler GD, eds. *Tintinalli's Emergency Medicine: A Comprehensive Study Guide.* 7th ed. New York: McGraw-Hill, 2011.

patients with findings concerning for spinal cord injury or ligamentous instability. All patients with abnormal imaging and/or neurological deficits require neurosurgical consultation. Transfer such patients to a higher level of care if necessary (Figure 86-8).

TREATMENT

All patients with suspected cervical spine injury require immediate immobilization on presentation. The collar can be temporarily removed to facilitate endotracheal intubation as necessary provided an additional health care provider can maintain appropriate in-line stabilization. If available, some of the newer fiber-optic devices permit endotracheal intubation with little to no movement of the cervical spine.

Patients who are either clinically or radiographically cleared can be managed with oral analgesics. Those who require parenteral pain control should have their diagnosis reconsidered.

The use of steroids in SCI remains highly controversial. The recent Consortium for Spinal Cord Medicine (2008) concluded that there is no current evidence to definitely recommend the use of steroids in the standard management of patients with blunt spinal cord injury. Furthermore, the most current American Association of Neurological Surgeons guidelines (2013) state that the use of steroids for acute spinal cord injury is not recommended and there is

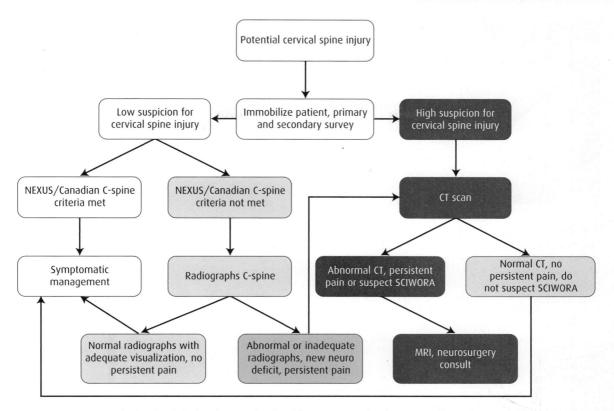

▲ **Figure 86-8.** Cervical spine injuries diagnostic algorithm. CT, computed tomography; MRI, magnetic resonance imaging; SCIWORA, spinal cord injury without radiologic abnormality.

no Class I or Class II evidence to suggest clinical benefit, while there is evidence to suggest harmful side-effects.

DISPOSITION

▶ Admission

Admit all patients with documented SCI to an intensive care unit (ICU) setting with neurosurgical consultation for frequent neurologic evaluations. In addition, all patients with unstable injuries regardless of the presence or absence of associated cord injury require ICU admission pending operative management. If the appropriate subspecialty services are unavailable, transfer to an institution that specializes in SCI. Patients with significant persistent pain despite negative imaging, the elderly, and those with poor social support may require admission for pain management and/or placement for rehabilitation.

▶ Discharge

Low-risk patients who have either been clinically cleared or complain only of minimal persistent pain with negative

imaging studies can be safely discharged. In addition, it is safe to discharge patients with stable fractures (eg, anterior wedge, spinous process) after neurosurgical consultation, provided they are given clear plans for outpatient follow-up.

▼ SUGGESTED READING

Baron BJ, McSherry KJ, Larson JL, TM Scalea. Spine and spinal cord trauma. In: Tintinalli JE, Stapczynski JS, Ma OJ, Cline DM, Cydulka RK, Meckler GD. *Tintinalli's Emergency Medicine: A Comprehensive Study Guide.* 7th ed. New York, NY: McGraw-Hill, 2011, pp. 1709–1730.

Hoffman JR, Mower WR, Wolfson AB, et al. Validity of a set of clinical criteria to rule out injury to the cervical spine in patients with blunt trauma. *N Engl J Med.* 2000;343:94.

Hurlbert RJ et al. Pharmacological therapy for acute spinal cord injury. Neurosurgery 2013;72(3):supplement 93–105.

Stiell IG, Wells GA, Vandemheen KL, et al. The Canadian C-spine rule for radiography in alert and stable patients. *JAMA.* 2001;286:1841.

Thoracic Trauma

Michael A. Schindlbeck, MD

Key Points

- Thoracic trauma is the second leading cause of traumatic death in the United States.

- All patients require a rapid primary survey focused on patient airway, breathing, and circulation and stabilization of any emergent life-threatening conditions.

- Emergent life threats in thoracic trauma include airway obstruction, tension pneumothorax, open pneumothorax, massive hemothorax, and pericardial tamponade.

- In select penetrating trauma victims who suffer witnessed loss of vital signs, emergent thoracotomy can be a lifesaving procedure.

INTRODUCTION

Thoracic trauma accounts for more than 16,000 deaths in the United States annually and constitutes approximately 25% of all trauma related mortality. For clinical purposes, patients can be divided into blunt and penetrating categories based on the mechanism of injury. Approximately 80% of cases of significant blunt thoracic trauma are secondary to motor vehicle collisions (MVC), whereas most cases of penetrating trauma in the United States are due to stab wounds and low-velocity handgun injuries.

▶ Blunt Thoracic Injuries

Injuries that occur after blunt thoracic trauma include fractures (sternum/ribs), flail chest, pulmonary contusion, myocardial injury, and aortic injury. Although fractures to the sternum and ribs are usually not life-threatening, displaced and/or multiple rib fractures are an exception. Evaluate for injury to underlying structures—the mediastinum and great vessels with ribs 1–3, the lungs with ribs 4–8, and the liver or spleen with ribs 9–12. Flail chest occurs when ≥3 contiguous ribs are fractured in ≥2 places, thereby creating a "free floating" segment of the chest wall.

Pulmonary contusions are focal regions of bruised lung parenchyma resulting in alveolar hemorrhage and edema, which can significantly impair normal respiratory function.

They typically develop over several hours post injury and are often missed on the initial patient assessment.

Blunt myocardial injury (BMI) should be considered in any patient with significant direct trauma to the anterior chest wall. Myocardial contusions present as regions of "stunned" tissue that clinically behave analogous to myocardial infarctions. Rarely, patients with significant BMI may progress to outright cardiogenic shock due to impaired pump function or dysrhythmia.

Blunt aortic injury (BAI) is seen in patients when a rapid decelerating force causes significant sheer strain and secondary rupture of the aorta. More than 80% of cases occur at the site of the ligamentum arteriosum just distal to the takeoff of the left subclavian artery. Roughly 20% of patients with BAI will survive to emergency department (ED) presentation because of the tamponading effects of an intact adventitia. As the presenting symptoms and clinical picture are highly variable, a high index of suspicion for BAI should be maintained for any patient with the appropriate mechanism of injury.

▶ Penetrating Thoracic Injuries

Injuries common after penetrating thoracic trauma include pneumothorax, hemothorax, cardiac injury, pericardial tamponade, great vessel injury, and tracheobronchial injury. Pneumothoraces (PTX) are rather common after penetrating thoracic trauma, but can also be seen in blunt injuries when a fractured rib lacerates the underlying pleura. A simple pneumothorax occurs when injured lung tissue creates an air leak in the potential space between the visceral and parietal pleura. An open or communicating PTX occurs when a large open defect in the thoracic wall allows communication between the intrapleural space and the environment. Defects greater than two thirds of the diameter of the trachea will lead to severe respiratory impairment. A tension pneumothorax arises when an injury to the thoracic wall and/or underlying bronchopulmonary structures allows the progressive accumulation of air into the intrapleural space. Rising intrathoracic pressure will eventually inhibit the venous return of circulating blood to the right atrium, resulting in cardiovascular collapse and ensuing pulseless electrical activity (PEA) arrest. Tension PTX is a clinical diagnosis that requires immediate intervention.

Hemothoraces (HTX) develop secondary to the accumulation of blood into the intrapleural space after injury to the lungs, heart, or thoracic vasculature. Each hemithorax can accommodate up to 40% of a patient's circulating blood volume. Massive HTX (accumulation >1,500 mL) is an emergent life-threatening condition that can induce severe hypoxia and systemic hypotension.

Penetrating cardiac injury (PCI) can be rapidly fatal. Occasionally patients, especially those with stab wounds to the anterior heart, will survive to ED presentation because of the tamponading effects of an intact pericardium. Accumulating fluid in the pericardial space will eventually collapse the right side of the heart, resulting in cardiac arrest. Pericardial tamponade is an emergent life threat requiring immediate intervention.

Penetrating great vessel injury (PGVI) presents with massive HTXs with persistent high-volume bloody chest tube effluent. Suspect venous air embolism (VAE) in patients with penetrating vascular trauma, especially involving the subclavian vein, who suddenly decompensate into PEA arrest without alternative explanation.

Tracheobronchial injury can be seen in both blunt and penetrating trauma and should be suspected in patients with an appropriate mechanism and either extensive subcutaneous emphysema or a persistent high-volume air leak after chest tube placement.

CLINICAL PRESENTATION

▶ History

A detailed history is usually deferred until the completion of the primary survey and stabilization of any evolving emergent life threats (Table 87-1). The severity of the mechanism should be estimated to determine the potential for underlying injury. Emergency medical service (EMS) personnel are an invaluable asset. Clues to significant injuries after an MVC include lack of seat-belt restraint, dashboard deformity, significant intrusion into the passenger compartment, prolonged extraction, ejection from the vehicle, and on-the-scene

Table 87-1. Emergent life threats in thoracic trauma.

Airway obstruction
Tension pneumothorax
Pericardial tamponade
Open pneumothorax
Massive hemothorax

death of other occupants. Sudden deceleration mechanisms, such as falls greater than 30 feet or an MVC greater than 30 mph, should raise concern for potential vascular shearing injuries. With penetrating trauma, the type of stabbing implement should be ascertained.

▶ Physical Examination

An assessment of patient vital signs is the cornerstone of the primary survey. Progressive sinus tachycardia and systemic hypotension indicates a serious cardiovascular derangement that should be addressed immediately. Significant hypoxia could indicate an underlying pulmonary contusion, HTX, or PTX.

Inspection of the patient's neck might reveal jugular venous distension indicative of pericardial tamponade or tension PTX or tracheal deviation indicative of an evolving tension PTX. Examination of the thorax should begin with gross observation. Chest wall asymmetry with regional paradoxical movement during respiration indicates underlying flail chest. A large open defect in the chest wall with audible air movement during respiration indicates a communicating PTX. Penetrating wounds either located within or transecting the "cardiac box" are most likely to involve the heart and surrounding mediastinal structures and require a more extensive work-up. The anterior cardiac box is defined as the region medial to the nipples extending between the suprasternal notch and xiphoid process. The posterior cardiac box is defined as the region between the medial borders of the scapulae extending from the superior border of the scapulae to the costal margin (Figure 87-1). Palpation of the chest wall can detect point tenderness indicative of an underlying fracture of the thoracic cage or soft tissue crepitus suggestive of an underlying PTX or tracheobronchial injury.

Auscultation of the chest will reveal absent or diminished breath sounds indicative of an underlying PTX or HTX, whereas inspiratory crackles suggests an evolving pulmonary contusion. Diminished heart sounds are heard in patients with pericardial bleeding and potential cardiac tamponade.

Patients with significant thoracic trauma often have concomitant abdominal injuries. A careful examination of the upper abdomen should be performed in patients with fractures of the lower ribs due to the potential for contusion or laceration of the underlying liver or spleen. Finally, distal pulses should be assessed, as marked asymmetry could indicate significant vascular injury.

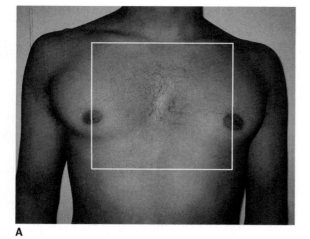

A

B

▲ **Figure 87-1. A, B.** Anterior and posterior cardiac box.

DIAGNOSTIC STUDIES

▶ Laboratory

There are no laboratory studies specific to the work-up of patients with thoracic trauma. Typical studies obtained include a complete blood count, electrolyte panel with renal function, serum and urine toxicology studies including an ethanol level, a serum lactate level, and a serum base deficit.

These tests should be used primarily to determine the severity of the traumatic insult and the adequacy of the patient's physiologic response.

▶ Imaging

All thoracic trauma patients, both blunt and penetrating, require an initial screening chest x-ray (CXR). Sternal and rib fractures are often difficult to detect, with ~50% missed on the initial CXR. This is especially true for fractures of the anterior and lateral portions of the first 5 ribs and sternal fractures when a lateral view is not obtained. Fortunately, it is the potential injury to any underlying structures that is of clinical significance. Pulmonary contusions will appear as focal opacifications within the lung parenchyma and typically manifest within the first 6 hours of presentation. A simple pneumothorax will appear as free air within the intrapleural space with an adjacent visible edge of visceral pleura. A good rule of thumb is that a PTX of 2.5 cm in an adult indicates a 40% loss of lung volume. Penetrating thoracic trauma patients with a normal initial CXR typically require repeat imaging several hours later to rule out the development of a delayed PTX. An HTX can be visualized on an upright CXR once ~200 mL of blood has accumulated and will initially appear as blunting of the ipsilateral costophrenic angle (Figure 87-2). On a supine CXR, a large HTX will appear as a diffuse haziness of the entire hemithorax due to posterior layering of the free-flowing intrapleural blood. Finally, chest radiography can be used as a screening study for BAI. Concerning findings include a widened superior mediastinum (>8 cm), an indistinct or obscured aortic knob, rightward displacement of an intraesophageal nasogastric tube, inferior displacement of the left mainstem bronchus, or an apical pleural cap (Figure 87-3). Because of a false-negative rate of ~10%, a normal initial CXR cannot reliably exclude BAI.

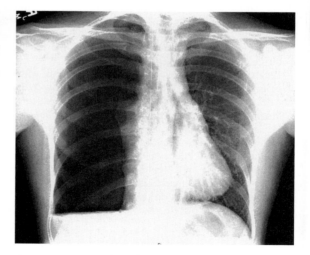

▲ **Figure 87-2.** Right-sided hemopneumothorax. Note the absence of lung markings in the right hemithorax, radio-opaque collapsed lung tissue adjacent to the right hilum, blunting of the costophrenic angle due to blood in the intrapleural space, and air fluid level pathognomonic for a hemopneumothorax. Reprinted with permission from Young Jr. WF. Chapter 71. Spontaneous and Iatrogenic Pneumothorax. In: Tintinalli JE, Stapczynski JS, Cline DM, Ma OJ, Cydulka RK, Meckler GD, eds. *Tintinalli's Emergency Medicine: A Comprehensive Study Guide.* 7th ed. New York: McGraw-Hill, 2011.

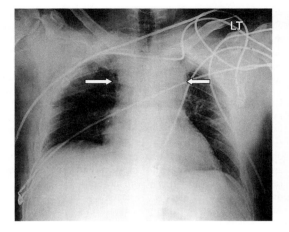

▲ **Figure 87-3.** Blunt aortic injury on CXR. Note the widened superior mediastinum (arrows).

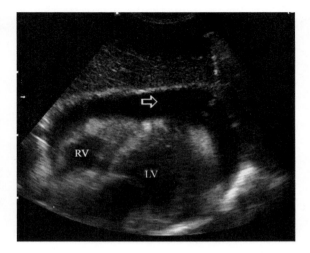

▲ **Figure 87-4.** Traumatic pericardial effusion on bedside FAST exam. Note the large collection of fluid within the pericardial space (arrow). Reprinted with permission from Ross C, Schwab TM. Chapter 259. Cardiac Trauma. In: Tintinalli JE, Stapczynski JS, Cline DM, Ma OJ, Cydulka RK, Meckler GD, eds. *Tintinalli's Emergency Medicine: A Comprehensive Study Guide.* 7th ed. New York: McGraw-Hill, 2011.

A standard 12-lead electrocardiogram (ECG) is the initial study of choice to work up patients with potential BMI. Because of its anterior location within the chest, the right ventricle is the most likely structure affected. Expected findings include ST-segment changes and/or T-wave inversions (typically in the inferior and anterior leads), conduction delays, and dysrhythmias. A normal initial ECG in an asymptomatic individual reliably excludes any future complications of BMI. A bedside echocardiogram (ECHO) can be a useful adjunct in patients with presumed symptomatic BMI and may demonstrate focal regions of myocardial contusion that have the potential to progress to subsequent cardiogenic shock. Furthermore, ECHO is indicated in the work-up of any patient with penetrating trauma to the cardiac box, with a qualified echocardiographer able to detect accumulations of blood as little as 20 mL within the pericardial sac (Figure 87-4). Finally, bedside ultrasound (US) does have a role in helping to diagnose PTX and can detect HTX with a volume as low as 50 mL.

Computed tomography angiography (CTA) has become the modality of choice in evaluating patients with potential BAI (Figure 87-5). Because of the high lethality associated with delayed diagnosis, any patient with a sudden deceleration mechanism (fall >30 ft or MVC >30 mph) and either an abnormal CXR or evidence of thoracic injury should undergo CTA. Given improvements in CTA technology, a normal study is essentially 100% sensitive to exclude BAI.

PROCEDURES

▶ Needle and Tube Thoracostomy

Needle decompression of a tension PTX is an emergently life-saving procedure and should be performed during the primary survey. Chest tube placement should be used for the management of nearly every traumatic PTX or HTX. See Chapter 7 for further details.

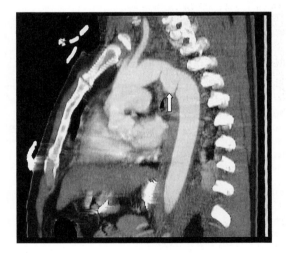

▲ **Figure 87-5.** Blunt aortic injury on CTA. Note the disrupted aortic lumen at the attachment site of the ligamentum arteriosum (arrow).

▶ Pericardiocentesis

Pericardiocentesis can be an emergently life-saving procedure for any patient exhibiting pericardial tamponade. A long large-gauge needle (eg, a 10-cm 18-gauge spinal needle) should be inserted at the subxiphoid space and directed toward the underlying pericardium. US guidance can facilitate proper placement. Aspiration of volumes as low as 10 mL of pericardial blood result in stroke volume increases between 25% and 50% and can stabilize the patient pending definitive operative treatment.

ED Thoracotomy

A resuscitative thoracotomy can be a life-saving procedure when performed on patients who lose signs of life either with EMS in route or in the ED. In the best possible circumstances, survival rates are <10% and usually highest for victims of penetrating trauma, especially those with anterior stab wounds. Once the decision is made to perform an ED thoracotomy, the procedure should be done expediently without delay. An incision should be made in the fourth or fifth intercostal space extending from the sternal border to the posterior axillary line. The intercostal muscles are incised and the ribs are retracted to expose the underlying thoracic viscera. The pericardium can be visualized by gently retracting the overlying lung, and any pericardial blood will be apparent. The pericardium should be opened with a vertical incision (to avoid trauma to the nearby phrenic nerves) and the heart lifted forward and "delivered" from the pericardial sac. Cardiac wounds are treated either with suture or staple closure (with care being made to avoid occluding an underlying coronary artery) or Foley catheter balloon tamponade. If the patient fails to respond, the descending aorta should be cross-clamped to direct any subsequent cardiac output into the cerebral and cardiopulmonary circulation.

MEDICAL DECISION MAKING

The management of the thoracic trauma patient should be algorithmic based on the mechanism and location of injury. Initial efforts should focus on a rapid primary survey and immediate aggressive intervention for any emergent life threats encountered. A more comprehensive secondary survey is then performed, aided by laboratory and imaging studies as outlined previously (Figure 87-6).

TREATMENT

Blunt Thoracic Injuries

Sternal and Rib Fractures

Provided there are no corresponding injuries to underlying viscera, care of these injuries should focus on adequate analgesia. Suboptimal pain control can result in impaired lung ventilation and the potential for secondary pneumonia. Intercostal nerve block can be an invaluable for pain control.

Pulmonary Contusions

These injuries are treated supportively with supplemental oxygen via a nonrebreather mask to maintain adequate systemic oxygenation. Patients with extensive contusions or those unresponsive to supplemental oxygen will require endotracheal intubation and positive pressure ventilation. Care must be taken to avoid overaggressively hydrating these patients to limit progressive alveolar edema and extension of the underlying contusion.

Blunt Myocardial Injury

Clinically significant injuries requiring aggressive intervention are very rare. Stable patients with normal initial ECGs can be discharged home without further evaluation. Patients with ECG anomalies should be observed for 12–24 hours on continuous telemetry to assess for the development of progressive dysrhythmias or cardiogenic shock. Patients who decompensate into cardiogenic shock should be managed via the appropriate Advanced Cardiac Life Support algorithms with the caveat that, for the most part, antiplatelet and anticoagulant medications should be avoided.

Blunt Aortic Injury

If possible, the systolic blood pressure (BP) should be aggressively lowered to ~110–120 mm Hg to reduce the shearing forces on the vessel wall and limit the potential for aortic rupture. Ideal agents include a combination of intravenous (IV) esmolol and either nitroprusside or nicardipine drips. Copious analgesia may be necessary to facilitate adequate BP control. Definitive treatment involves surgical repair or endovascular stenting.

Penetrating Thoracic Injuries

Pneumothorax

Almost all traumatic PTXs require tube thoracostomy within the ED. This is especially true of patients with bilateral PTXs or those undergoing positive pressure ventilation. Patients with an asymptomatic simple PTX smaller than 1 cm on CXR and no visible HTX or those with PTX visible only on CT imaging (occult PTX) can be observed on 100% supplemental oxygen, with tube thoracostomy reserved for those with evidence of increasing volume on serial imaging or the development of associated symptoms. Tension PTXs require immediate needle thoracostomy followed by chest tube placement. Open PTXs require placement of a 3-sided occlusive dressing over the wound to create a flutter valve and restore the integrity of the chest wall followed by subsequent tube thoracostomy.

Hemothorax

Almost all HTXs large enough to be detected on CXR should be drained with tube thoracostomy. Operative intervention is required in <5% of cases of HTX and should be reserved for cases of massive HTX with either initial volumes of evacuated blood >1,500 mL, persistent chest tube output of >200 mL/hr over the first 2–4 hours, or hemodynamic instability despite aggressive volume

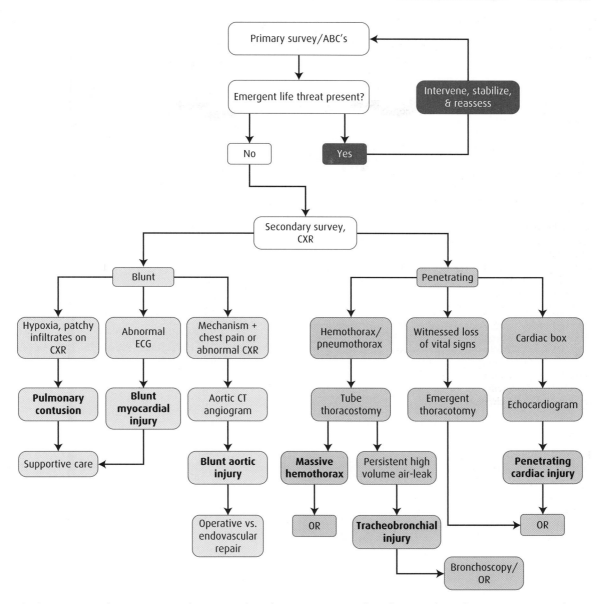

▲ **Figure 87-6.** Thoracic trauma diagnostic algorithm. ABCs, airway, breathing, and circulation; CT, computed tomography; CXR, chest x-ray; ECG, electrocardiogram; OR, operating room.

resuscitation. Autotransfusion should be considered in the majority of these patients.

Penetrating Cardiac Injury

Patients with loss of vital signs either in the field or ED should undergo emergent thoracotomy. Those with pericardial tamponade from an anterior cardiac stab wound have the highest likelihood of survival. Unstable patients with signs of pericardial tamponade either on physical exam or US should undergo emergent pericardiocentesis. Stable patients with evidence of bleeding in the pericardial sac on bedside ECHO should be taken to the operating room for either a pericardial window or an operative thoracotomy.

Penetrating Great Vessel Injury

The majority of these patients who survive to ED presentation will require emergent operative intervention. Early endotracheal intubation should be considered given the potential for significant mediastinal hematoma formation and secondary tracheal compromise. Any retained implements should be stabilized in place, and their removal should be performed only within the operating room.

Tracheobronchial Injury

All patients with presumed tracheobronchial trauma should undergo emergent bronchoscopy to determine the location and severity of injury. The majority of these patients will require operative repair. If necessary, endotracheal intubation should be performed under bronchoscopic guidance to limit any further trauma to the tracheobronchial tree and prevent the aberrant placement of the endotracheal tube into a false soft-tissue lumen.

DISPOSITION

▶ Admission

The majority of thoracic trauma patients will require hospital admission. Hemodynamically stable patients with an isolated PTX or small HTX can be admitted to a standard hospital bed after chest tube placement. Patients with BMI or pulmonary contusions should be admitted to either a telemetry unit or intensive care unit (ICU) setting depending on the severity of symptoms. Patients with BAI, PCI, PGVI, or tracheobronchial injury will require operative intervention followed by an ICU admission.

▶ Discharge

Patients with uncomplicated rib or sternal fractures can be safely discharged home provided that their pain can be adequately managed. Stable penetrating thoracic trauma patients with a normal initial CXR and otherwise negative work-up should have repeat imaging performed within 3–6 hours to check for the development of a delayed PTX. If negative, these patients can be safely discharged home.

▼ SUGGESTED READING

Bastos R et al. Penetrating thoracic trauma. *Semin Thorac Cardiovasc Surg.* 2008;20:19–25.

Brunett PH, Yarris LM, Cevik AA. Pulmonary trauma. In: Tintinalli JE, Stapczynski JS, Ma OJ, Cline DM, Cydulka RK, Meckler GD. *Tintinalli's Emergency Medicine: A Comprehensive Study Guide.* 7th ed. New York, NY: McGraw-Hill, 2011.

Keel M, Meier C. Chest injuries: What is new? *Curr Opin Crit Care.* 2007;13:674–679.

McGillicuddy D, Rosen P. Diagnostic dilemmas and current controversies in blunt trauma. *Emerg Med Clin North Am.* 2007;25:695–711.

Ross C, Schwab TM. Cardiac trauma. In: Tintinalli JE, Stapczynski JS, Ma OJ, Cline DM, Cydulka RK, Meckler GD. *Tintinalli's Emergency Medicine: A Comprehensive Study Guide.* 7th ed. New York, NY: McGraw-Hill, 2011.

Abdominal Trauma

Matthew T. Emery, MD

Key Points

- A normal physical examination cannot be used as the sole means to exclude significant injury in patients with abdominal trauma.

- Hemodynamically unstable patients with penetrating injuries into the peritoneal cavity or blunt abdominal trauma and evidence of intraperitoneal hemorrhage require emergent laparotomy.

- Gunshot wounds that violate the peritoneum require operative exploration because of the high likelihood of injury.

- In patients with blunt abdominal trauma, negative computed tomograhy imaging has an excellent negative predictive value for excluding significant injury.

INTRODUCTION

Victims of abdominal trauma can present with intraperitoneal, retroperitoneal, and intrathoracic injuries. Intraperitoneal structures at a high risk of injury include the solid organs (liver and spleen), hollow viscera (small and large intestines), and diaphragm, whereas commonly involved retroperitoneal structures include the kidneys and genitourinary (GU) tract, duodenum, pancreas, and portions of the large intestine. The initial evaluation and management of patients with abdominal trauma can be divided by the mechanism of injury into blunt and penetrating pathways. Motor vehicle collisions (MVC) and significant falls account for the majority of cases of blunt abdominal trauma, whereas stab wounds (SW) and gunshot wounds (GSW) account for most cases of penetrating trauma. Keep in mind that the location of an entrance wound can frequently be misleading. Although a wound located on the anterior abdomen is obviously a high-risk injury, alternative sites (lower chest, pelvis, back, or flank) can also result in significant intraperitoneal (or retroperitoneal) injury depending on the trajectory of the bullet, knife, or other wounding implement.

When evaluating patients with penetrating trauma, the abdomen can be divided up into 4 distinct zones to help predict which anatomic structures are at risk of injury. The **anterior abdomen** extends between the anterior axillary lines from the costal margins down to the inguinal ligaments (Figure 88-1). The **thoracoabdominal** region extends circumferentially around the entire trunk between the costal margins inferiorly and the nipple line or inferior scapular borders superiorly (Figure 88-2). Trauma to this region can injure intrathoracic and intraperitoneal structures as well as the diaphragm. The **flanks** compose the third anatomical zone and extend between the anterior and posterior axillary lines from the costal margins to the iliac crests. Consider injuries to both intraperitoneal and retroperitoneal structures in this region. The final anatomical zone is the **back**, which extends between the posterior axillary lines from the inferior scapular borders to the iliac crests. Trauma to this region is most likely to result in retroperitoneal injury.

MVCs account for the majority of cases of significant blunt abdominal trauma across all demographic groups, with the spleen by far the most commonly involved organ. With penetrating trauma, abdominal SWs are roughly 3 times more common than GSWs. That said, the latter accounts for roughly 90% of fatal injuries, as SWs are far less likely to violate the peritoneal cavity and cause significant injury. Abdominal GSWs most commonly

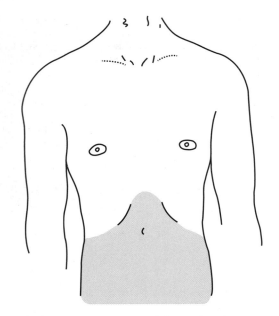

▲ **Figure 88-1.** Anterior abdominal region.

involve the small bowel, colon, and liver, as these organs take up the largest volume within the abdominal cavity. Abdominal SWs most commonly affect the liver, but laparotomy is required in only one quarter to one third of patients.

The severity of injury is proportional to the amount of energy transferred to target tissues. Blunt abdominal trauma causes injury primarily by the direct transmission of external forces to underlying organs. Solid viscera, namely the spleen and liver, are the most likely structures to be involved. Hollow viscera can be injured when sudden crushing forces induce a rapid spike in intraluminal pressure and secondary rupture. Blunt trauma can also transmit shearing forces to underlying structures. Significant injury is most commonly seen in areas of transition from fixed to mobile positions

such as the small bowel at the ligament of Treitz or the ileocolic junction.

In penetrating trauma, SWs result in low-energy mechanisms that cause injury only to those tissues directly impacted by the stabbing implement. As most assailants are right-hand dominant, the left upper quadrant is the most likely region to be affected. GSWs, on the other hand, transmit substantial amounts of energy and frequently result in significant intra-abdominal injury. Missile size, stability, and velocity all help to determine the amount of energy imparted. High-velocity projectiles (>2,000 ft/sec) as seen with combat wounds and hunting rifles can create waves of energy that result in temporary cavity formation and the disruption of tissues remote from the missile tract. In fact, intraperitoneal injury has been known to occur with high-velocity GSWs in the absence of peritoneal violation. Shotgun injuries are unique in that the velocity of the pellets decreases rapidly with the length of distance traveled. Furthermore, the spread of the pellets increases proportionally to the distance between the victim and the shooter. Wounds with a pellet spread of 10–25 cm most likely occurred at a distance of 3–7 yards and possess sufficient energy to penetrate into the peritoneal cavity. Finally, the potential for introducing contamination in the form of clothing or wadding further complicates GSW injuries.

CLINICAL PRESENTATION

▶ History

A rapid primary survey and patient stabilization should always take precedence over a thorough medical history. That said, obtain a quick AMPLE (Allergies, Medications, Past illnesses, Last meal, Events preceding injury) history as with all trauma patients and ask focused questions to delineate the potential severity of mechanism. Emergency medical service personnel can provide invaluable information about the mechanism of injury, initial scene evaluation, and response to interventions provided during transport. With patients from an MVC, inquire about the

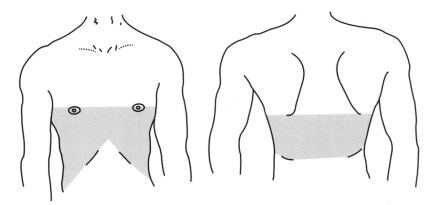

▲ **Figure 88-2.** Thoracoabdominal region.

severity of vehicular damage, seatbelt use, airbag deployment, need for patient extrication, and injuries to other occupants. For GSW victims, ask about the number of shots fired and the type of weapon involved.

Ask all patients about the presence of abdominal pain, vomiting, hematemesis, and rectal bleeding. Pain in the shoulder that is not associated with either tenderness on exam or discomfort with shoulder movement suggests that free intraperitoneal blood is irritating the diaphragm inducing referred pain (Kehr sign).

▶ Physical Examination

Check a complete set of vital signs and proceed with the primary survey. Any evidence of hemodynamic instability suggests hemorrhagic shock and requires aggressive intervention.

Perform a thorough examination of the chest and abdomen. Inspect the patient and note any contusions, hematomas, and abdominal distention. Lap-belt ecchymoses are highly concerning for underlying hollow viscus injuries or vertebral body (Chance) fractures. Note all open wounds and identify the zone of injury. GSWs may not follow a linear trajectory, and a thorough examination of the entire body is necessary to document all potential penetrating wounds. Look for retained implements and eviscerations as each require operative intervention. Carefully palpate all 4 quadrants to detect any point tenderness or signs of evolving peritonitis. Perform a rectal exam to assess for the presence of gross blood. Keep in mind that the abdominal examination in isolation lacks adequate sensitivity to identify all patients with significant injuries that require operative intervention.

DIAGNOSTIC STUDIES

▶ Laboratory

As with all victims of significant trauma, obtain a complete blood count, metabolic panel, coagulation studies, and type and screen. Serial hemoglobin measurements, and, if available, bedside lactate and base deficit analysis may help to determine the severity of injury and physiologic response to resuscitation. Obtain a urine sample for rapid pregnancy testing, urinalysis, and toxicology screening. Hemodynamically stable adults without evidence of gross blood on bedside urinary inspection do not require a urinalysis to search for microscopic hematuria, as significant GU injury is highly unlikely. Liver function tests and pancreatic enzymes are nonspecific and poorly predictive of injury severity. As such, they are of minimal clinical utility in the routine evaluation of patients with abdominal trauma.

▶ Imaging

Obtain an upright chest x-ray (CXR) in all patients to detect subdiaphragmatic free air suggestive of an underlying hollow viscus injury or the intrathoracic herniation of abdominal viscera indicative of a diaphragmatic rupture. In patients with penetrating thoracoabdominal trauma,

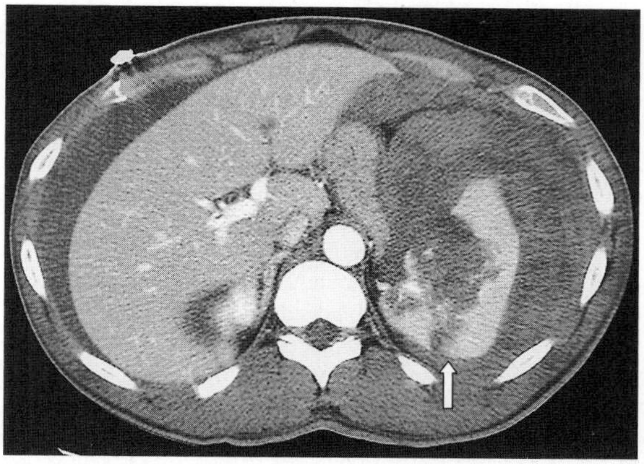

▲ **Figure 88-3.** CT scan demonstrating a splenic laceration (arrow). Note the free fluid around the liver.

carefully review the CXR to rule out an underlying pneumothorax. Obtain an anteroposterior film of the pelvis in blunt trauma victims to rule out unstable pelvic fractures and stabilize any visualized injuries by tightly securing a bed-sheet around the patient's waist to tamponade off any active pelvic bleeding. Place radiopaque markers (eg, electrocardiogram leads) over any open wounds in GSW victims before imaging to help determine the path of the projectile(s).

Pursue computed tomography (CT) imaging of the abdomen and pelvis in all stable blunt trauma patients to detect solid organ injury and hemoperitoneum (Figure 88-3). This modality is especially useful in patients whose exams are limited by distracting injuries or altered mental status. With penetrating trauma to the back and flank, order a "triple contrast" CT scan (by mouth, intravenous, and per rectum) to rule out intraperitoneal and retroperitoneal injury. CT imaging can also be used to diagnose peritoneal violation in patients with abdominal SWs. Of note, CT imaging is inadequately sensitive to exclude small diaphragmatic injuries with penetrating thoracoabdominal trauma and isolated hollow viscus injuries with significant blunt trauma.

PROCEDURES

▶ FAST Scan

Focused assessment with sonography for trauma (FAST) imaging is a widely available bedside procedure that can detect volumes of free intraperitoneal blood as low as 100 mL. It is easy to perform, quick (<5 minutes), noninvasive, and readily repeatable. The sensitivity of a FAST exam is directly proportional to the volume of free intraperitoneal blood, and this modality is highly sensitive in cases in which intraperitoneal hemorrhage is significant enough to produce hemodynamic instability. A positive FAST exam in an unstable patient with blunt abdominal trauma necessitates emergent laparotomy. See Chapter 8 for further details.

▶ Diagnostic Peritoneal Lavage (DPL)

Although largely supplanted by less invasive modalities such as CT and FAST, DPL may continue to play a role in the rapid bedside detection of free intraperitoneal blood in grossly unstable patients with equivocal FAST exams. This procedure can be broken down into 2 basic steps. Begin by inserting an 18-gauge needle into the peritoneal cavity and attempting to aspirate free intraperitoneal fluid. An aspirate of ≥10 mL of gross blood or obvious intestinal contents warrants operative laparotomy. In patients with negative aspirates, insert a guide-wire through the needle and place an intraperitoneal catheter via the Seldinger technique. Infuse 1 L of normal saline into the peritoneal cavity and then allow it to drain via gravity back into the empty saline bag. The collected fluid should then be sent to the lab for cell count analysis. In blunt abdominal trauma, a count >100,000 red blood cells (RBCs)/μL is considered the threshold for detecting significant visceral injury and the need for laparotomy. For abdominal GSWs, a count >5,000–10,000 RBCs/μL is considered positive. For patients with thoracoabdominal SWs, a similar count of 5,000–10,000 RBCs/μL is used to exclude diaphragmatic injuries. For all other abdominal SWs, a cut-off of >100,000 RBCs/μL is used.

▶ Local Wound Exploration (LWE)

This is a useful modality for excluding peritoneal violation in patients with anterior abdominal SWs. Carefully extend the margins of the injury as necessary to facilitate adequate visualization of the base of the wound. The use of copious local anesthetics is a must. This technique is far preferable to blindly probing the wound with blunt instruments. Assume peritoneal penetration in cases in which the base of the wound cannot be clearly identified. The deep exploration of thoracoabdominal wounds is generally avoided, although LWE may be reasonable to confirm the depth of very superficial slashing-type injuries.

MEDICAL DECISION MAKING

Begin all evaluations with a rapid primary survey and complete set of vital signs. Emergent laparotomy is generally indicated in all unstable patients with either penetrating abdominal trauma or blunt abdominal trauma and positive FAST imaging. Regardless of hemodynamic condition, patients with GSWs that clearly violate the peritoneal cavity require emergent laparotomy due to the high rate of significant underlying injury.

Hemodynamically stable patients warrant a work-up before deciding on the need for surgery. For victims of penetrating trauma, this might include LWE with anterior abdominal SWs, plain radiographs to localize radiopaque foreign bodies, FAST imaging to look for pericardial and intraperitoneal free fluid, CT imaging to help determine the need for and approach to any operative intervention, and DPL to rule out diaphragmatic injury or peritoneal violation. For victims of blunt trauma, the work-up

generally includes an upright CXR to look for intraperitoneal free air, gross diaphragmatic rupture, and pneumothorax/hemothorax along with plain films of the pelvis to rule out fracture. These images are usually followed by abdominal CT to exclude injuries to the solid abdominal viscera. Additional findings that warrant emergent laparotomy include retained foreign bodies, eviscerations, frank peritonitis, hematemesis or gross rectal bleeding, and imaging studies documenting hollow viscus or diaphragmatic perforation (Figures 88-4 and 88-5).

TREATMENT

Initiate aggressive volume resuscitation and address any emergent life threats encountered in the primary survey. Concurrently search for any sources of active hemorrhage to determine the need for operative intervention as described previously.

A growing percentage of solid organ injuries in hemodynamically stable patients are being managed nonoperatively. This decision should be made on a case-by-case basis in consultation with the trauma service. The conservative "watch and wait" approach has a failure rate of 10% for liver injuries and 20% for injuries to the spleen. The evolving use of angiographic embolization for bleeding vessels has decreased the need for laparotomy in many cases.

DISPOSITION

▶ Admission

Admit all patients who require laparotomy. Hemodynamically stable patients with CT evidence of liver or splenic injury warrant admission for serial physical exams and laboratory testing.

▶ Discharge

Patients with abdominal SWs and tangential low-velocity GSWs that clearly spare the peritoneal, retroperitoneal, and intrathoracic cavities can be safely discharged. Normal CT imaging in hemodynamically stable patients with blunt abdominal trauma has an excellent negative predictive value. In the absence of other injuries, these patients can be safely discharged.

▼ SUGGESTED READING

Isenhour JL, Marx JA. Abdominal trauma. In: Marx JA, Hockberger RS, Walls RM. *Rosen's Emergency Medicine: Concepts and Clinical Practice.* 7th ed. Philadelphia, PA: Mosby-Elsevier, 2010, pp. 414–434.

Nishijima DK, Simel DL, Wisner DH, et al. The rational clinical examination: Does this adult patient have a blunt intra-abdominal injury? *JAMA.* 2012;307:1517.

Scalea TM, Boswell SA. Abdominal injuries. In: Tintinalli JE, Stapczynski JS, Ma OJ, Cline DM, Cydulka RK, Meckler GD. *Tintinalli's Emergency Medicine: A Comprehensive Study Guide.* 7th ed. New York, McGraw-Hill, 2011, pp. 1699–1708.

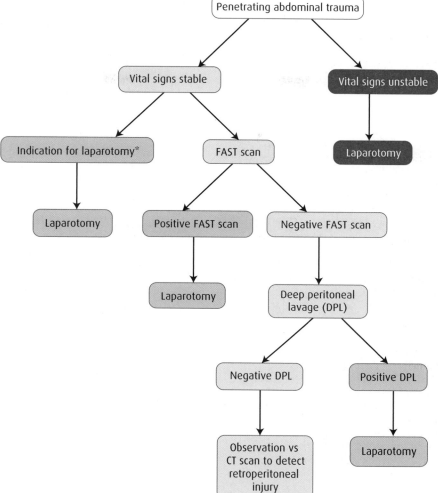

▲ **Figure 88-4.** Abdominal trauma diagnostic algorithm for penetrating abdominal trauma. CT, computed tomography; FAST, focused assessment with sonography for trauma.

*Peritonitis, free air, diaphragmatic injury, evisceration, gross blood from stomach or rectum, retained stabbing implement, positive diagnostic test, or any non-tangential GSW (intraperitoneal penetration).

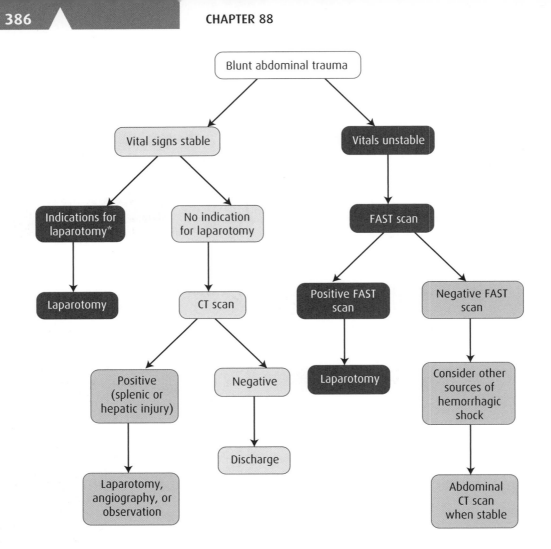

Figure 88-5. Abdominal trauma diagnostic algorithm for blunt abdominal trauma. CT, computed tomography; FAST, focused assessment with sonography for trauma.

*Peritonitis, free air, diaphragmatic injury, gross blood from stomach or rectum, positive diagnostic test.

Burns

Gim A. Tan, MBBS

Key Points

- Pursue early endotracheal intubation in patients with significant inhalation injuries.
- Emergency escharotomy may be a life- or limb-saving procedure in patients with evidence of respiratory compromise or limb ischemia.
- Consider concurrent carbon monoxide andcyanide poisoning in all fire victims.
- Never overlook the possibility of concomitant multisystem trauma, and always consider the possibility of abuse or neglect in burned children or the elderly.

INTRODUCTION

Burn injuries can occur from thermal, chemical, or electrical mechanisms. Of the 3, thermal burns are the most common and occur with either scalding or flame injuries. Chemical burns occur secondary to exposures to strong acids or alkali and account for 5–10% of all burn admissions. Electrical burns result from the flow of current through susceptible tissue and are frequently much more severe than initially visible.

The prevalence of burns is highest in patients between 18 and 35 years of age. Scald burns from hot liquids are most common in children under the age of 5 and the elderly, and approximately 20% of pediatric burns are attributable to either abuse or neglect. The American Burn Association estimates that burns account for more than 450,000 emergency department (ED) visits, 45,000 hospitalizations, and 3,500 deaths annually in the United States. There are currently 125 specialized burn centers in the United States that account for more than half of these admissions.

Burned skin classically undergoes a coagulative necrosis by which denatured skin proteins constrict to form a firm and potentially constricting eschar. A subsequent cascade of inflammatory reactions leads to the development of significant localized edema and the potential for further tissue loss. This inflammatory response becomes systemic when more than 30% of the patient's total body surface area is involved, resulting in multisystem organ injury.

Burns can be clinically classified as first, second, or third degree. **First-degree** burns are limited to the superficial epidermis and heal within 7 days without any long-term sequelae (eg, sunburn). **Second-degree** burns are partial-thickness injuries that extend into the dermis. They are further subdivided into **superficial** and **deep partial thickness** injuries. Deep partial thickness burns result in destruction of the deeper dermal structures including the hair follicles and sweat and sebaceous glands, whereas these tissues are spared with superficial partial thickness injuries. Superficial partial thickness burns tend to heal within a period of 2–3 weeks with minimal long-term scarring, whereas their deep counterparts often necessitate skin grafting for definitive care. **Third-degree** burns extend deep into the subcutaneous tissues and represent full-thickness injuries of the skin. All dermal structures including the capillary networks and neuronal tissues are destroyed, leaving behind an avascular and insensate skin. Skin grafting is invariably required.

From a physiologic standpoint, the skin functions to reduce evaporative water loss, in addition to creating a barrier to infection and controlling body temperature. Hypovolemic shock is common with severe burns as a result of a combination of increased peripheral blood flow with evaporative fluid losses and excessive capillary leak with circulating volume third-spacing. The decreased cardiac output that frequently complicates the systemic reaction to significant burns further exacerbates the circulatory insufficiency.

Inhalational injuries are common in fire victims who are found in enclosed spaces. They can be divided anatomically into supraglottic and infraglottic injuries. Supraglottic burns represent direct thermal injury to the face and pharyngeal tissues. They develop very rapidly, within minutes of exposure, and often necessitate emergent endotracheal intubation. Infraglottic burns represent chemically mediated injury to the bronchioles and alveoli. They develop much more slowly over the course of several hours and clinically mimic acute respiratory distress syndrome (ARDS).

CLINICAL PRESENTATION

▶ History

Details concerning the nature of the injury are extremely important. Identify the mechanism of injury, as this may provide a clue its severity. For example, scald injuries usually result in partial-thickness burns, whereas flash and flame exposures more commonly produce full-thickness injuries. Deeper injuries should be suspected in patients with electrical or chemical burns, especially those with high voltage or strong alkali exposures, respectively. Identify all victims of closed space fires, as they have an increased potential for inhalational injuries, carbon monoxide (CO) poisoning, and cyanide (CN^-) toxicity. Cyanide is formed by the combustion of nitrogen-containing compounds (eg, wool, silk, polyurethane, vinyl), and toxicity is not uncommon in victims of industrial fires. Obtain a very detailed history in all pediatric burn victims to uncover any possibility for abuse or neglect.

▶ Physical Examination

Always start with a primary survey and address any emergent life threats. Carefully document all vital signs, remembering that circumferential extremity burns may limit adequate blood pressure measurement. Assess the patient for any signs of inhalation injury, including singed facial hairs, carbonaceous sputum, stridor, wheezing, and dysphonia. Carefully assess the adequacy of respiration in all patients with significant thoracic burns to detect any evidence of an evolving compromise in chest wall compliance. Completely undress all patients and perform a comprehensive secondary survey, as concomitant traumatic injuries are common. Assume an occult C-spine injury until proven otherwise in all nonverbal or unreliable patients and immobilize appropriately. Ensure intact neurovascular function in all 4 extremities and take note of any circumferential burns.

Perform a detailed skin exam in all patients. First-degree burns are red in appearance and very tender. Skin blistering should not be present. Superficial second-degree burns present with red blistered skin, a moist

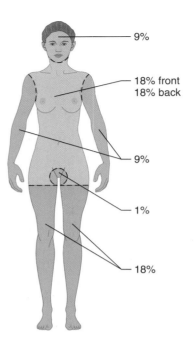

▲ **Figure 89-1.** The "rule of nines" to calculate the % total body surface area of the burn. Reprinted with permission from Schwartz LR, Balakrishnan C. Chapter 210. Thermal Burns. In: Tintinalli JE, Stapczynski JS, Cline DM, Ma OJ, Cydulka RK, Meckler GD, eds. *Tintinalli's Emergency Medicine: A Comprehensive Study Guide*. 7th ed. New York: McGraw-Hill, 2011.

exposed dermis, and good capillary refill. Deep second-degree burns, on the other hand, present with an exposed dermis that is a pale white to yellow in appearance with absent capillary refill. Third-degree burns are leathery, pale, and insensate with possible evidence of char formation.

Calculate the percentage of total body surface area (TBSA) involved with second- and third-degree burns. The "rule of nines" can help with this assessment (Figure 89-1). Immersion burns will appear as circumferential tissue damage with sparing of the flexor creases and are pathognomonic for abuse in pediatric patients.

DIAGNOSTIC STUDIES

▶ Laboratory

Obtain an electrolyte panel and renal function in all patients and calculate the anion gap. Significant metabolic acidosis suggests hemodynamic shock, carbon monoxide poisoning, or cyanide toxicity. Check an arterial blood gas in patients with potential CO poisoning to measure the carboxyhemoglobin level. Order a creatine phosphokinase to exclude rhabdomyolysis in patients with electrical injuries.

► Imaging

Obtain a chest x-ray (CXR) in patients with potential inhalation burns, keeping in mind that infraglottic burns may take several hours to evolve. Their appearance on CXR typically mimics ARDS.

PROCEDURES

Emergency escharotomy is indicated in all patients with circumferential burns and evidence of either impaired limb perfusion or restricted respiratory mechanics secondary to the development of an inflexible skin eschar with underlying edema. For the limbs, opposing mid-medial and mid-lateral incisions should be made down the entire length of the eschar, including the digits if necessary. For the chest, bilateral incisions should be made along the anterior axillary lines. An additional transverse horizontal incision is occasionally necessary to fully free the restricted chest wall. Regardless of location, the incisions must completely penetrate through the entire eschar and into the subcutaneous fat.

MEDICAL DECISION MAKING

Perform an appropriate primary survey and address any emergent life threats, including concomitant trauma. Secure the airway early in all patients with evidence of significant supraglottic inhalation injury. Rule out CO and CN⁻ poisoning in all seriously ill patients with any history of smoke exposure. Use the history and a comprehensive secondary survey to identify the extent and severity of injury. Calculate the TBSA involved and initiate aggressive volume resuscitation in patients with burns involving more than 20%. Consider early transfer to an appropriate burn center in such patients (Figure 89-2).

TREATMENT

Administer O_2 via a nonrebreather mask to all patients and administer pain medications as needed. If intubation is required, succinylcholine can be used safely within the first 24 hours after a burn, but its use should be avoided after this point to avoid precipitating life-threatening

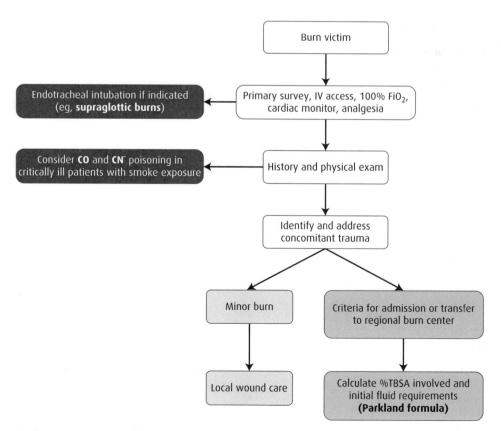

▲ **Figure 89-2.** Burns diagnostic algorithm. TBSA, total body surface area.

hyperkalemia. This can occur because significant burns drastically increase the number of postsynaptic acetylcholine receptors in the affected tissues, which can induce a massive efflux of potassium ions into the extracellular space in response to succinylcholine administration.

Treat CO poisoning with 100% oxygen and possibly hyperbaric O_2 (see Chapter 58) and CN^- toxicity with either the cyanide antidote kit (use only the sodium thiosulfate with concurrent CO poisoning) or hydroxocobalamin (5 g intravenously [IV] over 15 minutes).

Initiate aggressive volume resuscitation in all patients with burns that involve ≥20% TBSA. Use the Parkland formula (4 mL/kg × %TBSA given over 24 hours with the first half given over the initial 8 hours) to estimate initial volume needs, but titrate as necessary to maintain hemodynamic stability and a urine output of 0.5–1 mg/kg/hr. For example, an 80-kg patient with a 50% TBSA burn requires 16 L of total fluid over a 24-hour period with an initial rate of 1 L/hr for the first 8 hours. Use either Lactated Ringer's or isotonic saline, as colloid fluids have never been shown to improve survival.

Irrigate all thermal and chemical burns with cool running water to minimize further tissue injury, and remove affected clothing to limit ongoing chemical exposure. Brush off any adherent solid chemicals before irrigation. Apply nonadherent sterile dressings to all superficial injuries. Deeper burns will require debridement of necrotic tissue and protection with a topical antiseptic such as silver sulfadiazine. Most of these injuries will eventually require surgical excision and skin grafting. As local wound care is exceptionally painful, burn victims require aggressive analgesia with parenteral narcotics. Update your patient's tetanus status as necessary.

DISPOSITION

Admission

The criteria for admission or transfer to a burn center are listed in Table 89-1.

Table 89-1. Criteria for admission or transfer to a burn center.

Partial-thickness burns: >20% TBSA in all age groups, >10% TBSA for patients <10 or >50 years of age
Burns involving face, hands, feet, genitalia, perineum, or major joints
Third-degree burns >5% in any age group
Electrical burns (including lightning)
Chemical burns
Inhalational injury
Patients with preexisting medical disorders that could complicate management
Children when the originating hospital does not treat children

TBSA, total body surface area.

Discharge

Patients with minor burns can be safely discharged with appropriate follow-up arranged within 48 hours.

SUGGESTED READING

Kao LW, Nunagas KA. Carbon monoxide poisoning. *Emerg Med Clin North Am.* 2004;22:985–1018.
Monafo WW. Initial management of burns. *N Engl J Med.* 1996; 335:1581–1586.
Pomerantz WJ. Emergency management of paediatric burns. *Pediatric Emerg Care.* 2005;21:118–129.
Schwartz LR, Balakrishnan C. Thermal burns. In: Tintinalli JE, Stapczynski JS, Reed JL, Ma OJ, Cline DM, Cydulka RK, Meckler GD. *Tintinalli's Emergency Medicine: A Comprehensive Study Guide.* 7th ed. New York, NY: McGraw-Hill, 2011, pp. 1374–1380.

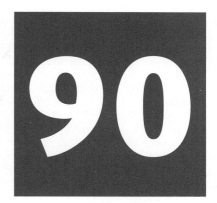

Upper Extremity Injuries

George Chiampas, DO

Matthew S. Patton, MD

Key Points

- When assessing a painful extremity, vascular compromise must be excluded first.
- A patient who has fallen on an outstretched hand and has tenderness in the anatomical snuffbox of the wrist and a negative radiograph should have a thumb spica splint placed until a scaphoid fracture is definitively excluded.
- Avoid nonsteroidal anti-inflammatory drugs after fractures. These medications inhibit bone healing.
- In the upper extremity, compartment syndrome is most common in the forearm, especially after displaced supracondylar fractures in children.

INTRODUCTION

Traumatic injuries to the upper extremity are common presenting emergency department (ED) complaints. It is the clinician's objective to distinguish benign (eg, sprains, contusions) from emergent injuries (eg, open fractures, dislocations, vascular compromise). A systematic approach to identifying and classifying orthopedic injuries is needed to properly manage, treat, and disposition patients. This requires a thorough knowledge of orthopedic anatomy and function. The upper extremity contains several important articulations and long bones, which are at risk for dislocations and fractures during falls or by direct force.

▶ Shoulder and Arm Injuries

The glenohumeral joint of the shoulder is the most mobile joint in the body and, unsurprisingly, the most commonly dislocated joint, accounting for 50% of all major dislocations seen in the ED. Anterior dislocations account for 95% of all shoulder dislocations (Figure 90-1). They occur most commonly when the arm is abducted, externally rotated, and extended and a posterior directed force is applied to the humerus. Axillary nerve injury is present in 12% of cases and is noted by testing sensation over the deltoid muscle and strength of abduction. Posterior dislocations are less common (5%) and present with inability to abduct and externally rotate. The classic mechanism that causes a posterior shoulder dislocation is a seizure.

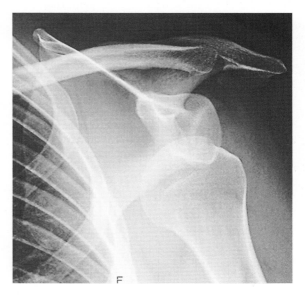

▲ **Figure 90-1.** AP view of an anterior shoulder dislocation.

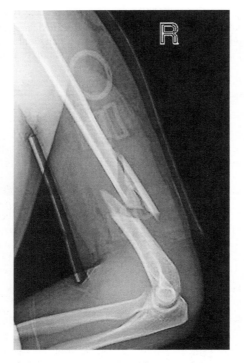

Figure 90-2. Humerus fracture. This fracture is described as a spiral, distal-third humerus fracture, with comminution, 100% displacement, and no angulation.

Shoulder separation is a soft tissue injury to the acromioclavicular and coracoclavicular ligaments, which provide stability to the acromioclavicular joint. These typically occur after a fall with direct impact onto the shoulder and are divided by severity into first-, second-, and third-degree injuries. First-degree injuries are sprains of the acromioclavicular ligament without significant separation of the acromion and clavicle. Second-degree injuries are the result of complete disruption of the acromioclavicular ligament but an intact coracoclavicular ligament. Widening of the acromioclavicular joint is present on radiographs. Third-degree injuries occur when both ligaments are disrupted, producing widening of the acromioclavicular joint and cephalad displacement of the clavicle.

Humerus fractures occur anywhere on the shaft of the humerus (Figure 90-2). Fractures of the distal third of the humerus are associated with radial nerve injuries in 5–15% of cases.

Elbow Injuries

The elbow is the second most common large joint dislocation, 80–90% of which are posterior. Common elbow fractures include the radial head and olecranon in adults and the supracondylar humerus in children. Displaced supracondylar fractures in children are prone to developing compartment syndrome.

Forearm Injuries

A nightstick fracture is an isolated fracture of the ulnar shaft that occurs when a patient is protecting the body from a blunt force to the upper torso or head. Both bone forearm fractures (radius and ulna) are common in children after a fall. In both children and adults, these are highly unstable fractures that require early orthopedic consultation. Galeazzi fracture-dislocation is a distal radius fracture with dislocation of the ulna at the distal radioulnar joint (wrist). Monteggia fracture-dislocation is a proximal ulna fracture with dislocation of the radial head at the proximal radioulnar joint (elbow). Both of these injuries require surgical reduction.

Wrist and Hand Injuries

Distal radius fractures account for up to 15% of upper extremity fractures and are classified by the pattern of injury. They are most commonly caused by a fall on an outstretched hand (FOOSH). A Colles fracture is an extra-articular metaphyseal fracture with dorsal angulation, as opposed to a Smith fracture, which is an extra-articular metaphyseal fracture with volar angulation (Figure 90-3). A Barton fracture involves the volar or dorsal rim of the distal radius with subluxation of the carpals. A Hutchinson fracture is an isolated fracture of the radial styloid.

Of the 8 carpal bones, the scaphoid accounts for 60–80% of all fractures (Figure 90-4). These fractures have a significant

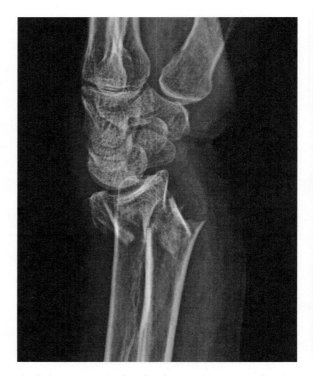

Figure 90-3. Distal radius fracture is an example of a Colles fracture.

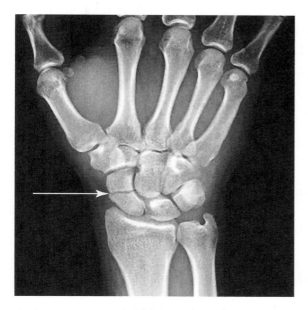

▲ **Figure 90-4.** Scaphoid fracture (arrow).

risk of avascular necrosis due to the pattern of blood supply in this area, and this risk increases with more proximal fractures. The false-negative rate of plain radiographs is as high as 20%, making conservative treatment in patients with tenderness over the scaphoid (anatomical snuffbox) appropriate.

Metacarpal fractures may occur in the base, shaft, neck, or head of the bone. The most common is a fracture to the neck of the fourth and/or fifth metacarpal, called a boxer's fracture (Figure 90-5). Angulation is acceptable if it is

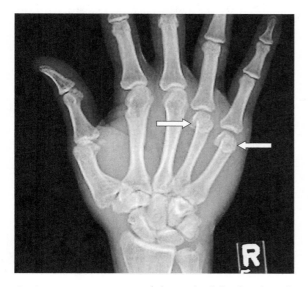

▲ **Figure 90-5.** Fracture of the neck of the fourth and fifth metacarpals—boxer's fracture (arrows).

<40 degrees. For fractures of the metacarpal shafts of the second and third metacarpal necks, less angulation (10–20 degrees) is acceptable because healing with significant angulation in these more anatomically fixed metacarpals may inhibit function.

Injury to the ligaments of the wrist produces several patterns of injury observed on plain radiographs. Progressive ligamentous injury results in a characteristic sequence of injuries, from scapholunate dissociation, to perilunate dislocation and, finally, lunate dislocation. Scapholunate dissociation occurs when the interosseous ligament between the scaphoid and lunate is disrupted. On the anteroposterior (AP) radiograph, the joint space between the scaphoid and lunate is ≥3 mm, a finding termed the Terry Thomas sign. The other 2 patterns are best seen on the lateral radiograph. On this view, a line drawn through the center of the radius should transect the lunate and capitate. In a perilunate dislocation, the capitate is malaligned, usually dorsally (Figure 90-6A). In a lunate dislocation, the lunate is in an anterior position and is tipped over like a "spilled teacup" (Figure 90-6B).

Tendon lacerations are common after lacerations of the hand. Examination should include testing the movement and strength of the digit, as well as inspection of the tendon through its full range of motion. Flexor tendons are tested by noting flexion at the distal interphalangeal joint (flexor digitorum profundus) and the proximal interphalangeal joint (flexor digitorum superficialis). Mallet finger is a closed extensor tendon injury due to forced flexion of an extended distal phalangeal joint. It may be associated with an avulsion fracture. This injury occurs commonly when a person attempts to catch a ball.

CLINICAL PRESENTATION

▶ History

The patient presenting with upper extremity injury must be assessed for other more urgent or life-threatening injuries such as head or torso trauma before focusing attention on the extremity. A detailed history should attempt to identify the mechanism of injury, as this is often helpful in determining the type of injury sustained. Careful attention should be paid to injuries associated with significant swelling and pain unresponsive to narcotic medications, as these may be signs of limb-threatening compartment syndrome.

▶ Physical Examination

A thorough neurovascular assessment will help characterize the urgency of a patient's injury. This includes assessing pulses, skin color, capillary refill, and nerve function. The radial nerve performs wrist extension and provides sensation to the dorsal web space between the first and second digits and may be damaged by mid-shaft

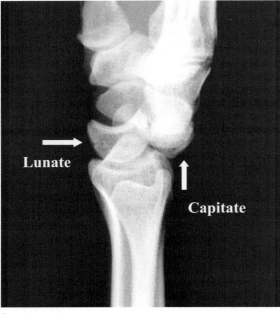

A

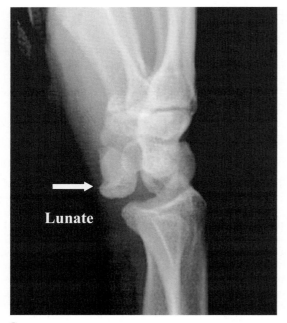

B

▲ **Figure 90-6. A.** Perilunate dislocation. Note that the lunate still articulates with the radius (horizontal arrow) but the capitate is dislocated dorsally (vertical arrow). **B.** Lunate dislocation. The lunate (arrow) is volarly dislocated and no longer articulates with the radius.

humerus fractures. The ulnar nerve travels posterior to the medial epicondyle of the elbow and abducts, or spreads apart, the digits, and provides sensation to the fifth digit. The median nerve allows opposition of the thumb and fifth digit and supplies sensation to the first 3 digits. It is most frequently injured in supracondylar humerus fractures.

After assessing for neurovascular integrity, evaluate for any gross deformities or swelling as well as any tenderness or "tenseness" that might suggest compartment swelling. Lacerations are noted, as these could represent open fractures. The entire extremity must be evaluated for secondary injuries that may be overlooked by a more "obvious" source of pain, paying particular attention to adjacent joints.

DIAGNOSTIC STUDIES

▶ Laboratory

Laboratory studies are usually unnecessary in the evaluation and management of extremity injuries.

IMAGING

In most cases, plain radiographs are sufficient to diagnose upper extremity trauma. Both an AP and lateral view of the bone must be viewed to fully understand and describe a fracture. Imaging the joint above and below the fracture is helpful to identify associated injuries.

Fractures must be described with a consistent language to properly manage and effectively communicate with consulting specialists. Common patterns include spiral, transverse, and oblique fractures. The degree of angulation, displacement, and level of comminution (see Figure 90-2) must be noted, in addition to the presence of intra-articular involvement, as these features frequently impact the definitive treatment plan.

Shoulder radiographs include AP films in internal and external rotation, a scapular "Y" view, and an axillary view. The axillary and "Y" view are especially helpful in diagnosing the posterior dislocation. Wrist radiographs consist of AP, lateral, and oblique views. The carpal bones are best scrutinized on the AP radiograph. Overlap of the bones suggests a carpal dislocation (ie, lunate or perilunate). The lateral view is best for detecting carpal dislocations and fractures of the distal radius and triquetrum. The oblique view allows for better visualization of the first metacarpal and the distal scaphoid. The scaphoid view, an AP view with ulnar deviation of the wrist, will increase the sensitivity for detecting scaphoid fractures.

Computed tomography (CT) and magnetic resonance imaging are not routinely ordered but have an improved sensitivity over plain radiographs for detecting occult fractures (eg, scaphoid fractures). CT scans can also better characterize complicated fractures seen on plain radiographs.

PROCEDURES

▶ Shoulder Dislocation Reduction

An anterior shoulder dislocation can be reduced by several techniques. The external rotation maneuver places the patient sitting upright or at 45 degrees. The patient's elbow is supported in adduction by one hand while the other hand is used to slowly and gently externally rotate the arm. The shoulder may reduce spontaneously. If not, the arm is slowly abducted and the humeral head is lifted into the socket. Scapular manipulation involves pushing the inferior portion of the scapular tip medially while the superior aspect is rotated laterally. This movement shifts the glenoid inferiorly toward the humeral head, allowing it to reduce spontaneously. The Stimson technique relies on gravity to slowly fatigue the shoulder musculature and allow spontaneous reduction of the humerus in 20–30 minutes. The patient is placed in the prone position with the arm hanging over the side of the bed with 10- to 15-lb weights suspended from the wrist.

MEDICAL DECISION MAKING

Most upper extremity injuries can be clinically diagnosed by a thorough history and physical exam. An accurate neurovascular exam is invaluable in rapidly identifying potentially limb-threatening injuries such as a vascular injury or compartment syndrome. When a fracture is suspected, radiographs are necessary to properly characterize fracture patterns, which will often dictate both the acute management and overall disposition of a patient (Figure 90-7).

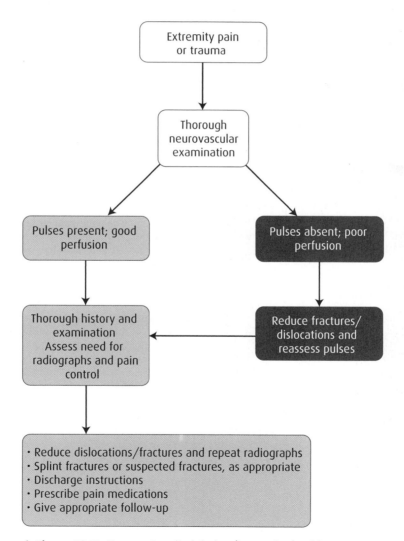

▲ **Figure 90-7.** Upper extremity injuries diagnostic algorithm.

CHAPTER 90

TREATMENT

The general treatment of most orthopedic injuries involves rest, ice, compression, and elevation (RICE). Most fractures should be immobilized with a splint that supports the joint above and below the injury. Ice should be applied 3–4 times daily for no more than 20 minutes at a time during the first 72 hours. Elevation of the injury will also help reduce swelling and pain. Gentle compression with elastic bandages can provide additional support to soft tissue injuries, though tight wrapping can induce compartment syndrome. Narcotic medications are preferred for fractures. Nonsteroidal anti-inflammatory drugs may inhibit bone healing and are therefore recommended only for soft-tissue injuries without underlying fractures.

Shoulder Dislocation

After successful reduction, apply a sling or shoulder immobilizer. The patient should be instructed to avoid external rotation of the arm, although early range of motion is often recommended for patients with shoulder injuries, especially in the elderly.

Shoulder Separation

Initial treatment of a first-, second-, or third-degree injury is a sling and pain control.

Humerus Fracture

A coaptation splint is applied for humeral shaft fractures, whereas a shoulder sling alone suffices for proximal fractures. Both injuries must be referred to an orthopedist for follow-up. Radial nerve injuries should be documented and are often managed conservatively.

Distal Radius Fracture

Closed reduction is recommended for displaced fractures with immobilization in a sugar tong splint.

Scaphoid Fracture

Because of the high risk of avascular necrosis with these fractures, a patient with wrist pain and anatomical snuffbox tenderness should be assumed to have a scaphoid fracture and immobilized with a thumb spica splint and referred for follow-up, even if radiographs are negative.

Metacarpal Fracture

These fractures will require reduction if significant angulation is present, followed by a radial or ulnar gutter splint.

Carpal Dislocation

Placement in a volar splint and orthopedic consultation for reduction and operative repair.

Mallet Finger

This injury must be splinted in extension for 6 weeks to allow for proper tendon healing.

Tendon Injury

Treatment of open tendon injuries in the ED includes thorough wound irrigation, laceration repair of skin wounds if indicated, and prophylactic antibiotics. Extensor tendon injuries should be splinted in extension, whereas flexor tendon injuries are splinted in flexion. Complete open tendon injuries require referral to a hand surgeon for tendon repair within a 7-day period.

DISPOSITION

Admission

Admission is indicated after orthopedic consultation for irreducible fractures or dislocations, open fractures, suspected compartment syndrome, or planned surgical repair. Admission for observation should also be considered for any injuries that are at high risk for early complications such as infection or compartment syndrome, or those that render patients unable to care for themselves.

Discharge

Most patients with upper extremity injuries are appropriate to discharge home after proper splinting and analgesia. Specific follow-up instructions and timing should be discussed if specialist referral is indicated. Discharge instructions should emphasize the importance of returning for signs of infection, neurovascular compromise, or compartment syndrome.

SUGGESTED READING

Carson S, Woolridge DP, Colletti J, et al. Pediatric upper extremity injuries. *Pediatr Clin North Am.* 2006;53:41–67.

Falcon-Chevere JL, Mathew D, Cabanas JG, et al. Management and treatment of elbow and forearm injuries. *Emerg Med Clin North Am.* 2010;28:765–787.

Menkes JS. Initial evaluation and management of orthopedic injuries. In: Tintinalli JE, Stapczynski JS, Ma OJ, Cline DM, Cydulka RK, Meckler GD. *Tintinalli's Emergency Medicine: A Comprehensive Study Guide.* 7th ed. New York, NY: McGraw-Hill, 2011, pp. 1783–1796.

Ufberg JW, Vilke GM, Chan TC, et al. Anterior shoulder dislocations: Beyond traction-countertraction. *J Emerg Med.* 2004;27:301–306.

Lower Extremity Injuries

Esther H. Chen, MD

91

Key Points

- If a hip fracture is suspected in an elderly patient, but plain radiographs are negative, obtain a computed tomography scan or magnetic resonance imaging.
- Delay in the reduction of a hip dislocation increases the likelihood of avascular necrosis of the femoral head.

- The presence of normal distal pulses after a knee dislocation does not exclude popliteal artery injury.
- A fracture at the base of the second metatarsal should raise suspicion for a Lisfranc fracture-dislocation.

INTRODUCTION

Lower extremity injuries are frequently caused by motor vehicle collisions (MVCs), pedestrian auto accidents, sports, and falls. These mechanisms often involve large forces, so concurrent torso injuries may be present. Fractures in patients with osteopenia and pathologic fractures occur after minor trauma. This chapter reviews lower extremity injuries from the hip to the foot and highlights some of the pitfalls in managing these orthopedic emergencies.

▶ Hip Injuries

Fractures at the hip are classified based on their location. Femoral neck (ie, subcapital) fractures are intracapsular and more likely to occur in elderly osteoporotic women. Displaced femoral neck fractures cause a hemarthrosis that compresses the femoral neck vessels and compromises the blood flow to the hip. This leads to avascular necrosis of the bone in 15–35% of cases and potential long-term disability. Intertrochanteric, subtrochanteric, and femoral shaft fractures are more likely to occur in young patients after a fall or direct blow to the knee (Figure 91-1).

Hip dislocations are posterior in 90% of cases. They are caused by high-energy trauma, such as striking the flexed knee on the dashboard during an MVC.

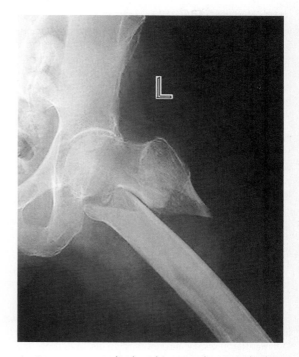

▲ **Figure 91-1.** A displaced intertrochanteric fracture of the hip.

Knee Injuries

The knee is stabilized by 4 ligaments, the anterior and posterior cruciates and the medial and lateral collateral ligaments. Maneuvers such as cutting, squatting, and twisting motions can cause ligamentous and meniscus injuries. The popliteal fossa contains the popliteal artery and vein, the common peroneal nerve, and the tibial nerve, so fractures involving the femoral condyles or proximal fibula may be associated with popliteal artery or deep peroneal nerve injury, respectively. Likewise, popliteal artery injuries may be seen with knee dislocations, even if distal pulses are palpable.

Tibial plateau fractures, seen more commonly in older patients even after minor trauma, can be difficult to detect on plain radiography. A proximal fibula fracture occurs from direct impact or when an external rotational force is applied to the foot or ankle that tears the interosseous membrane between the tibia and fibula, also called a Maisonneuve fracture.

Ankle and Foot Injuries

Anatomically, the foot is divided into the hindfoot (talus, calcaneus), midfoot (cuneiforms, navicular, cuboid), and forefoot (metatarsals, phalanges). The Chopart joint separates the hindfoot from the midfoot, whereas the Lisfranc joint divides the midfoot from the forefoot. A fracture of the second metatarsal base is associated with disruption of the ligaments that stabilize the Lisfranc joint. This results in dislocation of the other metatarsal bones. A Lisfranc fracture-dislocation occurs after severe plantar flexion of the foot with an abduction force, such as stepping off a sidewalk curb. Calcaneus fractures are often bilateral because the most frequent mechanism is a fall from height, landing on both feet. Lumbar spine fractures occur in 10% of patients with calcaneal fractures.

The ankle is stabilized by the deltoid ligament, lateral ligament complex (anterior and posterior talofibular, and calcaneofibular ligaments), and syndesmosis. The most common injury is an ankle sprain, 90% of which are inversion injuries. Ligamentous injuries and laxity is difficult to detect hours after an acute injury because of the surrounding ligamentous tension and muscle spasm.

Other important lower extremity injuries to diagnose include Achilles tendon rupture and patella and quadriceps tendon rupture.

CLINICAL PRESENTATION

Patients with lower extremity injuries present with pain over the injured site, swelling, ecchymosis, deformity, limited range of motion, and/or inability to ambulate. During the primary survey, stabilizing the limb may limit blood loss, and reducing a fracture/dislocation may restore neurovascular function. The joints above and below the injury should be examined for deformities,

shortening, rotation, lacerations, ligamentous instability, and neurovascular status. The physical exam can be very limited after an acute injury due to the pain associated with movement.

Intertrochanteric fractures of the hip may leave the leg shortened, abducted, and externally rotated because of traction on the iliopsoas. Patients with nondisplaced hip fractures may be ambulatory, so physicians should have a low threshold for obtaining imaging. A posterior hip dislocation presents with a shortened, adducted, and internally rotated leg.

A knee exam begins with inspecting for swelling, effusion, ecchymosis, and patella location, using the uninjured knee for comparison. Knee injuries, whether from a fracture, dislocation, or ligamentous injury, typically present with a hemarthrosis. Anterior cruciate ligament (ACL) tears cause the majority of hemarthrosis (75%), but other etiologies include meniscal tears and fractures. The mechanism of injury for an ACL tear is a deceleration, hyperextension, or internal rotation of the tibia on the femur, associated with a "pop" and swelling that develops within hours. Ligamentous testing of the knee is outlined in Table 91-1. A history of locking of the knee suggests a meniscal tear.

Knee dislocations are associated with tremendous ligamentous disruption. About half of all knee dislocations will have spontaneously reduced before presentation. Despite spontaneous reduction, there is still a high likelihood of popliteal artery and peroneal nerve injury. Palpation of the distal pulses is performed to assess the popliteal artery, but normal pulses are not sensitive enough to exclude arterial injury. In patients without evidence of vascular injury, an ankle brachial index (ABI) of >0.9 allows for safe observation without angiography. The deep peroneal nerve is assessed by testing sensation on the dorsal aspect of the foot between the first and second toes.

Table 91-1. Stress testing the ligaments of the knee.

Ligament	Stress Test	Description
Anterior cruciate ligament (ACL)	Lachman	Knee flexed to 30°, pull tibia forward; anterior displacement is positive
Posterior cruciate ligament (PCL)	Posterior drawer	Knee flexed to 90°, tibia pushed backwards; posterior displacement is positive
Medial collateral ligament (MCL)	Valgus stress test	Knee flexed 30° and hanging off lateral aspect of bed; valgus force applied to leg while palpating the MCL
Lateral collateral ligament (LCL)	Varus stress test	Knee flexed 30° and hanging off lateral aspect of bed; varus force applied to leg while palpating the LCL

Some lacerations overlying the knee may be deep enough to extend into the joint capsule (ie, traumatic arthrotomy). The knee is the most common joint to be affected. Once an underlying fracture has been excluded, the joint will need to be injected with saline or dilute methylene blue. If fluid flows out of the laceration when the joint is injected, then the joint has been violated and requires a wash out in the operating room.

Patients with patella fractures and patella and quadriceps tendon rupture may be able to ambulate normally, but the extensor function of the knee is affected (ie, the patient would not be able to perform a straight leg raise). The position of the patella is notably altered on exam in patients with tendon rupture, particularly after a patella tendon rupture.

Posttraumatic compartment syndrome causes severe pain that starts within a few hours after the injury (but can occur up to 48 hours), worsens with passive range of motion, and is associated with progressive swelling around the injured area. In the lower extremity, the most common location to develop compartment syndrome is the leg, usually after a tibia fracture. The 4 compartments of the leg are the anterior, lateral, posterior, and deep posterior.

The most common ankle injury is a lateral ankle sprain. Patients will present with tenderness and swelling around the anterolateral aspect of the ankle and difficulty bearing weight. Grade I ankle sprains present with minimal functional loss, pain, and swelling. Grade II and III sprains involve partial and complete tear of the ligaments and result in significant functional loss.

Achilles tendon rupture most commonly occurs after a weekend warrior (ie, middle-aged man who infrequently performs strenuous activities) applies a force to the dorsiflexed foot and then has sudden severe pain in the back of the leg. On examination, the calf is tender and swollen and there is a gap in the tendon about 2–6 cm proximal to the calcaneus. The Thompson test is performed with the patient lying prone, knees bent at 90 degrees. If the foot does not dorsiflex when the calf is squeezed, then the tendon is completely torn.

Fractures at the base of the fifth metatarsal have 2 common types—tuberosity avulsion fractures and Jones fractures. A tuberosity avulsion fracture occurs after an inversion injury to the ankle (Figure 91-2). Patients will present with pain in the lateral aspect of the foot that is worse with ambulation. By contrast, a Jones fracture is a more distal fracture of the fifth metatarsal shaft (within 1.5 cm of the tuberosity). It occurs when a laterally directed force is placed on the forefoot during plantar flexion of the ankle.

DIAGNOSTIC STUDIES

▶ Laboratory

Laboratory studies are usually not necessary when evaluating patients with lower extremity trauma, although they may be required for patients who need hospital admission or operative management for their injuries.

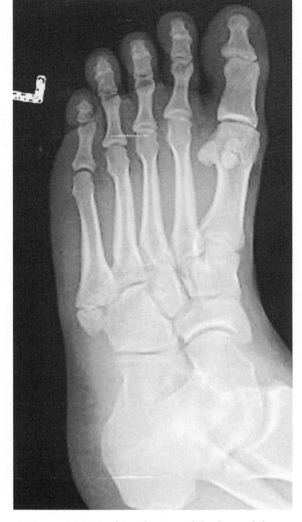

▲ **Figure 91-2.** Avulsion fracture of the base of the fifth metatarsal.

▶ Imaging

Plain radiography is the initial diagnostic imaging of choice for any lower extremity injury. If a hip fracture is suspected, adding an anteroposterior (AP) pelvis view to the routine hip AP, internal, and external rotation views enables the reader to compare the injured joint to the unaffected side. This is especially helpful in patients with severe degenerative joint disease. In elderly patients with normal radiographs and persistent significant pain with weight bearing, computed tomography (CT) or magnetic resonance imaging is useful for detecting an occult fracture.

Routine knee radiographs include the AP, lateral, and oblique views. In the setting of acute knee trauma, a patient meeting any of the criteria in the Ottawa knee rules (age >55 years, isolated patella tenderness, fibula head tenderness, inability to flex the knee to 90 degrees, and inability to ambulate 4 steps after the injury and in the emergency department [ED]) should receive knee radiographs. A high-riding patella on the lateral view indicates a possible patella tendon rupture. The presence of a fat-fluid level (ie, lipohemarthrosis) on the lateral view is an indirect sign of an intra-articular fracture. CT imaging may be required for determining the extent of tibial plateau fractures. An avulsion fracture at the site of the attachment of the lateral capsular ligament on the lateral tibial condyle (ie, Segond fracture) suggests an anterior cruciate ligament tear.

Ankle films include AP, lateral, and mortise views (AP with 15- to 20-degree internal rotation). The Ottawa ankle rules help dictate which patients need ankle radiographs. Any patient unable to ambulate 4 steps after the injury or in the ED or who is tender over the posterior aspect of the medial or lateral malleoli should have imaging. A lateral talar shift on the AP or mortise views indicates a deltoid ligament rupture (Figure 91-3). It is present when the space between the medial malleolus and talus is greater than the distance from the talar dome (superior aspect of the talus) to the tibial plafond (inferior aspect of the tibia). Fractures may be isolated distal lateral malleolus, bimalleolar, or trimalleolar (Figure 91-4).

Routine foot films are AP, lateral, and internal oblique views. For foot injuries, the Ottawa foot rules (ie, inability to ambulate 4 steps after the injury or in the ED; or tenderness at the base of the fifth metatarsal or the navicular) help determine which patients should be imaged. If a calcaneus fracture is suspected clinically, calculate Böhler angle on the lateral view to identify subtle fractures and measure the degree of fracture depression (Figure 91-5). The lines of this angle are formed from the superior margin of the posterior

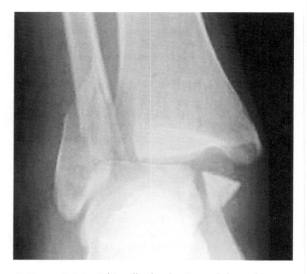

▲ **Figure 91-4.** A bimalleolar fracture of the ankle.

tuberosity of the calcaneus through the superior tip of the posterior facet and from the superior tip of the anterior facet to the superior tip of the posterior facet. Normally, this angle is 20–40 degrees. If the angle is <20 degrees, an occult depressed calcaneus fracture should be suspected.

On the AP view of the foot, the first 3 metatarsals should align with the 3 cuneiforms, the fourth and fifth metatarsals should align with the cuboid, and the medial portion of the middle cuneiform should align with the medial aspect of the second metacarpal. Any disruption to this alignment suggests a Lisfranc fracture-dislocation, and follow-up stress (weight-bearing) views should be obtained. A Lisfranc injury is present if there is any bony displacement greater than 1 mm between the bases of the first and second metatarsals.

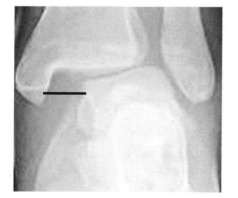

▲ **Figure 91-3.** Lateral talar shift indicating deltoid ligament disruption.

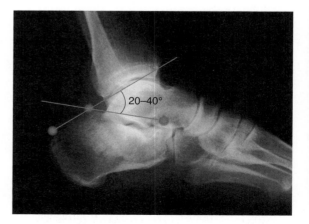

▲ **Figure 91-5.** The normal Böhler angle is between 20 and 40 degrees.

PROCEDURES

Joint dislocations and displaced fractures should be reduced in the ED to restore alignment and function. Procedural sedation is often required to relax the large muscle groups and facilitate manipulation of the bones and joints. Fractures or dislocations that are difficult to reduce with good alignment may require operative repair.

There are 2 common maneuvers for reducing hip dislocations: the Allis and Bigelow maneuvers. In the Allis maneuver, an assistant applies downward pressure to the anterior superior iliac spines while the physician flexes the knee and hip to 90 degrees. Grasping the knee with both hands, simultaneously pull and rotate the femur laterally and medially until the joint pops into place. In the Bigelow maneuver, the patient is also placed in a supine position with the affected hip and knee flexed to 90 degrees. Secure the knee with a flexed elbow and grab the foot with the opposite hand. Using the flexed elbow to apply traction to the femur, externally rotate and extend the hip until the femoral head reduces.

To reduce knee dislocations, apply gentle longitudinal traction to the lower leg while an assistant provides counter-traction on the thigh. Patella dislocations are treated by flexing the hip, hyperextending the knee, and sliding the patella back into place.

Arthrocentesis may be a therapeutic benefit in patients with large knee effusions, although there is no good evidence of its efficacy and recurrence of the effusion can occur. Diagnostically, the presence of blood and glistening fat globules is pathognomonic of lipohemarthrosis, a sign of an intra-articular fracture.

Ankle dislocation reduction is achieved by grasping the heel and foot with both hands and applying downward traction and rotation in the opposite direction to the mechanism of injury.

MEDICAL DECISION MAKING

With any limb injury, the integrity of the neurovascular status should be determined immediately (see Figure 90-7). As mentioned previously, knee dislocations or severely displaced tibia fractures may be associated with a popliteal artery injury, so patients with those injuries should undergo ABIs ± evaluation with CT angiography. There is poor collateral circulation around the knee, so the popliteal artery circulation must be restored within 8 hours to prevent amputation.

Compartment syndrome also should not be missed because it may develop after any traumatic injury. A tense, severely swollen limb should have its compartment pressures measured, along with serum creatinine phosphokinase and myoglobin levels. Patients placed in a splint after a sprain, nonoperative fracture, or reduced dislocation should be discharged with instructions to return for any signs or symptoms of compartment syndrome.

TREATMENT

Emergent orthopedic consultation should be obtained for compartment syndrome and all open fractures. Patients with open fractures should be copiously irrigated in the ED and given broad-spectrum antibiotics. For ligamentous and meniscus injuries, tendon ruptures, and most nondisplaced fractures, the joint or injured area should be immobilized with a splint. Patients should be given crutches for ambulation. Pain may be controlled with narcotic analgesia for fractures and nonsteroidal anti-inflammatory agents for soft-tissue injuries for several days. Swelling is decreased with rest, ice, compression, and elevation (RICE).

▶ Hip And Femur Fractures

Fractures of the femoral head, neck, intertrochanteric, and femoral shaft require admission for operative reduction and internal fixation (ORIF). Hare traction splints can be used temporarily to stabilize femoral shaft fractures during transport (eg, prehospital setting), but are contraindicated in femoral neck fractures because they can compromise femoral head blood flow and cause avascular necrosis.

▶ Knee Dislocation

In the setting of popliteal artery injury, operative repair within an 8-hour time period is recommended. When reduction has been achieved and vascular injury has been excluded, immobilization and referral for surgery is appropriate.

▶ Patella Fractures And Dislocation

Treated with analgesia, a knee immobilizer, and crutches with weight bearing as tolerated. Orthopedic referral for operative repair is indicated for displaced horizontal patella fractures.

▶ Patella And Quadriceps Tendon Rupture

Treated with analgesia, a knee immobilizer, and crutches with weight bearing as tolerated. Orthopedic referral for operative repair is indicated.

▶ Tibial Plateau Fracture

Tibial plateau fractures may be immobilized in a long leg posterior splint and referred for orthopedic evaluation within 24–48 hours. These patients should be given crutches and remain non–weight-bearing.

▶ Ligamentous And Meniscal Injuries

Treated with analgesia, a knee immobilizer, and crutches with weight bearing as tolerated. After 2–3 days of immobilization, patients should perform daily range of motion exercises (ie, 10–20 knee flexions and extensions 3–4 times a day) to prevent contractures and maintain mobility.

Orthopedic referral for possible operative repair is indicated.

Tibia Fractures

Because the tibia is the weight-bearing bone of the lower leg, many tibia fractures are admitted for operative repair. These patients have a high risk of developing compartment syndrome.

Ankle Sprain

Grade I ankle sprains should be immobilized for 1–2 days in an ankle brace followed by early range of motion and strength training exercises. Grade II and III ligamentous injuries should be stabilized in a short leg splint with the ankle in a neutral position.

Achilles Tendon Rupture

Support the ankle with a short leg posterior splint and refer to an orthopedist for operative repair, the preferred treatment for young or more active patients. The ankle is immobilized in slight plantarflexion.

Ankle Fractures And Dislocation

Operative repair is the preferred treatment for ankle dislocations and unstable ankle fractures. Bimalleolar and trimalleolar fractures are unstable injuries that are typically reduced in the ED, if needed, and referred for operative repair. An isolated distal lateral malleolus fracture is considered to be a stable injury that can be immobilized in a short leg posterior splint and referred for orthopedic follow-up.

Foot Fractures

Nondisplaced fractures of the navicular and cuboid bones require a short leg splint. Calcaneus fractures require a bulky compressive dressing and a posterior splint. The patient will remain non–weight-bearing for 6–8 weeks.

Metatarsal fractures should be immobilized in a posterior leg splint and treated nonoperatively, unless there is an associated Lisfranc dislocation, a displacement of more than 3–4 mm, or angulation of more than 10 degrees, all of which are managed operatively. Because of a tenuous blood supply, a Jones fracture requires a posterior leg splint and non–weight-bearing status for proper healing. Finally, phalangeal fractures are treated with buddy taping the injured toe to an adjacent toe and a hard-soled shoe.

DISPOSITION

Admission

Admission is required for patients with hemodynamic instability (from acute blood loss) and fractures that are open, associated with multiorgan trauma, or require early ORIF (eg, hip fractures).

Discharge

Most patients with nondisplaced fractures, ligamentous injury, or meniscus tears can be splinted and sent home with referral to orthopedics for further management (ie, cast or surgical repair). If non–weight-bearing status is required, patients must be able to ambulate with crutches or have home assistance with activities of daily living.

SUGGESTED READING

Newton EJ, Love J. Emergency department management of selected orthopedic injuries. *Emerg Med Clin North Am.* 2007;25:763–793.

Perron AD, Brady WJ. Evaluation and management of the high-risk orthopedic emergency. *Emerg Med Clin North Am.* 2003;21:159–204.

Menkes JS. Initial evaluation and management of orthopedic injuries. In: Tintinalli JE, Stapczynski JS, Ma OJ, Cline DM, Cydulka RK, Meckler GD. *Tintinalli's Emergency Medicine: A Comprehensive Study Guide.* 7th ed. New York, NY: McGraw-Hill, 2011, pp. 1783–1796.

Low Back Pain

Paul E. Casey, MD

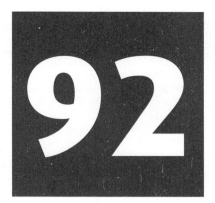

Key Points

- The diagnostic approach to lower back pain is facilitated by classifying back pain into (1) nonspecific low back pain, (2) back pain associated with radiculopathy, and (3) back pain due to a serious underlying cause.

- It is critical to screen for risk factors associated with serious back pathology as well as identify the presence of neurologic deficits.

- Imaging is indicated in select patients with significant risk factors and/or neurologic deficits.

INTRODUCTION

Acute low back pain may be due to a variety of conditions ranging from benign (eg, muscle strain) to devastating (eg, spinal cord compression from malignancy or abscess). For the clinician in the emergency department (ED), it is critical to develop a systematic approach that will allow one to differentiate and manage the minority of patients with conditions that threaten neurologic function from those with benign, self-limited etiologies. This chapter focuses primarily on the evaluation and management of acute (<4 weeks) low back pain.

An estimated 60–70% of adults in the United States will experience low back pain in their lifetime, and although only 25–30% will seek medical care, low back pain is an exceedingly common reason for ED visits in the United States. The economic impact of low back pain is substantial, estimated to account for $26.3 billion of direct health care costs in the United States in 1998.

The pathophysiology of nonspecific low back pain is usually indeterminate, as pain may arise from a number of sites including the vertebral column, surrounding muscles, tendons, ligaments, and fascia. The mechanism of injury to these structures varies from stretching, tearing, or contusion as a result of heavy lifting or torsion of the spinal column. In contrast, the pathophysiology of radicular low back pain is more clearly defined. Herniation of the nucleus pulposus through the annulus fibrosis causes compression of the dural lining around the spinal nerve root, resulting in radicular pain.

CLINICAL PRESENTATION

The history and physical examination serve as cornerstones in the evaluation of back pain. To facilitate a rational diagnostic approach, an attempt is made to classify low back pain into 1 of 3 categories:

1. Nonspecific low back pain: pain with no signs or symptoms of a serious underlying condition

2. Radicular back pain: pain with nerve root dysfunction associated with pain, sensory impairment, weakness, or impaired deep tendon reflexes in a specific nerve root distribution

3. Serious underlying etiology: pain with neurologic deficits or underlying conditions requiring prompt evaluation (eg, tumor, infection, fracture, cauda equina syndrome)

▶ History

The history should focus on the location of pain (including radiation of pain), frequency and duration of symptoms, and exacerbating and alleviating factors, as well as any

Table 92-1. Risk factors for serious pathology in back pain.

Risk factors for underlying malignancy
• Prior history of malignancy
• Age >50 years
• Unexplained weight loss
• Failure to improve after 4 weeks
Risk factors for vertebral infection
• Fever
• Intravenous drug use
• Recent infection
Risk factors for vertebral compression fracture
• Old age
• History of osteoporosis
• Corticosteroid use

previous episodes or treatments of back pain. Pain that radiates down the leg, usually past the knee, suggests a radiculopathy. Pain from a herniated disk is worse with movement, sitting, or Valsalva maneuver (eg, coughing). Pain worse at night or rest suggests malignancy or spinal infection. A past medical history of malignancy or immunocompromise is determined. Inquire about recent weight loss or fevers. Patients should also be asked about severe or progressive neurologic deficits including motor deficits, fecal incontinence, and bladder dysfunction. Bilateral leg pain and bowel/bladder dysfunction suggests cauda equina syndrome. Other warning signs of serious disease underlying low back pain are listed in Table 92-1.

Physical Examination

The musculoskeletal exam should include percussion of the spinous processes of the back. Pain with percussion suggests spinal infection, vertebral malignancy, or compression fracture. Tenderness and spasm of the paraspinal muscles frequently heralds muscle strain, but can also be seen in secondary condition (eg, epidural abscess). As a result, when other signs and symptoms for a serious back pain etiology are present, don't dismiss them just because the pain is reproduced by palpation of the paraspinal muscles.

Patients should also undergo a complete neurologic assessment. Neurologic deficits that suggest spinal cord compression include spasticity, bilateral weakness, positive Babinski sign, multiple dermatomes, and bilateral reflex abnormalities. Findings consistent with cauda equina syndrome are decreased sensation to light touch and pinprick in the inner thighs and perineum (saddle anesthesia), decreased rectal tone, and urinary retention with a post-void residual over 100 mL. Saddle anesthesia is seen in 75% of cases of cauda equina syndrome, whereas an elevated postvoid residual is present in 90%.

When a radiculopathy is suspected, perform the straight-leg raise and reverse straight-leg raise tests. A positive straight-leg raise (reproduction of the patient's radicular symptoms between 30 and 70 degrees of leg elevation) has a relatively high sensitivity (91%), but a low specificity (26%) for diagnosing a herniated disc. The reverse straight-leg raise is more specific (88%) but less sensitive (26%). Evaluate strength for nerve root dysfunction by testing knee strength (L4 nerve root), great toe/foot dorsiflexion (L5 nerve root), and foot plantarflexion (S1 nerve root). Sensory deficits in radiculopathy include decreased sensation between the first and second toes (L5 nerve root) and decreased sensation on the lateral aspect of the foot (S1 nerve root).

Lastly, assess the pulses and palpate the abdomen for possible vascular causes of the pain, including aortic aneurysm.

DIAGNOSTIC STUDIES

Laboratory

Laboratory testing generally plays a limited role in the evaluation of low back pain. Obtain a urine pregnancy test in females of reproductive age to exclude ectopic pregnancy and guide future decisions regarding imaging. A urinalysis may also be helpful to evaluate for nephrolithiasis or pyelonephritis as potential causes of low back pain. Although erythrocyte sedimentation rates and C-reactive protein may be elevated in some patients with back pain (eg, epidural abscess, malignancy), these studies are nonspecific and should not be routinely ordered as part of the work-up.

Imaging

Patients presenting with nonspecific low back pain with none of the high-risk features discussed previously do not warrant routine radiographic evaluation. Prompt evaluation with magnetic resonance imaging (MRI) or computed tomography (CT) is recommended when severe or progressive neurologic deficits are present or when serious underlying conditions are suspected on the basis of history and physical exam. If available, MRI is preferred over CT because it provides better visualization of soft tissues, vertebral marrow, and the spinal canal.

In patients suspected of a vertebral compression fracture (eg, osteoporosis, chronic steroid use), plain radiography is recommended (Figure 92-1). A CT should be considered if there is significant loss of height of the vertebral body or if any neurologic symptoms are present. Patients with an underlying malignancy with acute back pain should have an MRI on an urgent basis (within 24 hours) when no neurologic deficits are present. When neurologic deficits are present, the MRI is performed emergently. For patients with low back pain associated with radiculopathy, MRI (preferred) or CT are only recommended if the patient is a candidate for surgery or

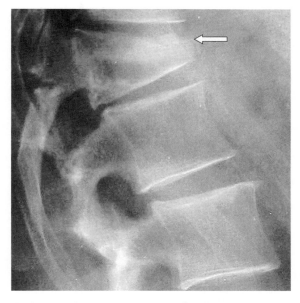

▲ **Figure 92-1.** T12 compression fracture.

epidural steroid injection, as the natural course of lumbar disc herniation with radiculopathy is improvement within 4 weeks.

MEDICAL DECISION MAKING

The history and physical exam serve as the cornerstones in the evaluation of low back pain. Eliciting risk factors indicative of a serious underlying condition (eg, urinary retention concerning for cauda equina syndrome) or identifying neurologic deficits on exam should prompt advanced imaging. In the absence of risk factors, neurologic deficits, or symptoms suggestive of a potentially serious cause, the source of the low back pain is most likely benign, and reassurance and symptomatic management with outpatient follow-up is recommended (Figure 92-2).

TREATMENT

The treatment of low back pain varies depending on the identified etiology. For those patients with nonspecific low back pain, symptomatic therapy should include advice to remain active and application of heat as needed. Acetaminophen and nonsteroidal anti-inflammatory drugs (NSAIDs) have shown short-term benefits. One must weigh the potential analgesic benefit from NSAIDs with the known risks of their use. Opioid analgesics or tramadol are an option for patients with severe, debilitating pain that is not controlled with acetaminophen or NSAIDs, but again, they should be prescribed judiciously and for very limited periods given the risk of medication interactions and potential for abuse. Musculoskeletal relaxants are approved by the

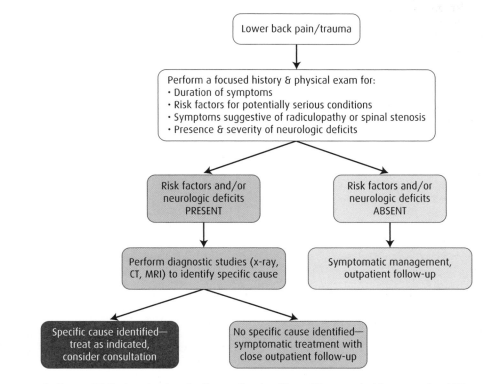

▲ **Figure 92-2.** Low back pain diagnostic algorithm. CT, computed tomography; MRI, magnetic resonance imaging.

Food and Drug Administration for treatment of musculo-skeletal conditions or spasticity and are another option for short-term use in acute low back pain.

When a specific etiology for low back pain is identified, the treatment varies depending on the underlying pathology. Low back pain with radiculopathy (in the absence of focal neurologic deficits) can be treated symptomatically, as most patients recover without surgery. Patients diagnosed with vertebral osteomyelitis require intravenous (IV) antibiotics, whereas an epidural abscess is treated with neurosurgical evaluation for potential drainage as well as parenteral antibiotics. Neurosurgical consultation should also be obtained immediately for patients with cauda equina syndrome. In patients with vertebral malignancy with new neurologic deficits, emergent radiation to shrink the tumor and relieve cord compression is advised. The administration of corticosteroids (dexamethasone 10 mg IV) for acute spinal cord compression should also be considered in consultation with neurosurgery.

DISPOSITION

▶ Admission

The patient disposition depends primarily on the etiology of the back pain as well as analgesic control of symptoms. Patients found to have a serious underlying etiology of low back pain (eg, cauda equina syndrome, epidural abscess) should be admitted in consultation with neurosurgery. It is also reasonable to consider observation for patients with nonspecific low back pain (with or without radiculopathy) when pain control cannot be achieved in the ED.

▶ Discharge

Patients with nonspecific low back pain or back pain with radiculopathy in whom pain is reasonably controlled can be discharged with outpatient follow-up. All patients should receive patient education regarding self-care and treatment for low back pain as well as indications to return to the emergency department (eg, development of neurologic deficit, change in urinary or bowel functions).

▼ SUGGESTED READING

Chou R, Huffman LH. Medications for acute and chronic lower back pain: A review of evidence for an American Pain Society/American College of Physicians clinical practice guideline. *Ann Intern Med*. 2007;147:505–514.

Chou R, Qaseem A, Snow V, et al. Diagnosis and treatment of low back pain: A joint clinical practice guideline from the American College of Physicians and the American Pain Society. *Ann Intern Med*. 2007;147:478–491.

Frohna WJ, Della-Giustina D. Neck and back pain. In: Tintinalli JE, Stapczynski JS, Ma OJ, Cline DM, Cydulka RK, Meckler GD. *Tintinalli's Emergency Medicine: A Comprehensive Study Guide*. 7th ed. New York, NY: McGraw-Hill, 2011, pp. 1885–1893.

Compartment Syndromes

Marc Doucette, MD

Key Points

- Compartment syndrome occurs when tissue pressure in a closed space rises, compromising perfusion to nerves and muscles.

- The leg and forearm compartments are most commonly involved, but compartment syndrome can also occur in the upper arm, thigh, hand, foot, gluteal region, or abdomen.

- Compartment syndrome is usually associated with long bone fracture, crush injuries, circumferential burn, or cast.

- Acute compartment syndrome is a surgical emergency, treated by fasciotomy to relieve pressure and restore circulation.

INTRODUCTION

Acute compartment syndrome is a surgical emergency. If unrecognized and untreated, it can lead to tissue ischemia, necrosis, and long-term functional impairment. Volkmann ischemic contracture is the end result of an ischemic injury to the muscles and nerves of a limb. Compartment syndrome is seen most commonly in the setting of trauma, including long bone fractures, crush injuries, and circumferential burns to the extremities. Males and young people are affected more commonly than females and elderly.

The pathophysiology of compartment syndrome involves increased pressure in a muscle compartment that is enclosed by a fascial structure with limited ability to expand. This increased pressure is caused by edema or bleeding, from compression of the compartment by a circumferential burn or a constricting cast, or a combination of both. Increased pressure leads to decreased venous outflow from the compartment, causing a decrease in the arteriovenous pressure gradient and ultimately cellular ischemia and tissue necrosis.

Cardinal signs and symptoms include severe pain over the involved area, pain with passive stretch of the muscles in the affected compartment, weakness, and paresthesias. Although commercially available devices can be used to measure compartment pressures, the diagnosis is often made on clinical grounds alone. Early recognition and orthopedic consultation are essential in preventing tissue necrosis and adverse outcome.

CLINICAL PRESENTATION

▶ History

Acute compartment syndrome is seen most commonly in the setting of trauma or long bone fracture. Significant blunt trauma or crush injury can lead to compartment syndrome, even in the absence of fracture. Symptom onset is usually within hours of injury, but can present up to 48 hours after the traumatic event.

Historically, the symptoms of compartment syndrome have been described by the "the five Ps": pain, pallor, paresthesias, pulselessness, and poikilothermia. However, all of these are not typically present, and many are late findings that signal irreversible injury. The primary complaint in the alert patient is usually of severe pain in the affected limb, often not controlled by opioid analgesics. The pain is often worsened by passive stretch of the muscles in the involved compartment. Nerve ischemia can lead to a burning sensation or dysesthesia.

Physical Examination

Detection of compartment syndrome requires a high clinical suspicion and an attentive exam. The involved compartment is swollen and tense. There is exquisite tenderness to palpation. Pain is intensified if the examiner passively stretches the muscles of the compartment. Sensory deficits may be present, but motor weakness is usually a later finding. Pulselessness is a rare and late finding, as the arterial pressure usually exceeds the tissue pressure. Thus, the limb often remains warm with normal color, pulses, and capillary refill. In the alert patient, the absence of pain, paresthesias, and pain with passive stretch excludes the diagnosis of compartment syndrome.

DIAGNOSTIC STUDIES

Laboratory

Laboratory testing is not helpful in making the diagnosis of compartment syndrome. In the setting of extensive muscle damage, creatine phosphokinase or myoglobin may be elevated.

Imaging

Although diagnostic imaging studies are routinely used to evaluate the traumatized limb for associated orthopedic fracture, they are not required to make the diagnosis of compartment syndrome. The presence of significant or comminuted long bone fractures should heighten the provider's concern for the development of compartment syndrome.

PROCEDURES

When there is doubt about the clinical diagnosis of compartment syndrome, such as in a patient with an unreliable exam due to altered mental status, compartment pressures should be measured. Pressures can be objectively measured using a commercially available handheld manometer, such as the Stryker device (Figure 93-1). These instruments contain a needle connected to a pressure monitor. The needle is inserted into the muscle compartment at the most tense point, or near the fracture site. A small amount of saline is injected into the compartment, and the manometer reads the resistance to injection created by the tissue. Pressure should be checked at a minimum of 2 locations within the affected compartment and can be checked in a normal compartment for comparison.

Normal tissue pressure in a muscle compartment is <10 mm Hg. Pressures up to 20 mm Hg are generally well tolerated. Pressures between 20–30 mm Hg may cause damage if they persist over multiple hours. Pressures >30 mm Hg are generally considered an indication for an emergent fasciotomy. More recent studies suggest that a more important number is the difference between the patient's diastolic blood pressure and the tissue pressure, or "delta pressure." These studies suggest that a delta

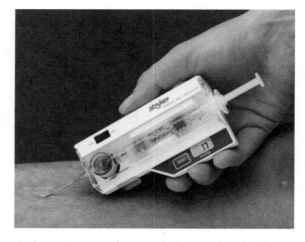

Figure 93-1. Stryker STIC device. Reprinted with permission from Hutson AM, Rovinsky D. Chapter 63. Compartment Pressure Measurement. In: Reichman EF, Simon RR, eds. *Emergency Medicine Procedures*. New York: McGraw-Hill, 2004.

pressure of >30 mm Hg is an indication for fasciotomy, whereas patients with delta pressure <30 mm Hg have a low likelihood of developing tissue damage if fasciotomy is withheld.

MEDICAL DECISION MAKING

History and physical exam along with a high index of suspicion may be all that is required to make the diagnosis of compartment syndrome. Measurement of compartment pressures can serve as a diagnostic tool. Failure to make the diagnosis and respond appropriately can lead to tissue damage and long-term functional deficits (Figure 93-2).

TREATMENT

The definitive treatment for an acute compartment syndrome is emergent fasciotomy. To minimize tissue damage, fasciotomy should be performed <8 hours and preferably <6 hours after the onset of symptoms. Emergency department (ED) management involves early orthopedic consultation as soon as the diagnosis is confirmed. The patient should be hydrated and hypotension should be avoided. The affected limb should be kept at the level of the heart and not elevated. Elevation of the limb above the level of the heart reduces the arterial pressure and may reduce perfusion. Generous analgesia is often required.

Fasciotomy is performed by an orthopedic or general surgeon in the operating room setting. A long incision is made in the skin and fascia, allowing the contents of the compartment to swell without increasing pressure. The incision is usually closed several days later, when the swelling has diminished. Sometimes skin grafting is necessary.

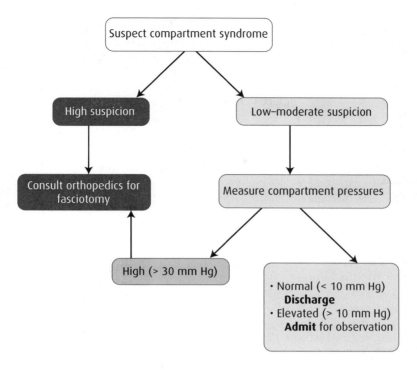

Figure 93-2. Compartment syndromes diagnostic algorithm.

DISPOSITION

▶ Admission

Patients with acute compartment syndrome require hospital admission and urgent surgical intervention. Patients with a high clinical concern for the development of compartment syndrome should receive orthopedic consultation in the ED, with consideration for admission and observation.

▶ Discharge

Patients who are being discharged with long bone fractures or blunt extremity trauma should be educated about the signs and symptoms of compartment syndrome and be given instructions to return if they develop worsening swelling, numbness, or pain that is not responsive to pain medications.

▼ SUGGESTED READING

Gourgioutis S, Villas C, Germanos S, et al. Acute limb compartment syndrome: A review. *J Surg Educ.* 2007;64:178.

Haller PR. Compartment syndrome. In: Tintinalli JE, Stapczynski JS, Ma OJ, Clince DM, Cydulka RK, Meckler GD. *Tintinalli's Emergency Medicine: A Comprehensive Study Guide.* 7th ed. New York, NY: McGraw-Hill, 2011, pp. 1880–1884.

Reichman EF, Simon RR. Compartment pressure measurement. In: *Emergency Medicine Procedures.* New York, NY: McGraw-Hill, 2004.

Septic Arthritis

Kim L. Askew, MD

Key Points

- Septic arthritis can lead to significant morbidity if not treated in a timely manner.
- Because the history and physical examination has limitations, arthrocentesis should be performed in anyone suspected of having a septic arthritis.

- A combination of the patient's presentation, risk factors, and synovial fluid tests determine appropriate management decisions.

INTRODUCTION

Emergency physicians' greatest concern and diagnostic dilemma when faced with patients presenting with nontraumatic acute joint pain is septic arthritis. The invasion by bacteria and the associated immune response can lead to rapid joint destruction and irreversible loss of function. Yet, despite the severity of the condition, misconceptions about patient presentations and the evaluation of patients with possible septic joints persist in all aspects of health care.

Septic arthritis affects approximately 2–10 people per 100,000 annually and is frequently encountered in the emergency department (ED) setting. Once infected, the joint cartilage is rapidly injured, with up to 30% of patients experiencing residual damage and up to 10% dying as a result of the septic joint. Septic arthritis typically affects young children and adults older than 55 years; however, any age group can be affected. The microbiology of septic joints can be divided into 2 groups: nongonococcal and gonococcal. Nongonococcal pathogens include *Staphylococcus aureus* (50%), *Streptococcus pneumoniae*, *Streptococcus pyogenes* (25%), and gram-negative bacilli (20%). Hematogenous spread is more common than contiguous extension from a local cellulitis or penetrating injury. Although the incidence of gonococcal arthritis has declined over the past 2 decades, it is the leading cause of septic arthritis among sexually active individuals and causes 5% of all septic joints.

CLINICAL PRESENTATION

▶ History

Nongonococcal Septic Arthritis

Patients typically develop symptoms over the span of hours to days. Symptoms present in more than half of patients with septic arthritis include joint pain, joint swelling, and fever. Sweats and rigors are less common findings. Patients will typically splint the joint and resist any active or passive range of motion. If patients have a history of similar episodes, the likelihood of septic arthritis decreases and the likelihood of other forms of arthritis increase. Although typically monoarticular and affecting the knee, polyarticular involvement occurs in 10% of cases. Risk factors for septic arthritis include immunosuppression (eg, diabetes), injection drug use, elderly, prosthetic joint, and previous joint injury (eg, rheumatoid arthritis).

Gonococcal Septic Arthritis

Gonococcal septic arthritis typically has a slightly different presentation. A prodromal phase with migratory arthritis and tenosynovitis is the major feature before one or more joints become involved. Patients may describe features of gonococcal disease such as vaginal discharge, pelvic pain, penile discharge, or pustules on the hands.

Physical Examination

Although patients can appear toxic, most patients will not have vital sign abnormalities, including fever. The goal of the examination is to attempt to distinguish a joint infection from inflammation or infection of the surrounding structures (bursa, tendons, skin). A septic joint typically has diffuse swelling, redness, and warmth. Pain severely limits both active and passive range of motion. This is in contradistinction to inflammation or infection of surrounding structures, in which pain is more severe with active range of motion.

Gonococcal arthritis may have more subtle signs. It commonly affects the wrist, knee, and/or ankle and is associated with tenosynovitis, rash, and migratory arthritis. Immunocompromised patients and those with prosthetic joints also have more subtle exam findings. In these patients, less of an immune response is generated with invasion of the joint. Therefore, the classic teaching of a red, hot, swollen, painful joint does not always predict septic arthritis.

DIAGNOSTIC STUDIES

Laboratory

There is no one laboratory test that can rule in or out a septic joint. Frequently ordered tests in the evaluation of patients with painful joints include a complete blood count, erythrocyte sedimentation rate, and C-reactive protein. However, these tests lack sensitivity and specificity and should not be used in determining the need for arthrocentesis.

Synovial Fluid Analysis

The synovial white blood cell (WBC) count has been shown to have a wide variety of sensitivity and specificity. Although one specific number cannot be used as a cutoff, patients with counts >50,000/µL should be considered septic until proven otherwise. The likelihood of a septic joint can be reduced with counts <25,000/µL (Table 94-1). Nonetheless, 10% of patients with septic arthritis have synovial fluid leukocyte counts <10,000/µL. A lower synovial WBC count is more common in immunocompromised patients and those with prosthetic joints. In prosthetic joints, a synovial WBC count >1,100/µL is concerning for an infectious etiology. Although the number of WBCs can be helpful, the type of WBCs is less helpful. Some reference a synovial polymorphonuclear cells count >90% as a rule-out criteria; however, its sensitivity has ranged from 60% to 70% in several studies.

Synovial lactate and lactate dehydrogenase (LDH) have been shown to be predictive of septic arthritis if their levels are greater than >5.6 mmol/L and >250 U/L, respectively. Gram stain and culture should always be performed; however, negative results can occur in septic arthritis, especially in the setting of gonococcal disease. Gram stain is positive in approximately 60–80% of cases on nongonococcal septic arthritis. Synovial crystals suggest a crystal-induced arthritis; however, a septic joint can be present in a patient with gout or pseudogout.

Table 94-1. Synovial fluid findings based on condition.

	Normal	Inflammatory	Septic
Synovial WBC	<25,000		>1100/µL if prosthetic >25,000/µL; LR 3.2 >50,000/µL; LR 4.7 >100,000/µL; LR 13.2
Synovial lactate	<5.6 mmol/L	<5.6 mmol/L	>5.6 mmol/L
Synovial LDH	<250 U/L	<250 U/L	>250 U/L
Culture	Negative	Negative	>50% Positive

LDH, lactate dehydrogenase; LR, likelihood ratio.

Adapted from Genes N, Chisolm-Straker M. Monoarticular arthritis update: current evidence for diagnosis and treatment in the emergency department. *Emerg Med Pract.* 2012 May;14(5):1–19.

Imaging

Radiographs have a limited role in the diagnosis of septic arthritis and are typically performed to exclude other disease processes.

PROCEDURES

Arthrocentesis

Once the area is cleansed with Betadine or chlorhexidine and anesthetized via local infiltration, an 18-gauge needle (for large joints) or 20- to 25-gauge needle (for smaller joints) is used to puncture and then aspirate the joint space. General principles to performing successful arthrocentesis include always inserting the needle over the extensor surface, applying approximately 20 degrees of joint flexion, and using slight distraction of the joint. Prosthetic joints benefit from orthopedic consultation before arthrocentesis. Hip arthrocentesis is associated with a high rate of complication and ultrasound or fluoroscopic guidance is useful. Overlying cellulitis and coagulopathy are relative contraindications to performing arthrocentesis.

MEDICAL DECISION MAKING

Table 94-2 includes a differential for the presentation of patients with joint pain. If a clinician suspects a septic joint, then an arthrocentesis should be performed with labs sent for synovial WBCs, LDH, lactate, crystals, Gram stain, and culture. Based on the results of these findings, appropriate disposition can be determined (Figure 94-1).

Table 94-2. Differential diagnosis for acute joint pain and swelling.

Number of Joints	Differential Diagnosis
Monarticular	Septic arthritis
	Crystal induced (gout, pseudogout)
	Osteoarthritis
	Lyme disease
	Avascular necrosis
	Tumor
Polyarticular	Lyme disease
	Reactive arthritis
	Gonococcal septic arthritis
	Rheumatic fever
	Rheumatoid arthritis
	Systemic lupus erythematosus
	Osteoarthritis
	Ankylosing spondylitis

Adapted from Burton JH. Chap. 281. Acute Disorders of the Joints and Bursae. In: Tintinalli JE, Stapczynski JS, Ma OJ, Cline DM, Cydulka RK, Meckler GD. *Tintinalli's Emergency Medicine: A Comprehensive Study Guide.* 7th ed. New York: McGraw-Hill, 2011.

TREATMENT

Emergency physicians must combine the clinical presentation with the synovial fluid results to determine whether the patient should be treated for a septic arthritis. Treatment includes administering intravenous antibiotics and providing adequate analgesia. There are no randomized controlled trials for antibiotic selection; therefore, choice of antibiotic is based on the suspected pathogen. Vancomycin should be given if *Staphylococcus* is suspected, especially with the rising prevalence of methicillin-resistant *S. aureus*. Additional treatment with ceftriaxone is suggested, especially in the setting of presumed gonococcal arthritis. Consultation with an orthopedic surgeon should also be obtained for consideration of open irrigation in the operating room.

DISPOSITION

▶ Admission

Patients who are presumed to have a septic joint based on presentation and laboratory evaluation should be admitted to the hospital for intravenous antibiotics and possible open irrigation. For patients with an undetermined cause and continued pain, consider possible admission or orthopedic consultation to monitor the cultures and symptoms.

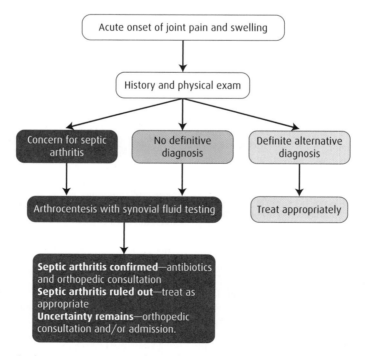

▲ **Figure 94-1.** Septic arthritis diagnostic algorithm.

▶ Discharge

Patients who are felt not to be suffering from septic arthritis can be treated with pain control and follow-up with an orthopedist, rheumatologist, or their primary care provider based on the suspected etiology of the joint pain.

▼ SUGGESTED READING

Burton JH. Acute disorders of the joints and bursae. In: Tintinalli JE, Stapczynski JS, Ma OJ, Cline DM, Cydulka RK, Meckler GD. *Tintinalli's Emergency Medicine: A Comprehensive Study Guide.* 7th ed. New York, NY: McGraw-Hill, 2011, pp. 1926–1933.

Carpenter CR, Schuur JD, Everett WW, Pines JM. Evidence based diagnostics: Adult septic arthritis. *Acad Emerg Med.* 2011;18:782–796.

Coakley G, et al. BSR & BHPR, BOA, RCPG and BSAC guidelines for the management of the hot swollen joint in adults. *Rheumatology.* 2006;45:1039–1041.

Genes N, Chisolm-Straker M. Monoarticular arthritis update: current evidence for diagnosis and treatment in the emergency department. *Emerg Med Pract.* 2012;14:1–19.

Splinting

Scott C. Sherman, MD

Key Points

- Splinting a fracture is useful to permit healing, relieve pain, and stabilize bony fragments.

- In acute injuries, splints are preferable to circumferential casts to limit the potential for iatrogenic compartment syndrome.

- The position of immobilization is important to facilitate proper healing and limit secondary joint stiffness.

- Always maintain a low threshold for splint application in situations with strong clinical concern but normal radiographs, as some fractures may be occult on initial imaging.

INDICATIONS

Fracture immobilization is extremely important to ensure proper healing, relieve pain, and stabilize bony fragments. Most acute injuries in the emergency department (ED) are immobilized with the use of splints (instead of casts) to prevent the consequent swelling from inducing a significant increase in tissue pressures. Of note, not all fractures require splinting, and in some situations, prolonged immobilization can lead to contracture formation and the long-term loss of function. In most cases, the extremity is placed in the position of function before immobilization (Table 95-1). The joints immediately distal

and proximal to the fracture should be included in the splint to ensure proper stabilization of the injury.

Splints are indicated for the majority of extremity fractures and certain soft tissue injuries such as reduced joint dislocations (Table 95-2). Splint placement is also warranted when

Table 95-1. Proper joint position for immobilization after most injuries.

Hand	DIP and PIP 5–10° flexion MCP 60–90° flexion
Wrist	20–30° extension
Elbow	90° flexion
Shoulder	Adducted and internally rotated
Knee	20–30° flexion
Ankle	Neutral position (90°)

DIP, distal interphalangeal; MCP, metacarpophalangeal; PIP, proximal interphalangeal.

Table 95-2. Recommended method of immobilization for common fractures seen in the ED.

Injury	Method of Immobilization
Phalanges	Finger or thumb splint
Metacarpals	Gutter or dorsal "clam digger" splint
Scaphoid (confirmed or suspected)	Thumb spica splint
Distal radius fracture	Sugar-tong splint
Elbow fractures	Long arm posterior splint
Humeral shaft fracture	Coaptation splint
Proximal humerus fractures	Sling
Clavicle fracture	Sling
Patella and tibial plateau fractures	Long leg splint or knee immobilizer
Tibia shaft fracture	Long leg splint
Ankle and foot fractures	Short leg splint

there is clinical evidence for a fracture despite equivocal or negative plain radiographs. In some cases, fractures that are not visible on the initial radiographs may become visible on repeat imaging performed several days to weeks later.

▶ Splints

Posterior Leg Splint

This splint extends along the posterior aspect of the leg from the toes to just below the knee (short leg) or to the middle of the thigh (long leg) (Figure 95-1). Fractures at the knee (ie, tibial plateau) require the placement of a long leg splint, whereas fractures of the ankle require only a short leg splint. Apply an additional U-shaped splint ("stirrup") for particularly unstable ankle fractures (eg, bimalleolar fracture). It should extend from the area just below the knee on the medial aspect of the leg, around the heel, to the same position on the lateral aspect of the leg.

Coaptation Splint

The coaptation splint is the preferred splint for fractures of the humeral shaft. This splint extends from above the

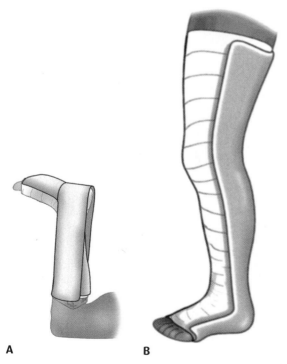

A   **B**

▲ **Figure 95-1.** Lower extremity splints. **A.** Short leg posterior splint with U-shaped splint for additional support. **B.** Long leg splint. Reprinted with permission from Simon RR, Sherman SC. Splints, Casts, and Other Techniques. In: Simon RR, Sherman SC, eds. *Emergency Orthopedics.* 6th ed. New York: McGraw-Hill, 2011.

shoulder joint down the lateral aspect of the arm, around the elbow, and then up the medial aspect of the arm to the axilla (Figure 95-2A). The weight of the splint applies gentle continuous traction to the fractured humerus to aid proper reduction and healing.

Sugar-Tong Splint

This splint is so named because it resembles the shape of the tongs used to grab a cube of sugar for coffee or tea. With the elbow positioned at 90 degrees of flexion, this splint extends from the dorsal aspect of the hand at the metacarpophalangeal (MCP) joints, around the elbow, to the flexor crease of the palm (Figure 95-2B). The sugartong splint is useful for both distal radius fractures and fractures of the radial and ulnar shafts.

Long Arm Posterior Splint

The long arm posterior splint extends along the ulnar aspect of the forearm from the palmar crease to the middle portion of the upper arm and functions to immobilize the wrist and elbow (Figure 95-2C). It is used for both forearm fractures and injuries to the elbow.

Gutter Splint (Radial And Ulnar)

These splints are positioned on either the radial or ulnar portion of the hand and forearm and extend two thirds of the way up the forearm (Figure 95-2D). Both splints include the fingers (fourth and fifth digits for an ulnar gutter, second and third digits for a radial gutter). For the radial gutter splint, a hole is cut out for the thumb. These splints are useful for fractures of the metacarpals and phalanges of digits 2 through 5.

Dorsal "Clam Digger" Splint

This splint is applied to the dorsal aspect of the hand and forearm and extends the length of the digits (Figure 95-2E). The hand is cupped in such a way that when the splint is applied, patients appear like they could go "digging for clams on the beach." The hand is kept in the "wine glass position," with care to ensure that the MCP joints are immobilized between 60 and 90 degrees of flexion. This splint is useful in cases of multiple hand bone fractures that a gutter splint cannot properly immobilize.

Thumb And Thumb Spica Splints

A thumb splint extends from the distal aspect of the first digit to two thirds of the way up the forearm and is used to immobilize the thumb. This splint is useful for thumb fractures and injuries to the ulnar collateral ligament of the first MCP (gamekeeper's thumb). A thumb spica splint is similar but includes the addition of a volar splint that extends from the palmar crease to two thirds of the way up the forearm. Further extending this volar splint beyond the elbow to the mid-upper arm ensures full immobilization of the thumb, wrist, and elbow. This splint is used to immobilize fractures of the scaphoid as it prevents both pronation and supination of the forearm (Figure 95-2F).

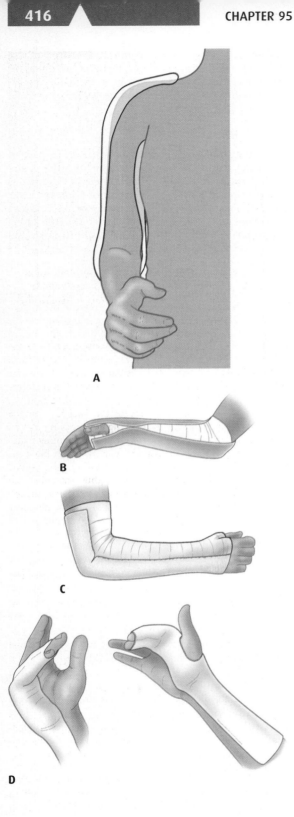

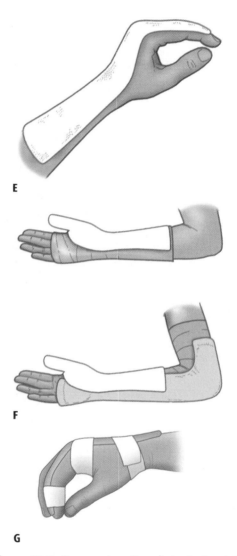

▲ **Figure 95-2.** Upper extremity splints. **A.** Coaptation splint. **B.** Sugar-tong splint. **C.** Long arm posterior splint. **D.** Gutter splints. **E.** Dorsal "Clam digger" splint. **F.** Thumb splint and thumb spica splint. **G.** Finger splint. Reprinted with permission from Simon RR, Sherman SC. Splints, Casts, and Other Techniques. In: Simon RR, Sherman SC, eds. *Emergency Orthopedics.* 6th ed. New York: McGraw-Hill, 2011.

Finger Splints

These splints can be rapidly placed using commercially available malleable padded materials (Figure 95-2G). Finger splints are used to protect the digits after phalangeal fractures. Alternatively, a dynamic finger splint can be used when a minor ligamentous sprain occurs at a proximal interphalangeal joint. Apply this functional splint by taping the proximal and middle phalanx of the injured digit to an uninjured neighboring finger (buddy taping).

CONTRAINDICATIONS

There are no absolute contraindications to splinting. Ensure proper wound care for all lacerations or open wounds before splint application. When re-evaluating such a patient, remove the splint to inspect for subsequent wound infection.

EQUIPMENT

Supplies include stockinette, cotton padding, fiberglass or plaster splint material, scissors, warm water, and elastic bandages.

PROCEDURE

Place a stockinette on the involved extremity extending beyond the proximal and distal limits of where the splint will be applied (optional). Use the patient's noninjured extremity to measure the correct length of necessary material. Cut either prefabricated fiberglass or approximately 10–15 sheets of plaster to the proper length.

▶ Fiberglass

Most EDs use fiberglass splinting material as its application is both easy and quick. It comes prefabricated with a layer of padding wrapped around the fiberglass. It should be placed on the injured extremity after lightly wetting the fiberglass component with warm water. Important tips when using fiberglass splint material include:

1. When working with fiberglass rolls, clamp the unused end of the protective covering immediately after cutting the splint material. This prevents prolonged air exposure and subsequent hardening of the entire roll.
2. Some prefabricated fiberglass splint material has a padded side and a nonpadded side. Remember to place the padded side against the skin.
3. Stretch the padding longitudinally to ensure that it covers the cut ends of the fiberglass, as exposed edges that remain in direct contact with the skin after hardening can induce skin injury (Figure 95-3).

▶ Plaster

When applying a plaster splint, start by circumferentially wrapping several layers of cotton padding around the affected extremity. Take special care to apply extra layers of padding over bony protuberances (eg, the malleoli) where excessive pressure might induce underlying skin necrosis. Finally, remember to place extra padding between all involved digits.

Briefly soak the premeasured plaster in a bath of warm water. Remove excess water by wringing the plaster between the hands and smooth out the sheets by holding them up with one hand while the thumb and index finger of the other

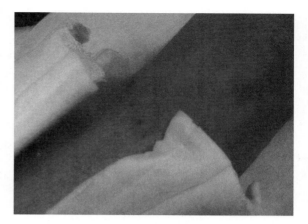

▲ **Figure 95-3.** Skin injury due to a fiberglass splint that was applied improperly. The padding should be stretched longitudinally to avoid contact between the hard, dried plaster and the skin.

hand gently squeeze out any folds and/or air pockets. As the calcium sulfate in the plaster reacts with the water it will produce heat as it cures, which the patient will notice as the splint is applied. Place the splint on the appropriate extremity and add an additional layer of cotton padding over the plaster (optional). This will prevent the final layer of the splint (elastic bandage) from adhering to the drying plaster.

Circumferentially wrap the extremity and splinting material (whether fiberglass or plaster) with an elastic bandage, taking care to ensure that the splint remains in the desired position when finished. Avoid over-tightly wrapping the extremity to prevent the development of a secondary compartment syndrome. Instruct the patient to not move the extremity until the splint has adequately hardened (5–10 minutes).

COMPLICATIONS

Circumferential bandages, especially when applied too tightly, may produce an iatrogenic compartment syndrome. Instruct the patient to return to the ED with the development of any worsening pain or new numbness or tingling of the extremity. Additionally, plaster splints will produce a significant amount of heat as they dry, which can result in thermal injuries when insufficient cotton padding is used.

▼ SUGGESTED READING

Menkes JS. Initial evaluation and management of orthopedic injuries. In: Tintinalli JE, Stapczynski JS, Ma OJ, Cline DM, Cydulka RK, Meckler GD. *Tintinalli's Emergency Medicine: A Comprehensive Study Guide.* 7th ed. New York, NY: McGraw-Hill, 2011, pp. 1783–1796.
Simon RR, Sherman SC. General principles and appendix. In: Simon RR, Sherman SC. *Emergency Orthopedics.* 6th ed. New York, NY: McGraw-Hill, 2011, pp. 1–31 and 563–579.

Life-Threatening Dermatoses

Henry Z. Pitzele, MD

Chad S. Kessler, MD

Key Points

- Rapid identification of life-threatening rashes and immediate treatment can be life-saving.

- If there is any uncertainty of etiology in a given case, treat presumptively for the most serious etiology, especially meningococcemia.

INTRODUCTION

Cutaneous lesions can be the first clinical sign of a serious systemic illness. It is important to recognize and treat these illnesses early. Life-threatening dermatoses can be grouped into 3 distinct categories: erythrodermas (diffuse red rashes), vesiculobullous lesions, and hemorrhagic lesions.

▶ Erythrodermas

Staphylococcal scalded skin syndrome (SSSS) is an exotoxin-producing Staphylococcal infection that causes shedding of the superficial layer of the epidermis. SSSS is most common in children and neonates; 98% of patients are <6 years of age.

Toxic shock syndrome (TSS) causes a diffuse red macular rash associated with fever, hypotension, and malfunction of at least 3 organ systems. It was originally diagnosed in menstruating women using vaginal tampons, but can also be seen in patients with surgical wounds and nasal packings. Incidence is about 10–20 cases per 100,000 persons. TSS is most often caused by a variant of *Staphylococcus aureus*, which produces the exotoxin TSST-1, which mediates the clinical effects. *Streptococcus pyogenes* may more rarely cause a similar syndrome.

Kawasaki disease is thought to be an immunologic disorder triggered by infection or toxin, leading to a generalized vasculitis. It causes nearly 3,000 hospital admissions annually and usually appears in children <9 years of age, with a peak incidence in children 18–24 months

of age. Epidemics occur primarily in the late winter and early spring. Approximately 20% of patients develop cardiovascular complications, and the most common cause of death is myocardial infarction secondary to coronary artery aneurysm, which can develop 2–8 weeks after fever.

▶ Vesiculobullous Lesions

Erythema multiforme (EM), as the name implies, presents with many simultaneous types of skin lesions, including macules, papules, and bullae. EM accounts for as many as 1% of dermatologic outpatient visits and is more common in spring and fall. The etiology is a hypersensitivity reaction precipitated by medications, infections, sarcoidosis, collagen vascular diseases, or malignancies. About 50% of cases are idiopathic.

Stevens-Johnson syndrome (SJS) is a more severe form of EM that involves ≥2 mucosal surfaces such as eyes, lips, mouth, urogenital area, or anus. SJS can progress to toxic epidermal necrolysis (TEN), with large bullae and sloughing of the epidermis in sheets. Frequency is up to 6 cases per 1 million persons annually. The etiology is similar to EM, but medications are more commonly associated with SJS.

TEN is the most severe end of the EM spectrum, with TEN affecting >30% of the body surface area. There is approximately 1 case per 1 million persons annually, with adults most commonly affected. TEN desquamates the entire thickness of the epidermis; therefore, mortality rates are 30–40% from hypovolemia and infection. TEN is thought to be provoked by drugs such as phenytoin, sulfas, penicillins, and nonsteroidal anti-inflammatory drugs. Onset is usually within the first 8 weeks of therapy.

Pemphigus vulgaris (PV) is characterized by flaccid bullae that begin in the mouth and spread to involve the skin. Frequency is approximately 3 cases per 100,000 persons. Peak age of onset is 50–60 years. The etiology is an autoimmune blistering reaction characterized by autoantibodies directed against keratinocyte cell surfaces; some cases are drug-induced. Bullous pemphigoid (BP) is a similar autoimmune blistering disease, but it usually only affects the elderly. Unlike PV, the bullae of BP are tense rather than flaccid, and oral involvement is uncommon.

▶ Hemorrhagic Lesions

Patients with disseminated gonococcal infection (DGI) are usually young, sexually active females with fever, skin lesions, arthritis, arthralgias, or migratory tenosynovitis. DGI occurs after approximately 1% of gonococcal genital infections. Certain subtypes of *Neisseria gonorrhoeae* are more likely to lead to disseminated infection.

Another Neisseria species, *Neisseria meningitidis*, can cause meningococcemia. Cutaneous manifestations are part of a hemorrhagic cascade resulting from systemic sepsis. The frequency is approximately 2 cases per 100,000 persons annually, although sporadic outbreaks with higher prevalence occur frequently. The mortality rate varies between 10% and 50%, depending on the severity of the systemic infection.

CLINICAL PRESENTATION

▶ Erythrodermas

SSSS generally begins on the face (perioral area) as red patches that are warm and tender. The erythema spreads and becomes flaccid clear bullae, which then desquamate in large sheets. The mucous membranes usually are not involved. Nikolsky sign is positive and can be elicited when gentle stroking of the skin produces peeling (Figure 96-1). Exfoliation begins on day 2 of the illness, and healing occurs within 10–14 days.

The TSS patient will present with fever, hypotension, and multisystem organ dysfunction. In addition to diffuse erythroderma, patients will have a strawberry-appearing tongue, red conjunctiva, and edema of the face, hands, and feet. The rash fades within 72 hours and is followed by acral desquamation within 1–2 weeks.

The rash of Kawasaki disease is erythematous and similar in morphology to Scarlet Fever. The clinical diagnosis of Kawasaki disease includes fever greater than 5 days' duration, plus 4 of 5 of the following criteria: conjunctivitis, oral mucous membrane involvement (strawberry tongue, cracked lips), edema/erythema of extremities, diffuse maculopapular rash, and cervical lymphadenopathy (usually >1.5 cm and unilateral). Patients often present with arthralgia and irritability and can have peripheral

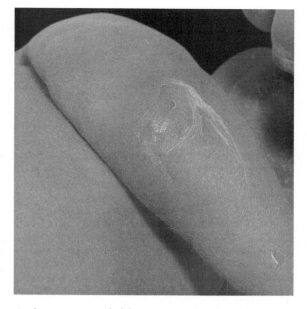

▲ **Figure 96-1.** Nikolsky sign. Reprinted with permission from Suurmond D. Section 24. Bacterial Infections Involving the Skin. In: Suurmond D, ed. *Fitzpatrick's Color Atlas & Synopsis of Clinical Dermatology.* 6th ed. New York: McGraw-Hill, 2009.

leukocytosis and elevated levels of acute-phase reactants and transaminases.

▶ Vesiculobullous Lesions

The typical lesion of EM is the "target lesion," described as erythematous plaques with dusky centers and bright red borders resembling the "bull's eye" of a target (Figure 96-2). The lesions are symmetric and are usually found on the extremities, palms, and soles and may also involve the oral mucosa. A burning sensation is present, and pruritus is notably absent.

Stevens-Johnson syndrome presents with lesions similar to those of EM, but has additional findings of blistering of <10% of the skin and mucosal involvement. Fever, malaise, myalgias, and arthralgias are common. Lesions begin on the dorsal surfaces of the hands and feet and spread centrally.

Toxic epidermal necrolysis begins with a prodrome of constitutional symptoms including fever, malaise, and myalgias. After 1–2 weeks, the skin becomes painful with hot red blisters and large areas of sloughing (>30% of skin), progressing to diffuse exfoliation and acute skin failure (Figure 96-3).

Pemphigus vulgaris may present with multiple scattered vesicles and bullae (scalp, face, chest, mucous membranes). However, since the bulla rupture easily, patients may present only with painful erosions. Almost all patients have mucosal involvement.

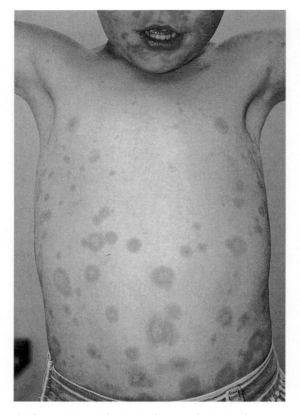

▲ **Figure 96-2.** The typical target lesions of erythema multiforme. Reprinted with permission from Hardin J. Chapter 13. Cutaneous Conditions. In: Knoop KJ, Stack LB, Storrow AB, Thurman RJ, eds. *The Atlas of Emergency Medicine*. 3rd ed. New York: McGraw-Hill, 2010. Photo contributor: Michael Redman, PA-C.

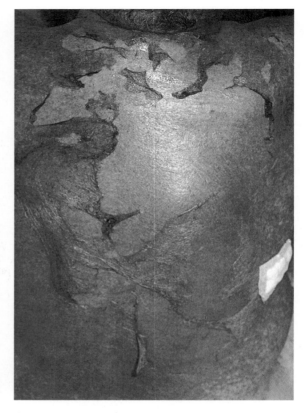

▲ **Figure 96-3.** Large surface skin sloughing in toxic epidermal necrolysis. Reprinted with permission from Suurmond D. Section 8. Severe and Life-Threatening Skin Eruptions in the Acutely Ill Patient. In: Suurmond D, ed. *Fitzpatrick's Color Atlas & Synopsis of Clinical Dermatology*. 6th ed. New York: McGraw-Hill, 2009.

▶ **Hemorrhagic Lesions**

DGI skin lesions are described as hemorrhagic gray necrotic pustules on an erythematous base, numbering between 10 and 30, and appearing on the extremities and resolving rapidly. The classic rash of meningococcemia can be petechial or macular, with pale gray vesicular centers, and may progress to a hemorrhagic rash (Figure 96-4). Fever, headache, and vomiting are present, although meningitis may or may not be present. It is rapidly progressive, with a 100% mortality rate without treatment.

DIAGNOSTIC STUDIES

Unfortunately, there are no diagnostic studies that can aid the emergency department (ED) diagnosis of these diseases. Patients with significant to severe systemic illness will receive routine blood tests and sometimes cultures,

immunoassays, and other specific testing. However, the results of none of these tests will be available or useful to guide the initial diagnosis in the ED.

MEDICAL DECISION MAKING

The initial diagnosis should be made clinically and will be centered on the evaluation for specific life-threatening conditions. It is easiest to first attempt to classify the patient's presenting skin lesion—erythroderma, vesiculobullous, or hemorrhagic lesion—and, once subclassified, to attempt to use a few clinical features to rule in or rule out specific diagnoses (Figure 96-5). However, because it is sometimes difficult to make a certain diagnosis in the initial presentation, the key to early treatment is to have a very high index of suspicion for the most immediately lethal of the syndromes, especially meningococcemia.

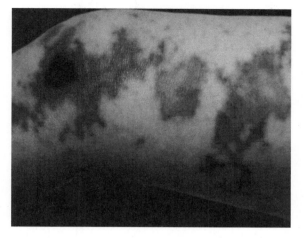

Figure 96-4. The petechial rash of meningococcemia. Reprinted with permission from Suurmond D. Section 24. Bacterial Infections Involving the Skin. In: Suurmond D, ed. *Fitzpatrick's Color Atlas & Synopsis of Clinical Dermatology*. 6th ed. New York: McGraw-Hill, 2009.

TREATMENT AND DISPOSITION

▶ Erythrodermas

Patients with SSSS should be treated with intravenous (IV) antistaphylococcal antibiotics (nafcillin or vancomycin) and IV fluids. They should be admitted to the hospital. Patients with TSS should first have the source (tampon, nasal packing) identified and removed. IV immunoglobulin G (IVIG) has been shown to be effective in neutralizing the TSS toxin and aids in recovery. These patients should also receive IV antibiotics (eg, nafcillin/vancomycin) and be admitted to an intensive care unit (ICU). When Kawasaki disease is diagnosed, high-dose aspirin therapy and IVIG should be administered. Patients should be admitted to the hospital for further monitoring and echocardiography.

▶ Vesiculobullous Lesions

Erythema multiforme is generally a benign, self-limited rash that resolves within 2–4 weeks. It requires no specific treatment except cool compresses and an attempt to identify and remove the precipitating cause.

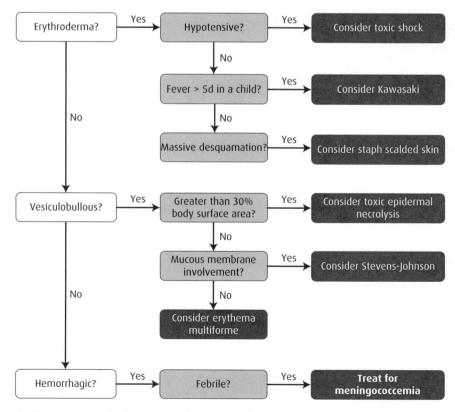

Figure 96-5. Life-threatening dermatoses diagnostic algorithm.

These patients do not require hospital admission. Patients with Stevens-Johnson syndrome will require IV fluids and debridement of large bullae. IV antibiotics should be administered for any coexisting infection. Patients should be admitted to a burn unit or ICU setting for wound care. TEN patients require care similar to that for SJS patients; however, they will require burn unit care because of the large amount of desquamation. Patients with pemphigus vulgaris should be treated with IV corticosteroids and fluid resuscitation. They should be admitted to the hospital.

▶ Hemorrhagic Lesions

Patients with DGI require IV ceftriaxone. Admission is required for systemically ill patients or those with involvement of weight-bearing joints. Patients with meningococcemia can deteriorate quickly over several hours, leading to hypotension, shock, renal failure, acute respiratory distress syndrome, and disseminated intravascular coagulation. Treatment consists of broad-spectrum IV antibiotics (ceftriaxone and vancomycin) and ICU admission.

▼ SUGGESTED READING

Rosenstein NE, Perkins BA, Stephens DS, Popovic T, Hughes J. Medical progress: Meningococcal disease. *N Engl J Med.* 2001;344:1378–1388.

Thomas J, Perron A, Brady W. Serious generalized skin disorders. In: Tintinalli JE, Stapczynski JS, Ma OJ, Cline DM, Cydulka RK, Meckler GD. *Tintinalli's Emergency Medicine: A Comprehensive Study Guide.* 7th ed. New York, NY: McGraw-Hill, 2011, pp. 1614–1624.

Weber DJ, Cohen MS, Morrell DS, Rutala WA. The acutely ill patient with fever and rash. In: Mandell GL, Bennett JE, Dolin R, eds. *Mandell, Douglas, and Bennett's Principles and Practice of Infectious Disease.* Philadelphia, PA: Elsevier Churchill Livingstone, 2009, pp. 791–807.

Allergic Reactions

Lisa R. Palivos, MD

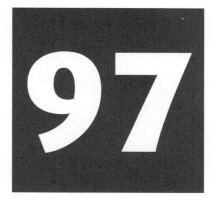

Key Points

- Epinephrine is the first-line medication for the treatment of anaphylaxis. Second-line treatment consists of antihistamines and corticosteroids.

- Urticaria may be the first sign of what might progress to angioedema or anaphylaxis.

- For patients with respiratory symptoms or throat swelling, perform a rapid assessment of the airway and intubate early.

- Attempt to determine and then discontinue the inciting agent.

INTRODUCTION

An allergic reaction is the body's way of responding to foreign substances that come in contact with the skin, nose, eyes, respiratory tract or gastrointestinal tract. Examples of allergens are dust, pollen, plants, medications, foods, latex, and insect bites. Anything can be an allergen. Allergic reactions can range from mild local urticarial eruptions to severe and life-threatening airway obstruction, respiratory failure, and circulatory collapse. Urticaria, or "hives," is an immunoglobulin E (IgE)-mediated hypersensitivity reaction to an allergen resulting in red, raised wheals that itch and sting. Circulating antibodies bind the allergen and IgE receptors on mast cells. In response, mast cells release inflammatory substances (histamine, bradykinin), which results in increased vascular permeability. Urticaria is one of the most common skin lesions seen in the emergency department (ED) in both young and older patients. About 20% of the population experiences at least 1 attack of urticaria in their lifetime.

Angioedema is nonpitting edema of the deeper layers of the skin owing to a loss of vascular integrity caused by inflammatory mediators. It is not pruritic but can cause burning, numbness, or pain, generally in the face or neck. Approximately 94% of the cases of angioedema presenting to the ED are drug-induced. Most drug-induced angioedema occurs in patients taking angiotensin-converting enzyme

(ACE) inhibitors. About 0.1–0.2% of the patients treated with ACE inhibitors will develop angioedema. There are 2 main types of angioedema based on the underlying mechanism. Mast cell angioedema is mediated by IgE, similar to urticaria. Bradykinin, an inflammatory mediator, is causal in both hereditary and ACE inhibitor–induced angioedema, although the mechanism for the bradykinin increase differs.

Anaphylaxis is a severe systemic allergic reaction that can present rapidly with hypotension, bronchospasm, and laryngeal edema. About 500–1,000 persons in the United States die every year as a result of anaphylaxis. Beta-lactam antibiotics and Hymenoptera stings constitute the most common causes of anaphylaxis. Anaphylaxis is IgE-mediated and results from release of histamine, leukotrienes, and prostaglandins from inflammatory cells. The result is a systemic increase in vascular permeability, vasodilation, and smooth muscle contraction.

CLINICAL PRESENTATION

▶ History

Patients with urticaria present with transient, pruritic, well-circumscribed lesions that are erythematous, nonpitting plaques (wheals) surrounded by an erythematous ring (flare) (Figure 97-1). Patients with angioedema present with swelling

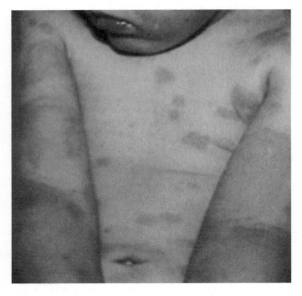

△ **Figure 97-1.** Urticaria. Reprinted with permission from Kane KS, Bissonette J, Baden HP, et al. *Color Atlas & Synopsis of Pediatric Dermatology*. New York: McGraw-Hill, 2002.

of the face, lips, tongue, eyelids, distal extremities, or genitalia. The swelling is nonpitting and may occur with urticaria. ACE inhibitor–induced angioedema has a predilection for the face (Figure 97-2). Patients with anaphylaxis present with a sensation of impending doom or "lump in the throat" followed by shortness of breath, chest pain, hypotension, nausea, vomiting, or diarrhea. More than 90% of patients have urticaria or angioedema. Most patients present with signs and symptoms within seconds of exposure to an allergen; however, symptoms may be delayed up to a few hours after exposure.

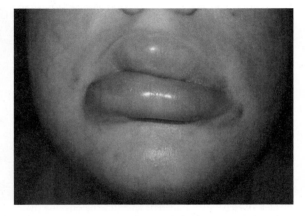

△ **Figure 97-2.** Angioedema of the lips. Reproduced with permission from Sarah M. Granlund.

If the patient is stable, try to identify the inciting factors. Ask about history of allergies, medications, exposures, contacts, underlying illness, diet, and family history of allergic reactions.

▶ Physical Examination

Initial evaluation of the patient should focus on airway, breathing, and circulation (ABCs). Airway obstruction is evidenced by swelling of the lips, tongue, or uvula. The patient may have hoarseness, stridor, wheezing, or respiratory distress. The patient may exhibit erythema, urticaria, pruritis, or angioedema of the face, neck, or extremities. In patients with ACE inhibitor angioedema, the face is involved in 86% of cases.

Once a patient is hemodynamically stable, a more detailed physical exam should be performed. Examine the skin while the patient is undressed and describe the rash. Include the type (macular, papular, vesicular), size, shape, number, and color of the rash. Remove the allergen if it can be identified. For example, remove stinging remnants from insect bites.

DIAGNOSTIC STUDIES

Diagnosis of urticaria, angioedema, and anaphylaxis is based on clinical symptoms, and no specific laboratory or imaging tests are necessary.

MEDICAL DECISION MAKING

History and physical examination should be sufficient to arrive at the diagnosis of acute allergic reactions, especially if there is clear history of an exposure, such as a bee sting. Diagnosis is not always obvious because anaphylaxis symptoms may mimic other presentations such as myocardial infarction, pulmonary embolism, syncope, status asthmaticus, or sepsis. Urticaria may be confused with a viral rash, erythema multiforme, or a vasculitis. Infection (cellulitis), contact dermatitis, and renal or liver disease may mimic angioedema (Figure 97-3).

TREATMENT

Anaphylaxis with airway compromise and hypotension is a true medical emergency and must be rapidly assessed and treated. The most important step in treatment is the rapid administration of epinephrine.

Initial stabilization consists of ABCs, cardiac monitoring, oxygen, and intravenous (IV) fluids. Further treatment depends on the severity and extent of the reaction. When the airway is threatened, early intubation is lifesaving. Epinephrine is indicated in patients with angioedema when the airway is compromised or in patients with bronchoconstriction or hypotension from anaphylaxis. If the patient is normotensive and without signs of cardiovascular collapse, administer 0.3–0.5 mg intramuscularly (IM) (0.3–0.5 mL of 1:1,000 [1 mg/1 mL] epinephrine every 5–10 minutes until

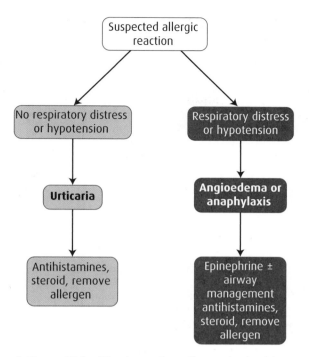

Figure 97-3. Allergic reactions diagnostic algorithm.

a positive response. IM dosing provides better blood epinephrine levels than subcutaneous administration. Injections into the thigh are more effective than injections into the deltoid area. If the patient does not respond or is hypotensive with signs of cardiovascular compromise, give epinephrine 0.1 mg IV slowly over 5 minutes (1 mL of 1:10,000 solution [1 mg/10 mL]). If the patient is refractory to the bolus, then an epinephrine infusion should be started.

Second-line treatments include corticosteroids and antihistamines. H1 blockers (diphenhydramine) should be administered by mouth (PO) or IM for mild reactions and IV for more severe reactions. An H2 blocker in combination with H1 blocker should be administered to patients with severe urticaria, angioedema, or anaphylaxis. Choices include famotidine 20 mg IV, ranitidine 50 mg IV, or cimetidine 300 mg IV. Corticosteroids should be administered for all moderate to severe reactions (prednisone 40–60 mg PO or methylprednisolone 125 mg IV). For treatment of bronchospasm, add an albuterol nebulizer, ipratropium bromide, and magnesium sulfate.

Patients with hereditary and ACE inhibitor–induced angioedema are usually refractory to treatment with epinephrine, antihistamines, and corticosteroids. However, it is difficult to distinguish these from angioedema due to an IgE-mediated reaction, which respond to these therapies. In the presence of an acutely ill patient, treatment of a presumed hypersensitivity reaction is necessary while considering other etiologies and treatments. None of the additional therapies work immediately, thus prophylactic intubation or cricothyrotomy should be performed when edema is progressive and there is evidence of airway compromise.

Discontinuation of ACE inhibitors leads to resolution within 24–48 hours. Fresh-frozen plasma or purified C1 inhibitor concentrate may be administered for suspected bradykinin mediated causes; however, improvement does not occur for 2–4 hours. Both agents replace the enzyme, kininase II, which breaks down excess bradykinin.

DISPOSITION

▶ Admission

Patients with systemic symptoms or potential airway compromise that does not resolve must be hospitalized in an intensive care setting.

▶ Discharge

Patients with resolution of symptoms may be discharged after several hours of ED observation. Refer the patient to an allergist or immunologist. Prescribe antihistamines and steroids for 3–5 days, and if the reaction was severe, prescribe an epinephrine autoinjector (EpiPen). Patients with known triggers should be advised about strict avoidance of those triggers. Advise patients about personal identification such as an allergy alert tag. Patients taking ACE inhibitors should be instructed to discontinue the medication and also avoid angiotensin receptor blockers.

▼ SUGGESTED READING

Bunney EB. Anaphylaxis. In: Wiebe RA, Ahrens WR, Strange GR, Schafermeyer RW, eds. *Pediatric Emergency Medicine*. 3rd ed. New York, NY: McGraw-Hill, 2009:589–591.

Rowe BH, Gaeta T, Gaeta TJ. Anaphylaxis, acute allergic reactions, and angioedema. In: Tintinalli JE, Stapczynski JS, Ma OJ, Cline DM, Cydulka, RK, Meckler GD. *Tintinalli's Emergency Medicine: A Comprehensive Study Guide*. 7th ed. New York, NY: McGraw-Hill, 2011:177–182.

Simons, FE. Anaphylaxis. *J Allerg Clin Immunol*. 2010; 125(suppl 2): S161–S181.

98

Approach to the Psychiatric Patient

Leslie S. Zun, MD

Key Points

- New-onset psychiatric illness requires a comprehensive emergency department work-up. Consider a medical etiology.
- Prior psychiatric illness with similar presentation does not require an extensive work-up.
- Agitated patients need immediate treatment in the emergency department.
- Patients with suicidal and homicidal plans or inability to care for themselves need psychiatric admission.

INTRODUCTION

Psychiatric illness is a common presentation to emergency departments (EDs). The number of psychiatric patients presenting to EDs has increased both in total number and in percentage of total ED visits, from 4.9% to 6.3% from 1992–2001. The main ED psychiatric diagnoses are substance-use disorders (22%), mood disorders (17%), and anxiety-related disorders (16%).

Patients with psychiatric illness may have various presentations depending on their underlying psychiatric diagnosis as well as their concurrent medical condition. Psychiatric patients may present with depressed affect, psychosis, agitation, suicidal or homicidal ideation, catatonia, delusions, or dementia.

Like other conditions presenting to the ED, the emergency physician must determine whether the patient has a life-threatening condition. The life-threatening conditions include suicidal or homicidal plans and medical condition masquerading as psychiatric illness (Table 98-1). Frequently identified medical causes of abnormal behavior include hypoglycemia, hypoxia, seizures, head trauma, and thyroid abnormalities. Patients should also be assessed for the presence of delirium or dementia, as both have potentially treatable causes. The primary role of the ED physician is to determine whether the psychiatric presentation is due to a medical or psychiatric etiology.

Table 98-1. Medical conditions that masquerade as psychiatric disease.

Alcohol intoxication or withdrawal
Anticholinergic poisoning
Drug intoxication or withdrawal
Electrolyte abnormality
Head injury
Hepatic failure
Hyperthyroidism
Hypoglycemia
Meningitis and encephalitis
Renal failure
Seizure
Stroke
Wernicke encephalopathy

This determination is often referred to as the medical clearance process. The secondary role of the ED physician is to evaluate the patient's coexisting medical conditions because many of these psychiatric patients have a high incidence of medical illnesses that have been neglected.

Some psychiatric patients present to the ED with acute agitation. These patients, like others in the ED, are acutely ill and need to be stabilized before definitive evaluation can be completed. Once the agitation has been reduced, the clinician must determine the cause of the agitation and the need for a psychiatric versus medical admission.

CLINICAL PRESENTATION

▶ History

A detailed history, including prior psychiatric history, is the most important step to determine whether the patient's presentation is due to a medical or psychiatric problem. It is important to determine whether the patient's current presentation is the same or similar to previous psychiatric presentations. Some psychiatric patients can provide a history of their condition, whereas others may require collateral information. History from family, bystanders, paramedics, police officers or medical records can provide valuable information. Medical and psychiatric history, medications, medication compliance, substance use, and recent stressors may provide insight into the patient's presentation.

Multiple factors cause a psychiatric patient to decompensate and present to the ED, including concomitant substance use and withdrawal, noncompliance with psychotropic medications, change in social situation, and environmental stressors. It is valuable to determine these factors to better address the patients' needs.

▶ Physical Examination

The physical examination can provide important clues into the etiology of the patient's presentation. The "red flags" indicating a possible medical etiology include age over 45 years, bowel or bladder incontinence, cognitive deficit, abnormal vital signs, and abnormal or focal examination (Table 98-2).

A psychiatric patient should have a thorough examination in the ED. A head-to-toe examination with focus on a neurologic and mental status examination is essential. The neurologic examination should assess for focal deficits by evaluating cranial nerves, sensation, strength, reflexes, and coordination. Every patient requires a mental status examination that should include

Table 98-2. Red flags of medical illness.

Age >45 years
Bowel or bladder incontinence
Focal neurologic examination
Cognitive deficit
Abnormal vital signs
Abnormal or focal physical examination

appearance, behavior and attitude, disorders of thought, disorder of perception, mood and affect, insight and judgment, sensorium, and intelligence. Patients also need an evaluation of their cognitive functioning because many times a deficit cannot be detected in a routine ED examination. Specific tests of cognitive function include the Mini-Mental State Examination, Clock Drawing Test, and the Cognitive Capacity Screening Examination. Patients with a psychiatric etiology for their symptoms usually have normal vital signs, a nonfocal examination, and a normal test of cognitive function, whereas patients with medical etiologies may have abnormal vital signs, a focal examination, or an abnormal cognitive deficit. Patients with abnormal level of arousal and cognition may have delirium, whereas patients with normal arousal, but impaired cognition may have dementia.

DIAGNOSTIC STUDIES

▶ Laboratory

Clinical judgment should determine the need for lab testing of patients presenting with psychiatric complaints. Rather than using clinical judgment, some institutions have a set of laboratory tests that are routinely performed on all patients with behavioral complaints. Patients with a first-time presentation of psychiatric illness or a change in the presentation of their psychiatric symptoms should have general laboratory studies (complete blood count [CBC], chemistry panel, urinalysis) performed. A CBC may indicate an infectious process, abnormal chemistries may reveal hypoglycemia or hypo/hypernatremia, and urinalysis may provide evidence of a urinary tract infection. Routine drug screens and alcohol levels are not useful and should be reserved for patients with altered mental status of unknown etiology. Patients with known psychiatric illness and a consistent psychiatric presentation usually do not require testing.

▶ Imaging

Imaging, like other testing, should be performed based on clinical judgment. A noncontrast head computed tomography scan is appropriate for patients with new symptoms. A chest radiograph is indicated when a patient has evidence of pneumonia or congestive heart failure. Other imaging should be determined by the patient's clinical condition.

PROCEDURES

Psychiatric patients are frequently agitated on presentation to the ED and may pose a threat to themselves or the staff. A stepwise progression of procedures is indicated to treat agitation with the goal of avoiding the use of restraints. The first step in treating the agitated patient is the process of de-escalation. The essentials of de-escalation include attempting to calm the patient, meeting their reasonable needs, and lessening environmental stimulation. The next step to reduce a patient's level of agitation is to medicate them with a benzodiazepine or anti-psychotic medication. These medications include haloperidol (5 mg administered intramuscularly [IM]), atypical antipsychotics (ziprasidone 10 mg IM), and lorazepam (1–2 mg IM), alone or in combination. The last step is restraining the patient in a supine position with a restraint on each limb. Restrained patients require frequent or continuous observation.

MEDICAL DECISION MAKING

History and physical examination, including a neurologic and mental status examination, may be sufficient to determine whether the patient has an acute psychiatric illness. However, any abnormality noted from the history and physical exam warrants further evaluation and treatment looking for a medical etiology. Once medical issues have been addressed, patients with ED presentation of psychosis, depression, anxiety, suicidal, or homicidal ideation need an appropriate psychiatric evaluation and disposition.

Patients with abnormal behavior from new-onset delirium, dementia, or other medical illness require further medical evaluation and admission (Figure 98-1).

TREATMENT

Treatment of the psychiatric patient in the ED varies. The patient may need a refill of their psychotropic medication, initiation of a new psychotropic medication, or emergent treatment for acute agitation. Most emergency physicians do not start patients on new psychotropic medications without psychiatric consultation or primary care communication. All active medical problems should also be addressed and treated.

DISPOSITION

Admission

There are 3 universally accepted criteria to admit patients with psychiatric illness: homicidal plan, suicidal plan, and the inability to care for oneself. Clinical judgment is often necessary to determine the need for admission in patients with chronic suicidal or homicidal ideation, and patients with other psychiatric illnesses and the potential inability to care for oneself.

Discharge

Patients discharged from the ED with psychiatric illness need close follow-up by a professional. In many communities there are limited psychiatric resources and professionals to care for these patients. In communities

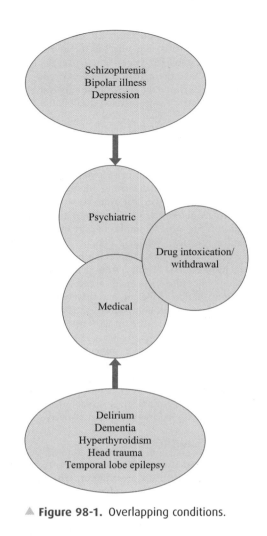

Figure 98-1. Overlapping conditions.

with limited psychiatric resources, these patients may be referred to a primary care physician, allied health professionals (nurse practitioner or physician assistant), or community resources (social worker, case manager).

SUGGESTED READING

Zun LS. Behavioral Disorders: Diagnostic Criteria. In *Tintinalli's Emergency Medicine: A Comprehensive Study Guide.* 7th ed. New York, NY: McGraw-Hill, 2011, pp. 1946–1952.
Zun LS. Evidence-based evaluation of psychiatric patients. *J Emerg Med.* 2005;28:35–39.
Zun LS. Evidence-based treatment of psychiatric patient. *J Emerg Med.* 2005;28:277–283.

Index

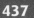